Animal and Translational Models for CNS Drug Discovery

Animal and Translational Models for CNS Drug Discovery
VOLUME I Psychiatric Disorders (ISBN: 978-0-12-373856-1)
VOLUME II Neurological Disorders (ISBN: 978-0-12-373855-4)
VOLUME III Reward Deficit Disorders (ISBN: 978-0-12-373860-8)

(ISBN set: 978-0-12-373861-5)

Animal and Translational Models for CNS Drug Discovery

VOLUME II
Neurological Disorders

Edited by

Robert A. McArthur, PhD
Associate Professor of Research
Consultant Behavioral Pharmacologist
McArthur and Associates GmbH, Basel, Switzerland

Franco Borsini, PhD
Head, Central & Peripheral Nervous System and
General Pharmacology Area – R&D Department
sigma-tau S.p.A., Pomezia (Rome), Italy

AMSTERDAM • BOSTON • HEIDELBERG • LONDON • NEW YORK • OXFORD
PARIS • SAN DIEGO • SAN FRANCISCO • SINGAPORE • SYDNEY • TOKYO
Academic Press is an imprint of Elsevier

Academic Press is an imprint of Elsevier
30 Corporate Drive, Suite 400, Burlington, MA 01803, USA
360 Park Avenue South, Newyork, NY 10010-1710, USA
525 B Street, Suite 1900, San Diego, CA 92101-4495, USA
32 Jamestown Road, London NW1 7BY, UK

⊗This book is printed on acid-free paper.

Library of Congress Cataloging-in-Publication Data
A catalog record for this book is available from the Library of Congress.

British Library Cataloguing-in-Publication Data
A catalogue record for this book is available from the British Library.

ISBN: 978-0-12-373861-5 (set)
ISBN: 978-0-12-373855-4 (vol 2)

For information on all Academic Press publications
visit our web site at www.elsevierdirect.com

Typeset by Charon Tec Ltd., A Macmillan Company.
(www.macmillansolutions.com)

Printed and bound by CPI Group (UK) Ltd, Croydon, CR0 4YY

Transferred to Digital Print 2011

This book is dedicated to that happy band of behavioral pharmacologists who over the generations have occasionally seen their compound progress into clinical development, and more rarely still seen it used to treat patients. New skills are being learned and new species creeping into the lab, including the ones "without tails." These offer new opportunities and challenges, but equally so greater satisfaction working at the interface. May all your compounds be winners!

Contents

Volume 2 Animal and Translational Models for CNS Drug Discovery: Neurological Disorders

Carrie Shilyansky, Weidong Li, M. Acosta, Y. Elgersma,
F. Hannan, M. Hardt, K. Hunter-Schaedle, L.C. Krab,
E. Legius, B. Wiltgen and Alcino J. Silva

CHAPTER 7   Translational Research in ALS 267

Jacqueline Montes, Caterina Bendotti, Massimo Tortarolo, Cristina Cheroni, Hussein Hallak, Zipora Speiser, Sari Goren, Eran Blaugrund and Paul H. Gordon

What Do *You* Mean by "Translational Research"? An Enquiry Through Animal and Translational Models for CNS Drug Discovery: Neurological Disorders

Robert A. McArthur[1] and Franco Borsini[2]

[1]McArthur and Associates GmbH, Basel, Switzerland
[2]Sigma-tau S.p.A, Pomezia (Rome), Italy

In the 50-odd years since the introduction of clinically effective medications for the treatment of behavioral disorders such as depression,[1] anxiety[2] or schizophrenia[3] there has recently been growing unease with a seeming lack of substantive progress in the development of truly innovative and effective drugs for behavioral disorders; an unease indicated by escalating research and development expenditure associated with diminishing returns (e.g.,[4]) and discussed by Hunter[5] in this book series. There are a number of reasons that may account for this lack of new drugs for CNS disorders (cf.,[6]), but according to the US Food and Drug Administration's (FDA) white paper on prospects for 21st century drug discovery and development,[7] one of the main causes for failure in the clinic is the discrepancy between positive outcomes of candidate drugs in animal models and apparent lack of efficacy in humans, that is, the predictive validity of animal models. Consequently, there have been a number of initiatives from the US National Institutes of Health (NIH) (http://nihroadmap.nih.gov/) and The European Medicines Agency (EMEA),[8] to bring interested parties from Academia and Industry together to discuss, examine and suggest ways of improving animal models of behavioral disorders[9-14]. The value of NIH-supported initiatives, even to the point of participating directly in drug discovery from screening to registration is not to be underestimated, as evidenced by the successful registration of buprenorphine (Subutex®) and buprenorphine/naloxone (Suboxone®) by Reckitt-Benckiser in collaboration with the National Institute on Drug Abuse[15], see also[16].[i]

Translational research and experimental medicine are closely related activities that have evolved in answer to the need of improving the attrition rate of novel drugs between the preclinical and clinical stage of development.[5,19-22] In general, translational research defines the *process* through which information and insights flow from clinical observations to refine the development of animal models *as well as* the complementary flow of information and insights gained from animal models to the clinical

---

[i]For a comprehensive discussion of NIH-sponsored initiatives and collaborations and opportunities, please refer to Winsky and colleagues[17] and Jones and colleagues[18], for specifics on NIH-Academic-Industrial collaborations in schizophrenia.

Animal and Translational Models for CNS Drug Discovery,
Vol. 2 of 3: Neurological Disorders
Robert McArthur and Franco Borsini (eds), Academic Press, 2008

setting, be it through improved diagnosis, disease management or treatment; including pharmacological treatment.[23] Experimental medicine, in terms of drug discovery, refers to studies in human volunteers to (1) obtain mechanistic and pharmacological information of compounds entering into development, (2) explore and define biological markers with which the state and progress of a disorder can be monitored, as well as the effects of pharmacological interventions on its progress and (3) establish models and procedures with which to obtain initial signals of efficacy test.[5,15,22] Though claimed as an innovative paradigm shift, translational research nevertheless, is not a new concept, as pointed out by Millan in this book series.[24] The origins of psychopharmacology abound with numerous examples of how pharmaceutical or medicinal chemists interacted directly with their clinical colleagues to "test their white powder", or clinicians who would knock at the chemists' door for anything new. Kuhn and Domenjoz, for example, describes the initial "Phase II" trials of the novel "sleeping pill" forerunner of imipramine.[25,26] Paul Janssen tells how the observation of the paranoid schizophrenia-like hallucinations experienced by cyclists who were consuming amphetamine to stay alert, led him to search for better amphetamine antagonists, one of which was haloperidol. This compound was subsequently given to a young lad in the midst of a psychotic episode by a local psychiatrist with good results.[27] Though largely overtaken in sales and prescription rates by 2nd generation atypical antipsychotics, Haloperidol (Haldol®) remains one of the standard drugs used in the treatment of schizophrenia.[18,28,29]

Translational research is a two-way process which, nonetheless can lead to differences in emphasis and agenda. We have gathered a number of definitions from different sources listed in Table 1 below to help us determine what one of our authors asked us to do when he was contacted to contribute to this book project, "What do *you* mean by 'translational research'?"

These definitions may emphasize the clinical, or top-down approach to translational research,[20,30] or the bottom-up approach of "bench-to-bedside".[21,31] It is clear though, that translational research has a purpose of integrating basic and clinical research for the benefit of the patient in need. While we welcome this as a general definition of translational research, we acknowledge, as do others (e.g.,[31,32]), that a more pragmatic, working definition is required. Consequently, we define translational research, in the context of drug discovery and research, as the partnership between preclinical and clinical research to align not only "… basic science discoveries into medications",[31] but also the information derived from the clinic during the development of those medications. The purpose of this reciprocal definition is to refine the model systems used to understand the disorder by identifying the right targets, interacting with those targets pharmacologically in both animals and humans and monitoring the responses in each throughout a compound's development (cf.,[5 and 15]). Central to this definition is the acknowledgement that the etiology of behavioral disorders and their description are too diffuse to attempt to model or simulate in their entirety. Consequently, emphasis must be placed on identifying specific symptoms or core features of the disorder to model, and to define biological as well as behavioral responses as indices of state, changes in state and response to pharmacological treatment. This process is made easier if, at the same time, greater effort is made to identify procedures used to measure these biological and behavioral responses that are consistent

Table 1 Selected definitions of translational research

Definition	Reference
Translational medicine may also refer to the wider spectrum of patient-oriented research that embraces innovations in technology and biomedical devices as well as the study of new therapies in clinical trials. It also includes epidemiological and health outcomes research and behavioral studies that can be brought to the bedside or ambulatory setting.	30
… connotes an attempt to bring information that has been confined to the laboratory into the realm of clinical medicine.	
To the extent that clinical studies could be designed to answer such questions (generated by information from the laboratory), they would represent types of translational clinical research.	20
… a two-way street where the drive to cure should be complemented by the pursuit to understand human diseases and their complexities.	21, 220
1. Basic science studies which define the biological effects of therapeutics in humans	
2. Investigations in humans which define the biology of disease and provide the scientific foundation for development of new or improved therapies for human disease	
3. Non-human or non-clinical studies conducted with the intent to advance therapies to the clinic or to develop principles for application of therapeutics to human disease	
4. Any clinical trial of a therapy that was initiated based on #1–3 with any endpoint including toxicity and/or efficacy.	M. Sznol cited by 21
…research efforts intended to apply advances in basic science to the clinical research setting. For drug discovery and development, the term refers to research intended to progress basic science discoveries into medications.	31
By bringing together top-down and bottom-up approaches, there is potential for a convergence of unifying explanatory constructs relating aetiology to brain dysfunction and treatment.	37, 221
… information gathered in animal studies can be translated into clinical relevance and vice versa, thus providing a conceptual basis for developing better drugs.	
… the application of scientific tools and method to drug discovery and development … taking a pragmatic or operational rather than a definitional approach, a key to a successful translation of non-human research to human clinical trials lies in the choice of biomarkers.	32
… two-way communication between clinical and discovery scientists during the drug development process are likely to help in the development of more relevant, predictive preclinical models and biomarkers, and ultimately a better concordance between preclinical and clinical efficacy.	82

within and between species.[23,24] Brain imaging is one technique that has cross-species consistency (e.g.,[33-36]), as do various operant conditioning procedures.[37,38]

There are at least two aspects of translational research to be considered as a result of the definition proposed above. First is the concept of specific symptoms, or core features of the disorder to model. Attempts to simulate core disturbances in behavior formed the basis of early models of behavioral disorders. McKinney and Bunney, for example, describe how they sought to "translate" the clinically observed changes in human depressed behavior (secondary symptoms) with analogous changes in animals induced by environmental or pharmacological manipulations.[39]

Whereas modelers have traditionally referred to diagnostic criteria such as DSM-IV[40] or ICD-10[41] the consensus to be found in this book series and other sources is that these diagnostic criteria do not lend themselves easily to basic or applied research. The etiology of behavioral disorders is unclear, and there is considerable heterogeneity between patients with different disorders but similar symptoms. Nevertheless, attempts to model particular behavioral patterns have been and are being done. Thus, for example, the construct of anhedonia (the loss of ability to derive pleasure), or the construct of social withdrawal, may be diagnostic criteria for a number of behavioral disorders including depression, schizophrenia, as well as a number of other disorders (cf.,[42]). There is considerable momentum to establish a dimension – rather than diagnostic-based classification or to "deconstruct" syndromes into "symptom-related clusters" that would help guide neurobiological research[ii].[18,43,44] In order to define these "symptom-based clusters", however, the symptoms have to be defined. Previously, these were identified as behavioral patterns, though lately they have been referred to variously as behavioral endophenotypes or exophenotypes (e.g.,[45-49]). It is appropriate here to review the definitions of both. Exophenotype and endophenotypes have been defined by Gottesman and Schields[50] as:

> *John and Lewis (1966) introduced the useful distinction between* exophenotype *(external phenotype)* and *endophenotype (internal),* with the latter only knowable after aid to the naked eye, e.g. a biochemical test or a microscopic examination of chromosome morphology (p. 19).[iii]

Subsequently, endophenotypes have been more rigorously defined[51] as:

1. *The endophenotype is associated with illness in the population.*
2. *The endophenotype is heritable.*
3. *The endophenotype is primarily state-independent (manifests in an individual whether or not illness is active).*
4. *Within families, endophenotype and illness co-segregate.*
5. *The endophenotype found in affected family members is found in nonaffected family members at a higher rate than in the general population. (p. 639)*

[ii] For reviews of the initiatives deconstructing a complex disorder like schizophrenia, the reader is invited to consult the following two issues of *Schizophrenia Bulletin*, where these initiatives are thoroughly discussed: *Schizophr Bull*, 2007, 33:1 and *Schizophr Bull*, 2007, 33:4.

[iii] See also Tannock *et al.*,[61] for definitions of endophenotypes and biomarkers.

And that "…The number of genes involved in a phenotype is theorized to be directly related to both the complexity of the phenotype and the difficulty of genetic analysis" (*op cit.*, p. 637). On the other hand, exophenotypes have been defined by Holzman[52] (and others) as:

> … *the external symptoms of a disorder that clinicians detect during an examination. An endophenotype, on the other hand, is a characteristic that requires special tools, tests, or instruments for detection. (p. 300)*

It behooves the unwary researcher to be careful with terminology and thus not fall into the trap of pretending greater accuracy by changing the name of the phenomenon being studied. Finally, to quote Hyman's *caveat*[43],

> *The term "endophenotype" has become popular for describing putatively simpler or at least objectively measurable phenotypes, such as neuropsychological measures that might enhance diagnostic homogeneity. I find this term less than ideal, because it implies that the current diagnostic classification is basically correct, and that all that is lacking is objective markers for these disorders. If, however, the lumping and splitting of symptoms that gave rise to the current classification was in error, then the search for biological correlates of these disorders will not prove fruitful. (p. 729)*

The second aspect to be considered in translational research is the concept of biomarkers. Biomarkers are crucial to translational research and serve as the interface between preclinical research, experimental medicine and clinical development. As with endophenotypes above, however, biomarkers also require some discussion. The FDA, NIH, and EMEA have been at the forefront in helping define and establish biomarkers, surrogate markers, and clinical endpoints[53-57] (http://ospp.od.nih.gov/biomarkers); an initiative now being carried out in partnership with private enterprise[58] (http://ppp.od.nih.gov/pppinfo/examples.asp). Lesko and Atkinson have provided summary definitions of various markers that are worth considering:[55]

> *A synthesis of some proposed working definitions is as follows:* (a) biological marker *(biomarker) - a physical sign or laboratory measurement that occurs in association with a pathological process and that has putative diagnostic and/or prognostic utility;* (b) surrogate endpoint - *a biomarker that is intended to serve as a substitute for a clinically meaningful endpoint and is expected to predict the effect of a therapeutic intervention; and* (c) clinical endpoint - *a clinically meaningful measure of how a patient feels, functions, or survives. The hierarchical distinction between biomarkers and surrogate endpoints is intended to indicate that relatively few biomarkers will meet the stringent criteria that are needed for them to serve as reliable substitutes for clinical endpoints (p. 348).*

An important characteristic of biomarkers is that they should also be capable of monitoring disease progression.[54] It is interesting more over that the establishment of biomarkers should also be subject to the same concepts of validity as defined by Willner initially for models of behavioral disorders, that is, face, construct and predictive validity.[59] Lesko and Atkinson further indicate that biomarkers must be evaluated and validated for (1) clinical relevance (face validity in being able to reflect physiologic/pathologic processes),

(2) sensitivity and specificity (construct validity that it is capable to measure changes though a given mechanism in a target population) and (3) must ultimately be validated in terms of clinical change, that is, predictive validity. Biomarkers also have other criteria that they need to fulfill such as: their accuracy, precision and reproducibility; an estimated rate of false positive and false negative probability; and practicality and simplicity of use. In addition, pharmacological isomorphism is used to establish a biomarker's predictive validity where response to a known clinically effective standard is ultimately required, especially if drugs of different mechanisms of action produce the same response in the biomarker. These criteria are very familiar to the animal modeler and highlight the shared interests and expertise that the preclinical researcher brings to the clinical arena. Biomarkers for behavioral disorders thus share many of the problems inherent to their animal models.[60] Nevertheless, it is among the most active pursuits in Pharma today (cf.,[61-70]).

It is clear from the previous discussion that translational research demands the combined efforts of a number of participants, each of which contributes a particular expertise to achieve a common goal. Translational research cannot be done effectively using the "tried and true" process of compartmentalization prevalent up to the end of the last century, that is, the splitting of R from D, or maintaining the preclinical from clinical, academic from industrial divides. For the past decade Pharma has fostered cross-disciplinary collaboration with the creation of Project teams in which participants from preclinical, clinical and marketing sections of the Industry are brought together in relation to the maturity of the Project. The concept of "pitching the compound over the fence" is no longer tolerated, and preclinical participation even in mature Projects is expected. This creates a much more stimulating environment for all the participants, who not only learn from the experiences of others, but also maintain a sense of ownership even when their particular expertise is no longer required for a Project's core activities. Nevertheless, creation of and participation in Project teams is not always an easy task as group dynamics evolve. Team members are assigned to a Project by line managers, and can be removed depending on priorities. Some team members contribute more than their share, while others coast. The skills of the Project Leader must go beyond scientific expertise in order to forge an effective team and deliver a successful drug.

The use of animal models is an essential step in the drug discovery and indeed the translational research process. Use of appropriate models can minimize the number of drug candidates that later fail in human trials by accurately predicting the pharmacokinetic and dynamic (PK/PD) characteristics, efficacy and the toxicity of each compound. Selection of the appropriate models is critical to the process. Primary diseases such as those caused by infections, genetic disorders or cancers are less problematic to model using both *in vitro* and *in vivo* techniques. Similarly some aspects of degenerative diseases have also been successfully modeled. However, modeling of disorders with a strong behavioral component has been less successful. This is not to say that there are no models for various aspects of these disorders. Many models have been proposed, validated pharmacologically with standard, clinically effective drugs and extensively reviewed. Indeed, these models have become so standardized that their use to characterize mechanisms of action and lead novel compounds in CNS drug discovery projects is mandatory, and positive outcomes are required before these compounds are considered for further development. However, it has become clear that positive outcome in these models is no guarantee that these new compounds will be efficacious medicines in humans. Refinements of existing models and development of new models relevant to drug discovery and clinical outcome are being pursued and documented (e.g.,[71-74]). Advancements in genetic aspects of disease are also being aided through the development and use of genetically modified animals as model systems. However, even though these techniques are more precise in modeling aspects of a disease such as amyloid overexpression in Alzheimer's disease, the ability of procedures used to assess the changes in behavior, and relating them to altered human behavior remains uncertain.

Books on animal models of psychiatric and neurological diseases have tended to be compendia of the so-called "standard" procedures developed over the years. Some of these books have formed part of classic reference texts for behavioral pharmacologists (e.g.,[75,76]). Others – more pragmatic in their approach – describe the application of these models and are useful as "cookbook" manuals (e.g.,[77,78]), while yet others have been very specific in their focus; for example, books entirely with models for a particular disorder, for example, depression or schizophrenia. It could be argued, however, that these books address a very circumscribed audience, and need not be necessarily so. Clinicians might and do claim that animal models are intellectually interesting, but of no relevance to their daily work of (1) demonstrating proof of concept, (2) showing efficacy or (3) treating their patients. Nevertheless, clinicians are constantly on the watch for potentially new pharmacological treatments with which to treat their patients, for example, new chemical entities that have reached their notice following extensive profiling in animal models. Academics develop a number of procedures or models to help them study neural substrates and disorders of behavior, and may use pharmacological compounds as tools to dissect behavior. The industrial scientist is charged with the application of these methods and models, establishing them in the lab at the request of the Project team and Leader. There is thus a shared interest in the development, use and ability of animal models to reflect the state of a disorder and predict changes in state following pharmacological manipulation. This shared interest has generated much collaboration between academics, clinicians and the industry (cf.,[79]).

Paradoxically in view of shared interest, close ties and general agreement on the need for bidirectional communication, the integration of the perspective and experience of the participants in the drug discovery and development process is not always apparent and is a source of concern (e.g.,[6,21,31,32,80-82]). Although we do not necessarily agree entirely with Horrobin's description of biomedical research scientists as latter day Castalians,[80] we suggest that there is a certain truth to the allusion that considerable segregation between the academic, clinician and industrial researcher exists (see also[21,81]). There have been numerous attempts to break down these barriers, such as having parallel sessions at conferences, or disorder-specific workshops organized by leading academics, clinicians and industrial scientists (e.g., *op. cit.*,[83]). With few exceptions, however, academics will talk to academics, clinicians to clinicians and industrial scientists will talk to either academics or clinicians; depending on which stage their Project in. Willner's influential book[84], "*Behavioral Models in Psychopharmacology: Theoretical, Industrial and Clinical Perspectives*" represents one of the first published attempts that brings together academics, pharmaceutical researchers and clinicians to discuss the various aspects of the animal models of behavioral disorders. Yet even in Willner's book with alternating chapters expounding the academic, industrial and clinical perspective on a subject, the temptation is always to go to the "more interesting", that is, directly relevant chapter and leave the others for later.

This three volume book series aims to bring objective and reasoned discussion of the relative utility of animal models to all participants in the process of discovery and development of new pharmaceuticals for the treatment of disorders with a strong behavioral component, that is, clearly psychiatric and reward deficits, but also neurodegenerative disorders in which changes in cognitive ability and mood are important characteristics. Participants include the applied research scientists in the Pharma industry as well as academics who carry out animal research, academic and industry clinicians involved in various aspects of clinical development, government officials and scientists setting funding priorities, and industrial, academic and clinical opinion leaders, who very clearly influence and help shape the decisions determining what therapeutic areas and molecular targets are to be pursued (or dropped) by Pharma. Rather than a catalog of existing animal models of behavioral disorders, the chapters of the book series seek to explore the role of these models within CNS drug discovery and development from the shared perspective of these participants in order to move beyond the concept of animal behavioral assays or "gut baths",[85,86] to stimulate the development of animal models to support present research of the genetic and biological basis of behavioral disorders and to improve the ability to translate findings and concepts between animal research and clinical therapeutics.

As indicated, the aim and scope of this book series has been to examine the contribution of the animal models of behavioral disorders to the process of CNS drug discovery and development rather than a simple compendium of techniques and methods. This book goes beyond the traditional models book presently published in that it is more a considered review of *how* animal models of behavioral disorders are used rather than *what* they are. In order to achieve this goal, leading preclinical and clinical investigators from both Industry and Academia involved in translational research were identified and asked to participate in the Project. First, a single author was asked to write an introductory chapter explaining the role of animal and translational models for CNS drug discovery from their particular perspective. Each volume thus starts with an industry perspective from a senior pharma research executive, which sets a framework. A leading academic author was contacted to provide a general theoretical framework of how animal and translational models are evolving to provide the tools for the study of the neural substrates of behavior and how more efficient CNS drug discovery may be fostered. Finally, leading clinicians involved in the changing environment of clinical trial conductance and design were asked to discuss how issues in clinical trial design and conductance have affected the development and registration of CNS drugs in their area of specialty, and how changes are likely to affect future clinical trials.

Following these 3 introductory chapters, there are therapeutic area chapters in which a working party of at least 3 (industrial preclinical, academic and clinical) authors were identified and asked to write a consensual chapter that reflects the view of the role of animal models in CNS translational research and drug development in their area of expertise. We deliberately created our chapter teams with participants who had not necessarily worked together before. This was done for three reasons. First, we were anxious to avoid establishing teams with participants who had already evolved a conceptual framework *a priori*. Second, we felt that by forcing people to "brainstorm" and develop new ideas and concepts would be more stimulating both for the participants and the readers. Thirdly, we wanted to simulate the conditions of the creation of an industrial Project team, where participants need not know each other initially or indeed may not even like each other, but who are all committed to achieving the goals set out by consensus. We sought to draw upon the experiences of industrial and academic preclinical and clinical investigators who are actively involved in CNS drug discovery and development, as well as translational research. These therapeutic chapter teams have contributed very exciting chapters reflecting the state of animal models used in drug discovery in their therapeutic areas, and their changing roles in translational research. For many, this has been a challenging and exhilarating experience, forcing a paradigm shift from how they have normally worked. For some teams, the experience has been a challenge for the same reason. One is used to write for one's audience and usually on topics with which one is comfortable. For some authors, it was not easy to be asked to write with other equally strong personalities with different perspectives, and then to allow someone else to integrate this work into a consensual chapter. Indeed, some therapeutic area chapter teams were not able to establish an effective team. As a consequence, not all the therapeutic areas envisioned to be covered initially in this Project were possible. Nevertheless, as translational research becomes more established, what appears to be a novel and unusual way of working will become the norm for the benefit not only of science, but for the patient in need.

VOLUME OVERVIEW AND CHAPTER SYNOPSES

This volume comprises contributions by different authors on some neurological disorders, such as neurofibromatosis type I, Alzheimer's disease, Parkinson's disease, Huntington's disease, amyotrophic lateral sclerosis (ALS) and the epilepsies. Animal models available for detecting potential compounds are satisfactory only to a limited extent and there are considerable unmet medical needs associated with all the neurological disorders surveyed. These are the non-motor aspects of neurological disorders such as changes in mood, affect and most of all, cognitive impairments.[87-89] Cognitive impairments and their treatment are major unmet needs in all of the neurological disorders surveyed as well as psychiatric disorders such as schizophrenia,[18] ADHD[61] or Autistic Spectrum Disorders,[90] for example.

Major efforts in the discovery and development of compounds that can improve or "enhance" cognition are evident in the number of drug targets being pursued by academic groups and the pharmaceutical industry (e.g.,[91-95]). However, issues have arisen with the development of compounds with cognitive enhancing potential because of failure to confirm positive preclinical results in clinical trials.[5,96] Failure to confirm preclinical results in humans may occur for a number of reasons including patient heterogeneity,[19,24] endpoint measures,[96] or variable preclinical methodology ([88]cf.,[6] for further discussion). Two factors have been identified and discussed in this Volume; pharmacokinetic/dynamic assessment[5,88] and clinical trial design.[19,88,96,97]

Correct PK/PD assessment in animals and humans, for example, is crucial to determine whether the compound is present at the right receptors at a concentration sufficient to have the desired effect.[5,24,61,87,98-102] Pharmacodynamic assessment not only in healthy volunteers, but in a patient population can be very important as well in determining the fate of a candidate drug. Klitgaard *et al.* cite the example of D-CPPene, which induced severe adverse effects in refractory complex partial epilepsy patients at a quarter of the dose tolerated in healthy volunteers.[103] These differences were attributed to higher exposure levels following administration of similar doses of D-CPPene in the epilepsy patients.

Montes and colleagues, in their examination of animal and translational models in ALS research discuss the lack of translatability of experimental compounds from preclinical research to clinical effectiveness.[88] Among the reasons identified were the use of transgenic animal models of familial ALS, which may not be representative of the sporadic and heterogeneous aspect of the disorder, and methodological issues. In their analysis of preclinical and clinical discrepancies of candidate drugs for ALS, they examined the history of Riluzole (Rilutek®, the clinical gold standard), celecoxib (Celebrex®) and gabapentin (Neurontin®); these latter compounds advanced for the treatment of ALS. Their analysis was made within the framework and analytical criteria outlined by Cudkowicz and colleagues in their examination of a celecoxib trial.[104] These criteria have tremendous heuristic value not only for ALS, but for all the disorders surveyed in this book series, regardless of therapeutic indication. Consequently, we have reproduced (with slight modification having substituted "ALS" for "disorders" and using the present tense) Montes *et al.*'s summary of Cudkowicz's criteria:

> *Criterion 1: Is there sufficient underlying rationale, as well as experimental evidence from preclinical studies?*
> *Criterion 2: Is the dose level used in the clinical trial sufficient to reach the plasma concentrations required for efficacy based on the preclinical models?*
> *Criterion 3: Is the CNS penetration of the drug sufficient to exert the expected pharmacologic response?*
> *Criterion 4: How well do preclinical models predict the effect of treatment in humans?*
> *Criterion 5: What is the response of the marker of drug effect or a disease biomarker (that reflects a compound's mechanism of action) relative to efficacy?*
> *Criterion 6: Is the clinical study design and execution acceptable?*

Over the past decade there has been a concerted shift in neurology to progress beyond symptomatic treatment of the disorders to the development of disease modifying therapeutic agents,[13,105-107] which has been stimulated by tremendous advances in understanding of genetic substrates of the various disorders, and molecular biological techniques developed to exploit those advances.[5,87-89,91,96] Indeed, it would be difficult now to find a drug discovery project without its complement of transgenic mice used to validate their target, and the chapters in this Volume describe various mutant mice strains used for this purpose. Nevertheless, there is an underlying assumption that the halting of a neurodegenerative process or the restoration of a compromised system will translate to a maintained or improved level of behavioral functioning, which requires a certain *caveat*.

In Volume 1 of this book series, Miczek[86] proposes eight conceptual principles for translational research. Principle 8 is particularly germane to this discussion: "*It is more productive to focus on behaviorally defined symptoms when translating clinical to preclinical measures, and vice versa. Psychological processes pertinent to affect and cognition are hypothetical constructs that need to be defined in behavioral and neural terms* as it reminds us we are ultimately referring to hypothetical constructs when we talk about cognition, mood, affect, etc. (cf.,[108]). These may well be operationally defined in terms of changes in behavior, or electrical signals, but are still subject to philosophical debate (cf.,[109] and references within). The amyloid hypothesis, for example has been the driving force behind disease modifying drug discovery strategies for the treatment of Alzheimer's disease and related cognitive impairments.[96,110] This hypothesis is the conceptual basis for the emphasis of therapeutic intervention on amyloid synthesis, accumulation and clearance; although it is not without its problems.[111-114] Transgenic mouse models suggest that amyloid and its fragments may be related to cognitive impairments,[115] and that these impairments may be ameliorated by clinically active symptomatic treatments for Alzheimer's (e.g.,[116,117]), or immunization (e.g.,[118-120]); though not invariably (e.g.,[121]). There is also a suggestion that cognitive ability in immunized Alzheimer subjects was also maintained by immunization ([122], but see[123]).

The relationship between abnormal amyloid synthesis, secretion and deposition and cell death *in vivo* and subsequently on impaired cognition is still not definite.[111] It is not uncommon to identify subjects *post-mortem* with amyloid loads that would have qualified them as Alzheimer's, notwithstanding age relative normal cognitive functions whilst alive (e.g.,[124-130]). Hardy and Selkoe and others argue that the diffuse plaques observed in these subjects are not associated with pathology and that soluble β amyloid species correlates better with cognitive decline than plaque deposits ([111,115,131] and references within). In order to see whether the development of amyloid plaques in the olfactory bulb and tract of Tg_{2576} transgenic mice, would have functional consequences, that is, impair the mouse from discriminating between three odors, McArthur and colleagues trained mice to associate a particular odor with food reward in a Y-maze. When required to choose between three odors (two of which were previously unrewarded), the transgenic mice were capable of selecting the arm with the odor associated with food; notwithstanding extensive plaque build up in the olfactory tract, hippocampus and other brain regions.[132] In other words, any presumed neurotoxic effect of amyloid plaques (and also presumably neurotoxic amyloid species[133-135]) did not have any functional effect on the mouse's ability to smell. Furthermore, not all aspects of cognition are impaired in transgenic mice models of the cognitive impairments of Alzheimer's (cf.,[136]). Lindner and colleagues[96] indicate that the aged Tg_{2576} transgenic mice tested previously for odor discrimination ability[132] are quite capable of learning complex second order operant conditioning procedures based upon olfactory discrimination, and also capable of reversing their behavior when the initial discriminatory stimulus was changed. There is presently great hope and expectation that anti-amyloid treatment options may not only will stop or reverse the deposition of amyloid and its fragments, but that they may also restore cognitive ability in Alzheimer's patients. Unfortunately, as indicated by Millan[24] in Volume 1, our models still await clinical confirmation (see also[89, 103]).

It is clear that disease modifying approaches to neurological disorders requires methods to determine (1) the state of neurodegeneration of patients, (2) the rate of neurodegeneration and (3) the effect of a candidate drug on both state and rate of change of the disorder. In most of these disorders the process of neurodegeneration begins long before symptoms are noted, at which point extensive damage is already present.[87,96] Differences in timing of experimental compound testing in animals and patients may also account for lack of translatability in certain therapeutic areas. Montes and colleagues point out that testing in ALS mutant mice, for example, is usually done at the prodromal or presymptomatic stage. These compounds, alas, can be tested in patients only after motor symptoms occur and ALS is diagnosed.[88] The search for valid and reliable biomarkers, therefore, is an extremely important part of drug discovery and development.[64,87,137,138] Brain imaging the most effective technique being used extensively in early development[5,24,68] not only in neurology,[17,87,96,103,139], but psychiatry[18,61,90,98,99,140,141] and reward deficit disorders.[101,102,142-144] These are techniques that lend themselves very well to translational research (e.g.,[82,145-149]). Notwithstanding the problems of adapting imaging techniques to animals,[iv] we can expect to see further developments in the future. Neuropsychological testing has traditionally been used to determine state and progress of neurodegeneration. Neuropsychological procedures that can be used both in animals and humans can be very powerful translational techniques. The development of the Cambridge Neuropsychological Test Automated Battery (CANTAB) by Robbins and his colleagues[150-153] represents one such technique. CANTAB appears capable, for example, of identifying prodromal Alzheimer or HIV patients and to monitoring their rate of cognitive decline,[153-155] can be combined with imaging techniques,[156-158] has been used to monitor drugs in clinical trials,[159,160] and is particularly adaptable for use in primates.[96,161-167] Other biological markers such as cerebrospinal fluid phosphorylated Tau proteins and amyloid $\beta_{(1-42)}$, or hippocampal volume are used as diagnostic and patient selection criteria in Alzheimer's.[97,168] In general, however, biomarker development has been slow and uncertain, and clinical evaluation remains the main tool to evaluate progression and treatment efficacy.[87-89,96,97,103,169,170] Measurement of plaque density, for example, is a putative biomarker[5] whose robustness/validity is uncertain, however, considering the dissociation between amyloid load and cognitive decline discussed above (see also[97]). Similarly, clinically diagnosed Parkinsonian patients may show no evidence of dopaminergic deficit.[87] Even brain imaging techniques such as EEG may be insensitive. Klitgaard and colleagues indicate that over half of epileptic patients may show normal EEG.[103]

Hunter examines the role of animal models and experimental medicine within the context of neurological drug discovery and development. Drug discovery begins with the identification of a molecular target that may or not be "drugable", that is, amenable to physico-chemical manipulation, validation, screening and development (cf.,[171, 172]).

---

iv See Brain Imaging Special Issue. *Psychopharmacology* (Berlin), 2005, Volume 180.

Transgenic mice strains, knockout,[173] and lately sRNAi interference technology[89,98,174,175] are being used extensively in neurological drug research. These mutant mice models represent a major advancement over lesion or pharmacological models, which are used to produce symptomatic changes in animals.[89,96,98]

As described above, there is a major concern within neurology to move beyond symptomatic treatment. Brain imaging is one of the principle tools used to monitor disease progression. Although clinical endpoints are still defined in terms of rating scales[88,97] and/or symptomatic changes,[87,103] imaging is being used more frequently in clinical trials offering more sensitive measures of treatment effects. Animals are also being used to model disease progression and as mechanistic screens for early pharmacodynamic/pharmacokinetic effects of drug candidates. Hunter indicates the use of APP-transgenic mice as models of amyloidosis rather than Alzheimer's disease (see above and also Lindner and colleagues[96] on this subject). Being able to monitor the rate of progression of amyloid deposition, or the rate of amyloid clearance is an important parameter in the development of potential anti-amyloid therapies presently being pursued.[176]

Littman and Williams[22] cogent discussion on experimental medicine and the search for biomarkers indicate their view that, "Humans are the ultimate model" is based upon their opinion that preclinical animal models are poorly predictive. Naturally we do not subscribe to this view and would suggest that although positive results in one, two or more animal models of a disorder will not necessarily be translated into a megasales drug, proper use of animal models at different stages of the drug discovery process will provide experimental medicine with the crucial information that is needed before first entry into human studies.[5] For example, the development of mechanistic animal pharmacodynamic models is providing crucial information on whether a candidate drug is active and can be ranked in terms of efficacy and potency. Mechanistic models such as the induction of drinking by histamine described by Hunter[5] need not relate to the intended therapeutic indication of the candidate drug (e.g., symptomatic treatment of Alzheimer's disease), but is indicative of the interaction of the molecule with its target (e.g., histamine H_3 receptor antagonism). Similarly, the use of animals in safety pharmacology to identify potential or actual adverse side-effects is a mandatory step in drug development,[177] and side-effect assessment is built into every discovery project.[5,15–17,101,103]

Schneider Cognitive impairments are major unmet needs in many of the therapeutic areas surveyed in this book series. Deterioration in cognitive abilities can range from the "mild forgetfulness" associated with advancing age to the selective or global impairments of neurological or psychiatric pathological conditions. While diagnostic and clinical trial endpoint criteria of dementia in Alzheimer's disease is widely accepted, the heterogeneity within "pre-Alzheimer" states such as mild-cognitive impairment, early Alzheimer's Disease, age-associated cognitive impairments, or vascular cognitive impairments makes similar diagnosis and study in these disorders more difficult. Furthermore, the reliability and validity of biochemical and imaging biomarkers of Alzheimer's are still not fully established (cf.,[178]), so clinical trials for cognitive enhancers for Alzheimer's and other indications continue to rely on rating scales to assess cognition, global assessment, and activities of daily living. The cognitive subscale of the Alzheimer's Disease Assessment Scale (ADAS-cog[179,180]), has become the *de facto* standard for nearly all recent clinical trials, where a four-point improvement relative to either baseline or the placebo group defines a clinical "responder" (see also[96]). Positive, or even significant changes in secondary endpoints like hippocampal volume[181] or neuropsychological test performance,[182] may be encouraging results, but if ADAS-cog changes are not significantly different, the trial will be deemed either failed (where there is no difference between the placebo and positive control) or negative (where the positive control group is significantly different from placebo, but the candidate drug is not significantly different from placebo[19]). Variable rates of placebo-treated decline is a major problem not only for clinical trials of cognitive enhancers, but also for psychiatric indications (cf.,[19,24,98,99,102]). In addition, the choice of positive control in clinical trials for cognitive enhancers may be problematic.[96] Donepezil (Aricept®) is a commonly used clinically effective standard, but one that is associated with a variable response and limited effectiveness.

Patient heterogeneity and selection are issues in clinical trial designs.[19] Schneider points out that an additional complication in clinical trials for cognitive enhancers is that the state of neurodegeneration is difficult to determine, and there may be a built-in bias of selection. Subjects volunteering for clinical trials are: (1) usually on a cholinesterase inhibitor already, (2) on psychotropic or other medications and (3) not representative of Alzheimer patients that are not in care. Genotyping and use of biomarkers for patient selection is presently of limited value. Both Schneider and Merchant *et al.*[87] discuss the two clinical trials designs used to demonstrate disease modification; a randomized withdrawal design and randomized start design. These designs have limitations, such as the need to increase sample size to compensate for subject drop-out, duration of the trial, effectiveness of the comparator and by the indirect, rather than direct, indication of disease modification. Finally, both Schneider and McEvoy and Freudenreich[19] discuss the conductance of clinical trials, especially in the context of international trials in many centers of variable quality. Such trials for potential cognitive enhancers are particularly problematic because of differences in language and culture influencing patient selection and outcome measures.

Shilyansky *et al.* Cognitive impairments are common in the neurological disorders,[88,89,96,97,183] as well as the psychiatric (e.g.,[18,61,90,99]) or reward deficit disorders (e.g.,[102,144]) surveyed. Shilyansky and colleagues refer to their work on neurofibromatosis type I, which is a neurological disorder associated with learning disabilities as one example of how the study of a single gene disorder not only may suggest drug targets for the development of drugs for its treatment, but also to provide insights into the neurobiology of cognition. Their work is also an example of "back translation" where the understanding of some of the mechanisms of action of clinically available drugs like statins may be used as pharmacological tools combined with a transgenic mouse model to explore the neurobiology of complex behaviors.[86,184,185] Cross-species validation is a central theme in translational research and Shilyansky *et al.* outline the types of tasks that assess working memory manipulation and maintenance that could be used in a human laboratory setting and their animal equivalents (see also Linder et al., below). Shilyansky and colleagues further introduce a novel interpretation of "forward" pharmacological isomorphism;[18,24,96,100,143,186] that is, designing a battery of cognitive tasks with which to assess patients based upon the activity of a drug's activity on animal's performance.

Lindner *et al*. Alzheimer's disease is a very important therapeutic indication for many pharmaceutical companies and society. Since the registration of the first cholinesterase inhibitors, there have been a number of compounds that have failed in clinical trials notwithstanding demonstrations of cognitive enhancing potential in preclinical models. In order to maximize the predictive validity of preclinical assessments, novel treatments should be evaluated preclinically with models that best simulate the overall pattern of disease pathology and the overall pattern and severity of cognitive/behavioral deficits; that is, in accordance to Miczek's fourth conceptual principle, *"The progression from a simple screen to a theoretically adequate model depends on the incorporation of a cardinal symptom characterizing the disorder under investigation. The closer the model approximates a symptom of clinical significance, the more likely will its use generate data that can be translated to clinical benefits"*.[86] Lindner and colleagues, more over, suggest that a ninth conceptual principle for translational psychopharmacology research could be added. *Principle 9: Therapeutic effects should also be produced on measures of cognitive and behavioral/functional abilities most similar to the procedures and primary endpoints required for establishing efficacy in clinical trials.* Procedures to test clinically relevant behavioral/cognitive functions exist to assess spatial mapping (e.g.,[187-189]), working memory (e.g.,[190-192]) and attention (e.g.,[193-195]) across species. However, it is clear that selective use of models, procedures, and lack of replication of results may bias the advancement of compounds without adequate confirmation.[196] Closer adherence to good laboratory practice (GLP) and the use of more careful controls would help control for this bias (see also[89]).

Merchant *et al*. The discovery of the dopaminergic basis of Parkinson's disease,[197] the efficacy of replacement therapy with L-Dopa,[198] and the use of neurotoxin lesion models, both to study the neurobiology of the disorder and as test beds for drug discovery were important milestones for neurological disorders. However, as important as these breakthroughs were, treatment for Parkinson's disease remains symptomatic, and the treatments themselves are not without their problems.[199] Furthermore, the notable failure of some compounds to show clinical efficacy calls into question the use of dopamine mechanistic models in which to evaluate compounds with novel mechanisms of action.

The discovery of Parkinson's-related mutations such as α-synuclein,[200,201] *parkin*,[202] PINK1[203] and DJ-1[204] offer new, but difficult drug targets for Parkinson's (*cf.* Hunter's discussion on target druggability[5]). Also, as discussed, the relationship of these mutations to sporadic, that is, non-familial forms of neurological disorders is yet unclear.[88]

The description of use of genetic models of Parkinson's disease by Merchant and her colleagues illustrate well Miczek's third and fifth conceptual principle for translational psychopharmacology research[86] in terms of the construct validity of the models (see above). Though individual genetic models presented may not recapitulate all of the characteristics of human Parkinson's disease, the combination of these models will help develop a more complete picture. *Principle 3: Preclinical data are more readily translated to the clinical situation when they are based on converging evidence from at least two, and preferably more, experimental procedures, each capturing cardinal features of the modeled disorder.* Environmental susceptibility and genetic vulnerability are very important factors to model not only in neurological disorders, but in psychiatric and reward deficit disorders as well (see[18,98,108,143,144,205]). *Principle 5: The inducing*

conditions for modeling a cardinal symptom or cluster of symptoms may be environ-
mental, genetic, physiological or a combination of these factors. The choice of the type
of manipulation that induces the behavioral and physiological symptoms reveals the
theoretical approach to the model construction.

Wagner *et al*. Huntington's disease (HD) is an autosomal dominant neurodegenerative disorder characterized by the insidious development of progressive motor,
cognitive, and neuropsychiatric symptoms. The underlying genetic defect in HD is an
expansion of CAG trinucleotide repeats in the first exon of the *HD* gene (also called
IT-15) that produces a mutant huntingtin protein with an expanded polyglutamine
tract. The identification of the abnormal HD gene encoding for mutant huntingtin, has
enabled the development of multiple HD mouse models that have been engineered to
express either fragments of human mutant huntingtin, full-length human mutant huntingtin, or pathogenic CAG expansions in the murine HD gene (Hdh). These mouse
models are currently being used for pre-clinical therapeutic trials and target validation
of experimental compounds.

Notwithstanding the availability of a number of animal models, consistency in
results between laboratories, and even within laboratories, is difficult to achieve
(cf.,[196,206]). Genetic background of animals, living and testing environment are only
some of the factors that must be carefully controlled to improve reproducible results.
Wagner *et al*. also stress the need to include a series of cognitive and motor tests over
extended periods of time in order to develop a full profile of the mouse's behavior
and to monitor how that behavior is being changed by pharmacological treatments.
This approach illustrates Miczek's third conceptual principle discussed previously.
Considering the sheer numbers of mice needed, and the length of time required to
test these animals, Wagner and colleagues suggest it best also to consider mutant
mouse testing as mini-clinical trials, and to borrow from clinical investigators; including the use of Bayesian statistics[207] to plan large scale preclinical studies.

Montes *et al*. As discussed above ALS and other neurological disorders have a
strong genetic component (see also[87, 89, 208, 209]). Familial forms of neurodegenerative
disorders affects a relatively small number of affected subjects (e.g.,[87,96], but see[89]). ALS
affects some 10% of ALS patients,[210] which is related to Cu/Zn-binding superoxide dismutase (SOD1) mutations,[211] and is the most fulminant of ALS. The transgenic modeling
of SOD1 overexpression[212] has been a significant boost to the study of ALS neurobiology, but which has not led to clinically effective drugs. Riluzole, a drug with glutamate
release inhibitor properties,[213] is the clinical standard with modest effects. Montes and
colleagues discuss the need to develop animal models more representative of the sporadic and heterogeneous nature of the disorder, and underline important methodological considerations in preclinical research with mutant models.[214] Montes and colleagues
indicate that the rapidly progressive disease course of ALS could be used to expedite the
testing and registration of compounds that are shown to slow the rate of neurodegeneration in ALS other neurodegenerative disorders.

Klitgaard *et al*. Animal models of acute seizure activity have been very successful
in the discovery and development of anti-epileptic drugs (AEDs[215]). Nevertheless, it is
necessary to use a battery of procedures to identify and profile the clinical utility of individual drugs. These drugs are very effective in 60% of patients with epilepsy. However,
existing AEDs are associated with adverse effects – which affect compliance – and there

are a significant 30% of patients that are treatment resistant.[216,217]v Furthermore, present AEDs are symptomatic treatments rather than disease modifying.[13] Treatment resistance, adverse side-effect profile and disease modifying strategies represent the three main challenges to AED drug discovery and development. Klitgaard and colleagues have chosen to focus on models of pharmaco-resistance in their chapter (see also[5, 18, 19, 24, 88, 98, 99] in this book series for further discussion on pharmaco-resistance).

REFERENCES

1. Kline, N.S. (1958). Clinical experience with iproniazid (marsilid). *J Clin Exp Psychopathol*, 19(2, Suppl 1):72–78.
2. Selling, L.S. (1955). Clinical study of a new tranquilizing drug; use of miltown (2-methyl-2-n-propyl-1,3-propanediol dicarbamate). *JAMA*, 157(18):1594–1596.
3. Delay, J. and Deniker, P. (1955). Neuroleptic effects of chlorpromazine in therapeutics of neuropsychiatry. *J Clin Exp Psychopathol*, 16(2):104–112.
4. Kola, I. and Landis, J. (2004). Can the pharmaceutical industry reduce attrition rates?. *Nat Rev Drug Discov*, 3(8):711–715.
5. Hunter, A.J. (2008). Animal and translational models of neurological disorders: An industrial perspective. In McArthur, R.A. and Borsini, F. (eds.), *Animal and Translational Models for CNS Drug Discovery: Neurologic Disorders*. Academic Press: Elsevier, New York.
6. McArthur, R. and Borsini, F. (2006). Animal models of depression in drug discovery: A historical perspective. *Pharmacol Biochem Behav*, 84(3):436–452.
7. FDA (2004) Innovation or Stagnation: Challenge and Opportunity on the Critical Path to New Medical Products. US Department of Health and Human Services, Food and Drug Administration, Washington, DC.
8. EMEA. (2005). *The European Medicines Agency Road Map to 2010: Preparing the Ground for the Future*. The European Medicines Agency, London.
9. Nestler, E.J., Gould, E., Manji, H., Buncan, M., Duman, R.S., Greshenfeld, H.K. *et al.* (2002). Preclinical models: Status of basic research in depression. *Biol Psychiatry*, 52(6):503–528.
10. Shekhar, A., McCann, U.D., Meaney, M.J., Blanchard, D.C., Davis, M., Frey, K.A. *et al.* (2001). Summary of a National Institute of Mental Health workshop: Developing animal models of anxiety disorders. *Psychopharmacology (Berl)*, 157(4):327–339.
11. Bromley, E. (2005). A Collaborative Approach to Targeted Treatment Development for Schizophrenia: A Qualitative Evaluation of the NIMH-MATRICS Project. Schizophr Bull, 31(4):954–961.
12. Winsky, L. and Brady, L. (2005). Perspective on the status of preclinical models for psychiatric disorders. *Drug Discov Today: Disease Models*, 2(4):279–283.
13. Stables, J.P., Bertram, E., Dudek, F.E., Holmes, G., Mathern, G., Pitkanen, A. *et al.* (2003). Therapy discovery for pharmacoresistant epilepsy and for disease-modifying therapeutics: Summary of the NIH/NINDS/AES models II workshop. *Epilepsia*, 44(12):1472–1478.
14. Stables, J.P., Bertram, E.H., White, H.S., Coulter, D.A., Dichter, M.A., Jacobs, M.P. *et al.* (2002). Models for epilepsy and epileptogenesis: report from the NIH workshop, Bethesda, Maryland. *Epilepsia*, 43(11):1410–1420.
15. McCann, D.J., Acri, J.B., and Vocci, F.J. (2008). Drug discovery and development for reward disorders. In McArthur, R.A. and Borsini, F. (eds.), *Animal and Translational Models for CNS Drug Discovery: Reward Deficit Disorders*. Academic Press: Elsevier, New York.

---

v Treatment or pharmacoresistance is not only a concern in the treatment of the epilepsies, but also one within psychiatric disorders. See [98] or [218, 219] for further discussion.

16. Rocha, B., Bergman, J., Comer, S.D., Haney, M., and Spealman, R.D. (2008). Development of medications for heroin and cocaine addiction and Regulatory aspects of abuse liability testing. In McArthur, R.A. and Borsini, F. (eds.), *Animal and Translational Models for CNS Drug Discovery: Reward Deficit Disorders*. Academic Press: Elsevier, New York.

17. Winsky, L., Driscoll, J., and Brady, L. (2008). Drug discovery and development initiatives at the National Institute of Mental Health: From cell-based systems to Proof-of-Concept. In McArthur, R.A. and Borsini, F. (eds.), *Animal and Translational Models for CNS Drug Discovery: Psychiatric Disorders*. Academic Press: Elsevier, New York.

18. Jones, D.N.C., Gartlon, J.E., Minassian, A., Perry, W., and Geyer, M.A. (2008). Developing new drugs for schizophrenia: From animals to the clinic. In McArthur, R.A. and Borsini, F. (eds.), *Animal and Translational Models for CNS Drug Discovery: Psychiatric Disorders*. Academic Press: Elsevier, New York.

19. McEvoy, J.P. and Freudenreich, O. (2008). Issues in the design and conductance of clinical trials. In McArthur, R.A. and Borsini, F. (eds.), *Animal and Translational Models for CNS Drug Discovery: Psychiatric Disorders*. Academic Press: Elsevier, New York.

20. Schuster, D.P. and Powers, W.J. (2005). *Translational and Experimental Clinical Research*. Lippincott Williams & Wilkins, Philadelphia, PA.

21. Mankoff, S.P., Brander, C., Ferrone, S., and Marincola, F.M. (2004). Lost in translation: Obstacles to translational medicine. *J Transl Med*, 2(1):14.

22. Littman, B.H. and Williams, S.A. (2005). The ultimate model organism: Progress in experimental medicine. *Nat Rev Drug Discov*, 4(8):631–638.

23. Robbins, T.W. (1998). Homology in behavioural pharmacology: An approach to animal models of human cognition. *Behav Pharmacol*, 9(7):509–519.

24. Millan, M.J. (2008). The discovery and development of pharmacotherapy for psychiatric disorders: A critical survey of animal and translational models, and perspectives for their improvement. In McArthur, R.A. and Borsini, F. (eds.), *Animal and Translational Models for CNS Drug Discovery: Psychiatric Disorders*. Academic Press: Elsevier, New York.

25. Domenjoz, R. (2000). From DDT to imipramine. In Healey, D. (ed.), *The Psychopharmacologists III: Interviews with David Healy*. Arnold, London, pp. 93–118.

26. Kuhn, R. (1999). From imipramine to levoprotiline: The discovery of antidepressants. In Healey, D. (ed.), *The Psychopharmacologists II: Interviews with David Healy*. Arnold, London, pp. 93–118.

27. Janssen, P. (1999). From haloperidol to risperidone. In Healy, D. (ed.), *The Psychopharmacologists II: Interviews by David Healy*. Arnold, London, pp. 39–70.

28. Almond, S. and O'Donnell, O. (2000). Cost analysis of the treatment of schizophrenia in the UK. A simulation model comparing olanzapine, risperidone and haloperidol. *Pharmacoeconomics*, 17(4):383–389.

29. Gasquet, I., Gury, C., Tcherny-Lessenot, S., Quesnot, A., and Gaudebout, P. (2005). Patterns of prescription of four major antipsychotics: A retrospective study based on medical records of psychiatric inpatients. *Pharmacoepidemiol Drug Safety*, 14(11):805–811.

30. Pizzo, P. (2002). Letter from the Dean, *Stanford Medicine Magazine*. Stanford University School of Medicine.

31. Lerman, C., LeSage, M.G., Perkins, K.A., O'Malley, S.S., Siegel, S.J., Benowitz, N.L. *et al.* (2007). Translational research in medication development for nicotine dependence. *Nat Rev Drug Discov*, 6(9):746–762.

32. Horig, H. and Pullman, W. (2004). From bench to clinic and back: Perspective on the 1st IQPC Translational Research conference. *J Transl Med*, 2(1):44.

33. Beckmann, N., Kneuer, R., Gremlich, H.U., Karmouty-Quintana, H., Ble, F.X., and Muller, M. (2007). In vivo mouse imaging and spectroscopy in drug discovery. *NMR Biomed*, 20(3):154–185.

34. Risterucci, C., Jeanneau, K., Schoppenthau, S., Bielser, T., Kunnecke, B., von Kienlin, M. *et al.* (2005). Functional magnetic resonance imaging reveals similar brain activity changes in two different animal models of schizophrenia. *Psychopharmacology (Berl)*, 180(4):724-734.
35. Tamminga, C.A., Lahti, A.C., Medoff, D.R., Gao, X.-M., and Holcomb, H.H. (2003). Evaluating Glutamatergic Transmission in Schizophrenia. *Ann NY Acad Sci*, 1003(1):113-118.
36. Shah, Y.B. and Marsden, C.A. (2004). The application of functional magnetic resonance imaging to neuropharmacology. *Curr Opin Pharmacol*, 4(5):517-521.
37. Robbins, T.W. (2005). Synthesizing schizophrenia: A bottom-up, symptomatic approach. *Schizophr Bull*, 31(4):854-864.
38. Porrino, L.J., Daunais, J.B., Rogers, G.A., Hampson, R.E., and Deadwyler, S.A. (2005). Facilitation of task performance and removal of the effects of sleep deprivation by an ampakine (CX717) in nonhuman primates. *PLoS Biol*, 3(9):e299.
39. McKinney, W.T.J. and Bunney, W.E.J. (1969). Animal model of depression I: Review of evidence: Implications for research. *Arch Gen Psychiatry*, 21(2):240-248.
40. American Psychiatric Association. (1994). Diagnostic and Statistical Manual of Mental Disorders, 4th edition. American Psychiatric Association, Washington, DC.
41. World Health Organization. (2007). International Statistical Classification of Diseases, 10th Revision, 2nd Edition. World Health Organization, Geneva.
42. Silverstone, P.H. (1991). Is anhedonia a good measure of depression?. *Acta Psychiatr Scand*, 83(4):249-250.
43. Hyman, S.E. (2007). Can neuroscience be integrated into the DSM-V? *Nat Rev Neurosci*, 8(9):725-732.
44. Kupfer, D.J., First, M.B., and Regier, D.A. (2002). *A Research Agenda for DSM-V*. American Psychiatric Association, Washington, DC.
45. Eisenberg, D.T., Mackillop, J., Modi, M., Beauchemin, J., Dang, D., Lisman, S.A. *et al.* (2007). Examining impulsivity as an endophenotype using a behavioral approach: A DRD2 TaqI A and DRD4 48-bp VNTR association study. *Behav Brain Funct*, 3:2.
46. Hasler, G., Drevets, W.C., Manji, H.K., and Charney, D.S. (2004). Discovering endophenotypes for major depression. *Neuropsychopharmacology*, 29(10):1765-1781.
47. Cannon, T.D. and Keller, M.C. (2006). Endophenotypes in the genetic analyses of mental disorders. *Ann Rev Clin Psychol*, 2(1):267-290.
48. Meehl, P.E. (1972). A critical afterword. In Gottesman, I.I. and Schields, J. (eds.), *Schizophrenia and Genetics: A Twin Study Vantage Point*. Academic Press, New York, pp. 367-415.
49. Breiter, H., Gasic, G., and Makris, N. (2006). Imaging the neural systems for motivated behavior and their dysfunction in neuropsychiatric illness. In Deisboeck, T.S. and Kresh, J.Y. (eds.), *Complex Systems Science in Biomedicine*. Springer, New York, pp. 763-810.
50. Gottesman, I.I. and Shields, J. (1973). Genetic theorizing and schizophrenia. *Br J Psychiatry*, 122(566):15-30.
51. Gottesman, I.I. and Gould, T.D. (2003/4/1). The endophenotype concept in psychiatry: Etymology and strategic intentions. *Am J Psychiatry*, 160(4):636-645.
52. Holzman, P.S. (2001). Seymour, S. Kety and the genetics of schizophrenia. *Neuropsychopharmacology*, 25(3):299-304.
53. Biomarkers Definitions Working Group. (2001). Biomarkers and surrogate endpoints: Preferred definitions and conceptual framework. *Clin Pharmacol Ther*, 69(3):89-95.
54. Katz, R. (2004). Biomarkers and surrogate markers: An FDA perspective. *NeuroRx*, 1(2):189-195.
55. Lesko, L.J. and Atkinson, A.J.J. (2001). Use of biomarkers and surrogate endpoints in drug development and regulatory decision making: Criteria, validation, strategies. *Ann Rev Pharmacol Toxicol*, 41:347-366.

56. De Gruttola, V.G., Clax, P., DeMets, D.L., Downing, G.J., Ellenberg, S.S., Friedman, L. *et al.* (2001). Considerations in the evaluation of surrogate endpoints in clinical trials. Summary of a National Institutes of Health workshop. *Control Clin Trials*, 22(5):485–502.

57. EMEA. (2007). *Innovative Drug Development Approaches: Final Report from the EMEA/ CHMP-Think-Tank Group on Innovative Drug Development*. The European Medicines Agency, London.

58. Zerhouni, E.A., Sanders, C.A., and von Eschenbach, A.C. (2007). The biomarkers consortium: Public and private sectors working in partnership to improve the public health. *Oncologist*, 12(3):250–252.

59. Willner, P. (1991). Methods for assessing the validity of animal models of human psychopathology. In Boulton, A., Baker, G., and Martin-Iverson, M. (eds.), *Neuromethods Vol 18:Animal Models in Psychiatry I*. Humana Press, Inc., pp. 1–23.

60. Kraemer, H.C., Schultz, S.K., and Arndt, S. (2002). Biomarkers in psychiatry: Methodological issues. *Am J Geriatr Psychiatry*, 10(6):653–659.

61. Tannock, R., Campbell, B., Seymour, P., Ouellet, D., Soares, H., Wang, P. *et al.* (2008). Towards a biological understanding of ADHD and the discovery of novel therapeutic approaches. In McArthur, R.A. and Borsini, F. (eds.), *Animal and Translational Models for CNS Drug Discovery: Psychiatric Disorders*. Academic Press: Elsevier, New York.

62. Gordon, E., Liddell, B.J., Brown, K.J., Bryant, R., Clark, C.R., Das, P. *et al.* (2007). Integrating objective gene-brain-behavior markers of psychiatric disorders. *J Integr Neurosci*, 6(1):1–34.

63. Turck, C.W., Maccarrone, G., Sayan-Ayata, E., Jacob, A.M., Ditzen, C., Kronsbein, H. *et al.* (2005). The quest for brain disorder biomarkers. *J Med Invest*, 52(Suppl):231–235.

64. Gomez-Mancilla, B., Marrer, E., Kehren, J., Kinnunen, A., Imbert, G., Hillebrand, R. *et al.* (2005). Central nervous system drug development: An integrative biomarker approach toward individualized medicine. *NeuroRx*, 2(4):683–695.

65. Javitt, D.C., Spencer, K.M., Thaker, G.K., Winterer, G., and Hajos, M. (2008). Neurophysiological biomarkers for drug development in schizophrenia. *Nat Rev Drug Discov*, 7(1):68–83.

66. Cho, R.Y., Ford, J.M., Krystal, J.H., Laruelle, M., Cuthbert, B., and Carter, C.S. (2005). Functional neuroimaging and electrophysiology biomarkers for clinical trials for cognition in schizophrenia. *Schizophr Bull*, 31(4):865–869.

67. Choi, D.W. (2002). Exploratory clinical testing of neuroscience drugs. *Nat Neurosci*, 5(Suppl):1023–1025.

68. Pien, H.H., Fischman, A.J., Thrall, J.H., and Sorensen, A.G. (2005). Using imaging biomarkers to accelerate drug development and clinical trials. *Drug Discov Today*, 10(4):259–266.

69. Thal, L.J., Kantarci, K., Reiman, E.M., Klunk, W.E., Weiner, M.W., Zetterberg, H. *et al.* (2006). The role of biomarkers in clinical trials for Alzheimer disease. *Alzheimer Dis Assoc Disord*, 20(1):6–15.

70. Phillips, M.L. and Vieta, E. (2007). Identifying functional neuroimaging biomarkers of bipolar disorder: toward DSM-V. *Schizophr Bull*, 33(4):893–904.

71. Schaller, B. (ed.) (2004). *Cerebral Ischemic Tolerance: From Animal Models to Clinical Relevance*. Nova Science Publishers, Hauppauge, NY.

72. Carroll, P.M. and Fitzgerald, K. (eds.) (2003). *Model Organisms in Drug Discovery*. John Wiley and Sons, Chichester, UK.

73. Offermanns, S. and Hein, L. (eds.) (2003). *Transgenic Models in Pharmacology (Handbook of Experimental Pharmacology)*. Springer, Heidelberg, Germany.

74. Levin, E.D. and Buccafusco, J.J. (eds.) (2006). *Animal Models of Cognitive Impairment*. Taylor & Francis CRC Press.

75. Boulton, A.A., Baker, G.B., and Martin-Iverson, M.T. (eds.) (1991). *Neuromethods: Animal Models in Psychiatry I*. The Humana Press, Clifton, New Jersey.

76. Olivier, B., Mos, J., and Slangen, J.L. (eds.) (1991). *Animal Models in Psychophramacology*. Birkhaüser-Verlag, Basel.
77. Myers, R.D. (ed.) (1971). *Methods in Psychobiology: Laboratory Techniques in Neuropsychology and Neurobiology*. Academic Press, New York.
78. Svartengren, J., Modiri, A.-R., and McArthur, R.A. (2005). Measurement and characterization of energy intake in the mouse. *Curr Protocols Pharmacol*, 5(Supplement 28). 5.40.1–5.19
79. Chin-Dusting, J., Mizrahi, J., Jennings, G., Fitzgerald, D. (2005). Finding improved medicines: The role of academic–industrial collaboration, *Nat Rev Drug Discov*, 4(11):891-7.
80. Horrobin, D.F. (2003). Modern biomedical research: An internally self-consistent universe with little contact with medical reality? *Nat Rev Drug Discov*, 2(2):151-154.
81. FitzGerald, G.A. (2005). Anticipating change in drug development:The emerging era of translational medicine and therapeutics, *Nat Rev Drug Discov* 4(10):815-8.
82. Pangalos, M.N., Schechter, L.E., and Hurko, O. (2007). Drug development for CNS disorders: Strategies for balancing risk and reducing attrition. *Nat Rev Drug Discov*, 6(7):521-532.
83. Agid, Y., Buzsaki, G., Diamond, D.M., Frackowiak, R., Giedd, J., Girault, J.-A. *et al.* (2007). How can drug discovery for psychiatric disorders be improved? *Nat Rev Drug Discov*, 6(3):189-201.
84. Willner, P. (ed.) (1991). *Behavioural Models in Psychopharmacology: Theoretical, Industrial and Clinical Perspectives*. Cambridge University Press, Cambridge.
85. Willner, P. (1991). Behavioural models in psychopharmacology. In Willner, P. (ed.), *Behavioural models in psychopharmacology: Theoretical, industrial and clinical perspectives*. Cambridge University Press, Cambridge, pp. 3–18
86. Miczek, K.A. (2008). Challenges for translational psychopharmacology research – the need for conceptual principles. In McArthur, R.A. and Borsini, F. (eds.), *Animal and Translational Models for CNS Drug Discovery: Psychiatric Disorders*. Academic Press: Elsevier, New York.
87. Merchant, K.M., Chesselet, M.-F., Hu, S.-C., and Fahn, S. (2008). Animal models of Parkinson's disease to aid drug discovery and development. In McArthur, R.A. and Borsini, F. (eds.), *Animal and Translational Models for CNS Drug Discovery: Neurologic Disorders*. Academic Press: Elsevier, New York.
88. Montes, J., Bendotti, C., Tortarolo, M., Cheroni, C., Hallak, H., Speiser, Z. *et al.* (2008). Translational research in ALS. In McArthur, R.A. and Borsini, F. (eds.), *Animal and Translational Models for CNS Drug Discovery: Neurologic Disorders*. Academic Press: Elsevier, New York.
89. Wagner, L.A., Menalled, L., Goumeniouk, A.D., Brunner, D.P., and Leavitt, B.R. (2008). Huntington disease. In McArthur, R.A. and Borsini, F. (eds.), *Animal and Translational Models for CNS Drug Discovery: Neurologic Disorders*. Academic Press: Elsevier, New York.
90. Bartz, J., Young, L.J., Hollander, E., Buxbaum, J.D., and Ring, R.H. (2008). Preclinical animal models of Autistic Spectrum Disorders (ASD). In McArthur, R.A. and Borsini, F. (eds.), *Animal and Translational Models for CNS Drug Discovery: Psychiatric Disorders*. Academic Press: Elsevier, New York.
91. Shilyansky, C., Li, W., Acosta, M., Elgersma, Y., Hannan, F., Hardt, M. *et al.* (2008). Molecular and cellular mechanisms of learning disabilities: A focus on neurofibromastosis type I. In McArthur, R.A. and Borsini, F. (eds.), *Animal and Translational Models for CNS Drug Discovery: Neurologic Disorders*. Academic Press: Elsevier, New York.
92. Medhurst, A.D., Atkins, A.R., Beresford, I.J., Brackenborough, K., Briggs, M.A., Calver, A.R. *et al.* (2007). GSK189254, a novel H3 receptor antagonist that binds to histamine H3 receptors in Alzheimer's disease brain and improves cognitive performance in preclinical models. *J Pharmacol Exp Ther*, 321(3):1032-1045.

93. Sanacora, G., Zarate, C.A., Krystal, J.H., and Manji, H.K. (2008). Targeting the glutamatergic system to develop novel, improved therapeutics for mood disorders. *Nat Rev Drug Discov*, 7(5):426–437.

94. Thomas, G.M. and Huganir, R.L. (2004). MAPK cascade signalling and synaptic plasticity. *Nat Rev Neurosci*, 5(3):173–183.

95. O'Neill, M.J., Bleakman, D., Zimmerman, D.M., and Nisenbaum, E.S. (2004). AMPA receptor potentiators for the treatment of CNS disorders. *Curr Drug Targets CNS Neurol Disord*, 3(3):181–194.

96. Lindner, M.D., McArthur, R.A., Deadwyler, S.A., Hampson, R.E., and Tariot, P.N. (2008). Development, optimization and use of preclinical behavioral models to maximise the productivity of drug discovery for Alzheimer's disease. In McArthur, R.A. and Borsini, F. (eds.), *Animal and Translational Models for CNS Drug Discovery: Neurologic Disorders*. Academic Press: Elsevier, New York.

97. Schneider, L.S. (2008). Issues in design and conduct of clinical trials for cognitive-enhancing drugs. In McArthur, R.A. and Borsini, F. (eds.), *Animal and Translational Models for CNS Drug Discovery: Neurologic Disorders*. Academic Press: Elsevier, New York.

98. Cryan, J.F., Sánchez, C., Dinan, T.G., and Borsini, F. (2008). Developing more efficacious antidepressant medications: Improving and aligning preclinical and clinical assessment tools. In McArthur, R.A. and Borsini, F. (eds.), *Animal and Translational Models for CNS Drug Discovery: Psychiatric Disorders*. Academic Press: Elsevier, New York.

99. Large, C.H., Einat, H., and Mahableshshwarkar, A.R. (2008). Developing new drugs for bipolar disorder (BPD): From animal models to the clinic. In McArthur, R.A. and Borsini, F. (eds.), *Animal and Translational Models for CNS Drug Discovery: Psychiatric Disorders*. Academic Press: Elsevier, New York.

100. Markou, A., Chiamulera, C., and West, R.J. (2008). Contribution of animal models and preclinical human studies to medication development for nicotine dependence. In McArthur, R.A. and Borsini, F. (eds.), *Animal and Translational Models for CNS Drug Discovery: Reward Deficit Disorders*. Academic Press: Elsevier, New York.

101. Dourish, C.T., Wilding, J.P.H., and Halford, J.C.G. (2008). Anti-obesity drugs: From animal models to clinical efficacy. In McArthur, R.A. and Borsini, F. (eds.), *Animal and Translational Models for CNS Drug Discovery: Reward Deficit Disorders*. Academic Press: Elsevier, New York.

102. Heidbreder, C. (2008). Impulse and reward deficit disorders: Drug discovery and development. In McArthur, R.A. and Borsini, F. (eds.), *Animal and Translational Models for CNS Drug Discovery: Reward Deficit Disorders*. Academic Press: Elsevier, New York.

103. Klitgaard, H., Matagne, A., Schachter, S.C., and White, H.S. (2008). Animal and translational models of the epilepsies. In McArthur, R.A. and Borsini, F. (eds.), *Animal and Translational Models for CNS Drug Discovery: Neurologic Disorders*. Academic Press: Elsevier, New York.

104. Cudkowicz, M.E., Shefner, J.M., Schoenfeld, D.A., Zhang, H., Andreasson, K.I., Rothstein, J.D. et al. (2006). Trial of celecoxib in amyotrophic lateral sclerosis. *Ann Neurol*, 60(1):22–31.

105. Wolfe, M.S. (2002). Therapeutic strategies for Alzheimer's disease. *Nat Rev Drug Discov*, 1(11):859–866.

106. Bowers, W.J., Howard, D.F., and Federoff, H.J. (1997). Gene therapeutic strategies for neuroprotection: Implications for Parkinson's disease. *Exp Neurol*, 144(1):58–68.

107. Stefan, H., Lopes da Silva, F.H., Loscher, W., Schmidt, D., Perucca, E., Brodie, M.J. et al. (2006). Epileptogenesis and rational therapeutic strategies. *Acta Neurol Scand*, 113(3):139–155.

108. Steckler, T., Stein, M.B., and Holmes, A. (2008). Developing novel anxiolytics: Improving preclinical detection and clinical assessment. In McArthur, R.A. and Borsini, F. (eds.), *Animal and Translational Models for CNS Drug Discovery: Psychiatric Disorders*. Academic Press: Elsevier, New York.

109. Kandel, E.R. (2006). *In search of memory: The emergence of a new science of mind.* W.W. Norton & Company, New York.

110. Hardy, J.A. and Higgins, G.A. (1992). Alzheimer's disease: The amyloid cascade hypothesis. *Science*, 256(5054):184-185.

111. Hardy, J. and Selkoe, D.J. (2002). The amyloid hypothesis of Alzheimer's disease: Progress and problems on the road to therapeutics. *Science*, 297(5580):353-356.

112. Schenk, D. (2002). Amyloid-beta immunotherapy for Alzheimer's disease: The end of the beginning. *Nat Rev Neurosci*, 3(10):824-828.

113. Aisen, P.S. (2005). The development of anti-amyloid therapy for Alzheimer's disease: From secretase modulators to polymerisation inhibitors. *CNS Drugs*, 19(12):989-996.

114. Wang, Y.J., Zhou, H.D., and Zhou, X.F. (2006). Clearance of amyloid-beta in Alzheimer's disease: Progress, problems and perspectives. *Drug Discov Today*, 11(19-20):931-938.

115. Ashe, K.H. (2001). Learning and Memory in Transgenic Mice Modeling Alzheimer's Disease. *Learn Mem*, 8(6):301-308.

116. Van Dam, D., Coen, K., and De Deyn, P.P. (2008). Cognitive evaluation of disease-modifying efficacy of donepezil in the APP23 mouse model for Alzheimer's disease. *Psychopharmacology (Berl)*, 197(1):37-43.

117. Dong, H., Csernansky, C.A., Martin, M.V., Bertchume, A., Vallera, D., and Csernansky, J.G. (2005). Acetylcholinesterase inhibitors ameliorate behavioral deficits in the Tg2576 mouse model of Alzheimer's disease. *Psychopharmacology (Berl)*, 181(1):145-152.

118. Arendash, G.W., Gordon, M.N., Diamond, D.M., Austin, L.A., Hatcher, J.M., Jantzen, P. et al. (2001). Behavioral assessment of Alzheimer's transgenic mice following long-term Abeta vaccination: task specificity and correlations between Abeta deposition and spatial memory. *DNA Cell Biol*, 20(11):737-744.

119. Wilcock, D.M., Rojiani, A., Rosenthal, A., Subbarao, S., Freeman, M.J., Gordon, M.N. et al. (2004). Passive immunotherapy against Abeta in aged APP-transgenic mice reverses cognitive deficits and depletes parenchymal amyloid deposits in spite of increased vascular amyloid and microhemorrhage. *J Neuroinflammation*, 1(1):24.

120. Janus, C., Pearson, J., McLaurin, J., Mathews, P.M., Jiang, Y., Schmidt, S.D. et al. (2000). A beta peptide immunization reduces behavioural impairment and plaques in a model of Alzheimer's disease. *Nature*, 408(6815):979-982.

121. Austin, L., Arendash, G.W., Gordon, M.N., Diamond, D.M., DiCarlo, G., Dickey, C. et al. (2003). Short-term beta-amyloid vaccinations do not improve cognitive performance in cognitively impaired APP + PS1 mice. *Behav Neurosci*, 117(3):478-484.

122. Hock, C., Konietzko, U., Streffer, J.R., Tracy, J., Signorell, A., Muller-Tillmanns, B. et al. (2003). Antibodies against beta-amyloid slow cognitive decline in Alzheimer's disease. *Neuron*, 38(4):547-554.

123. Gilman, S., Koller, M., Black, R.S., Jenkins, L., Griffith, S.G., Fox, N.C. et al. (2005). Clinical effects of Abeta immunization (AN1792) in patients with AD in an interrupted trial. *Neurology*, 64(9):1553-1562.

124. Dickson, D.W., Crystal, H.A., Mattiace, L.A., Masur, D.M., Blau, A.D., Davies, P. et al. (1992). Identification of normal and pathological aging in prospectively studied nondemented elderly humans. *Neurobiol Aging*, 13(1):179-189.

125. Arriagada, P.V., Marzloff, K., and Hyman, B.T. (1992). Distribution of Alzheimer-type pathologic changes in nondemented elderly individuals matches the pattern in Alzheimer's disease. *Neurology*, 42(9):1681-1688.

126. Lue, L.F., Brachova, L., Civin, W.H., and Rogers, J. (1996). Inflammation, A beta deposition, and neurofibrillary tangle formation as correlates of Alzheimer's disease neurodegeneration. *J Neuropathol Exp Neurol*, 55(10):1083-1088.

127. Davis, D.G., Schmitt, F.A., Wekstein, D.R., and Markesbery, W.R. (1999). Alzheimer neuropathologic alterations in aged cognitively normal subjects. *J Neuropathol Exp Neurol*, 58(4):376–388.

128. Mufson, E.J., Chen, E.Y., Cochran, E.J., Beckett, L.A., Bennett, D.A., and Kordower, J.H. (1999). Entorhinal cortex beta-amyloid load in individuals with mild cognitive impairment. *Exp Neurol*, 158(2):469–490.

129. Crystal, H., Dickson, D., Fuld, P., Masur, D., Scott, R., Mehler, M. *et al.* (1988). Clinico-pathologic studies in dementia: Nondemented subjects with pathologically confirmed Alzheimer's disease. *Neurology*, 38(11):1682–1687.

130. Geddes, J.W., Tekirian, T.L., Soultanian, N.S., Ashford, J.W., Davis, D.G., and Markesbery, W. R. (1997). Comparison of neuropathologic criteria for the diagnosis of Alzheimer's disease. *Neurobiol Aging*, 18(4 Suppl):S99–105.

131. Hardy, J. (2006). Has the amyloid cascade hypothesis for Alzheimer's disease been proved?. *Curr Alzheimer Res*, 3(1):71–73.

132. McArthur, R.A., Franklin, S.R., Goodwin, A., Oostveen, J., Buhl, A. (2000). APP-overexpressing transgenic mice (TG2576) are not impaired in acquisition of an olfactory discrimination. *Society for Neurosciences 30th Annual Meeting*, November 4–9, 2000, New Orleans, LA, p. 275.3.

133. Westerman, M.A., Cooper-Blacketer, D., Mariash, A., Kotilinek, L., Kawarabayashi, T., Younkin, L.H. *et al.* (2002). The relationship between Abeta and memory in the Tg2576 mouse model of Alzheimer's disease. *J Neurosci*, 22(5):1858–1867.

134. Lesne, S., Koh, M.T., Kotilinek, L., Kayed, R., Glabe, C.G., Yang, A. *et al.* (2006). A specific amyloid-[beta] protein assembly in the brain impairs memory. *Nature*, 440(7082):352–357.

135. Urbanc, B., Cruz, L., Le, R., Sanders, J., Ashe, K.H., Duff, K. *et al.* (2002). Neurotoxic effects of thioflavin S-positive amyloid deposits in transgenic mice and Alzheimer's disease. *Proc Natl Acad Sci USA*, 99(22):13990–13995.

136. Dodart, J.C., Mathis, C., Bales, K.R., and Paul, S.M. (2002). Does my mouse have Alzheimer's disease? *Genes Brain Behav*, 1(3):142–155.

137. Fehniger, T.E., Laurell, T., and Marko-Varga, G. (2005). Integrating disease knowledge and technology to deliver protein targets and biomarkers into drug discovery projects. *Drug Discov Today: Technologies*, 2(4):345–351.

138. Frank, R. and Hargreaves, R. (2003). Clinical biomarkers in drug discovery and development. *Nat Rev Drug Discov*, 2(7):566–580.

139. Brooks, D.J., Frey, K.A., Marek, K.L., Oakes, D., Paty, D., Prentice, R. *et al.* (2003). Assessment of neuroimaging techniques as biomarkers of the progression of Parkinson's disease. *Exp Neurol*, 184(Suppl 1):S68–S79.

140. Doran, S.M., Wessel, T., Kilduff, T.S., Turek, F.W., and Renger, J.J. (2008). Translational models of sleep and sleep disorders. In McArthur, R.A. and Borsini, F. (eds.), *Animal and Translational Models for CNS Drug Discovery: Psychiatric Disorders*. Academic Press: Elsevier, New York.

141. Airan, R.D., Meltzer, L.A., Roy, M., Gong, Y., Chen, H., and Deisseroth, K. (2007). High-speed imaging reveals neurophysiological links to behavior in an animal model of depression. *Science*, 317(5839):819–823.

142. Gardner, T.J., Kosten, T.A., and Kosten, T.R. (2008). Issues in designing and conducting clinical trials for reward disorders. In McArthur, R.A. and Borsini, F. (eds.), *Animal and Translational Models for CNS Drug Discovery: Reward Deficit Disorders*. Academic Press: Elsevier, New York.

143. Koob, G.F. (2008). The role of animal models in reward deficit disorders: Views from Academia. In McArthur, R.A. and Borsini, F. (eds.), *Animal and Translational Models for CNS Drug Discovery: Reward Deficit Disorders*. Academic Press: Elsevier, New York.

144. Williams, W.A., Grant, J.E., Winstanley, C.A., and Potenza, M.N. (2008). Currect concepts in the classification, treatment and modelling of pathological gambling and other impulse control disorders. In McArthur, R.A. and Borsini, F. (eds.), *Animal and Translational Models for CNS Drug Discovery: Reward Deficit Disorders*. Academic Press: Elsevier, New York.

145. Rauch, S.L. and Savage, C.R. (1997). Neuroimaging and neuropsychology of the striatum. Bridging basic science and clinical practice. *Psychiatr Clin North Am*, 20(4):741-768.

146. Andreasen, N.C. (1997). Linking mind and brain in the study of mental illnesses: A project for a scientific psychopathology. *Science*, 275(5306):1586-1593.

147. Karitzky, J. and Ludolph, A.C. (2001). Imaging and neurochemical markers for diagnosis and disease progression ALS in. *J Neurol Sci*, 191(1-2):35-41.

148. Wise, R.G. and Tracey, I. (2006). The role of fMRI in drug discovery. *J Magn Reson Imaging*, 23(6):862-876.

149. Bacskai, B.J., Kajdasz, S.T., Christie, R.H., Carter, C., Games, D., Seubert, P. *et al.* (2007). Imaging of amyloid-beta deposits in brains of living mice permits direct observation of clearance of plaques with immunotherapy. *Nat Med*, 7(3):369-372.

150. De Luca, C.R., Wood, S.J., Anderson, V., Buchanan, J.A., Proffitt, T.M., Mahony, K. *et al.* (2003). Normative data from CANTAB I: Development of executive function over the lifespan. *J Clin Exp Neuropsychol*, 25(2):242-254.

151. Robbins, T.W., James, M., Owen, A.M., Lange, K.W., Lees, A.J., Leigh, P.N. *et al.* (1994). Cognitive deficits in progressive supranuclear palsy, Parkinson's disease, and multiple system atrophy in tests sensitive to frontal lobe dysfunction. *J Neurol Neurosurg Psychiatry*, 57(1).79-88.

152. Robbins, T.W., James, M., Owen, A.M., Sahakian, B.J., McInnes, L., and Rabbitt, P. (1994). Cambridge Neuropsychological Test Automated Battery (CANTAB): A factor analytic study of a large sample of normal elderly volunteers. *Dementia*, 5(5):266-281.

153. Blackwell, A.D., Sahakian, B.J., Vesey, R., Semple, J.M., Robbins, T.W., and Hodges, J.R. (2004). Detecting dementia: Novel neuropsychological markers of preclinical Alzheimer's disease. *Dement Geriatr Cogn Disord*, 17(1-2):42-48.

154. Swainson, R., Hodges, J.R., Galton, C.J., Semple, J., Michael, A., Dunn, B.D. *et al.* (2001). Early detection and differential diagnosis of Alzheimer's disease and depression with neuropsychological tasks. *Dement Geriatr Cogn Disord*, 12(4):265-280.

155. Sahakian, B.J., Elliott, R., Low, N., Mehta, M., Clark, R.T., and Pozniak, A.L. (1995). Neuropsychological deficits in tests of executive function in asymptomatic and symptomatic HIV-1 seropositive men. *Psychol Med*, 25(6):1233-1246.

156. Owen, A.M. and Doyon, J. (1999). The cognitive neuropsychology of Parkinson's disease: A functional neuroimaging perspective. *Adv Neurol*, 80:49-56.

157. Owen, A.M., Doyon, J., Dagher, A., Sadikot, A., and Evans, A.C. (1998). Abnormal basal ganglia outflow in Parkinson's disease identified with PET. Implications for higher cortical functions. *Brain*, 121(Pt 5):949-965.

158. Reeves, S.J., Grasby, P.M., Howard, R.J., Bantick, R.A., Asselin, M.C., and Mehta, M.A. (2005). A positron emission tomography (PET) investigation of the role of striatal dopamine (D2) receptor availability in spatial cognition. *Neuroimage*, 28(1):216-226.

159. Greig, N.H., Sambamurti, K., Yu, Q.-S., Brossi, A., Bruinsma, G., and Lahiri, D.K. (2005). An Overview of Phenserine Tartrate, A Novel Acetylcholinesterase Inhibitor for the Treatment of Alzheimer's Disease. *Current Alzheimer Research*, 2(3):281-290.

160. Froestl, W., Gallagher, M., Jenkins, H., Madrid, A., Melcher, T., Teichman, S. *et al.* (2004). SGS742: The first GABA(B) receptor antagonist in clinical trials. *Biochem Pharmacol*, 68(8):1479-1487.

161. Spinelli, S., Pennanen, L., Dettling, A.C., Feldon, J., Higgins, G.A., and Pryce, C.R. (2004). Performance of the marmoset monkey on computerized tasks of attention and working memory. *Brain Res Cogn Brain Res*, 19(2):123-137.

162. Weed, M.R., Taffe, M.A., Polis, I., Roberts, A.C., Robbins, T.W., Koob, G.F. *et al.* (1999). Performance norms for a rhesus monkey neuropsychological testing battery: Acquisition and long-term performance. *Brain Res Cogn Brain Res*, 8(3):185–201.

163. Spinelli, S., Ballard, T., Gatti-McArthur, S., Richards, G.J., Kapps, M., Woltering, T. *et al.* (2005). Effects of the mGluR2/3 agonist LY354740 on computerized tasks of attention and working memory in marmoset monkeys. *Psychopharmacology (Berl)*, 179(1): 292–302.

164. Taffe, M.A., Davis, S.A., Gutierrez, T., and Gold, L.H. (2002). Ketamine impairs multiple cognitive domains in rhesus monkeys. *Drug Alcohol Depend*, 68(2):175–187.

165. Taffe M.A., Weed M.A., Gold L.H. (2000). Disruption of visuo-spatial paired-associate learning in rhesus monkeys. Society for Neurocience, *30th Annual Meeting*, New Orleans, LA.

166. Taffe, M.A., Weed, M.R., and Gold, L.H. (1999). Scopolamine alters rhesus monkey performance on a novel neuropsychological test battery. *Brain Res Cogn Brain Res*, 8(3):203–212.

167. Weed, M.R., Gold, L.H., Polis, I., Koob, G.F., Fox, H.S., and Taffe, M.A. (2004). Impaired performance on a rhesus monkey neuropsychological testing battery following simian immunodeficiency virus infection. *AIDS Res Hum Retroviruses*, 20(1):77–89.

168. Bailey, P. (2007). Biological markers in Alzheimer's disease. *Can J Neurol Sci*, 34(Suppl 1): S72–S76.

169. Ledford, H. (2008). Drug markers questioned. *Nature*, 452(7187):510–511.

170. Henley, S.M., Bates, G.P., and Tabrizi, S.J. (2005). Biomarkers for neurodegenerative diseases. *Curr Opin Neurol*, 18(6):698–705.

171. Imming, P., Sinning, C., and Meyer, A. (2006). Drugs, their targets and the nature and number of drug targets. *Nat Rev Drug Discov*:821–834.

172. Bartfai, T and Lees, G.V. (2006). *Drug Discovery: from bedside to wall Street*. Elsevier Academic Press, Burkington, MA.

173. Picciotto, M.R. and Wickman, K. (1998). Using knockout and transgenic mice to study neurophysiology and behavior. *Physiol Rev*, 78(4):1131–1163.

174. de Fougerolles, A.R. (2008). Delivery vehicles for small interfering RNA in vivo. *Hum Gene Ther*, 19(2):125–132.

175. Lundstrom, K. (2007). Prospects of treating neurological diseases by gene therapy. *Curr Opin Investig Drugs*, 8(1):34–40.

176. Brendza, R.P., Bacskai, B.J., Cirrito, J.R., Simmons, K.A., Skoch, J.M., Klunk, W.E. *et al.* (2005). Anti-Abeta antibody treatment promotes the rapid recovery of amyloid-associated neuritic dystrophy in PDAPP transgenic mice. *J Clin Invest*, 115(2):428–433.

177. ICH. (1993). Guidance for Industry: Safety Pharmacology Studies for Human Pharmaceuticals S7A. p. 1–4.

178. De Leon, M.J., Snider, D.A., and Federoff, H. (eds.) (2007). *Imaging and the Aging Brain*. New York Academy of Sciences, New York.

179. Rosen, W.G., Mohs, R.C., and Davis, K.L. (1984). A new rating scale for Alzheimer's disease. *Am J Psychiatry*, 141(11):1356–1364.

180. Mohs, R.C., Knopman, D., Petersen, R.C., Ferris, S.H., Ernesto, C., Grundman, M. *et al.* (1997). Development of cognitive instruments for use in clinical trials of antidementia drugs: additions to the Alzheimer's Disease Assessment Scale that broaden its scope. The Alzheimer's Disease Cooperative Study. *Alzheimer Dis Assoc Disord*, 11(Suppl 2):S13–21.

181. Silcoff, S. (2007). Neurochem CEO Bellini still confident about Alzhemed despite FDA setback. November 09.

182. Greig, N.H., Sambamurthi, K., Yu, Q.S., Brossi, A., Bruinsma, G., and Lahiri, D.K. (2005). An Overview of phenserine tartrate, a novel acetylcholinesterase inhibitor for the treatment of Alzheimer's disease. *Current Alzheimer Research*, 2(3): 281–290.

183. Lyketsos, C.G., Kozauer, N., and Rabins, P.V. (2007). Psychiatric manifestations of neurologic disease: Where are we headed? *Dialogues Clin Neurosci.*, 9(2):111-124.

184. Kelleher, R.T. and Morse, W.H. (1968). Determinants of the specificity of behavioral effects of drugs. *Ergeb Physiol*, 60:1-56.

185. Blundell, J.E. and Latham, C.J. (1982). Behavioural Pharmacology of Feeding. In Silversone, T. (ed.), *Drugs and Appetite*. Academic Press, London, pp. 41-80.

186. Matthysse, S. (1986). Animal models in psychiatric research. *Prog Brain Res*, 65:259-270.

187. Morris, R. (1984). Developments of a water-maze procedure for studying spatial learning in the rat. *J Neurosci Methods*, 11(1):47-60.

188. Ludvig, N., Tang, H.M., Eichenbaum, H., and Gohil, B.C. (2003). Spatial memory performance of freely-moving squirrel monkeys. *Behav Brain Res*, 140(1-2):175-183.

189. Ekstrom, A.D., Kahana, M.J., Caplan, J.B., Fields, T.A., Isham, E.A., Newman, E.L. *et al.* (2003). Cellular networks underlying human spatial navigation. *Nature*, 425(6954):184-188.

190. Dunnett, S.B. (1985). Comparative effects of cholinergic drugs and lesions of nucleus basalis or fimbria-fornix on delayed matching in rats. *Psychopharmacology (Berl)*, 87(3):357-363.

191. Murphy, B.L., Arnsten, A.F., Jentsch, J.D., and Roth, R.H. (1996). Dopamine and spatial working memory in rats and monkeys: Pharmacological reversal of stress-induced impairment. *J Neurosci*, 16(23):7768-7775.

192. Smith, E.E. and Jonides, J. (1998). Neuroimaging analyses of human working memory. *Proc Natl Acad Sci*, 95(20):12061-12068.

193. Birrell, J.M. and Brown, V.J. (2000). Medial frontal cortex mediates perceptual attentional set shifting in the rat. *J Neurosci*, 20(11):4320-4324.

194. Dias, R., Robbins, T.W., and Roberts, A.C. (1996). Dissociation in prefrontal cortex of affective and attentional shifts. *Nature*, 380(6569):69-72.

195. Lawrence, A.D., Sahakian, B.J., Hodges, J.R., Rosser, A.E., Lange, K.W., and Robbins, T.W. (1996). Executive and mnemonic functions in early Huntington's disease. *Brain*, 119(Pt 5): 1633-1645.

196. Lindner, M.D. (2007). Clinical attrition due to biased preclinical assessments of potential efficacy. *Pharmacol Ther*, 115(1):148-175.

197. Hornykiewicz, O. (1966). Dopamine (3-hydroxytyramine) and brain function. *Pharmacol Rev*, 18(2):925-964.

198. Hornykiewicz, O. (2002). L-DOPA: From a biologically inactive amino acid to a successful therapeutic agent. *Amino Acids*, 23(1-3):65-70.

199. Koller, W.C. and Tse, W. (2004). Unmet medical needs in Parkinson's disease. *Neurology*, 62(90011):1S-8S.

200. Polymeropoulos, M.H., Lavedan, C., Leroy, E., Ide, S.E., Dehejia, A., Dutra, A. *et al.* (1997). Mutation in the alpha-synuclein gene identified in families with Parkinson's disease. *Science*, 276(5321):2045-2047.

201. Spillantini, M.G., Schmidt, M.L., Lee, V.M., Trojanowski, J.Q., Jakes, R., and Goedert, M. (1997). Alpha-synuclein in Lewy bodies. *Nature*, 388(6645):839-840.

202. Kitada, T., Asakawa, S., Hattori, N., Matsumine, H., Yamamura, Y., Minoshima, S. *et al.* (1998). Mutations in the parkin gene cause autosomal recessive juvenile parkinsonism. *Nature*, 392(6676):605-608.

203. Valente, E.M., Abou-Sleiman, P.M., Caputo, V., Muqit, M.M.K., Harvey, K., Gispert, S. *et al.* (2004). Hereditary early-onset Parkinson's disease caused by mutations in PINK1. *Science*, 304(5674):1158-1160.

204. Bonifati, V., Rizzu, P., van Baren, M.J., Schaap, O., Breedveld, G.J., Krieger, E. *et al.* (2003). Mutations in DJ-1 gene associated with autosomal recessive early-onset parkinsonism. *Science*, 299(5604):256-259.

205. Little, H.J., McKinzie, D.L., Setnik, B., Shram, M.J., and Sellers, E.M. (2008). Pharmacotherapy of alcohol dependence: Improving translation from the bench to the clinic. In McArthur, R.A. and Borsini, F. (eds.), *Animal and Translational Models CNS for Drug Discovery: Reward Deficit Disorders*. Academic Press: Elsevier, New York.

206. Crabbe, J.C., Wahlsten, D., and Dudek, B.C. (1999). Genetics of Mouse Behavior: Interactions with Laboratory Environment. *Science*, 284:1670–1672.

207. Berry, D.A. (2006). Bayesian clinical trials. *Nat Rev Drug Discov*, 5(1):27–36.

208. Price, D.L. and Sisodia, S.S. (1998). Mutant genes in familial Alzheimer's disease and transgenic models. *Annu Rev Neurosci*, 21:479–505.

209. Gasser, T. (2005). Genetics of Parkinson's disease. *Curr Opin Neurol*, 18(4):363–369.

210. Deng, H.X., Hentati, A., Tainer, J.A., Iqbal, Z., Cayabyab, A., Hung, W.Y. *et al.* (1993). Amyotrophic lateral sclerosis and structural defects in Cu,Zn superoxide dismutase. *Science*, 261(5124):1047–1051.

211. Rosen, D.R., Siddique, T., Patterson, D., Figlewicz, D.A., Sapp, P., Hentati, A. *et al.* (1993). Mutations in Cu/Zn superoxide dismutase gene are associated with familial amyotrophic lateral sclerosis. *Nature*, 362(6415):59–62.

212. Gurney, M.E. (1994). Transgenic-mouse model of amyotrophic lateral sclerosis. *N Engl J Med*, 331(25):1721–1722.

213. Doble, A. (1996). The pharmacology and mechanism of action of riluzole. *Neurology*, 47(6_Suppl_4):233S–234S.

214. Benatar, M. (2007). Lost in translation: treatment trials in the SOD1 mouse and in human ALS. *Neurobiol Dis*, 26(1):1–13.

215. Smith, M., Wilcox, K.S., and White, H.S. (2007). Discovery of antiepileptic drugs. *Neurotherapeutics*, 4(1):12–17.

216. French, J.A., Kanner, A.M., Bautista, J., Abou-Khalil, B., Browne, T., Harden, C.L. *et al.* (2004). Efficacy and tolerability of the new antiepileptic drugs II: Treatment of refractory epilepsy: Report of the Therapeutics and Technology Assessment Subcommittee and Quality Standards Subcommittee of the American Academy of Neurology and the American Epilepsy Society. *Neurology*, 62(8):1261–1273.

217. French, J.A., Kanner, A.M., Bautista, J., Abou-Khalil, B., Browne, T., Harden, C.L. *et al.* (2004). Efficacy and tolerability of the new antiepileptic drugs I: Treatment of new onset epilepsy: Report of the Therapeutics and Technology Assessment Subcommittee and Quality Standards Subcommittee of the American Academy of Neurology and the American Epilepsy Society. *Neurology*, 62(8):1252–1260.

218. Keller, M.B. (2005). Issues in treatment-resistant depression. *J Clin Psychiatry*, 66(Suppl 8): 5–12.

219. Souery, D., Oswald, P., Massat, I., Bailer, U., Bollen, J., Demyttenaere, K. *et al.* (2007). Clinical factors associated with treatment resistance in major depressive disorder: Results from a European multicenter study. *J Clin Psychiatry*, 68(7):1062–1070.

220. Marincola, F.M. (2003). Translational Medicine: A two-way road. *J Transl Med*, 1(1):1.

221. Fray, P.J., Robbins, T.W., and Sahakian, B.J. (1996). Neuropsychiatric applications of CANTAB. *Int J Geriatr Psychiatry*, 11(4):329–336.

Acknowledgements

We would like to thank our many colleagues who have pooled their knowledge and who have contributed to the creation of this book. We have enjoyed this experience of working with them on a "Global Project Team." Hopefully this sharing of our experiences will "translate" into a more efficient and fruitful use of animals to model the devastating disorders we are trying to understand, and to help us discover and develop the drugs needed to alleviate them.

We would especially like to thank Stephanie Diment, Keri Witman, Kirsten Funk and Renske van Dijk of Elsevier for their cheerful encouragement throughout this project, and without their help this book would have never been completed. We thank as well the members of our "advisory board": Professors Trevor Robbins, Tamas Bartfai, Bill Deakin; and Doctors Danny Hoyer, David Sanger, Julian Gray and Markus Heilig for their productive interventions and thoughtful discussions at various times over the past 18 months.

Finally we would like to thank all those who provided the space and opportunity so that this book could become a reality. You know who you are....

List of Contributors

M. Acosta, MD Department of Neurology, Children's National Medical Center, Washington, DC

Caterina Bendotti, PhD Laboratory of Molecular Neurobiology, Department of Neuroscience, Istituto di Ricerche Farmacologiche, Mario Negri, Via G.La Masa 19, 201567 Milano, Italia

Eran Blaugrund, PhD Project Evaluation & Pre Clinical Development, Teva Innovative Ventures, Teva Pharmaceuticals Industries Ltd, 5 Basel St, Petach Tikva 49131, Israel

Daniela Brunner, PhD Behavioral Research and Development, PsychoGenics Inc., 765 Old Saw Mill River Road, Tarrytown, NY 10591, USA and Biopsychology Department, New York State Psychiatric Institute/Columbia University, New York, USA

Franco Borsini, PhD sigma-tau Industrie Farmaceutiche Riunite S.p.A., Via Pontina km 30,400, 00040 Pomezia (Rome), Italy

Cristina Cheroni, PhD Laboratory of Moleculor Biology, Department of Neuroscience, Istituto di Ricerche Farmacologiche, Mario Negri, Via G.La Masa 19, 201567 Milano, Italia

Marie-Françoise Chesselet, MD, PhD The David Geffen School of Medicine at UCLA, 710 Westwood Plaza, Los Angeles, CA 90095-1769, USA

Sam A. Deadwyler, PhD Department of Physiology and Pharmacology, Wake Forest University School of Medicine, Medical Center Boulevard, Winston Salem, NC 27157-1083, USA

Y. Elgersma, PhD Neuroscience Institute, Erasmus University, Rotterdam

Stanley Fahn, MD Chief and H. Houston Merritt Professor of Neurology, Neurological Institute, Columbia University Medical Center, Movement Disorders Division, 710 W 168th St, New York, NY 10032, USA

Paul H. Gordon, MD Department of Neurology, Columbia University, 710 W.168th St., New York, NY 10032, USA

Sari Goren, PhD Medical Assessment and Planning, Global Innovative Pipeline Management, Teva Pharmaceuticals Industries Ltd, 5 Basel St, Petach Tikva 49131, Israel

Alexander D. Goumeniouk, MD, FRCP(C), FAPA Department of Anesthesiology, Pharmacology & Therapeutics, Faculty of Medicine, University of British Columbia, 2176 Health Sciences Mall, Vancouver, British Columbia, Canada V6T 1Z3

Hussein Hallak, PhD Non-Clinical PK Leader, Metabolism, PK & Drug Screening, Project Evaluation & Pre Clinical Development, Teva Innovative Ventures, Teva Pharmaceuticals Industries Ltd, 5 Basel St, Petach Tikva 49131, Israel

Robert E. Hampson, PhD   Department of Physiology and Pharmacology, Wake Forest University School of Medicine, Medical Center Boulevard, Winston Salem, NC 27157-1083, USA

F. Hannan, PhD   Cell Biology and Anatomy Department, New York Medical College, New York

M. Hardt, BSc   Department of Psychology and Clinical Neuroscience Laboratory, University of California, Los Angeles

Shu-Ching Hu, MD, PhD   Department of Neurology, Columbia University Medical Center, New York, NY, USA

A. Jackie Hunter, PhD   GlaxoSmithKline plc, Neurology and Gastro-Intestinal (GI) Centre of Excellence for Drug Discovery, New Frontiers Science Park (north), Third Avenue, Harlow, Essex CM19 5AW, UK

K. Hunter-Schaedle, PhD   Children's Tumor Foundation, New Jersey

Henrik Klitgaard, PhD   UCB Pharma SA, Preclinical CNS Research, Chemin du Foriest, Braine-l'Alleud, Belgium

L.C. Krab, MSc   Neuroscience Institute, Erasmus University, Rotterdam

Blair R. Leavitt, MD, CM, FRCP(C)   Centre for Molecular Medicine and Therapeutics, British Colombia Research Institute for Children's and Women's Health, Department of Medical Genetics, University of British Columbia, Vancouver British Columbia, Canada

E. Legius, MD, PhD   Department of Human Genetics, Catholic University of Leuven, Leuven

Weidong Li, MD, PhD   Department of Neurobiology, University of California, Los Angeles

Mark D. Lindner, PhD   McArthur and Associates GmbH, Basel, Switzerland

Alain Matagne, MSc   UCB Pharma SA, Preclinical CNS Research, Chemin du Foriest, Braine-l'Alleud, Belgium

Robert A. McArthur, PhD   McArthur and Associates, GmbH, Ramsteinerstrasse 28, CH-4052, Basel, Switzerland

Liliana Menalled, PhD   PsychoGenics Inc., 765 Old Saw Mill River Road, Tarrytown, NY 10591, USA; Biopsychology Department, NYSPI/Columbia University, 1051 Riverside Dr., New York, NY 10032, USA

Kalpana M. Merchant, PhD   Neuroscience Division, Eli Lilly and Company, Lilly Corporate Center, Indianapolis, Indiana 46285, USA

Jacqueline Montes, PT, MA, NCS   Department of Neurology, Columbia University, 710 W. 168th Street, New York, NY 10032, USA

Steven C. Schachter, MD Professor of Neurology and Director of Research, Department of Neurology, Beth Israel Deaconess Medical Center, 330 Brookline Avenue-KS 478, Boston, MA 02215, USA

Lon S. Schneider, MD Professor of Psychiatry, Neurology, and Gerontology, Keck School of Medicine, University of Southern California, 1510 San Pablo St., HCC 600, Los Angeles, CA 90033, USA

Carrie Shilyansky, PhD Department of Neurobiology, University of California, Los Angeles

Alcino J. Silva, PhD Department of Neurobiology, Psychiatry and Biobehavioral Sciences, Psychology and Brain Research Institute, UCLA, 695 Young Drive South, Room 235, Box 951761, Los Angeles, CA 90095-1761, USA

Zipora Speiser, PhD Consultant to TEVA, Pharmacology unit, CNS Project Evaluation & Pre Clinical Development, Teva Innovative Ventures, Teva Pharmaceuticals Industries Ltd, 5 Basel St, Petach Tikva 49131, Israel

Pierre N. Tariot, MD Director, Memory Disorders Center, Banner Alzheimer's Institute, Research Professor of Psychiatry, University of Arizona College of Medicine, 901 E Willetta St., Phoenix, AZ 85006, USA

Massimo Tortarolo, PhD Laboratory of Molecular Neurobiology, Department of Neuroscience, Istituto di Ricerche Farmacologiche, Mario Negri, Via G.La Masa 19, 201567 Milano, Italia

Laura A. Wagner, MSc Centre for Molecular Medicine and Therapeutics, Child and Family Research Institute, BC Children's Hospital, Department of Medical Genetics, University of British Columbia, Vancouver, BC, Canada

H. Steve White, PhD Anticonvulsant Drug Development Program, Department of Pharmacology and Toxicology, Room 408, 20 S. 2030 E., Salt Lake City, UT 84112, USA

B. Wiltgen, PhD Department of Neurobiology, University of California, Los Angeles

Paul Willner, PhD, DSc Department of Psychology, University of Swansea, Singleton Park, Swansea, Wales SA2 8D, UK

Animal and Translational Models of Neurological Disorders: An Industrial Perspective

A. Jackie Hunter

GlaxoSmithKline plc, Neurology Centre of Excellence for Drug Discovery, New Frontiers Science Park (North), Harlow, Essex, UK

INTRODUCTION

It has been well documented for over a decade that the productivity of the pharmaceutical industry as a whole has declined despite an increase in investment in Research and Development.[1,2] This is even more true for medicines to treat CNS disorders, where the chances of success for delivering a therapeutic are much lower than for other therapeutic disorders (Figure 1.1). Yet recent advances in biomedical technology, in genetics, translational science and in experimental medicine offer real promise that this situation is about to change. Such a change will ultimately offer real benefits for patients with serious neurological conditions that currently have few, if any, treatment options.

Animal and Translational Models for CNS Drug Discovery,
Vol. 2 of 3: Neurological Disorders
Robert McArthur and Franco Borsini (eds), Academic Press, 2008

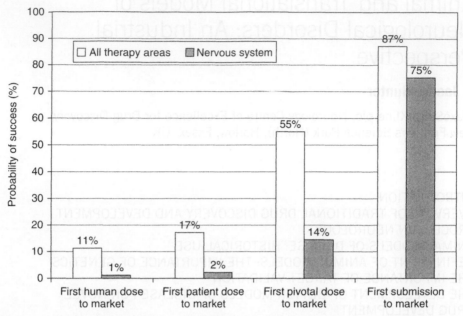

Figure 1.1   Cumulative probability of success to market nervous system versus all therapy areas. Probabilities of success were calculated using the proportion of decisions resulting in progression for each phase, based on NASs entering phase between 1997 and 1999. (*Source*: CMR International http://www.cmr.org/.)

OVERVIEW OF TRADITIONAL DRUG DISCOVERY AND DEVELOPMENT PROCESS IN NEUROLOGY

Discovering drugs for neurological disorders is challenging but the overall process is similar in nature to that for other disease areas. A very simplified diagram illustrates the sequential nature of the process for a small molecule (Figure 1.2). A protein target is selected for research based on any one or a combination of the following pieces of data: – disease association (e.g., linkage, altered expression in disease), involvement in a key pathway known to be important in the disease or disease-related process, or through observations of relevant changes in physiology or behavior due to drug action or genetic manipulation (e.g., sRNAi interference). This initial target selection step is a key point for investment for a company, whether large or small, and it could be argued that companies have historically paid too little attention to the early stages of target selection and validation.

Once the target has been chosen, it is cloned and expressed, assays are developed and screens run – either large high-throughput screens (HTSs) with millions of compounds, or smaller, more targeted, arrays or compound sets. To get to this point takes a minimum of several years work for each target and many millions of pounds will have already been spent. Even at this early stage up to 50% of projects can fail as assays may not be reproducibly configured and screens do not always produce hits. One particular issue for neurology is that many of the targets for which there is good validation

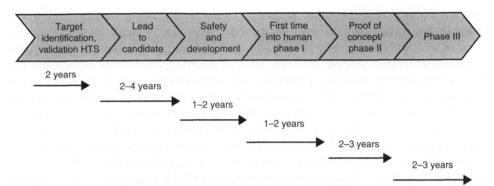

Figure 1.2 Timelines and process flow in drug discovery and development. The overall process can take anything from 11 to 16 years from picking a target to actually being able to file a drug for a neurological indication. Mean development cycle times in 2000–2002 were approximately 2.6 years longer for CNS drugs than other therapeutic areas. (*Source*: CMR international http://www. cmr.org/.)

through disease association, such as alpha-synuclein in Parkinson's disease (PD), are also the least tractable, and as such cannot be configured for screening. In other cases pathway expansion studies have identified tractable nodes for drug intervention such as the secretases on the amyloid processing pathway in Alzheimer's disease (AD). Even then there may still be issues. The secretase, BACE-1, an enzyme involved in the processing of amyloid precursor protein (APP) and a key target for disease modification, has a very restricted pharmacophore that limits chemical tractability.[3] However, other targets can be highly amenable to screening and an HTS can produce several different lead series.

If screening does produce hits, then a lead optimization program is initiated that can take anything from 2 to 4 years to come up with a candidate molecule. Such a molecule should have the right pharmacokinetic properties, demonstrate activity in animal models, possess a good therapeutic index and have appropriate selectivity for the target. By this point some initial toxicology testing (e.g., 4-day toxicology in a rodent and non-rodent species) will usually have been carried out. Once selected, the candidate enters preclinical development for a more extensive range of *in vitro* and *in vivo* safety assessment tests prior to first time in human (FTIH). During this time large amounts of time and money will be spent on developing the synthetic route for scaling up the production of the candidate molecule and optimizing its formulation in order to provide the large quantities of compound needed for toxicology testing and FTIH. More extensive pharmacokinetic studies of the parent compound and its metabolites are also initiated. In general, somewhere between 30% and 40% of molecules are lost at this stage due to unexpected toxicity.[4,5]

This preclinical phase lasts from 9 months to a year on average, but, if problems occur, it can be much longer. For example, solubility issues (which frequently occur due to the need for high lipophilicity to enable brain penetration) can limit exposure in toxicology studies. This means additional time must be spent on formulation to enable the true toxicological potential of a molecule to be explored at high doses.

Candidates that pass through this stage enter into clinical studies. FTIH Phase I studies are traditionally carried out in normal volunteers but in some instances patients are used as, for example, in FTIH vaccination approaches for disease modification in neurodegenerative disease. In many areas of neurology there has been a growing use of experimental medicine paradigms and other studies to look for pharmacodynamic markers of efficacy. The aims of such studies are to reduce attrition in Phase II by either improving dose selection or allowing the selection of the most appropriate patient group for efficacy testing. Phase IIa studies are generally small, single dose studies to look for signals of efficacy prior to moving to a larger dose ranging Phase IIb study.[i] There is good rationale for doing this as a single Phase IIb study for examining the efficacy of novel symptomatic treatments in AD, for example, can cost over £10 million.[ii] A positive Phase IIb study will trigger two much larger Phase III studies that will not only examine efficacy in a broader sample of patients, but also examine safety in the more general population. In parallel to all this clinical activity, longer term toxicology studies are carried out together with other development activities. The worst scenario is a Phase III failure when a company has already spent hundreds of millions on the compound. Memric® (Sabcomeline, SB 202026), a muscarinic M_1 receptor agonist, was just such a compound – promising Phase II results failed to translate into significance in two Phase III trials in AD in the 1990s.[iii] The situation becomes even more critical when disease modification is the ultimate goal – not only are such trials long and time-consuming but many of the end-points have yet to be defined from a regulatory perspective.

Today, lack of efficacy and safety issues are the major causes of attrition in Phase II studies,[6] in part because many of the targets that are now being worked on are clinically unprecedented. It is important that Phase II clinical studies of efficacy are designed such that a negative finding ensures that the target is invalidated. To do this one must be sure that the right amount of compound was delivered to the target site for the right duration of time. In many cases for neurological disorders, this means the brain and the spinal cord, and industry is currently expending a significant amount of resource in assessing brain penetration and duration of occupancy of molecules both clinically and preclinically to demonstrate that this is the case.

So how can animal models contribute to this process? *In vivo* models play an important role in many stages – they contribute to target validation, to demonstration of efficacy, provide pharmacodynamic assessments for screening and translation to man, mechanistic and disease understanding and safety profiling. Their impact continues long after the initial phase of drug discovery has completed and a compound

---

[i] Please refer to Schneider, Issues in design and conduct of clinical trials for cognitive-enhancing drugs, in this Volume or to McEvoy and Freudenreich, Issues in the design and conductance of clinical trials of psychiatric candidate drugs in Volume 1, Psychiatric Disorders for overviews of clinical development phases.
[ii] Please see Lindner *et al.,* Development, optimization and use of preclinical behavioral models to maximize the productivity of drug discovery for Alzheimer's disease in this volume for distinctions between symptomatic and disease modification approaches to the treatment of neurological disorders.
[iii] Please refer to McEvoy and Freudenreich, Issues in the design and conductance of clinical trials of psychiatric candidate drugs in Volume 1, Psychiatric Disorders for an overview of failed and negative clinical trials.

moves into development when further supportive evidence of safety, mechanism or differentiation may be required.

ANIMAL MODELS OF DISEASE: HISTORICAL USE

There are very few true animal models of neurological disease – that is, ones that are identical in cause, pathology and symptomatology – although much time, effort and money has been spent by behavioral scientists trying to develop these. In the late 1970s and 1980s, scientists relied on naturally occurring mutations (e.g., seizure prone mice and rats[7]), or on lesion models (e.g., 6-OH-dopamine lesioned rat as a model of the motor deficits in PD[iv][8]), or challenge models such as scopolamine-induced amnesia to mimic the memory deficits in AD.[9][v] Animal models such as these only reproduce certain aspects of the disease phenotype at best and were mainly focused on symptoms. Other models focused on symptoms and pathology, for example, the experimental allergic/autoimmune encephalitis (EAE) models have driven new research approaches to multiple sclerosis (MS). However, many aspects of pathology and immunology differ between MS and EAE.[10] This is not surprising as the general immunological profile in normal rodents is very different from that in normal humans.

These limited animal models actually were quite successful in developing symptomatic therapies, for example, sodium channel blockers for epilepsy, dopamine D2 receptor agonists for PD and cholinesterase inhibitors for AD.[11-13] They were much more limited in their ability to produce novel therapeutics for indications such as stroke and pain. A number of therapeutic agents were taken to the clinic on the basis of their activity in animal models of focal ischemia but they all failed. The potential reasons for this have been reviewed extensively but one thing is clear – the conditions in terms of time course under which the drugs were shown to work in animals (1–2 h) was not the same as the conditions under which they were tested in man (6–12 h[14]). Thus one could argue that the predictive validity of the stroke models in terms of target has not necessarily been invalidated. Indeed the one agent that is used therapeutically, tPA, only works if given within 3 h in animals and also if given within 3 h in man. These examples point to the importance of realistically understanding how the animal model relates to the human situation, not just in terms of the model itself, but also the timing of drug intervention.

In terms of pain most models appear to have good face validity but in reality are still only modeling symptomatology. Although the symptoms appear to be the same as in the disease in question, the etiology is quite different. Inflammatory pain is a good example – injection of Freuds Complete Adjuvant (FCA) into the paw of an animal causes inflammation but this is very different to that seen in rheumatoid arthritis where there is chronic inflammation of the joint. Likewise models of neuropathic pain

---

[iv] Please see Merchant et al., Animal models of Parkinson's disease to aid drug discovery and development in this Volume for a discussion of lesion and other animal models of Parkinson's disease.

[v] Please see Lindner et al., Development, optimization and use of preclinical behavioral models to maximize the productivity of drug discovery for Alzheimer's disease in this Volume for a discussion of pharmacological challenge and other animal models of Alzheimer's disease.

such as the Seltzer model do not reflect the etiology of back pain or post-herpetic neuralgia. Such models have been used extensively to test for novel anti-inflammatory drugs and analgesics but have not extrapolated to clinical efficacy.

More recently the lack of novel therapeutics, even in areas where such models have traditional been seen as valuable, has driven the development of new animal models of disease for efficacy screening. In the case of pain, for example, development of models of central sensitization have been driven by a better understanding of the contribution of higher centers to the modulation of pain perception.

REFINEMENT OF ANIMAL MODELS: THE IMPORTANCE OF GENETICS

As our knowledge of the genetic basis of disease increased in the late 1980s and 1990s, animal models became available that used manipulations of genes identified as causal in human disease. This is best exemplified by the SOD mouse model of amyotrophic lateral sclerosis (ALS) characterized by Gurney and others.[15] In this mouse the genetic mutation in superoxide dismutase seen in about 6% of ALS patients has been over-expressed and the result is a pathology and symptomatology that reproduces most, if not all, of the sequaele of ALS in man.[vi] Clearly this defect only represents a small percentage of the ALS patient population so its relevance for sporadic ALS remains to be defined.

A major advance in AD drug discovery came with the discovery that mutations in APP were a causal factor in the disease along with other mutations that were subsequently identified to be in genes involved in APP processing. This led to the creation of transgenic animals expressing human mutated APP or double transgenics with mutations in both APP and presenillin.[16] These models, whilst showing increased amyloid deposition and cognitive deficits, do not show the neurofibrillary tangles and cell loss that are also characteristic of AD. More recently triple transgenics have been made (APP × presenillin × tau) which reproduce more of the pathology of AD and show synapse loss before the development of plaques and tangles,[17] but routine use of these animals for drug screening and discovery is limited by a number of factors, not least the amount of space required to generate such a triple transgenic line.[vii] Despite the lack of true pathology, the discovery of the genetic link to APP in AD and the generation of APP transgenic mice has made possible the discovery and development of antibodies and small molecules that are targeting disease progression, although there are clearly still issues here in terms of rate of deposition, etc. (see "Pharmacodynamic" section below).

Many more transgenic mouse models have been created to follow up on the genetic findings from humans – this is especially true in PD where there have been

---

[vi] Please see Montes *et al.*, Translational research in ALS in this Volume for a discussion of pharmacological challenge and other animal models of ALS.

[vii] Please see Lindner *et al.*, Development, optimization and use of preclinical behavioral models to maximize the productivity of drug discovery for Alzheimer's disease in this Volume for a discussion of transgenic animal models of Alzheimer's disease and their limitations.

a number of important advances in our genetic understanding of the disorder.[18] [viii] Given the relatively discrete location of pathology, at least early on in the disease, it is feasible not only to make transgenic models to try to create better PD disease models, but also regionally to overexpress mutated genes in rats and other species, in either the substantia nigra or the striatum.[19] These may not only provide better models for drug development, but also models that can be used to understand the disease pathology better, leading ultimately to better target validation. The development of regional brain-specific promoters will become more important as our knowledge of the genetic basis of disease progresses. There are a number of initiatives to look at enhancing regional expression, for example, the Pleiades consortium in Canada (www.pleiades.org) to look for brain-specific promoters (see also Table 1.2).

Models where the gene of interest has been deleted (knockouts, KOs) have also been used extensively to create models of disease. There are issues with KO animals in terms of compensatory mechanisms and redundancy (e.g.,[20]), but they have provided some vital information about gene function and target validation.

THE IMPORTANCE OF TARGET VALIDATION

As mentioned earlier choosing the best target is crucial for drug discovery as once a choice is made, it triggers a chain of commitment that ultimately will end up with a molecule to test in the clinic. In the 1980s and 1990s target validation was usually carried out by looking at changes in the expression of the gene or protein of interest in a relevant disease animal model. Stroke models provide a good example of how a range of different therapeutic mechanisms and targets were prioritized. Numerous studies were carried out that demonstrated the importance of inflammatory mediators[21] as well as apoptotic pathways. Many of these findings were shown to be mirrored in post-mortem studies in human stroke patients. However, these studies to date have failed to produce an effective neuroprotective agent.

Animal models of pain have been used to show increases or decreases in the expression of particular genes. An example is the upregulation of the vanilloid receptor-1 (TRPV1) in animals and man.[22] In inflammatory pain states and following experimental nerve injury and in animal models of diabetic neuropathy TRPV1 is present on neurons that do not normally express TRPV1.[23] Likewise a number of different sodium channels have been shown to be upregulated in several different models of neuropathic pain, for example, Nav1.3 is upregulated in chronic constriction injury[24] and diabetic neuropathy.[25] However, expression analysis alone is unlikely to give sufficient confidence in a target to initiate a large scale drug discovery program.

The development of transgenic and KO technology allows further validation in mice of the critical role of a particular gene product in the disease or process of interest. Clearly this is only possible at present where the mechanism or model can be generated in mice and has been particularly useful in areas such as pain, epilepsy and

---

[viii] Please see also Merchant *et al.*, Animal models of Parkinson's disease to aid drug discovery and development in this Volume for a discussion of genetic models of Parkinson's disease.

neurodegeneration. In pain, for example, a range of ion channels have been knocked out in mice and shown either an exacerbation of or reduction in, inflammatory or neuropathic pain responses. Sodium channels have been particularly well studied in this regard,[26] although the data has not always been consistent with the results of expression analyses, for example, both global and conditional KO of NaV1.3 has not lead to changes in neuropathic pain responses.[26,27] More recently other means of reducing gene expression, for example, RNAi have also been used to overcome some of the potential limitations of KO technology such as developmental compensation. Many of these targets have also been further validated by selective pharmacological agents.[28]

Clinical experience with use-dependent sodium channel blockers such as topiramate (Topamax®) and lamotrigine (Lamictal®) has produced mixed results in trials in neuropathic pain.[29-31] However, on the basis of the types of studies described above a number of companies are pursuing the development of selective sodium ion channel blockers for pain and a number of these targets have now reached early clinical development. One example is ralfinamide, a mixed sodium channel blocker that has activity in preclinical models of neuropathic and inflammatory pain.[32] Ralfinamide appears to be well tolerated in man in both healthy individuals and patients with neuropathic pain. It is currently in Phase II studies in patients which have a mixture of neuropathic pain syndromes.

More powerful support for a target comes with the combination of animal and human genetic data. Perhaps one of the best examples of this is the linkage of orexin to control of the sleep–wake cycle. Orexin neuropeptides act on two receptors, OX_1 and OX_2. OX_2 receptor KO animals have disturbed wakefulness and abnormal attacks of non-REM sleep. A similar pattern of disturbed wakefulness and sleep is seen in orexin $-/-$ mice but these mice also have severe cataplexy.[33] This had been previously suggested by the discovery that a narcolepsy-like syndrome in Doberman dogs was due of a natural mutation in the OX_2 receptor.[34] Biomarker studies in rodents, monkeys and humans showed variations in orexin levels during the circadian cycle with levels being highest at the end of the wake–active cycle and lowest toward the end of the sleep period. Central injections of orexin also stimulated wakefulness and maintained cortical activation.[35] These findings led to drug discovery programs at GSK, Actelion and others for orexin receptor antagonists for the treatment of sleep disorders. Recently published data with a brain penetrant antagonist of both OX_1 and OX_2 receptors, ACT-078573, has provided further support for the crucial role of the orexin system in the maintenance of wakefulness. When ACT-078573 was tested in rats it produced an increase in non-REM sleep and REM-sleep – thus differing from a benzodiazepine, zolpidem (Ambien®), which only increases non-REM sleep. Furthermore it also increased sleep in dogs and reduced latency to sleep stage 2 in humans. In addition it showed increases in theta and delta power in EEG power spectrum analyses, whereas zolpidem did not.[35] This is one of the clearest examples of genetic validation in preclinical species leading to small molecule studies in animals that translate to a similar pharmacological effect in man.[ix]

[ix] For further discussion on the hypocretin/orexin system, please refer to Doran *et al.,* Translational models of sleep and sleep disorders in Volume 1, Psychiatric Disorders.

THE DEVELOPMENT OF BETTER MODELS OF DISEASE FOR NOVEL DRUG DEVELOPMENT

Alongside the advances in the use of genetically engineered mice, there has been a continued effort to develop better animal models for efficacy evaluation. These models are also important for the exploitation of genetics. Clearly any information of the role of a particular gene is only as good as the phenotypic test or model that is carried out. The characterization of these models for their relevance to the disease state in man is a vital step in showing improved relevance. This is where the translation back from human studies to animals is so crucial and is a key area of focus for translational science, for example, comparison of biomarkers such as plasma proteins or imaging in the preclinical model and the human disease. One relatively new model of migraine and other head pain has been developed by Burstein and others whereby chemical stimulation of the dura mater with an "inflammatory soup" produces trigeminal stimulation.[36] The GSK TRPV1 receptor antagonist, SB705498 was tested in this model and shown to be effective in reducing this sensitization to sensory input following inflammation of the trigeminovascular distribution.[37] However, this compound was ineffective in a clinical trial in acute migraine (unpublished data) suggesting that this model may not be a good predictor of efficacy in man. Furthermore it suggests that central sensitization of the trigeminal system may not be as crucial as has been thought to migraine pain.

A MOVE TOWARD PHARMACODYNAMIC MODELS AND MODELS OF MECHANISM

In recent years more emphasis has been placed on developing better mechanistic or pharmacodynamic models for drug discovery rather than better disease models *per se*. It is clear that *in vivo* models are required for ranking compounds in efficacy and potency at the native target as part of a screening cascade. These data are required to calculate the exposures needed for a compound to have efficacy in man and also to calculate a therapeutic index as biologically active compounds may have unwanted side effects at higher doses (most very efficacious compounds do have side effects at higher doses e.g., aspirin, benzodiazepines). Thus even in the absence of a validated disease model, some form of *in vivo* testing is required.

Pharmacodynamic screens do not necessarily have to have any face validity for the ultimate disease in question but can answer whether the drug gets to the required target, is active and has the required potency and duration of effect. Pharmacokinetics is no substitute for this as frequently the pharmacodynamic half-life can be very different from the observed pharmacokinetic half-life. In addition pharmacokinetics may lead to optimization on parameters (volume of distribution, plasma half-life) that are irrelevant to the target organ (i.e., brain). Although the use of *ex-vivo* binding to brain tissue can compensate for this to some extent, a functional measure is preferable. One example of this is the use of R-α-methylhistamine-induced drinking behavior to optimize histamine H_3 receptor antagonists for brain penetration, potency and duration of action. The ultimate aim of the H_3 antagonist program at GSK was to develop compounds for cognitive enhancement in AD – R-α-methylhistamine-induced drinking bore no relevance to this target in a therapeutic sense but was extremely useful in selecting potent antagonists for further behavioral testing in cognition paradigms. Not only was the program successful in selecting compounds that were active in the $\mu g\,kg^{-1}$ range, this was also achieved in a relatively short space of time (approximately 18 months). The screening cascade is shown in Table 1.1. The data from the pharmacodynamic assay was complemented by further *ex vivo* receptor binding assays and pharmacokinetic studies to give a profile of brain occupancy at a given concentration.

Table 1.1 Criticality of *in vivo* models in the screening cascade for H₃ receptor antagonist program

Test	Comment
Functional activity at human H₃ receptor	
⬇	
Rat native tissue binding and *in vitro* selectivity	Check for species differences in affinity
⬇	
In vitro DMPK	Cytochrome P450 assays
⬇	
R-α-methylhistamine induced drinking	*In vivo* pharmacodynamic assay for antagonism of central H₃ receptors
⬇	
Ex vivo binding and pharmacokinetic sampling	*In vivo* CNS receptor occupancy and PK profile in periphery and brain
⬇	
Cognitive testing – novel object recognition	*In vivo* activity in model of therapeutic relevance
⬇	
Irwin test	Side effect testing to give approximate therapeutic index
⬇	
Candidate selection work up	

To some extent the APP transgenic mice models described earlier should be viewed as pharmacodynamic models of amyloid deposition rather than disease models of AD. They have been especially useful as pharmacodynamic assays for the development of therapeutic antibodies and secretase inhibitors.[38] However, extrapolation from such rodent transgenic models is complicated by the potential differences in the type, amount and rate of amyloid deposition across species. Thus the ability of a transgenic amyloidosis model to predict dose and efficacy in man is still the subject of much debate.

PHARMACODYNAMIC MODELS AND TRANSLATION TO MAN

Apart from the use of pharmacodynamic models for mechanistic efficacy testing, they offer the opportunity of developing assays that assess mechanism that can be translated into the clinical setting to ensure that the drug is acting at the mechanistic target. This is clearly somewhat easier if one is looking at an antihypertensive agent that is targeting the vasculature rather than targeting a CNS mechanism for a neurological disease. However, the advent of imaging and other technology has made this easier for neurological conditions and there is intensive work ongoing to search for peripheral biomarkers that may be of relevance to disease progression for a range of neurodegenerative disorders. For immunological-based therapies (e.g., for MS) there are a number of peripheral biomarkers that can be used such as the measurement of particular subsets of lymphocytes or subsets of lymphocytes in plasma (cf.,[39]).

Although the rodent is very different from the human, attempts have been made to develop pharmacodynamic assays in rodents and extrapolate them to man. A good example of this use of pharmacodynamic challenge models in animals that can be translated to man is the use of capsaicin challenge in the development of TRPV1 receptor antagonists for pain. Capsaicin is an agonist of the TRPV1 receptor and causes pain and central sensitization in man. Several companies have used capsaicin challenge in their screening program for novel compounds. A good example of the use of this model preclinically was recently published by Amgen to select a TRPV1 antagonist, AMG 517, to move into clinical trials.[40] AMG 517 was maximally active at 3 mg/kg in this model and produced a 100% reversal of the capsaicin-induced behavior. Interestingly AMG 517 only produced a 35% maximal reduction in thermal hyperalgesia in an inflammatory pain model suggesting that TRPV1 receptors may only have limited involvement in this model.

These data can be translated into similar effects in man. Thus SB 705498, a novel TRPV1 antagonist, has been shown to antagonized capsaicin-induced flare in a FTIH study,[41] although there was no effect on the decrease in heat pain threshold caused by sensitization with capsaicin.

NEUROLOGICAL SIDE EFFECT PROFILING AND SAFETY

Animal models will continue to be very valuable for screening for the unwanted effects of potential neurological medicines. Studies of sedation, cognitive impairment, abuse liability, etc. are vital in determining the therapeutic index of a drug (e.g.,[42]). This integrated, whole system, approach is especially important where one is targeting the central nervous system as unwanted effects are unlikely to be predicted from any isolated tissue experiment. Thus prior to selecting a candidate molecule for further drug development, a number of *in vivo* pharmacology screens will be carried out – at the very least a modified Irwin test would be carried out for comparison of doses producing gross side effects.[x]

EXPERIMENTAL MEDICINE AND TRANSLATIONAL SCIENCE

Both experimental medicine and translational science, if applied and executed appropriately, have the potential to make a real impact on neurological drug discovery. Translational science is described by Fitzgerald in a recent article[43] as a discipline which integrates preclinical information to inform human pharmacology. Such studies can derive a range of indices in man including pharmacodynamic markers, biochemical markers and genetic markers which can inform both the potential for safety issues as well as efficacy determinations. Central to this is a basic understanding of clinical pharmacology and pharmacokinetics as well as an appreciation of whole animal physiology. The drive here is to move away from animal models of disease and more to animal models of mechanism that can then inform clinical studies and their design.

An example of such translational science can be seen in experiments carried out with the novel immunosuppressant drug FTY720. Early studies in animals showed that the compound accelerated lymphocyte homing and thereby decreased the number of lymphocytes in peripheral blood.[44] Subsequently studies were carried out in man that also showed a similar modulation of lymphocyte trafficking, which was transient at all but the highest doses tested.[45] Further studies have demonstrated that FTY720 traps primarily naïve and central memory T-cells but spares peripheral effector memory T-cells.[46] This demonstrates the usefulness of such markers to aid mechanism of action data for compounds in development. Clinical studies using other immunomodulator therapies for MS have used peripheral lymphocyte counts to guide dose selection in Phase II, for example, for VLA4 integrin antagonists and antibodies such as natalizumab (Tysabri®). There has been an extensive search for peripheral biomarkers for other neurodegenerative diseases such as AD but to date no peripheral marker has been thoroughly validated.[xi] Although many groups have published data on promising markers, none have demonstrated rigorous replication.[47,48] In the future, data from animal models and human samples such as cerebrospinal fluid[49] or plasma may be pooled to yield information about particular pathways.[50] Such studies will probably need to combine imaging data and genetic data to give more homogenous phenotypes for biomarker characterization.

---

[x] Please see Rocha *et al.*, Development of medication for heroin and cocaine addition and regulatory aspects of abuse liability testing chapter in Volume 3, Reward Deficits, for a discussion of Regulatory agency stipulations and the use of animal models to evaluate abuse liability of novel drugs.

[xi] Please see Lindner *et al.*, Development, optimization and use of preclinical behavioral models to maximize the productivity of drug discovery for Alzheimer's disease in this Volume for a discussion of biomarkers of Alzheimer's disease and their limitations.

There has been an elegant combination of human genetics and transgenic validation with regard to the alpha subunit of the sodium channel subtype Nav1.7. Recent genetic studies have shown that gain of function mutations cause pain syndromes in man and loss of function mutations cause an inability to experience pain.[51-53] Interestingly, these different mutations cause separate syndromes, and give rise to differential responses to the sodium channel blocker carbamazepine (Tegretol®). These studies have given much more confidence that antagonism of Nav1.7 is a viable strategy for pain and demonstrate the two-way nature of translational science (i.e., patient to preclinical as well as preclinical to patient). Subsequent genetic studies will hopefully allow the stratification of patients on the basis of mechanism. Other studies have shown a clear relationship between genetic variation and pain sensitivity.[54] Polymorphisms in GTP-cyclohydrolase give rise to a reduced pain phenotype following surgical diskectomy for lumbar root pain[55] and others have shown variants of the COMT gene affect opiate responses to a pain stressor.[56] Pain is an area where this stratification would be of great value as pain studies are plagued with large placebo effects which can easily confound small Phase II studies.

THE IMPORTANCE OF IMAGING

As well as being important as a translational technology from preclinical experiments to the clinic, imaging is beginning to make a real difference to the ability to carry out clinical trials of disease modifying agents in neurological disorders (cf ,[57]). The most extensive technology developments have occurred in positron emission tomography (PET) imaging and in structural and functional magnetic resonance imaging (fMRI). PET imaging has had a major impact in the diagnosis and development of treatments for PD.[xii] ^{18}F-dopa was developed as a ligand for imaging functional dopaminergic neurons and was initially used for the diagnosis of PD. An initial pilot trial with the dopamine receptor agonist ropinirol (Requip®) had suggested that progression rates in terms of dopaminergic cell loss were reduced with treatment with this dopamine agonist compared to L-DOPA. This was subsequently confirmed in a 2-year, randomized, double-blind, multinational study. This study compared the rates of loss of dopamine-terminal function in patients with clinical and ^{18}F-dopa PET evidence of early PD. Patients treated with ropinirol or L-Dopa showed a decrease in putamen ^{18}F-dopa uptake (Ki) between baseline and 2-years but the decrease was lower in the ropinirol treated patients.[58] This type of imaging will be essential to facilitate trials of disease modifying agents that will be developed from the genetic association studies of the disease. However, there is still a need to develop more sensitive ligands that could not only detect a reduction in function but also cell loss.

In MS, MRI imaging is a standard tool for diagnosis and its use is routine in Phase II and III clinical trials where it is an accepted end-point. A 2-year long Phase III trial of natalizumab, an antibody directed against VLA4 receptor demonstrated an 83%

[xii] Please refer to Merchant *et al.*, Animal models of Parkinson's disease to aid drug discovery and development in this Volume for a discussion of brain imaging in Parkinson's disease.

decrease in new lesions as detected by T2-weighted MRI. Natalizumab also reduced lesions as detected by gadolinium-enhanced MRI by approximately 90%.[59] This data in conjunction with functional outcome measures speeded the approval for natalizumab and allowed it to show clear differentiation in terms of benefit from the existing treatments such as the interferons. Such differentiation for new agents compared to standard treatment is now an important component in registration packages both in the United States of America, Europe and elsewhere. Other agents in development for MS have also used imaging outcomes, for example, the sphingosine 1-phosphate (S1P1) receptor agonist FTY720 (Fingolimod).[60]

Clearly assessment of disease progression in other neurodegenerative disorders such as AD and the ability to detect a change in disease progression when disease modifying agents are given is a real challenge. For AD existing functional tools such as the ADAS-cog are not sufficiently sensitive to detect changes over shorter periods of time. For example, there is evidence from our own and other studies that ADAS-cog does not now show the expected decline in placebo-treated patients with mild AD over 6 months.[xiii] There have been some studies that have used structural brain imaging and shown changes in hippocampal volume over a several years. These volumetric analyses have been used recently in a failed trial of a disease modifying agent, Alzhemed. ([61]Neurochem communication November 2007 http://www.neurochem.com/ResearchActivities.htm), and did hint at some efficacy in the absence of a signal on functional end-points. Agents that can image amyloid deposits in the brains of AD would clearly be better than purely structural imaging of brain regions, especially in the early phase of the disease, but these would need to have sufficient sensitivity to detect changes after treatment. Several groups have developed agents which look promising. The Pittsburg agent B (^{11}C-PIB) has been shown to retained in areas shown to have large amounts of amyloid deposits in AD patients compared to controls whilst areas that are relatively unaffected in AD have little retention.[62] Importantly PIB retention correlated inversely with cerebral glucose metabolism as determined by ^{18}F-flurodeoxyglucose. There are several other classes of imaging agent that are being developed (e.g., F-18-FDDNP[63]), but much more information needs to be gained on the nature of the interaction of these and PIB with the various amyloid species in the brain of AD patients.[64] In terms of the translational aspects of neuroimaging, the adaptation of these techniques to rodent models is particularly germane (e.g.,[65]).[xiv]

Stroke is another neurodegenerative disease where progress has been made in imaging which may help stratify patients for clinical trials.

One of the major reasons for the higher attrition in CNS programs is the need for adequate brain penetration. PET imaging allows for the development of tracer ligands to assess biodistribution and pharamacokinetics both in the periphery and centrally of the drug of interest. These measures will aid the interpretation of clinical studies

---

[xiii] Please see Schneider, Issues in design and conduct of clinical trials for cognitive-enhancing drugs in this Volume for a thorough discussion of this topic.

[xiv] Please refer to Millan, The discovery and development of pharmacotherapy for psychiatric disorders: A critical survey of animal and translational models, and perspectives for their improvement, in Volume 1, Psychiatric Disorders for further discussion regarding the prominence of brain imaging in drug discovery and development.

of efficacy and dose selection for such studies. Initial studies begin with animals to develop a labeled form of the compound of interest and many drugs can be labeled with ^{18}F or ^{11}C which means that physicochemical and pharmacological properties of the compound are minimally, if at all, affected. Some compounds cannot be labeled and in this case a radioligand has to be developed specially with the appropriate characteristics for taking into displacement studies with the molecule of interest in the clinic. For example, GSK has developed a specific ligand for the $5HT_6$ receptor, GSK-215083, as the lead molecule GSK-742457 could not be radiolabeled (cf.,[66]). Over the past 6 years GSK has developed a number of tracer ligands for a range of neurological target programs e.g., ^{11}C GW-406381, a brain penetrant Cox2 inhibitor and ^{11}C GSK-189254, a H_3 receptor antagonist. These novel PET ligands will also be useful in exploring the role of receptors in a range of neurological diseases and should be useful tools in enhancing our understanding of disease.

THE ROLE OF EXPERIMENTAL MEDICINE

Experimental medicine is "the use of innovative measurements, models and designs in studying human subjects for establishing proof of mechanism and concept of new drugs, for exploring the potential for market differentiation for successful drug candidates, and for efficiently terminating the development of unsuccessful ones".[67] These paradigms are being developed to allow early reads on efficacy with using patients, or more commonly, studies of mechanism in volunteers. For example, a number of models of pain and sensitization have been established that can be used on either patients or volunteers to allow an early read on potential for clinical efficacy.[68] These include electrical hyperalgesia and UV burn to the skin. These can be used in addition to the routine measurement of normal pain threshold to mechanical or thermal sensation after chronic or acute drug treatment. Currently, these models mostly rely on psychophysical markers; further progress in this area will involve refinement of pain markers and end-points, including fMRI and EEG/evoked potentials.[69] There remains much validation to be done with these pain models with standard agents before they can become decision-making in drug discovery and development. A longer term objective would be to correlate efficacy in the disease with efficacy in volunteer models and in preclinical pain models although sufficient data with a range of compounds for this comprehensive analysis does not yet exist.

Cognitive enhancement is also amenable to experimental medicine studies. Particularly powerful is a combination of imaging with tests of memory and attention. These studies can be done in young or old volunteers under normal conditions or where performance is impaired either by the use of a pharmaceutical agent such as the muscarinic antagonist scopolamine or a stressor such as sleep deprivation. Under these conditions cholinesterase inhibitors such as donepezil (Aricept®) have been shown to reverse deficits caused by scopolamine or sleep deprivation. Recently Gregory et al.[70] demonstrated that a combination of fMRI and cognitive assessment could detect changes after the administration of an H_3 antagonist compared to placebo. A single dose of GSK-189254 could produce discreet changes in brain activity during associative learning and paired attention tasks probably via effects on histaminergic neurons in the posterior hypothalamus.

Table 1.2 List of some relevant precompetitive consortia/initiatives

Initiative	URL
Innovative Medicines Initiative in Europe	http://www.imi-europe.org
FDA Critical path	http://www.fda.gov/oc/initiatives/criticalpath http://www.fda.gov/oc/initiatives/criticalpath/opportunities06.html
A collaboration platform for proteomics biomarker analysis (US)	http://www.genome.gov/page.cfm?pageID =17015407&display_abstract=on&query_ grantid=R44HG04537&cr_yr
Critical Markers of Disease (US)	http://www.cmod.org/
NCI consortium (US)	http://deainfo.nci.nih.gov/concepts/edrnRFA.htm
Preventative Health Flagship (Australia): research areas for Flagship Collaboration Fund projects 2007–2008	http://www.csiro.au/partnerships/ps2y0.html
Scottish Enterprise and Wyeth in biomarkers collaboration	http://bulletin.sciencebusiness.net/ebulletins/showissue.php3?page=/548/1774/5344 http://www.scottish-enterprise.com/sedotcom_home/sig/life-sciences.htm

THE FUTURE

If the important advances in technology, genetics, translational science and experimental medicine are to be of value to patients, more work needs to be done to move them from confidence building tools to end-points acceptable to regulatory bodies. There is a need for companies to work together in a precompetitive manner with the regulatory agencies to establish a framework for accelerating the utility of these biomarkers. This need has been recognized in a number of ongoing or proposed precompetitive initiatives in the United States of America, Europe and Asia-Pacific. Some of these initiatives are listed in Table 1.2.

REFERENCES

1. DiMasi, J.A., Hansen, R.W., and Grabowski, H. (2003). The price of innovation: New estimates of drug development costs. *J Health Econ*, 22(2):151–185.
2. Mervis, J. (2005). Productivity counts – But the definition is key. *Science*, 309:726.
3. Beswick, P., Charrier, N., Clarke, B., Demont, E., Dingwall, C., Dunsdon, R., Faller, A., *et al.* (2007). BACE-1 inihbitors Part 3: Idenitfcation of hyroxyethylamines with nanomolar potency in cells. BMCL.
4. Kola, I. and Landis, J. (2004). Can the pharmaceutical industry reduce attrition rates? *Nat Rev Drug Discov*, 3(8):711–715.

5. Kramer, J.A., Sagartz, J.E. *et al.* (2007). The application of discovery toxicology and pathology towards the design of safer pharmaceutical lead candidates. *Nat Rev Drug Discov*, 6(8):636–649.
6. DiMasi, J.A. (2001). Risks in new drug development: Approval success rates for investigational drugs. *Clin Pharmacol Ther*, 69:297–307.
7. Jackson, H.C., Hansen, H.C., Kristiansen, M., Suzdak, P., Klitgaard, H., Judge, M., and Swedberg, M.D.B. (1996). Anticonvulsant profile of the imidazoquinazolines NNC 14-0185 and NNC 14-0189 in rats and mice. *EJP*, 308(1):21–30.
8. Gnanalingham, K.K., Hunter, A.J., Jenner, P., and Marsden, C.D. (1995). Selective dopamine antagonist pre-treatment on the antiparkinsonian effects of benzazepine D_1 and DA agonists in rodent and primate models of Parkinson's disease-the differential effects of D_1 dopamine antagonists in the primate. *Psychopharmacology*, 117:403–412.
9. Hunter, A.J. (1991). The effects of cholinergic drugs on memory in animals. In Weinman, J. and Hunter, A.J. (eds.) *Memory: Neurochemical and Abnormal Perspectives*, Harwood, pp. 43–63.
10. Friese *et al.* (2006).
11. Eden, R.J., Costall, B., Domeney, A.M., Gerrard, P., Harvey, C.A., Kelly, M.E. *et al.* (1991). Preclinical pharmacology of ropinirole (SK&F 101468-A) a novel dopamine D2 agonist. *Pharmacol Biochem Behav*, 38(1):147–154.
12. Miller, A.A., Wheatley, P., Sawyer, D.A., Baxter, M.G., and Roth, B. (1986). Pharmacological studies on lamotrigine, a novel potential antiepileptic drug: I. Anticonvulsant profile in mice and rats. *Epilepsia*, 27(5):483–489.
13. Snape, M., Misra, A., Murray, T.K., DeSouza, R.J., Williams, J.L., Cross, A.J., and Green, A.R. (1999). A comparative study in rats of the in vitro and in vivo pharmacology of the acetylcholinesterase inhibitors tacrine, donepezil and NXX-066. *Neuropharmacology*, 38(1):181–193.
14. Hunter, A.J., Mackay, K.B., and Rogers, D.C. (1998). To what extent have functional studies of ischaemia in animals been useful in the assessment of potential neuroprotective agents? *TIPS*, 19:59–66.
15. Gurney, M.E. (1997). The use of transgenic mouse models of amyotrophic lateral sclerosis in preclinical drug studies. *J Neurol Sci*, 152(Suppl 1):S67–S73.
16. Borchelt, D.R., Ratovitski, T., van Lare, J., Lee, M.K., Gonzales, V., Jenkins, N.A. *et al.* (1997). Accelerated amyloid deposition in the brains of transgenic mice coexpressing mutant presenilin 1 and amyloid precursor proteins. *Neuron*, 4:939–945.
17. Oddo, S., Caccamo, A., Shepherd, J.D., Murphy, M.P., Golde, T.E., Kayed, R., Metherate, R., Mattson, M.P., Akbari, Y., and LaFerla, F.M. (2003). Triple-transgenic model of Alzheimer's disease with plaques and tangles: Intracellular Abeta and synaptic dysfunction. *Neuron*, 39:409–421.
18. Gandhi, S. and Wood, N.W. (2005). Molecular pathogenesis of Parkinson's disease. *Hum Mol Genet*, 14(18):2749–2755.
19. Kirik, D., Annett, L.E., Burger, C., Muzyczka, N., Mandel, R.J., and Björklund, A. (2003). Nigrostriatal α-synucleinopathy induced by viral vector-mediated overexpression of human α-synuclein: A new primate model of Parkinson's disease. *PNAS*, 100(5):2884–2889.
20. Picciotto, M.R. and Wickman, K. (1998). Using knockout and transgenic mice to study neurophysiology and behavior. *Physiol Rev*, 78(4):1131–1163.
21. del Zoppo, G., Ginis, I., Hallenbeck, J., Iadecola, C., Wang, X., and Feuerstein, G.Z. (2000). Inflammation and stroke: Putative role for cytokines, adhesion molecules and iNOS in brain response to ischemia. *Brain Pathol*, 10(1):95–112.
22. Gopinath, P., Wan, E., Holdcroft, A., Facer, P., Davis, J.B., Smith, G.S., *et al.* (2005). Increased capsaicin receptor TRPV1 in skin nerve fibres and related vanilloid receptors TRPV3 and TRPV4 in keratinocytes in human breast pain. *BMC Women's Health*, 5.

23. Cortright, D.N. and Szallasi, A. (2004). Biochemical pharmacology of the vanilloid receptor TRPV1. An update. *Eur J Biochem*, 271(10):1814–1819.
24. Dib-Hajj *et al.* (1999).
25. Hong, S., Morrow, T.J., Paulson, P.E., Isom, L.L., and Wiley, J.W. (2004). Early painful diabetic neuropathy is associated with differential changes in tetrodotoxin-sensitive and – resistant sodium channels in dorsal root ganglion neurons in the rat. *J Biol Chem*, 279:29341–29350.
26. Rogers, M., Tang, L., Madge, D.J., and Stevens, E.B. (2006). The role of sodium channels in neuropathic pain. *Sem Cell Develop Biol*, 17:571–581.
27. Nassar, M.A., Baker, M.D., Levato, A., Ingram, Mallucci, R., and McMahon, S.B. (2006). Nerve injury induces robust allodynia and actopic discharges in Na1.3 null mutant mice. *Mol Pain*, 2:33–43.
28. Yogeeswari, P., Ragavendran, J.V., and Sriram, D. (2007). Neuropathic pain: strategies in drug discovery and treatment. *Expert Opin Drug Disc*, 2(2):169–184.
29. McCleane, G. (1999). 200 mg daily of lamotrigine has no analgesic effect in neuropathic pain: A randomized, double blind, placebo controlled trial. *Pain*, 83:105–107.
30. Eisenberg, E., Lurie, Y., Braker, C., Daoud, D., and Ishay, A. (2001). Lamotriginne reduces painful diabetic neuropathy: A randomized controlled trial. *Neurology*, 56:184–190.
31. Dib, J.G. (2004). Focus on topiramate in neuropathic pain. *Curr Med Res Opin*, 20:1857–1861.
32. Cattabeni, F. (2004). Ralfinamide Newron Pharmaceuticals. *Idrugs*, 7(10):935–939.
33. Willie, J.T., Chemelli, R.M., Sinton, C.M., Tokita, S., Williams, C., Kisanuki, Y.Y. *et al.* (2003). Dinstinct narcolepsy syndromes in Orexin Receptor-2 and orexin null mice: Molecular genetic dissection of non-Rem and REM sleep regulatory processes. *Neuron*, 38:715–730.
34. Lin, L., Faraco, J., Li, R., Kadotani, H., Rogers, W., Lin, X. *et al.* (1999). The sleep disorder canine narcolepsy is caused by a mutation in the hypocretin (orexin) receptor 2 gene. *Cell*, 98:365–376.
35. Brisbare-Roch, C., Dingemanse, J., Koberstein, R., Hoever, P., Aissaoui, H., Flores, S. *et al.* (2007). Promotion of sleep by targeting the orexin system in rats, dogs and humans. *Nat Med*, 13(2):150–155.
36. Burstein, R., Yamamura, H., Malick, A., and Strassman, A.M. (1998). Chemical stimulation of the intracranial dura induces enhanced responses to facial stimulation in brain stem trigeminal neurons. *J Neurophysiol*, 79:964–982.
37. Lambert, G.A., Appleby, J.A., Chizh, B.A., Metcalf, A., del Carmen Osuna, M., Hoskin, K.L., Zagami, A.S. (2007). Reversal of inflammation induced trigeminovascular second order neurons by SB705798, a TRPV1 antagonist.
38. Beher, D., Graham, S.L. (2005). Protease Inhibitors as potential disease modifying therapis for Alzheimer's Disease. *Exp Opin Investig Drugs*, 1385–1409.
39. O'Hara, R.M. Jr., Benoit, S.E., Groves, C.J., and Collins, M. (2006). Cell-surface and cytokine biomarkers in autoimmune and inflammatory diseases. *Drug Discov Today*, 11:342–347.
40. Doherty, E., Fotsch, C., Bannon, A.W., Bo, Y., Chen, N., Dominguez, C., *et al.* (2007). Novel vanilloid receptor antagonists: 2. Structure-activity relationships of 4-oxopyrimidines leading to the selection of a clinical candidate. *J Am Chem Soc*.
41. Chizh, B.A., O'Donnell, M.B., Napolitano, A., Wang, J., Brooke, A.C., Aylott, M.C., Bullman, J.N., Gray, E.J., Lai, R.Y., Williams, P.M., and Appleby, J.M. (2007). The effects of the TRPV1 antagonist SB-705498 on TRPV1 receptor-mediated activity and inflammatory hyperalgesia in humans. *Pain*, 132:132–141.
42. Blokland, A., Hinz, V., and Schmidt, B.H. (1995). Effects of metrifonate and tacrine in the spatial morris task and modified Irwin test: Evaluation of the efficacy/safety profile in rats. *Drug Dev Res*, 36:166–179.

43. Fitzgerald, G.A. (2005). Anticipating change in drug development: The emerging era of translational medicine and therapeutics. *Nat Rev Drug Discov*, 4:815-818.

44. Chiba, K., Yanagawa, Y., Masubuchi, Y., Kataoka, H., Kawaguchi, T., Ohtsuki, M., and Hoshino, Y. (1998). FTY720, a novel immunosuppressant, induces sequenstration of circulating mature lymphocytes be acceleration of lymphocyte homing in rats. I. FTY720 selectively decreases the number of circulating mature lymphocytes by acceleration of lymphocyte homing. *J Immunol*, 160:5037-5044.

45. Budde, K., Schmouder, R.L., Brunkhorst, R., Nashan, B., Lucker, P.W., Mayer, T. *et al.* (2002). First human trial of FTY720, a novel immunomodulator, in stable renal transplant patients. *J Am Soc Nephrol*, 13:1073-1083.

46. Brinkmann, V. (2007). Sphingosine 1-phosphate receptors in health and disease: mechanistic insights from gene deletion studies and reverses pharmacology. *Pharmacol Therap* (in press).

47. Ray, S., Britschgi, M., Herbert, C., Takeda-Uchimura, Y., Boxer, A., Blennow, K. *et al.* (2007). Classification and prediction of clinical Alzheimer's diagnosis based on plasma signalling proteins. *Nat Med*, 13(11):1359-1362.

48. Lovestone, S. (2006). Biomarkers in Alzheimer's disease. *J Nutr Health Aging*, 10:118-122.

49. Finehout, E.J., Franck, Z., Choe, L.H., Relkin, N., and Lee, K.H. (2007). Cerebrospinal fluid proteomic markers for Alzheimer's disease. *Ann Neurol*, 61:120-129.

50. Cutler, P., Akuffo, E., Bodna, W., Briggs, D., Davis, J., Debouck, *et al.* (2008). Identification of biomarkers for early Alzheimer's disease by proteomic analysis of plasma. *Brain* (in press)

51. Cox, J.J., Reimann, F., Nicholas, A.K., Thornton, G., Roberts, E., Springell, K. *et al.* (2006). An *SCN9A* channelopathy causes congenital inability to experience pain. *Nature*, 444:894-898.

52. Yang, Y., Wang, Y., Li, S., Xu, Z., Li, H., Ma, L. *et al.* (2004). Mutations in SCN9A, encoding a sodium channel alpha subunit, in patients with primary erythermalgia. *J Med Gen*, 41:171-174.

53. Fertleman, C.R., Baker, M.D., Parker, K.A., Moffatt, S., Elmslie, F.V., Abrahamsen, B., Ostman, J., Klugbauer, N., Wood, J.N., Gardiner, R.M., and Rees, M. (2006). SCN9A mutations in paroxysmal extreme pain disorder: Allelic variants underlie distinct channel defects and phenotypes. *Neuron*, 52:767-774.

54. Fillingim, R.B., Kaplan, L., Staud, R., Ness, T.J., Glover, T.L., Campbell, C.M. *et al.* (2005). The A118G single nucleotide polymorphism of the mu-opioid receptor gene (OPRM1) is associated with pressure pain sensitivity in humans. *J Pain*, 6(3):159-167.

55. Tegeder, I., Costigan, M., Griffin, R.S., Abele, A., Belfer, I., Schmidt, H., Ehnert, C., Nejim, J., Marian, C., Scholz, J., Wu, T., Allchorne, A., Diatchenko, L., Binshtok, A.M., Goldman, D., Adolph, J., Sama, S., Atlas, S.J., Carlezon, W.A., Parsegian, A., Lotsch, J., Fillingim, R.B., Maixner, W., Geisslinger, G., Max, M.B., and Woolf, C.J. (2006). GTP cyclohydrolase and tetrahydrobiopterin regulate pain sensitivity and persistence. *Nat Med*, 12:1269-1277.

56. Zubieta, J-K., Heitzeg, M.M., Smith, Y.R., Bueller, J.A., Xu, Y., Koeppe, R.A., *et al.* (2003). COMT val[158] genotype affects μ-opioid neurotransmitter responses to a pain stressor. *Science*, 299.

57. Chizh, B.A. and Hobson, A.R. (2007). Using objective markers and imaging in the development of novel treatments of chronic pain. *Expert Rev Neurother*, 7:443-447.

58. Whone, A.L., Watts, R.L., Stoessl, A.J., Davis, M., Reske, S., Nahmias, C., Lang, A.E., Rascol, O., Ribeiro, M.J., Remy, P., Poewe, W.H., Hauser, R.A., and Brooks, D.J. (2003). Slower progression of Parkinson's disease with ropinirole versus levodopa: The REAL-PET study. *Ann Neurol*, 54:93-101.

59. Polman, C.H., O'Connor, P.W., Havrdova, E., Hutchinson, M., Kappos, L., Miller, D.H. *et al.* (2006). A randomized, placebo-controlled trial of natalizumab for relapsing multiple sclerosis. *New Engl J Med*, 354:899-910.

60. Kappos, L. *et al.* (2006). For the FTY720 D2201 Study Group. Oral fingolimod (FTY720) for relapsing multiple sclerosis. *N Engl J Med*, 335(11):1124-1140.

61. Aisen, P.S., Gauthier, S., Vellas, B., Briand, R., Saumier, D., Lauroin, J., and Garceau, D. (2007). Alzhemed: A potential treatment for Alzheimer's disease. *Curr Alz Res*, 4:473–478.

62. Klunk, W.E., Engler, H., Nordberg, A., Wang, Y., Blomqvist, G., Holt, D.P. *et al.* (2004). Imaging brain amyloid in Alzheimer's disease with Pittsburgh Compound-B. *Ann Neurol*, 55(3):306–319.

63. De Leon, M., Mosconi, L., and Logan, J. (2007). Seeing what Alzheimer saw. *Nat Med*, 13(2):129–130.

64. Lockhart, A., Ye, L., Judd, D.B., Merritt, A.P., Lowe, P.N., Morgenstern, J.L. *et al.* (2005). Evidence for the presence of three distinct binding sites for the thioflavin T Class of Alzheimer's disease PET imaging agents on β-amyloid peptide fibrils. *J Biol Chem*, 280(9):7677–7684.

65. Maeda, J., Ji, B. *et al.* (2007). Longitudinal, quantitative assessment of amyloid, neuroinflammation, and anti-amyloid treatment in a living mouse model of Alzheimer's disease enabled by positron emission tomography. *J Neurosci*, 27(41):10957–10968.

66. Johnson, C.N. (2006). The Impact of PET on the Discovery of 742457, a Brain Penetrant 5-HT6 Receptor Antagonist for the Symptomatic Treatment of Alzheimer's Disease. Lecture presented to the CHI 13th International Molecular Medicine Triconference, San Francisco, USA, 21–24 February 2006.

67. Littman, B.H. and Williams, S.A. (2005). The ultimate model organism: Progress in experimental medicine. *Nat Rev Drug Discov*, 4:631–638.

68. Arendt-Nielsen, L., Curatolo, M., and Drewes, A. (2007). Human experimental pain models in drug development: Translational pain research. *Curr Opin Investig Drugs*, 8:41–53.

69. Klein, T., Magerl, W., Rolke, R. *et al.* (2005). Human surrogate models of neuropathic pain. *Pain*, 115:227–233.

70. Gregory, S.L., Hall, D.L., Kenny, G., Caceres, A., Lai, R., Libri, V., *et al.* (2007). A novel potent histamine H3 antagonist produces discrete changes in brain activity during learning and sustained attention: Implications for cognitive enhancement. Brit Assoc Pychopharm Meeting.

CHAPTER 2

Issues in Design and Conduct of Clinical Trials for Cognitive-Enhancing Drugs

Lon S. Schneider

Departments of Psychiatry and Neurology, Keck School of Medicine and
Leonard Davis School of Gerontology, University of Southern California,
Los Angeles, CA, USA

Animal and Translational Models for CNS Drug Discovery,
Vol. 2 of 3: Neurological Disorders
Robert McArthur and Franco Borsini (eds), Academic Press, 2008

INTRODUCTION

This chapter is arranged in three sections: (1) current designs of clinical trials for cognitive enhancement and cognitive disorders; (2) clinical trials designs needs in order to better demonstrate efficacy and effectiveness in cognitive impairment syndromes; (3) current and future conduct of clinical trials including prevention trials.

Section 1 reviews current regulatory guidelines for cognitive impairment clinical trials where they exist, principally for Alzheimer's dementia, then the *de facto* guidelines or trial designs for other syndromes with cognitive impairment including vascular dementia, Parkinson's disease, mild cognitive impairment, and age-associated memory impairment.

Section 2 discusses research design needs. In part it addresses the controversy over the currently approved cognitive enhancers by demonstrating that, by design, the clinical trials that were the basis for approval of current drugs could not speak to pragmatic effectiveness, utility, or worthwhileness of the marketed drugs. It critiques the basic sample selections, study conduct, and outcomes, pointing out that simply making the trials longer or using different statistical techniques will not address effectiveness. Putting new drugs that are putative neurodegenerative disease modifiers into longer studies will not necessarily demonstrate disease modification.

Yet it is obvious that an effective cognitive enhancer for various neurodegenerative illnesses must substantially modify the disease processes, and to such an extent that it is clinically meaningful. Therefore, discussions of the idea of symptomatic versus disease-modifying trials, and prevention trials will follow. This section will end by pointing out that if new drugs are developed using the current "standard" paradigms, then the potential for effective drugs to not be recognized as such would be great with consequent failure to find effective treatments.

Section 3, on trial conduct, reviews Good Clinical Practice (GCP) from the viewpoint that perceptions of GCP may impair study conduct and international drug development. It reviews what is involved in conducting clinical trials of cognitive enhancers, including the sites, sample selection, samples of convenience, monitoring that may lead only to the potential to demonstrate internal validity but not external validity, outcome measures applied to multi-site trials and internationally, the issues of randomization and blinding, and the practical distinctions between Phase II and III trials in this area.

SECTION 1: CURRENT CLINICAL TRIALS DESIGN AND REGULATORY GUIDELINES

This section reviews cognitive impairment syndromes, therapeutic targets, inclusion criteria for trials, typical trials outcomes, current regulatory guidelines, principally for Alzheimer's dementia, and the *de facto* guidelines or trial designs for other syndromes with cognitive impairment including vascular dementia, Parkinson's disease, mild cognitive impairment (MCI), and age-associated memory impairment (AAMI).

History and Background

Prior to the 1970s, various medications were evaluated for the treatment of dementia based on clinical experience or prevailing theories of dementia and aging. These included psychostimulants, vasodilators, ergoloids, and medication "cocktails." In the United States only one drug, a combination of ergoloid mesylates (dihydroergotoxin mesylates, Hydergine®) was and continues to be approved for an ill-defined condition, senile mental decline.

By the late 1980s, the advent and general acceptance of research-based diagnostic criteria for the dementia of Alzheimer's disease (AD),[1] an initial understanding of the underlying pathology of AD, mechanism-based pharmacological therapeutics, and the feasibility and availability of one longer acting cholinesterase inhibitor (ChI), tacrine (tetrahydroaminoacridine, THA, Cognex®), provided the framework for clinical trials to exploit new treatment strategies. The initial research, and now clinical, criteria for AD are included in Table 2.1.[1,2] These criteria have enabled the progression of drug development from a regulatory and commercial basis, because a key general regulatory requirement is that the target of the therapeutic claim be straightforward to recognize and accepted by experts in the field.

Table 2.1 Potential "categorical" cognitive impairment therapeutic indications

- Alzheimer's disease (dementia)
- Early Alzheimer's disease (pre-dementia)
- Mild cognitive impairment
- Age-associated memory impairment
- Dementia with Lewy bodies
- Parkinson's disease dementia
- Frontotemporal dementia
- Cerebrovascular cognitive impairment and dementia
  - Ischemic, small vessel, and large vessel
- Stroke syndromes
  - For example, anterior communicating artery syndrome
- Cognitive impairment associated with schizophrenia
- Depression
- Bipolar disorder
- Attention deficit hyperactivity disorder (adults and children)
- Post traumatic stress disorder
- Cognitive impairment associated with multiple sclerosis
- Cognitive impairment subsequent to post-coronary artery bypass graft
- HIV neurocognitive disorder
- Cognitive impairment associated with diabetes mellitus
- Developmental disability, mental retardation
- Cognitively normal people
- Other conditions

Cognitive Impairment Syndromes and Potential Therapeutic Targets

A range of cognitive impairment syndromes could be considered as potential therapeutic targets. Many are listed in Table 2.1. A few are discussed below, including AD,[1,2] MCI[3] and early AD.[4,5] During the 1990s, research- and consensus-based criteria were proposed for many and include vascular dementia,[6,7] dementia with Lewy bodies,[8] frontotemporal dementia syndrome. More recently Parkinson/s disease dementia criteria[9] and research criteria for early AD[5] have been offered. These latter criteria are evolving, have not been as well-accepted as AD, and thus clinical trials including these populations have been limited.

Alzheimer's Disease

AD is the most common and best described dementia of old age. The clinical description is associated with a relatively well-described neuropathology. Criteria for AD are straightforward and can be applied by general practitioners. It is the most important dementia for drug development because its pragmatic, consensus-based criteria have been broadly accepted and drugs for AD have received regulatory approval. Thus it has become the prototypical clinical condition for the development of cognitive enhancers.

Table 2.2 Diagnostic criteria for Alzheimer's disease*

- The criteria for the clinical diagnosis of probable AD include:
  - Dementia established by clinical examination and documented by the Mini-Mental Test, Blessed Dementia Scale, or some similar examination, and confirmed by neuropsychological tests;
  - Deficits in two or more areas of cognition;
  - Progressive worsening of memory and other cognitive functions;
  - No disturbance of consciousness;
  - Onset between 40 and 90 years of age (most often after 65);
  - Absence of systemic disorders or other brain disease that in and of themselves could account for the progressive deficits in memory and cognition.
- Other clinical features consistent with the diagnosis of probable AD, after exclusion of causes of dementia other than AD, include:
  - Plateaus in the course of progression of the illness;
  - Associated symptoms depression, insomnia, incontinence, delusions, illusions, hallucinations, catastrophic verbal, emotional, or physical outbursts, sexual disorders, and weight loss;
  - Other neurologic abnormalities in some patients, especially with more advanced disease and including motor signs such as increased muscle tone, myoclonus, or gait disorder, seizures in advanced disease; and CT normal for age.
- *DSM-IV-TR criteria are essentially similar but deficits must be sufficient to interfere with social or occupational function.*

Modified from [1] and [2]
*Frequently referred to as "NINCDS-ADRDA criteria" or "McKhann criteria" for probable AD.

An essential criterion for the diagnosis of AD is the presence of dementia (see Table 2.2). The presence of AD in the absence of dementia cannot be currently diagnosed with sufficient accuracy and consensus to satisfy regulatory or indeed clinicians. Because AD is currently defined by the presence of dementia, attempts have been made to identify a predementia state of cognitive impairment likely to lead to AD. These include MCI[3] and early AD.[4,5]

Age-Associated Memory Impairment

Criteria for "age-associated memory impairment" (AAMI), an attempt to recognize functionally significant, although mild and probably non-progressive cognitive impairment have not been generally recognized as a diagnostic construct, although DSM-IV-TR includes a code for "age-related cognitive decline," equivalent to AAMI. In effect, AAMI consists of a memory complaint coupled with performance on unspecified neuropsychological tests below 1 SD of a 30-year-old person.[10] Arguments against including AAMI as a therapeutic target include that it is vague, over inclusive of most people over 55 with a memory complaint, does not define a medical condition, and there is a lack of consensus about its validity. Arguments for AAMI include that it defines an age-related condition, which although non-progressive, still impairs function and quality of life (QoL).

Mild Cognitive Impairment

Mild cognitive impairment (MCI) has been a therapeutic target for several clinical trials of cholinesterase inhibitor medications marketed for AD and the methodology of MCI trials is discussed below. The criteria for MCI are generally taken to include: a subjective cognitive (memory) complaint; MMSE within normal limits; neuropsychological test results for memory of greater than 1.5 standard deviation below age-appropriate norms; activities of daily living (ADL) within normal limits; and a Clinical Dementia Rating (CDR) of 0.5.

The evolving validity of MCI will rest mainly on its clinical homogeneity, relevance, and ability to predict the onset of the dementia of AD. For example, although all MCI trials use the Petersen or Mayo Clinic criteria for MCI[11] the criteria were applied somewhat differently. When the Janssen, Novartis, and the ADCS criteria were applied to the same clinic cohort differing prevalences were found of 51%, 21%, and 17% depending on the criteria.[12]

In research clinics a diagnosis of "amnestic MCI" or "MCI of the amnestic type," implies a conversion rate to AD of about 12–15% per year.[13] However, MCI is not necessarily a predementia stage of AD, since many people who fulfill criteria do not progress to dementia and some improve to not being cognitively impaired.[14,15] MCI is viewed also as a transitional state on the road to the development of AD, as an "at risk" state with an increased likelihood for the development of dementia over a specified time, or as the very early diagnosis of AD before the full dementia syndrome is recognized.[16] Although criteria for MCI can be defined by consensus, the diagnosis as variously used suffers from vagueness in conceptualization, with the condition overlapping with AD.

"MCI of the amnestic type," characterized primarily by memory impairment, may more closely resemble early AD. Just as in more moderate dementia, some patients may show very little decline or a stabilization of symptoms, there may be similar stabilization or even the failure of a progression to further cognitive symptoms or to dementia among people with the neuropathology of AD.

Early AD

Recently, a group formed on an *ad hoc* basis proposed new research criteria for AD that attempts to recognize AD before the onset of dementia; essentially recognizing an early AD syndrome. The core feature is progressive episodic memory loss over 6 months without the requirement for dementia. Additional requirements, however, are for biological evidence such as hippocampal atrophy viewed by MRI imaging or changes in a biological markers such as β-amyloid protein fragments, tau or phospho-tau proteins.[5] As with other newly proposed diagnostic criteria, there are issues of validity, context, generality, and consensus that are barriers to their acceptance. Their offering, however, indicates the desire to make an AD diagnosis earlier than the onset of the dementia.

Parkinson's Disease Dementia (PDD)

Patients with Parkinson's disease have an increased risk for dementia and about 25% may develop dementia after the onset of their Parkinson's disease. Operationalized criteria for patients with PDD have been proposed recently, although, validity, adequate sensitivity and specificity have not been fully established.[9] The dementia, occurring after the onset of Parkinsonian motor symptoms can be characterized by a particular pattern of impairments in executive function, memory, and attention that is different from other dementias such as AD.

From a US Food and Drug Administration (FDA) regulatory perspective, however, a diagnosis of the PDD is made in patients in whom "a progressive dementia syndrome occurs at least 2 years after a diagnosis of Parkinson's disease" in the absence of other causes of the dementia. The criteria for the dementia diagnosis are the DSM-IV-TR dementia syndrome criteria, "Dementia Due To Other General Medical Condition" (code 294.1x). This definition serves the purpose of defining a clinical condition for a therapeutic drug claim that can be recognized, agreed to by consensus, and is straightforward to recognize, without the risk of over-specifying the characteristics of the dementia. It came about as a result of FDA approving the cholinesterase inhibitor, rivastigmine (Exelon®), for "mild to moderate dementia associated with Parkinson's disease".[16]

Vascular Cognitive Impairment and Dementia

The NINDS-AIRENS criteria[7] have been applied most commonly in published clinical trials. The criteria for the diagnosis of probable vascular dementia include: (1) dementia defined by cognitive decline from a previously higher level of functioning and manifested by impairment of memory and of two or more cognitive domains with deficits severe enough to interfere with ADL; (2) cerebrovascular disease defined by the presence of focal signs on neurologic examination or brain imaging; (3) a relationship between the dementia and cerebrovascular disease manifested by dementia onset within 3 months following a stroke or abrupt deterioration in cognitive functions; or fluctuating, stepwise progression of cognitive deficits.

The issue is that vascular dementia and the use of the criteria do not lead to a sufficiently homogeneous clinical entity that can serve as a therapeutic claim (FDA Peripheral and Central Nervous System Drugs Advisory Committee, March 14, 2001, http://www.fda.gov/ohrms/dockets/ac/01/minutes/3724m2.pdf). Thus far, no drugs have been approved for treating either vascular dementia or cognitive impairment in the context of cerebrovascular disease. In particular neither cholinesterase inhibitors nor memantine (Ebixa®/Axura®)/Namenda®) have shown sufficient efficacy and safety in 3-, 6-month donepezil (Aricept®) trials, two galantamine (formerly Reminyl® and currently Razadyne®) trials, one rivastigmine trial, and two memantine trials.[17] There were modest cognitive changes in some trials but no overall significant effects on global assessments or ADLs.

Dementia with Lewy Bodies

The criteria of McKeith *et al.*, 2005[18] have become a *de facto* standard for studies in DLB, but they show a very high specificity but low sensitivity. Core clinical features of DLB consist of rapid fluctuations in cognition, recurrent visual hallucinations and spontaneous and fluctuating features of Parkinsonism; these are further supported by high sensitivity for extrapyramidal side effects to antipsychotic medications and rapid eye movement sleep behavior disorder.

In part because of availability of the drug, pharmaceutical company sponsorship, and the rationale that DLB is associated with markedly reduced acetylcholinergic function, one smaller multicenter trial was carried out with rivastigmine, modeled on the typical 6-month placebo controlled AD trial methodology.[19] The trial showed significant effects on a summary behavior rating scale and speed of response.

Summary

There are a range of cognitive impairment syndromes that could be considered as clinical conditions for therapeutic intervention. A number, such as AD, PDD, HIV neurocognitive disorder, and cognitive impairment associated with schizophrenia are sufficiently describable and accepted, and with clear enough criteria that they can be considered clinical targets for drug indications. Others, such as MCI and vascular dementia are considered too heterogeneous and less well accepted. AD is the drug indication most commonly pursued by far and is the focus of this chapter.

Typical Inclusion Criteria for AD Clinical Trials

Typical inclusion criteria for clinical trials include the presence of probable AD (NINCDS-ADRDA workshop criteria),[1] a specified Mini-Mental State Examination (MMSE)[20] score (e.g., typically from 10 or 12 to 24 or 26 for "mild to moderate AD;" more recently from 16 or 20 to 26 for longer term trials; or under 11 for "severe AD"); a score of less than 4 on the Modified Hachinski Scale;[21] a CT scan or MRI consistent with AD and showing no evidence of significant focal lesions; generally good physical health other than the dementia (confirmed by medical history, physical examination, neurological examination, ECG, and laboratory tests); normal blood pressure or controlled with antihypertension medications; and having a reliable caregiver to ensure medication compliance and to participate in clinical evaluations.

Exclusion criteria typically consist of a history of other psychiatric or neurological disorders, a stroke, imaging evidence of a stroke, significant concurrent physical illness, or abnormal clinical laboratory findings. Therefore, dementia samples studied in clinical trials consist mainly of mildly to moderately impaired outpatients living at home with their families, who are otherwise medically healthy and lack significant behavioral symptoms. To this extent, therefore, they are samples of convenience and do not represent the broad distribution of people with AD in the population.

Recently, some trials of putative disease-modifying drugs, or of drugs thought to exert their clinical actions by affecting metabolic or pathological processes in AD, have expanded inclusion criteria to allow the concurrent use of approved antidementia therapies such as cholinesterase inhibitors or memantine. The allowance of the use of marketed drugs is intended to address the prospects that a successful disease-modifying drug may be used in addition to a symptomatic drug and that it is difficult to recruit AD patients who are not taking marketed drugs into clinical trials.

Typical Outcomes and Endpoints for AD Clinical Trials

Three main domains have been assessed in AD and dementia clinical trials: cognition, global assessment, and ADL. More recently behavior, caregiver burden, QoL,

Table 2.3 Cognitive/neuropsychological outcome measures used in Phase II and III clinical trials of approved anti-dementia drugs

Alzheimer's Disease Assessment Scale – cognitive subscale (ADAS-cog)
- A battery of brief individual tests. Includes word recall, naming, commands, constructional and ideational praxis, orientation, word recognition, spoken language and comprehension, word-finding, and recall of test instructions
- Requires approximately 45–60 min to administer
- Error scores range from 70 (lowest) to 0.

Mini-Mental State Examination (MMSE)
- Brief, structured bedside mental status examination
- Screens orientation, memory, attention, naming, comprehension, and praxis
- Requires 10–15 min to administer
- Scores range from 0 (lowest) to 30
- Also used to screen for entry into studies; scores from 10 to 26 or 12 to 24 represent "mild to moderate AD," 10 or below "severe AD".

Severe Impairment Battery (SIB)
- Intended for use with severely impaired patients
- Items are single words or one-step commands combined with gestures
- Nine areas are assessed: social interaction, memory, orientation, language, attention, praxis, visuospatial ability, construction, and orientation to name
- Scored on a 0 to 100 range.

Adapted from [35,36]

health care resource use, and economics have been assessed in Phase II and III clinical trials.

Key rating scales are listed and described in Tables 2.3 and 2.4 and include the cognitive subscale of the Alzheimer's Disease Assessment Scale (ADAS-cog), the standard instrument for the measurement of efficacy in dementia trials; scales that assess AD patients' abilities to perform ADL, including the Disability Assessment for Dementia (DAD) scale and the AD Cooperative Study – Activities of Daily Living Inventory (ADCS-ADL); scales to assess behavioral symptoms in dementia, including the Neuropsychiatric Inventory (NPI) and the Behavioral Pathology in Alzheimer's Disease Rating Scale (BEHAVE-AD); scales for assessing global clinical change; and methods for assessing caregiver time, QoL, and health economics.

From both a pragmatic and regulatory standpoint, a drug for AD must show efficacy by improving at least cognition or retarding its deterioration, largely because impaired cognition is the first and core manifestation of AD and can be measured objectively. In addition, the FDA requires that a clinically meaningful effect determined by a clinician independently from psychometric assessment should be observed, creating a requirement for two co-primary outcomes or the "dual outcome criterion."

To gain a true overview of the impact of AD on patients, caregivers and society, areas such as cognition, ADL, behavior, caregiver burden and QoL need to be adequately assessed (Table 2.4). Changes in these domains are currently considered to be of secondary importance by US standards for regulatory approval compared with cognitive, global or ADL outcomes. However, European regulatory criteria require

Table 2.4 Functional activity measures used in clinical trials

Progressive Deterioration Scale (PDS)
- Assesses quality of life changes or activities of daily living on 29 items
- Rated by caregiver on a visual analog scale
- Scores range from 0 to 100.

Alzheimer's Disease Cooperative Study – Activities of Daily Living (ADCS-ADL)
- Assesses functional performance, 24 items
- Structured interview and ratings by an informant
- Scores range from 0 to 54.

Disability Assessment in Dementia Scale (DAD)
- Assess ability to initiate and perform basic and instrumental activities of daily living and leisure activities, 17 items
- Conducted as either a questionnaire completed by caregiver or as a structured interview of the caregiver
- Scores range from 0 to 46.

Functional Assessment Staging (FAST)
- 16-items that consist of physical and instrumental ADL, intended to project the progression of loss of function in AD
- Interview of caregiver.

Adapted from [35,36].

improvement in ADL as the co-primary outcome with global assessment secondary[22] (http://www.emea.europa.eu/pdfs/human/ewp/055395en.pdf).

No guidelines recognize improvement in behavior, functional activities or caregiver burden *alone* as legitimate therapeutic goals for regulatory purposes. Rather, these domains must complement demonstrated cognitive improvement. An exception, however, is FDA's potential recognition of specific behavioral syndromes associated with AD, including psychosis of AD and depression of AD, both characterized in large part by the onset of the psychosis and depression after the onset of the dementia.[23]

Cognitive Function

Assessment of cognitive function is the essential primary measure of efficacy in clinical trials. Prevalent thinking is that treatments that improve, or reduce the decline of, cognition would be expected to provide important benefits to patients with AD and their caregivers, and that even maintenance of baseline levels of cognitive function should mean an improvement in QoL and autonomy for patients (compared to placebo-treated patients). However, the idea that cognitive improvement as measured by point differences on cognitive tests in AD clinical trials necessarily translates into meaningful clinical improvement has been challenged from when the drugs were first approved in the mid 1990s, and more recently from the UK's National Institute for Health and Clinical Excellence (NICE), especially from the point of view of overall effectiveness, QoL, and health economics.[24,25]

The two cognitive instruments most commonly used in AD trials have been the ADAS-cog and the MMSE.[20] [In Phase I and some Phase IIa trials, computer-assisted assessments such as the Cognitive Drug Research computerized assessment system

(CDR; http://www.cognitivedrugresearch.com/newcdr/index.php?cat=5) and similar have been used to gain initial evidence of efficacy. But these assessment measures have been infrequently used in Phase IIb and III trials]. Only recently and in longer term trials have additional cognitive batteries been employed based mainly on established neuropsychological scales used clinically (Section 2, below).

The ADAS-cog assesses various cognitive abilities including memory, comprehension, orientation in time and place and spontaneous speech.[26] It has become a *de facto* standard, and nearly all recent clinical trials have used ADAS-cog as the primary index of cognitive change. Versions in numerous languages have been developed, although other than the French versions, validity testing has been lacking. The National Institute of Aging (NIA) ADCS has been developing an expanded ADAS-cog to assess attention and executive function more directly[27] and this expanded ADAS-cog has been used in several AD and MCI trials.[28]

Compared with other cognitive scales, the ADAS-cog is more sensitive to a wider range of disease severity and has greater specificity to the major dysfunctions experienced by patients within the moderate range of AD. However, it lacks an episodic memory component, an attention component, and is less sensitive to change in mild AD (MMSE about 21 and above) than in more moderate AD.

Prescribing information approved by regulatory authorities often defines a 4-point improvement on ADAS-cog relative to either baseline or the placebo group as a clinical "responder." Over 6, 12, and 18 months, placebo-treated clinical trials patients with mild to moderate AD, as a group, may be expected to deteriorate on the ADAS-cog by a little less than 2 points; 4–5 points, or 6–7 points, respectively. However, this is highly variable and the precise rate of deterioration depends on the baseline disease severity, sample selection, language, and number of ADAS-cog administrations, and most strongly on sample size.

The ADAS-cog is not an interval scale and, for example, decline in absolute scores is less in the milder and more severe stages of cognitive impairment than in the middle stages. Therefore, in any clinical trial there will be a degree of variation in baseline scores and in change scores over time.

In randomized clinical trials of marketed cholinesterase inhibitors, the significant improvement in cognition results from the combination of slight improvement or stabilization in ADAS-cog score in the medication group and a worsening in the placebo group compared with baseline over the 6- to 12-month trials durations. A limitation in current trials methodology is that if the placebo group does not show decline on the ADAS-cog, perhaps because of small sample size, then the effects of a medication that might maintain or improve cognition over several months would not be apparent.

The MMSE is commonly used as a secondary cognitive outcome measure, in large part because it is brief and easy to use in a clinical situation.[20] It was meant to be a physician-administered, "bedside" examination of cognitive function and was not intended to be used other than as a clinical screening instrument. Nonetheless it has been incorporated into clinical trials as a staging criterion for entry and as a secondary measure of cognitive outcomes.

It was initially deemed to be relatively crude and insensitive to change, and showed reduced sensitivity and increased variability compared with more comprehensive tests such as the ADAS-cog.[29] But like the ADAS-cog, the MMSE is sensitive to change in cognitive performance over time in trials of mild to moderate AD. It covers relatively few domains, although it includes attention and concentration that the ADAS-cog does not. Over 12 months, untreated patients with mild to moderate AD are expected to decline by approximately 2 points.

The Severe Impairment Battery (SIB) is noteworthy since most patients who are beyond moderate–severely impaired (e.g., MMSE less than about 10) cannot complete cognitive testing with an instrument such as the ADAS-cog because of progressive deterioration in expressive and receptive language, and are excluded from clinical trials. The SIB can be used to assess patients who cannot complete conventional testing.[30,31] It measures nine different cognitive domains relying on single word or one-step commands along with gestures as well as behavioral responses. The SIB has been used as a component of the ADCS instrument protocol and in memantine trials, one rivastigmine trial, and three donepezil trials. A further advantage is that it appears sensitive to change in patients with only moderate cognitive impairment as well. The SIB is the cognitive assessment that was the efficacy basis for the approval of memantine and donepezil for moderate to severe and for severe AD, respectively.

Daily Function and ADL

The maintenance or improvement of functional abilities compared with placebo treatment – as with cognitive improvement – is also considered to be clinically meaningful from both a clinical and regulatory perspective. The perspective here is that the maintenance of ADL may allow a patient to live more independently and for longer, and may delay institutionalization (although this assumption has not been proven).

A number of scales exist to assess patients' abilities to perform basic and instrumental ADL (Table 2.4). However, not all of them adequately measure all functional domains and many of them were not specifically designed for evaluating ADL in patients with dementia. The most commonly used ADL rating scales were initially the Progressive Deterioration Scale (PDS), and currently the DAD (Feldman[32,33]) and the ADCS-ADL inventory.[34]

The Blessed-Roth Dementia Scale had been used widely in dementia research in senile dementia.[37] The scale consists of 22 items, half of which measure changes in functional abilities: 8 items measure changes in performance of everyday activities, 3 measure changes in self-care habits, and 11 assess behavioral changes. It has been shown to be a valid measure of the severity of dementia in that it is correlated with cognitive performance and aspects of the pathology of AD.[37] The behavioral items, however, may influence overall scores and the limited range per item may be reasons why it is not used commonly.

The PDS had been used frequently in AD trials with cholinesterase inhibitors – rivastigmine, donepezil, and tacrine (Table 2.4). It is composed of 29 items rated by a caregiver, largely addressing ADL but also including items reflecting behavior and QoL.[38] Scores per item range from 0 to 100 scaling on a visual analog scale. Trials using this scale as a measure of ADL have been criticized because the scale measures a range of domains and the resulting score does not necessarily assess solely changes in ADL.[39] Nevertheless, the PDS was demonstrated to be sensitive to the effects of three marketed cholinesterase inhibitors and accepted as a clinical measure by both the FDA and the European Medicines Agency (EMEA) as indicated by its inclusion in the prescribing information. In later trials other ADL scales replaced it perhaps also because it requires a proprietary scoring system.

The Interview for Deterioration in Daily living activities in Dementia (IDDD) was designed as a severity instrument for quantifying impairment of patients' ADL. It is a 33-item structured interview of caregivers consisting of self-care items (e.g., washing, dressing, eating) and complex activity items (e.g., shopping, writing, answering the telephone) performed by men and women.[40] Descriptions are elicited and frequency of assistance is rated on a 3-point scale for each item, for an overall range of 33–99 (most severe) points. In a donepezil study[41] using a modified version of the IDDD, the complex activity scale, but not the self-care scale was sensitive to the effects of the higher dose medication, showing a marginally lesser decline.

The ADCS-ADL inventory was developed by the ADCS to assess functional performance in patients with AD.[34] In a structured interview format that takes less than 15 min to administer, informants are asked whether patients attempted each of 24 items in the inventory during the previous 4 weeks and, if so, to comment on their levels of performance. The ADCS-ADL scale has good test–retest reliability and it clearly distinguishes the stages of severity of AD patients, from very mild to severely impaired. It includes items from traditional basic ADL items (e.g., grooming, dressing, walking, bathing, feeding, and toileting) as well as instrumental ADL items (e.g., shopping, preparing meals, using household appliances, keeping appointments, and reading). The ADCS-ADL inventory has been used as an outcome measure in AD clinical trials and versions suitable for assessing mild or very severe patients have been developed by the ADCS.

As with the ADCS-ADL, the DAD scale was developed specifically for use in AD patients.[32,42] The DAD scale includes 17 items related to basic self-care and 23 to instrumental ADL, including hygiene, dressing, undressing, continence, eating, meal preparation, telephone use, going on an outing, finance and correspondence, medications, and leisure and housework. The ability of patients to initiate, plan, organize, and perform ADL is assessed either by questionnaire or as a structured interview with the caregiver.[32] A maximum score of 15 for initiation, 11 for planning and organizing, and 20 for performing activities yields a maximum score of 46. Untreated AD patients have been expected to deteriorate by 11–13 points on the DAD scale over 12 months. The DAD scale has been used to assess ADL in several trials of cholinesterase inhibitors and longer term trials.

Global Interview-Based Severity Scales Assessment

There are a variety of global ratings (Table 2.5). Included in this broad category are the Clinicians' Global Impressions – Severity of Illness scale (CGIS),[43] Clinical Dementia Rating Scale (CDR)[44] and the Global Deterioration Scale (GDS).[45]

The CGIS is an unanchored 7-point scale, performed by an experienced clinician. The clinician is asked, "considering your total clinical experience with this particular population, how ill is the patient at this time?" The patient is rated on a 7-point scale ranging from 1 (normal) through 4 (moderately ill) to 7 (among the most extremely ill). There are virtually no other guidelines. By contrast other severity scales use extensive anchoring for their ratings.

Table 2.5 Interview-based global severity and change scales

Clinical Dementia Rating scale (CDR)
- Structured interview with both patient and informant
- Performance is rated in six domains: memory, orientation, judgment and problem solving, community activities, home and hobbies, and personal care
- A 5-point scale: 0 = no impairment, 0.5 = questionable, 1 = mild, 2 = moderate, and 3 = severe dementia
- The six domains are often summed to create a 0 – 18 "sum of the boxes" score.

Global Deterioration Scale (GDS)
- A 7-point scale of severity or stage of dementia: 1 = normal; 3 = late confusion; 5 = middle dementia; 7 = late dementia
- Assessed by a clinician who has access to all sources of information.

Clinicians' Global Impression of Change (CGIC)
- Also used as a general term for various impressionistic measures, rated by the clinician, based on interviews with or without a collateral source, with or without reference to mental status examination, and with or without reference to cognitive assessment results
- Rated on 7 points: 1 = very much improved; 2 = much improved; 3 = minimally improved; 4 = no change; 5 = minimally worse; 6 = much worse; 7 = very much worse.

FDA Clinicians' Interview-Based Impression of Change (CIBIC) (Leber 1992, personal communication)
- FDA modifications to the CGIC suggested that clinical change should be patient interview only
- Access to other sources of information is prevented to minimize bias and maintain independence. During a 10-minute interview, the clinician should systematically assess the domains ordinarily considered part of a clinical examination
- Rationale: if an experienced clinician can perceive clinical change on the basis of an interview, then such change is likely to be clinically meaningful
- Various constructions have been made by different companies
- Clinicians' Interview-Based Impression of Change-Plus (CIBIC+)
- A CIBIC as described above except conducted by interviewing both the patient and informant has come to be known as a CIBIC+.

Alzheimer's Disease Cooperative Study-Clinicians Global Impression of Change (ADCS-CGIC)
- Assesses 15 areas under the domains of cognition, behavior, and social and daily functioning
- Using a form as a guideline, both patient and caregiver are interviewed; order is not specified
- Under each area list of sample probes and space for notes with few requirements for the interviews–an assessment of mental status must be made; clinicians not permitted to ask about side effects, nor to discuss patient with others
- Change rating is made on the 7-point CGIC scale
- Operationalized example of a CIBIC+.

Adapted from [35,36].

The CDR[i] score is based on a comprehensive structured interview using worksheets. It assesses dementia severity by staging, and includes cognitive, functional and social domains in the overall staging. The CDR structured interview can also be used as a diagnostic tool. In some clinical trials the CDR is used as a more quantitative "sum-of-the-boxes" numerical rating. This sums up the scores of the six individual domains and expresses it on a range from 0 to 18 and is more sensitive than the 4-point CDR staging from 0.5, to 1, 2, and 3.[44]

The GDS rates seven stages of dementia, scored from 1 to 7, assessing the phenomenological global progression of AD cognitively, functionally, and behaviorally, based on interview with the patient.[45]

Limitations of Severity Scales

Severity measures help to provide a structure by which the clinician can assess a patient's dementia. Staging a dementia on the basis of severity alone, however, does not necessarily assist management or predict future course. For example, although increased severity of dementia certainly correlates with institutionalization, it is not the sole predictor of institutionalization. Assessing dementia severity might help to understand when particular symptoms might be expected or have prognostic importance. For example, Forstl was able to show through severity ratings that AD patients with hallucinations and delusions who were more mildly impaired (on the basis of a CDR rating of 1) had a more rapid progression, while hallucinations and delusions occurring in more severe stages did not have prognostic significance.[46]

On the other hand, some global severity measures may be useful in diagnosis or in clinical trials which follow patients for a year or more, since change in severity can be more readily appreciated over a longer time course. As a method of tracking disease progression, global severity measures are broader in range than neuropsychological tests and are less subject to bottoming or topping out. Nominally, at least, they include the use of more information for making ratings than cognitive assessments alone.

As with other ratings, differences on severity scales between one time point and another may be difficult to interpret clinically, but, when these severity outcomes are assessed within the context of the outcome of other measures including cognitive and global change scales, their significance becomes clearer.

Global Interview-Based Change Scales

This broad category includes the Clinicians' Global Impression of Change (CGIC),[43] the FDA Clinicians' Interview-Based Impression of Change (CIBIC) (FDA CIBIC),[47] ADCS-CGIC,[48,49] and others (Table 2.5). They are different from other scales in that they assess only change from the trial baseline.

Global change scales have been used extensively as primary outcome criteria in early clinical trials for antidementia drugs. The rationale for their use is that a skilled clinician should be able to see the clinical effect of a treatment after a brief interview. The original CGIC used in dementia trials, however, showed little sensitivity

---

[i]Not to be confused with the computerised cognitive assessment battery provided by Cognitive Drug Research (http://www.cognitivedrugresearch.com) discussed above.

to the treatment effects of putative medications. The addition of modest structuring has enhanced the details provided by CGICs (providing cues and direction, or requiring documentation by the clinician). CGICs are most frequently used in shorter term clinical trials.

The CGIC[43] has been the most commonly used and most basic assessment of global change in neuropsychopharmacological trials. It consists of 7-point ratings of severity (CGIS) and change (CGIC), and an "index of efficacy" that contrasts change with side effects (although the latter part is not commonly used). An overarching but implicit assumption in its use is that clinicians are sufficiently skilled to make appropriate clinical inferences and assess meaningful change in patients. Therefore, there are only minimal guidelines; there are no instructions about the kind of interview to be conducted or the method for rating change. The instructions state: "As determined by the physician *relative* to baseline. Rate *total improvement* whether or not, in your judgment, it is due entirely to drug treatment. Choose *ONE* response ranging from 1, very much improved; 2, much improved; 3, minimally improved; 4, no change; 5 minimally worse; 6, much worse; 7, very much worse." This basic framework has been applied to subsequent, derivative CGIC instruments.

Originally detailed in a letter to pharmaceutical companies in November 1991, the rationale for the FDA-CIBIC[47] was that most experts will readily accept a drug inducing effects of sufficient size to be detected during a clinical interview as clinically meaningful. This example of a CGIC, therefore, is intended to determine whether the effects of a drug are large enough to allow their detection by an experienced clinician. The CIBIC was intended to be based entirely upon information collected during an interview with the patient, alone, without input from third parties in order to capture this global or holistic assessment. When caregiver-input is allowed the CIBIC is referred to as the CIBIC+. Ratings were done on the same unanchored 7-point scale used for the CGIC.

The ADCS-CGIC was developed for the NIA's ADCS Instrument Development Project as a method to examine the processes and determinants of making change scores.[48] It consists of a format with which a clinician may address clinically relevant overall change, including 15 areas under the domains of cognition, behavior, and social and daily functioning, and has been used in many regulatory trials of AD drugs over the last 15 years. In this way a CIBIC+ is assessed under relatively systematic conditions.

Limitations of CGICs

The construct underlying a CGIC score is that it is an instrument whose intended use is to measure *clinically meaningful* change, as distinct from an instrument's use to assess any change. CGICs are not intended as sensitive measures of small changes that are unlikely to be clinically meaningful. In principle, a clinician rating a subject as changed on a global change scale is determining clinically meaningful and distinct change. Therefore, any change recorded on a CGIC is considered clinically significant by definition.

Although a CGIC is simpler to interpret than sensitive psychometric instruments, its inherent lack of structure limits the precision with which ratings can be made. Despite this disadvantage, there is a general opinion that CGIC ratings are potentially sensitive to clinically meaningful effects. Indeed, in numerous trials of various cholinesterase inhibitors, CGICs have proven sensitive enough to detect clinical effects. CGICs, however, are not the only instruments that can fulfill this role. The rationale above has been extended to interview-based severity ratings, and changes in functional activities and QoL may also indicate clinically meaningful change.

Regulatory Considerations

The US FDA, among other functions, regulates how drugs are developed, advertised, and sold. It receives its authority from the Food, Drug and Cosmetic Act. "The provisions of the FD&C Act are intended to insure that all drug products marketed within the United States will be 'safe for use' and 'effective in use,' under the 'conditions of use' described in their approved labeling".[50]

In effect, the FDA's mission is to protect consumers against false and misleading claims and advertising by regulating the corporate free speech of pharmaceutical sponsors. In developing cognitive enhancers the regulatory questions may be as follows: (1) Are there cognitive enhancing claims that can be considered "conditions of use?" (2) Are outcomes used in cognitive enhancer trials meaningful enough to assess whether the drug itself is "effective in use?" (3) Is the drug "safe and effective" for the population to which it will be prescribed? (4) Are there "adequate and well-controlled studies" demonstrating its safety and effect? (5) What is proposed for the labeling of the drug, are the health claims, and the instructions for use?

However for this evidence to be substantial, and in particular that there be substantial evidence for cognitive enhancement in a given condition, the evidence must be such that it would allow scientific experts to conclude, "fairly and responsibly that the drug will have the effect it purports or is represented to have under the conditions of use prescribed, recommended, or suggested in the labeling or proposed labeling…".[50]

FDA's actions are guided under Title 21 *Code of Federal Regulations* part 312 (http://www.access.gpo.gov/nara/cfr/waisidx_03/21cfr312_03.html). In addition specific procedures are discussed in individual formal and *ad hoc* guidelines, bilateral discussions with drug developers, and through advisory committees. With respect to cognitive enhancers there are no formal guidelines for drug development. Guidelines for conditions that do not have a previously approved drug would depend on the specific condition for which the drug is intended. Any future guidelines, of necessity will include the definition of the clinical condition, the acceptable outcomes, the duration of trials, and safety standards. During the last decade the FDA has held advisory committees to address, MCI (March 13, 2001, http://www.fda.gov/ohrms/dockets/ac/01/minutes/3724m1.pdf), vascular dementia (March 14, 2001, http://www.fda.gov/ohrms/dockets/ac/01/minutes/3724m2.pdf), and behavioral disorders in dementia (March 9, 2000, http://www.fda.gov/ohrms/dockets/ac/00/minutes/3590m.htm). No regulatory actions were taken at these meetings.

By comparison EMEA promotes guidelines both for symptomatic drugs[51,52] and slowing the progression of neurodegenerative diseases, and has addressed other indications and methodological issues.[53]

It is notable that only draft guidelines from the FDA exist for the clinical evaluation of antidementia drugs, a draft circulated in 1990 (Leber P, unpublished). In effect for

AD the pragmatic guidelines are the development plans for the previously approved drugs. Thus for the development of new cognitive indications there is no clear road map and development plans have to be individualized. To do this requires obtaining consensus from experts and discussing the conditions needed to define the clinical claim and the acceptable outcomes with the FDA.

It is likely that a request for approval of a cognitive enhancer for other than AD would involve a review by an FDA advisory committee. Questions that would be asked at such an advisory committee would include: (1) Can the clinical entity be clearly defined in a clinical setting? (2) Are there valid criteria for the diagnosis of the condition? (3) Is there sufficient sensitivity and specificity, and is there predictive validity to the diagnosis? (4) Is there a known etiology or pathogenesis? (5) Is there a characteristic clinical course? And finally, (6) does the treatment improve the essential condition? (7) Were the studies adequate and well controlled? (8) Is the drug safe and effective?

Sponsors' Perspectives

For potential indications where the above may not have been established, these questions or requirements present an obvious disincentive to drug development in that pharmaceutical companies would like to know in advance what patient sample or clinical condition would be acceptable and the criteria that will be used to evaluate their drug. Thus, they are reluctant to develop drugs for therapeutic claims for which there are not drugs that have been approved previously. This imposes an obvious limit on drug discovery efforts. However, other barriers would arise if the FDA or EMEA were to create a list of "approvable" conditions and the required methods to demonstrate efficacy and safety. Thus, to some degree there is an impasse that is approached mainly by direct consultation between the sponsor and the regulator.

Companies are understandably reluctant to pursue treatments for clinical indications before the diagnostic criteria for the clinical disorder have been recognized and approved. As one example, sponsors will now consider limited development programs for cognitive impairment associated with schizophrenia (CIAS) in part because of a general acceptance among sponsors, regulators, and academics of the *definitions* of the condition and the ranges of outcomes that can be used to assess it. Diagnostic criteria, however, cannot be imposed by a regulatory authority and rather must be fundamentally described and validated by researchers and clinicians. Such validated criteria are very helpful in attracting pharmaceutical companies to work on these indications.[ii]

Regulatory Guidelines for AD

The FDA uses *de facto* guidelines for establishing that a drug has antidementia efficacy.[50] These require, in part, that: (1) clinical trials be double-blind and placebo-controlled; (2) patients fulfill generally accepted criteria for a primary dementia

---

[ii] See to Jones *et al.*, Developing new drugs for schizophrenia: From animals to the clinic, in Volume 1, Psychiatric Disorders, for a comprehensive discussion regarding government, academic and industry initiatives do define diagnostic criteria and methods of assessing cognitive impairments in schizophrenia, and development of animal models.

such as AD (e.g., DSM-IV-TR or NINCDS-ADRDA (National Institute of Neurological and communicative Disorders and Stroke-Alzheimer's Disease and Related Disorders Association) Work Group Criteria);[1] and (3) appropriate efficacy outcomes be used. Further, a putative antidementia drug must show efficacy at improving memory or retarding its deterioration since memory impairment is one of the primary features of dementia. The drug also must have an effect, determined independently from neuro-psychological assessment, using a global clinical measure or a measure of functional incapacity in order to address the concern that drug-related memory improvement may be observed with psychometric testing but not be clinically meaningful. Changes in behavior are considered to be of secondary importance for regulatory purposes (Table 2.6).

Most clinical trials of antidementia drugs undertaken in the United States to seek regulatory approval for mild to moderate AD have used the ADAS-cog as the index of cognitive change and a version of a CGIC as the "global" clinical measure.[48] Trials conducted in people with moderate and severe dementia have used other cognitive measures, such as the SIB and/or the ADCS-ADL Scale to assess aspects of daily functioning.[30,31]

Limitations of Current Guidelines

Limitations to the current guidelines include the lack of recognition of improvement in ADLs or behavior as legitimate therapeutic indications in the prescribing information, despite the fact that behavioral symptoms occur in the majority of dementia patients. The existing guidelines are also oriented toward shorter term trials to demonstrate symptomatic effects and not trials methods that might be used to demonstrate disease-modifying or preventative effects. The FDA draft guidelines criterion that patients fulfill established criteria for a primary dementia is an attempt to avoid the inclusion of ill-defined dementia syndromes in clinical trials, to obtain sample homogeneity, and to achieve consensus that the medication is effective in a specific group of patients with an illness such as AD accepted by a substantial number of experts.

De facto Guidelines for Other Dementia and Cognitive Impairment Syndromes

De facto guidelines for PDD exist because one drug, rivastigmine, is approved for the condition. The FDA-approved prescribing information essentially details the requirements in the clinical studies section of the label. In the case of PDD this essentially includes a clinical definition of PDD and cognitive and clinical efficacy demonstrated with the ADAS-cog and ADCS-CGIC in a 6-month long clinical trial as with AD.

It is important to consider that guidelines do not exist for drugs to treat AAMI, MCI, or for improving cognitive function in unimpaired individuals since there is insufficient agreement about the existence or recognition of these conditions. MCI has been a particular concern both because of the clinical heterogeneity as discussed above, but also because at least four MCI trials were undertaken by pharmaceutical sponsors in an effort to attain some form of regulatory approval or recognition. As it resulted, all the trials did not achieve their protocol-specified endpoints, mainly a delay in the onset of dementia or AD so the issue was moot.

Table 2.6 Guidelines on approval of antidementia drugs by regulatory authorities

---

EMEA, Europe (1997, http://www.emea.europa.eu/pdfs/human/ewp/05539en.pdf)
Based on the guidelines formulated by the FDA
May be applicable to dementias other than AD

Diagnosis, grading of severity and patient selection for trials discussed
- Diagnosis of dementia based on DSM, ICD or NINCDS/ADRDA criteria of probable AD considered most appropriate for testing drugs.

Efficacy assessment
- Concentrate on symptomatic improvement
- Cognitive, functional and global endpoints are key
- Statistically significant differences in two primary variables, one of which must be cognitive, followed by analysis of proportion who achieve a meaningful benefit
- For a claim in behavioral symptoms, a specific trial required with this as the primary endpoint
- In advanced disease, robust differences in functional and global endpoints (without cognition) may be sufficient.

Design issues
- Six months duration for efficacy
- One year for maintenance of efficacy
- Twelve-month open label for long-term safety, with at least 100 good-quality cases
- Appropriate follow-up to detect withdrawal phenomena (at least 2 months, mentioned in previous draft)
- Instruments not specified, though required to be valid and reliable.

FDA, US (www.fda.gov)
Advice provided in planning, design, conduct and interpretation of anti dementia trials with Investigational New Drug application.
Broadly similar to the EMEA guidelines.

Efficacy
- Statistically significant differences in two primary variables, one of which must be cognitive, and the other a global assessment or ADL (added with memantine approval in 2003)
- Global measure chosen is a clinical interview-based impression of change
- Cognitive instrument not specified, though the ADAS-cog is most commonly used.

Design issues
- Three months duration is sufficient
- Minimum of 1000 patients exposed for several weeks to relevant dose range
- Minimum of 300 patients exposed to doses above the median for 6 months to a year
- Maintenance of efficacy in chronic use or withdrawal, encouraged but, not essential.

(In effect, however, FDA guidelines and requirements change over time, and closely reflect the basis for the last drug to be approved.)

Notes: All regulatory authorities require evidence of quality, safety and efficacy based on laboratory, animal and human toxicology, and Phase I, II, and III human studies. Quality of life or economic evaluations are not currently required by regulatory authorities.
Adapted from [50].

If any of the trials had demonstrated safety and efficacy then the trials methods and results may have been included in the drug labeling. The indication, however, may not have changed from AD. FDA might have allowed reference to early or very mild AD because retrospectively about half of MCI patients had AD before the dementia and the endpoint of the studies was a delay in the onset of the dementia of AD, which is similar to a delay or attenuation in the signs and symptoms of AD. There would not have been an approved indication for MCI itself. The results from the NIH ADCS MCI trial with vitamin E and donepezil, although failing to achieve its primary outcome delaying onset of dementia, added a wrinkle to clinical interpretation by demonstrating cognitive effects for donepezil compared to placebo over the first 12–18 months of the trial that were no longer apparent over the last 12 months of the trial. This observation raised the possibility that the efficacy of donepezil very early in the course of AD may not be enduring and raised the question of when and for how long should donepezil be given during the course of AD.

Similarly, regulatory guidelines do not exist for treating the cognitive components of vascular dementia, DLB, or for cognitive impairment associated with schizophrenia or depression because of the lack of generally accepted diagnostic standards for these conditions. Not only did the cholinesterase inhibitors, memantine, and the xanthine derivative and phosphodiesterase inhibitor, propentofylline trials for vascular dementia not show significant effects on all their primary outcomes, but the diagnosis of vascular dementia was too heterogeneous to be recognized or described in the product labeling. Thus the conditions of use for vascular dementia could not be described.

Current Clinical Trials Designs

Current clinical trials designs for AD Phase IIb and III trials for symptomatic treatments are rather tightly defined and mainly limited to the confirmation of efficacy and safety alone. Specifically, inclusion criteria for Phase III trials are often as restricted as they are in Phase IIa; the same outcome instruments are often used in both Phase II and III, and study designs are very similar. Current inclusion/exclusion criteria tend to create a fairly homogeneous group of patients with AD of only mild to moderate severity, who are generally physically healthy, who usually do not have significant concomitant behavioral problems, and are living as outpatients with caregivers. Although these are not typical AD patients living in the community they are probably representative enough of the AD patients who would receive the drug if it were marketed.

Rather than exploring differing durations, these Phase III studies are of limited, fixed duration. Generally 6-month long clinical trials are offered to regulatory agencies as evidence of efficacy for symptomatic drugs; and the experiences of about 2000 patients, including those from Phases I and II are offered for evidence of safety, with about 100 followed for 1 year or more. Trials durations are becoming longer, however, with the introduction of putative disease-modifying drugs into clinical trials.

The primary outcome criteria among the Phase IIb and III trials tend to be similar: the ADAS-cog, CGIC, and an assessment of function, either the ADCS-ADL or the DAD. In addition to these outcomes, other supplementary outcomes may be added, including the MMSE, caregiver burden scales, behavior and mood assessments, instruments designed to capture service utilization and costs, health utilities, as well as other cognitive tests. The purpose of the primary outcome ratings is to fulfill FDA's and EMEA's criteria, that an effective drug for the symptoms of dementia must show both cognitive improvement and clinically meaningful change. EMEA goes further, and requires also the demonstration of change in ADLs for a medication to be considered effective in AD.[51,52] Thus the main areas in which Phase IIb and III trials tend to vary both within and among proprietary medication development programs are in the use of secondary outcome measures and sample sizes. There may be somewhat more dose-ranging in Phase II but many Phase III trials are dose-ranging as well.

The advent of drugs in development that are expected to be taken over the long term or to have direct effects on the pathological processes of AD have led to even Phase II trials being extended to 12 and 18 months in length. The trials are otherwise similar to the 6 months trials and tend to enroll patients with mild to moderate AD, use the ADAS-cog as the cognitive outcome and now the CDR as the global outcome. The rationale is that these newer drugs are not expected to have symptomatic effects but rather are expected to attenuate the cognitive and clinical decline expected over 18 months.

These trials are also characterized by the use of biomarkers in a subset of patients. The markers may include hippocampal volume estimates, cerebrospinal fluid (CSF) β-amyloid peptides, and tau and phospho-tau levels. The intent here is to demonstrate salutary changes in the markers correlating with the expected clinical changes.[iii]

The trials try to take advantage of the expected deteriorating clinical course of AD in the placebo patients, while hypothesizing that the test drug will maintain function or lessen deterioration. The methods presuppose that AD patients entered into trials decline more or less in parallel with each other, and do not dropout in excessive numbers. Inspection of available individual patient data shows that, although on average the placebo patients worsen by about 6–7 ADAS-cog points over 18 months, they do not so much worsen in parallel as a group but rather "fan out" or show great intra- and inter-subject variation with some not worsening at all, and others worsening considerably [unpublished observations].

The standard deviation around the 6- to 7-point change is about 6 or 7 points; thus about 30% of placebo-treated patients may not worsen over this time. Trial sponsors also hope that any significant clinical ratings at 18 months will be interpreted as long-term effects, and if supported by a salutary effect with biomarkers, might be further interpreted as the drugs exerting disease-modifying effects. The study designs of the current 18-month clinical trials, however, cannot distinguish between effects on AD symptoms and effects on progression of the underlying illness.

Descriptions of ongoing or recently completed 18-month long trials and their current status are listed in Table 2.7. Many of the drugs used thus far are already marketed, such as cholesterol-lowering drugs, vitamins and nutraceuticals. These trials were

---

[iii] For further discussion regarding the search for and use/limitations of biomarkers, see Lindner *et al.*, Development, optimization and use of preclinical behavioral models to maximize the productivity of drug discovery for Alzheimer's Disease, in this Volume; Tannock *et al.*, Towards a biological understanding of ADHD and the discovery of novel therapeutic approaches, in Volume 1, Psychiatric Disorders or Dourish *et al.*, Anti-obesity drugs: From animal models to clinical efficacy, in Volume 3, Reward Deficit Disorders, among others in the Series.

Table 2.7 18-month long placebo-controlled trials*

Trial Name/Drug/Sponsor/ Mechanism	Characteristics	Primary outcomes	Status
EFC 2724 and EFC 2946/ xaliproden/Sanofi-Aventis/ neurotrophic	N (both trials) ≈ 2761 Mild to moderate AD, may or may not be on ChI treatment One drug dose	ADASc, CDR, hippocampal atrophy (subset)	Completed October 2006 No significant effects in both trials; less atrophy in the EFC2724?
VITAL/B vitamins/NIH ADCS/ homocysteine lowering	N ≈ 409 Mild to moderate AD, may or may not be on ChI treatment	ADASc, CDR	Completed February 2007 No significant effects; (presented)
Tramiprosate/North American trial/Neurochem/amyloid fibrillogenesis inhibitor	N ≈ 1050 Mild to moderate AD	ADASc, CDR	Completed February 2007 No significant effects
Tramiprosate/European trial	N ≈ 930 Mild to moderate AD	ADASc, CDR	Discontinued November 2007
CLASP/simvastatin/NIH ADCS/ cholesterol lowering	N ≈ 400 Mild to moderate AD, may or may not be on ChI treatment	ADASc, CDR	Completed June 2007 No significant effects
LEADe/atorvastatin plus donepezil versus donepezil/ Pfizer/cholesterol lowering	N ≈ 641 Mild to moderate AD	ADASc, CDR	Completed July 2007 No significant effects
R-flurbiprofen (tarenflurbil)/ Myriad Pharma/US trial/ β-amyloid lowering agent	N ≈ 1684 Mild AD	ADASc, ADLs	Completed March 2008 No significant effects

(continued)

Table 2.7 (Continued)

Trial Name/Drug/Sponsor/Mechanism	Characteristics	Primary outcomes	Status
R-flurbiprofen/international trial	$N \approx 840$ Mild AD	ADASc, ADLs	Last patient to complete September 2008
DHA trial/docosahexaenoic acid/NIH ADCS with Martek Biosci/antioxidant, anti-β-amyloid	$N \approx 400$ Mild to moderate AD, may or may not be on ChI treatment	ADASc, CDR	Last patient to complete March 2009
Bapineuzumab (AAB-001)/Elan/β-amyloid antibody	$N \approx 240$ Mild to moderate AD Phase II trial	NTB, ADASc, ADLs	Completed Spring 2008 Primary efficacy endpoints not significant overall
Bapineuzumab (AAB-001)/Elan/β-amyloid antibody	N (four trials) ≈ 4000 total Separate trials with APOE4 and non-APOE4	NTB, ADASc, ADLs	Ongoing
PF 4494700 (TTP 488)/Pfizer with NIH ADCS support/RAGE inhibitor	$N \approx 400$	ADASc, CDR	Ongoing

N = sample size; NIH ADCS, NIH AD Cooperative Study; CDR, Clinical Dementia Rating scale; NTB, neuropsychological battery; RAGE, receptor for advanced glycation end products.
*Most allowed the concomitant use of cholinesterase inhibitors and often memantine. Adapted from[54].

started earlier than those for the drugs in development such as tramiprosate (homo-taurine, Alzhemed™),[iv] tarenflurbil (R-flurbiprofen, Flurizan™), and bapineuzumab, and thus served as *de facto* precedent for the proprietary drugs.

Thus far, none of the trials have shown efficacy or statistical significance. Many obtained biomarkers such as hippocampal and whole brain volumes by MRI and β-amyloid and tau from CSF from subsets of patients. Nevertheless, their designs represent the current predominant methodology for approaching AD drugs.

In sum, the designs of current regulatory trials of putative disease modifiers are not so much trials for disease modification as incrementally longer symptomatic trials, often enhanced with biomarkers such as CSF β-amyloid and tau proteins levels or brain volume changes taken from a subset of the trials sample. If any of the trials do show favorable statistical significance on their primary outcomes, then there will emerge issues involved in their interpretation, the most important of which is whether regulators will consider the results as demonstrating disease modification. This would mainly involve a discussion of the meaning of the biological markers or the particular statistical analysis used.

SECTION 2: RESEARCH DESIGN NEEDS AND CONTROVERSIES

The controversy over the currently approved cognitive enhancers results in large part because, by design, the clinical trials and development programs that were used as the basis for demonstrating their safety and efficacy and their subsequent approval, could not speak to pragmatic effectiveness, utility, or "worthwhileness" of the marketed drugs. The lack of trials data on effectiveness measures, health-related QoL, health economics, and individual patient outcomes contributed to the United Kingdom's National Institute for Health Care Excellence (NICE) to recommend against the use of memantine and against the use of cholinesterase inhibitors in mild and severe AD (in effect, in patients with MMSE scores greater than 20 or less than 10). Although the NICE guidance was based on cost-effectiveness modeling of Phase III clinical trials data and considerations, the difficulty in interpreting the clinical meanings of mean differences between drugs and placebos observed on the ADAS-cog, global, and ADL scales played a large part in informing the NICE's guidance. It should be noted, however, that regulators currently require evidence for clinical efficacy and do not require health economics assessments in order to approve AD drugs for marketing.

Most drugs in development failed in Phase II and III 3-month and 6-month trials using the ADAS-cog and a global scale as primary outcomes; and this high failure rate contributes to the controversy about effectiveness. The health economics and

---

[iv]Alzhemed™ (tramiprosate, homotaurine) has since failed to reach its primary endpoint, although its sponsor, Neurochem, Inc. claims that a reduction in hippocampal volume was noted (see biomarkers below) prompting an interest by this company to develop a prodrug of tramiprosate (NRM-8499) and to market tramiprosate as a "nutraceutical" http://72.232.136.18/~neurochem/PressReleases.php Neurochem Inc. (2007) We are Neurochem Quarterly Report Third Quarter ended September 30, 2007, Laval, Quebec, Canada. See also Hunter, Animal and translational models of neurological disorders: An industrial perspective, in this Volume.

effectiveness of marketed drugs is important for drugs in development to the extent that similar questions will be raised if these new drugs are marketed.

Diagnosis and Clarity of Therapeutic Conditions

In principle, any of a number of clinical conditions could be considered as a therapeutic claim. For dementia or cognitive impairment trials to proceed on a regulatory basis there needs to be more refined conceptualization of diagnosis and the clarity of the therapeutic conditions being treated. This discussion focuses on AD because it is an established clinical diagnostic target and therapeutic claim.

As noted, however, the actual clinical diagnosis of AD occurs late in the pathological processes of AD. Attempts to diagnose AD earlier before the dementia has manifested have been constrained by the greater difficulty in recognizing the clinical phenotype of the disease process earlier on. The concept of MCI is limited in that it does not identify or predict only AD. The concept of very early AD before the dementia, similar to MCI, is currently hard to define in such a way that it can be recognized with accuracy and may be difficult for general physicians to recognize.

Other cognitive impairment diagnoses related to AD also obscure the clinical picture and provide both barriers and opportunity for drug development. For example, AD coexists with cerebrovascular disease. The coexistent cerebrovascular disease might involve large or small vessel disease and ischemic or hemorrhagic pathology. Moreover, the ischemia may be mainly subcortical or periventricular, leading to differing clinical expression more similar to AD than to stroke syndromes. The uncertainties involved in diagnosing various cerebrovascular cognitive impairment conditions, difficulties are only multiplied when including AD.

In sum there is a need to be able to recognize very mild AD, and mixed AD and vascular cognitive impairment. There is a need to develop cognitive enhancers for other cognitive impairment conditions as well, especially when the science and drug mechanisms suggest it.

Sample Selection

Sample selections for AD clinical trials have been problematic. Although they have evolved somewhat over the years they remain samples of convenience in which available patients who fulfill nominal criteria for probable AD or Dementia of the Alzheimer's type[1,2] are recruited. These trials, whether Phase II or III, generally require the patients be relatively free of concomitant medical illnesses or that they at least show stable medical illnesses that do not themselves impair cognition, and that they live as outpatients usually in family settings. There is often an age limitation to preclude the youngest or the oldest from participating.

Early in the development of cholinesterase inhibitors, patients were not allowed to be on drugs that might be cognitive enhancing or impairing. After cholinesterase inhibitors established themselves in the market, and after expert committees declared their prescriptions to be standards of practice[55,56] patients have been included in trials of some drugs while either being maintained on the cholinesterase inhibitor or only after having been exposed to a cholinesterase inhibitor and deciding not to continue medication. The allowance of patients into trials who were on cholines-terase inhibitors is as much a pragmatic consideration as a design feature. It is much harder to recruit patients into North American and European trials if concomitant cholinesterase inhibitor use is precluded. It was also framed as an ethical issue in that depriving study patients of a marketed treatment would be harmful to them. On the other hand, there are probably substantial clinical differences between research participants maintained on cholinesterase inhibitors and those not taking them.

The NMDA receptor antagonist memantine (Ebixa®/Axura®/Namenda®) was approved for US marketing based on one pivotal study that required patients with moderate to severe AD to have been maintained on donepezil for at least 6 months before being randomized to memantine or placebo.[57] The FDA rightly interpreted the results of the trial as demonstrating the effects of memantine compared to placebo since that was the only randomized intervention. Some consumers and advocates however incorrectly interpreted the results as that the effect of memantine and donepezil combined was superior to donepezil alone.

This interpretation allowed for easier marketing of the medications as "combination" treatment when no such evidence existed. The fact that a similar placebo-controlled memantine trial in mild to moderate AD also requiring cholinesterase inhibitor background therapy did not show efficacy evidence did not dissuade a prevalent use of memantine in mild to moderate AD.

Difficulties in interpreting such add-on or augmentation trials (as compared to combination trials which would require factorial or Latin square clinical trials designs) are whether or not the drug being "added on" to, for example, donepezil, was having any therapeutic effect at all, or for that matter possibly having a counter-therapeutic effect. The average length of donepezil treatment prior to randomization in the moderate to severe memantine trial was 2¼ years, and the memantine-placebo group continued to deteriorate at a rapid rate. Since no trial has demonstrated the effectiveness of donepezil for more than 2 years, and that trial was rather controversial,[58] it is questionable whether the drug was having a therapeutic effect and it is not known whether the effect of memantine required the background of donepezil. However, one memantine trial, MD-12, thus far unpublished, in mild to moderate AD allowed background treatment with cholinesterase inhibitors and did not show significant effects (http://www.forestclinicaltrials.com/CTR/CTRController/CTRViewPdf?_file_id=scsr/ SCSR_MEM-MD-12_final.pdf).

To a large extent this question was resolved with memantine in particular, in that one pivotal trial in patients who had not received cholinesterase inhibitors showed memantine to be effective.[59] Thus, it was these two trials together that provided the basis for the FDA's approval of memantine. Currently, there are development programs of investigational drugs based mainly on patients who are continuing to take cholinesterase inhibitors and memantine. The implications of this "add-on" approach for drug approval and labeling have yet to be addressed.

Notably, and perhaps as an example of a sliding scale of regulatory standards and politics, memantine received EU marketing approval for moderately severe to severe AD on the basis of the latter monotherapy trial[59] and a smaller and shorter 12-week trial of patients with both AD and vascular dementia performed in mainly nursing homes in Latvia and that did not use a cognitive outcome.[60] Later, EMEA expanded memantine's indication to moderate to severe AD on the basis of a meta-analysis that included two additional moderate to severe AD trials (one of which was not statistically significant) and subsets of three mild to moderate AD trials, two of which were not statistically significant on their primary and secondary outcomes (http://www. emea.europa.eu/humandocs/PDFs/EPAR/axura/Axura-H-378–II-11–SD.pdf).

Other aspects of sample selection include the requirement that patients be cooperative and able to perform the cognitive outcomes, that psychotropic medications are allowed to various extents, and that there be an active caregiver to provide information. In the United States many AD patients live alone, perhaps with relatives or neighbors looking in occasionally, and such patients would not be candidates for trials. The substantial majority of patients with AD develop behavioral disorders and symptoms such as aggression, delusions, depression, significant irritability or apathy, and non-specific agitation. Many are precluded from studies of cognitive enhancers by protocol design or because they cannot participate in the outcomes testing. Many others have been treated with antipsychotics and antidepressants, can participate in testing, and are often included in clinical trials in North America and Europe. In many Phase II and III trials a quarter to a half of patients are maintained on psychotropics, but the effects of these medications on response to the cognitive enhancer have not been determined. Thus, in current and future trials patients may be receiving cholinesterase inhibitors, memantine, antipsychotics and antidepressants in various combinations as they are randomized to the study drug or placebo. This poses unresolved issues to the extent that concomitant medications may affect outcomes.

Over the years, the severity bounds for inclusion into trials have changed somewhat. Early in the development of symptomatic drugs, patients were chosen to be in a mild to moderate AD severity range based on MMSE scores between approximately 10 and 26 or some subset within that range. Because it was recognized that some patients with more severe dementia might not be able to perform the main cognitive outcome, the ADAS-cog, the lower severity limit was sometimes raised to 12. When it was recognized that patients who were more mildly impaired may not worsen cognitively as much as patients who were more moderately impaired on the ADAS-cog, inclusion criteria for mild AD was constrained to top MMSE scores of 23–24 rather than 26. In the current 18-month trials there has been a further limiting of the more moderate AD range to MMSE scores of 14–20 as many of the trials try to balance the lesser cognitive worsening in mild AD with a longer trials length and to take into consideration the metrical characteristics of the ADAS-cog. Thus, in many respects inclusion criteria have been shaped to fit the expected characteristics of the outcome instruments and their sensitivity to measuring change over the length of the trials.

Genotyping and Biomarkers for Sample Selection

APOE4 genotyping has been used for sample selection and stratification in recent trials. Biomarkers such as β-amyloid peptides, tau protein, and hippocampal volumes have been suggested as potential selection factors and stratification factors.[5]

In the case of genotyping, APOE alleles have been used prospectively in rosiglitazone (Avandia®) trials as a stratification factor for a hypothesis of a differential response to treatment based on the presence or not of an APOE4 allele (unpublished).

Elan Pharmaceuticals launched a Phase III trials program of bapineuzumab, a β-amyloid antibody that included separate trials for APOE4 patients and patients who did not have the APOE4 allele, apparently expecting differential efficacy and adverse events by genetic variant (www.clinicaltrials.gov).

Because of observations that patients with relatively smaller hippocampal volumes who have early or mild AD deteriorate cognitively more rapidly, suggestions have been made to enrich sample selection in Phase II and III trials by considering inclusion of only patients with relatively smaller hippocampal volumes. Similar suggestions have been made with respect to CSF β-amyloid protein and tau levels based on the hypotheses that patients with the relevant biological markers will more likely have AD.

Despite these observations, hippocampal, other brain volumes and APOE genotype did not predict onset of AD to a greater or additional extent than did the baseline cognitive test scores in a retrospective analysis of an MCI trial.[88] Caution in the broad or premature use of such markers is advised.

Stratification by genotyping or biomarker levels, however, opens the possibility of limited claims for marketing approval based not only on the presence and severity of AD but also on a genetic variant or biological characteristic that might influence course of illness or drug response. Stratification or sample enrichment by biomarkers is additionally complex because the genetic variants might influence clinical state and the biomarkers may be indexing a level of disease severity rather than a trait characteristic.

Clinically Relevant and Stage-Specific Outcomes

Traditionally, outcomes in AD trials include cognitive, global, and functional outcomes as described above, the triad having been largely encouraged by regulatory guidance for Phase II and III trials and reinforced by expert opinion. These broad clinical outcomes however are lacking in a number of ways.

In Phase II broader outcomes are less important compared to the need to demonstrate that the experimental drugs have the cognitive effects that they are expected to have. Change on a cognitive test may represent both a pharmacodynamic measure of a cognitive enhancer's or disease modifier's effect and a clinical outcome, but still may not easily translate into a clinically meaningful effect. In Phase III and IV trials, however, broader outcomes are more important as they facilitate and allow further description of overall clinical effects. These outcomes include less sensitive cognitive tests such as the ADAS-cog or NTI, ADLs, global assessments, health-related QoL, other QoL assessments, resource use, and utilities, mood and pain scales, and on the caregiver's side, caregiver time, burden, stress.

Depending on the course or severity of a particular dementia syndrome, expectations of response in symptoms would be expected to vary. Clinically relevant outcomes need to be stage or severity specific. A one size fits all cognitive outcomes or general overall global outcome may not suffice. For example, patients with mild or very mild dementia may show very little or no impairments in most ADL or in QoL ratings scales. Moreover, by definition, their cognitive impairment is relatively mild; there may be little room for improvement on the ratings. A CGIC also may not be as clinically relevant as presumed, and depending on the severity of the cognitive impairment, the amount of kind of change observed, the skill and experience of the person doing the ratings, and what that person values, the assessment of CGIC change can vary markedly (see below).

Nevertheless, the small amount of improvement that could be shown with an effective drug in very early AD should not be overlooked or under-appreciated. By comparison, people with more moderate to severe dementia might show rather large, at least statistically large, improvements on cognitive rating scales. However, these larger statistical improvements should not be overvalued as they may not be indicating a substantial clinical difference.

One reason for inconsistent outcomes in mild to moderate AD trials may be because the outcomes are particularly sensitive to one strata of severity or another. For example, the ADAS-cog is relatively insensitive to change in more mild AD. In part this may be because of the lack of a delayed recall, working memory, or executive function component and to a testing-interval period of only 6 months that may be too short to detect clinical progression of mild AD. Moreover, it may be harder to appreciate global clinical change in patients with very mild AD; ADL scales may emphasize impairments that occur farther along in the Alzheimer's dementia process than are of interest in mild AD. Given the relatively slow rates of cognitive and functional decline in AD clinically relevant measures may be less sensitive to change over short periods of time. Neuropsychological and other outcomes need to be customized for patients based on severity of illness.

Examples of customizing cognitive measures include a battery of tests used in an MCI trial[28] and a grouping of cognitive scales called the "Neuropsychological Test Battery (NTB)," an attempt to develop an assessment battery sensitive to both early, mild AD and more moderate AD.[61] The latter consists of nine components: Wechsler Memory Scale (WMS) visual immediate, WMS verbal immediate, Rey Auditory Verbal Learning Test (RAVLT) immediate, WMS Digit Span, Controlled Word Association Test (COWAT), Category Fluency Test (CFT), WMS visual delayed, WMS verbal delayed, and RAVLT delayed. A z-score is calculated for each component based on the sample means and standard deviations, and then they are averaged to obtain an overall composite score. In addition composite executive function, immediate and delayed memory scores can be calculated. This battery is an example of using "off the shelf" established neuropsychological scales combined in such a way as to take advantage of the known cognitive deficits in mild to moderate AD in an effort to assess a drug effect. Based on one trial the composite z-score was shown to be more sensitive to change in mild AD than the ADAS-cog, but about the same as the ADAS-cog in moderate AD.[61]

Time to Event Trials ("Survival Trials")

Initially implemented in a trial comparing selegiline (Eldepryl®) to vitamin E in moderate to severely impaired AD patients,[62] this methodology was employed in two donepezil trials, and most recently and broadly in MCI trials of several marketed cholinesterase inhibitors.[63-66] In the first trial, the "event" was a composite of time to nursing home placement, a sharply lower ADL score, a change in CDR score, or death. The MCI trials used the Petersen or Mayo Clinic criteria for MCI for trial entry and time to diagnosis of AD and dementia as the event. As mentioned above, each trial operationalized MCI criteria slightly differently and had differing incidences of MCI in the placebo group. Survival trial designs also characterize prevention trials methodology as discussed below.

Time to endpoint studies or survival analyses are parallel group trials that are considered by some[67] to support a claim for disease modification on the basis that the intervention would delay the onset of the illness. However, a significant outcome in such a trial can just as easily be interpreted as symptomatic and as not providing information on any effect on the underlying pathophysiology, especially when the endpoint of "diagnosis of dementia" rests on a continuum and no information is obtained on symptoms prior to the endpoint or clinical course afterword.

In considering endpoints for cognitive impairment survival studies, the appropriateness of the milestone needs to be considered. In the prototypical trial above,[62] the endpoint was a composite of four markers – death, institutionalization, loss of ability to perform ADLs, or a worsening of one level on the CDR. On further consideration, none of these endpoints are intimately related with a neurodegenerative process. Death is not a direct consequence of the illness, and moreover, other milestones in the progression of cognitive impairment can be reached before death. Institutionalization or nursing home placement, the timing of which is determined by multiple medical, social, psychological, cultural, and economic factors, is not a reasonable index for illness progression, although it may be a useful health-economics and QoL index for Phase IV studies. Using cutting scores for loss of ability to perform ADLs may be useful but may not have an advantage over assessing outcomes as a continuum across ordinal ADL scale. Certain measures of dementia severity such as the CDR, which itself are composite measures are highly dependent on cognitive change alone. In prevention trials or MCI trials, deciding on the time to make the dementia diagnosis is subject to considerable judgment and could vary greatly.

It may not matter as much if a drug delays an AD diagnosis if the course of illness before diagnosis or afterward is no different than with non-treatment, or if the course of AD after the delayed diagnosis is more rapid than with no treatment. Another difficulty with these ratings as endpoints in survival trials, involve how close patients may be to the endpoint before entry into a trial. Finally, confounding variables play a larger role than with focused outcomes such as cognitive change alone.

Current Issues in Phase II and III Symptomatic Trials

Past and current AD Phase II and III trials for symptomatic benefit are rather tightly defined and tend to be limited to the confirmation of efficacy and potential safety. Both Phase II and III trials may include additional measures such as economics or QoL but they tend not to explore various conditions of efficacy. Inclusion criteria for Phase III trials are often as limited as they are in Phase II; the same outcome instruments are used, and study designs are very similar.

The main areas in which Phase II and III studies tend to vary both within and among proprietary medication development programs are in sample size, dose-ranging groups, and the use of secondary outcome measures. These assessments include a selection of additional functional or daily activities scales, QoL scales, behavioral rating scales, caregiver symptoms or burden scales, or scales purporting to measure health services use or pharmacoeconomic outcomes. When the Phase II and III clinical trials designs of the various cholinergic medications under development are compared, it is the range of drug dosage and the choice of secondary outcome scales that tend to differentiate their designs.

Obvious concerns in designing Phase II and III clinical trials are that excessive variability in the characteristics of patients selected for trials may mask potential drug effects, patients might be included who do not have AD, and extensive medical comorbidity or concomitant medications may complicate the clinical presentation or affect outcome. Sponsors of clinical trials have attempted to reduce the clinical heterogeneity by using relatively restrictive selection criteria for patients entering them to greater or lesser extents. But given that dementia is a diagnosis based on clinical phenotypes such attempts will likely not reduce heterogeneity.

Phase IIa Trials

Recent and current Phase IIa trials have tended to be small versions of later Phase IIb or III trials. Selection criteria tend to be for mild to moderate AD patients without significant physical problems, and essentially identical with patients who will later be enrolled in Phase III. The trials tend to use a broader dosage range of typically two or three doses, and fewer patients per group than Phase III trials. With drugs expected to act more symptomatically they have tended to be 12 weeks in duration. Yet, outcomes scales have been similar to Phase III, typically using the ADAS-cog as the primary outcome. Twelve-week and shorter Phase IIa trials were characteristic of the cholinesterase inhibitors, and are currently used with some current symptomatic drugs such as those active on nicotinic receptor subtypes or serotonin receptor subtypes.

More recently, the essentially same short-term trial design using 2–3 doses and placebo has been employed as a proof of concept trial for disease-modifying drugs such as γ-secretase inhibitors or other putative β-amyloid lowering drugs. These Phase IIa studies, although also assessing cognition either with an ADAS-cog or with other cognitive assessments, have focused more on pharmacokinetics and pharmacodynamics in that outcomes involve drug penetration into the CSF and a change in CSF or blood putative biomarkers, such as β-amyloid$_{40}$ and β-amyloid$_{42}$.

A recent change in Phase IIa has been 12- and 18-month long placebo-controlled dose-ranging trials that use typical Phase III outcomes. The main distinction between these Phase IIa trials and the subsequent pivotal trials largely reduce to smaller sample sizes, somewhat different and more liberal hypothesis testing, exploratory subgroup analyses, and the obtaining of frequent blood levels and biomarkers in the Phase II trials.

The obvious issues with current Phase IIa trials are that they are not sensitive to subtle changes, that their designs may not be appropriate for disease-modifying studies, they do not explore a full dosing range and that they are profoundly underpowered with respect to the expected therapeutic effect of the drug if it were to be marketed. Any reliance on biomarkers or markers thought to be the equivalent of surrogate markers will likely to be misleading. Rather than focus on obtaining the kind of clinical efficacy signal expected in standard Phase III trials, Phase II trials can be improved substantially by assessing whether the drug in development has the expected pharmacokinetic and pharmacodynamic characteristics predicted from preclinical research, and the judicious use of cognitive tests similar to those used in preclinical development of the drug. For drugs with effects that occur fairly soon after administration, repeated measures designs and crossover designs should be considered as ways of gaining more precise outcomes in Phase IIa.

The practical consequence is that otherwise effective drugs are not recognized as effective, and some ineffective drugs are incorrectly identified as potentially effective because of an underpowered study.

Interpretation of Phase III Trials

Some symptomatic trials have been extended to 12-month durations in an effort to better take advantage of the expected decline of placebo-treated patients and to provide evidence of longer durations of treatment effects. Interpretation and generalization of outcomes from 6- to 12-month symptomatic trials have been controversial as well. The trials are intended to take advantage of an expected cognitive worsening of the placebo group and thus the drug effect is an offset of the progression. If the placebo group should fail to progress then the likelihood of determining a clinical effect diminishes. In clinical trials placebo-treated patients decline cognitively at less than half the rate reported in clinic-based populations (e.g., approximately ½ to 3 MMSE points per year, and approximately 4 ADAS-cog points per year compared to 3-4, and 7-8 points per year, respectively reported in clinics. Some subgroups such as those with delusions, extrapyramidal signs may comprise 10-30% of the AD population and have a different natural history from other patients, possibly deteriorating more rapidly than others. Thus, as represented in Figure 2.1, placebo treatment perhaps as a result of the selection criteria may be destined to have better outcomes than those ordinary patients in ordinary clinical practice.

The interpretation of the effect becomes an issue as it is comprised of some degree of cognitive improvement in some patients and worsening in others over time. This difference, "a" in the figure is one expression of the effect, a mean difference in performance scores at any given time point. Another expression is a potential time

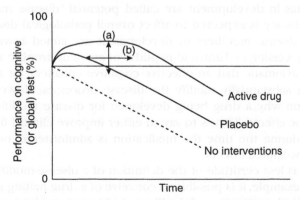

Figure 2.1 Diagram of symptomatic effects in a clinical trial showing that the slopes of placebo, intervention, and active drug are the same after time (*x*). (a) magnitude of maximum improvement from baseline with respect to placebo, (b) delay of symptomatic decline. Other measures of the effect could be the proportion improving by a given level of performance on a cognitive (or global) test. From.[68,69]

effect, "b," the time delay or lag for the mean drug effect to reach a previous mean performance score for a given placebo point. This latter metric has been interpreted by some as an index of delay in *clinical* progression, and sometimes mis-interpreted as disease-modifying effects.

One compensation in these trials designs has been to increase the duration and sample sizes of the trials. This in turn requires an increase in the number of sites and countries involved in trials such that some current 12- to 18-month long trials include over 100 to 200 sites and 1000 to 1600 patients (see below).

There are pragmatic limits to this however, notwithstanding the considerable issue of accounting for dropouts and missing values, at some point the rate of decline of the active drug group will be greater than that of placebo as the placebo group approaches the floor of the outcomes measures used or the drug looses effect and there will be no difference between the groups. During the time that the rates of decline are equal a clinical consideration is whether or not the delay in time is long enough to be clinically meaningful.

Disease-Modification Trials

The terms "disease-modifying" and "slowing progression" of cognitive impairment sometimes are used interchangeably. It is useful, however, to consider that slowing progression mainly describes the apparent slowing of the progression of clinical symptoms and the expression of illness while "disease-modifying" implies an effect on the underlying pathophysiological processes of the illness. A symptomatic drug such as a cholinesterase inhibitor could be considered to slow progression of illness, at least over a limited time.

Advances in understanding of the pathogenesis of the illness leads to new therapeutic strategies intended for disease modification that would also slow the progression of AD are in development. These advances provide a means to develop and test medications that are intended to target-specific mechanisms involved in neuronal death. Many drugs in development are called potential "disease modifiers" because their potential efficacy is expected to affect overall pathological disease progression. Currently, most disease modifiers in development are aimed toward affecting the production or processing of β-amyloid peptides or are neurotrophic agents.

It should be axiomatic that an effective cognitive enhancer for a neurodegenerative illness must substantially modify the disease processes. However, in principle, there is no reason why a drug being developed for disease modification could not have symptomatic effects. That is to say, to either improve clinical function or lessen clinical decline during the time the medication is administered, or otherwise have temporary or time-limited effects.

Indeed there is less certitude of the definition of a disease-modifying drug than it might seem. For example, it is possible to conceive of a drug halting neuronal loss and thus slowing clinical progression of the illness and symptoms for a period of time, but then this effect is lost with the disease process continuing. The longer the delay in progression caused by the drug, the easier it is to consider the medication a disease modifier; but the shorter the delay in progression, the more the drug's efficacy will have the characteristics of a symptomatic medication.

There is an intimate relationship between the advancing knowledge of the illness and the potential drugs in development that can be thought of as disease modifiers. As knowledge progresses drug targets increases and each can be considered potentially disease-modifying. Thus, it may be difficult to define a disease-modifying drug in the absence of a particular drug that has already been proven to be clinically efficacious.

Both disease-modifying and symptomatic drugs could have greater or lesser efficacy on cognitive function depending on the stage of the illness in which it is used. Moreover, the differing magnitudes of efficacy in different stages may appear paradoxical, in part, because of the disease processes and in part because of the characteristics of the outcome scales used. For example, a drug that clearly would work best as a disease modifier early in the course of AD, before the dementia, might have very small or clinically undetectable effects in the early stages of illness because disease progression is slow and the outcome scales insensitive to small changes; but when given in a more moderate stage of illness after the onset of dementia, the measurable clinical effects would appear to be larger because clinical progression is more rapid and the scales more sensitive.

There is an underlying assumption that the loss of cognitive function is causally related to neuronal changes, including cell death. One overarching hope for anti-amyloid strategies such as amyloid vaccines, antibodies, or "plaque busters" is that a dementia patient will regain cognitive function and stabilize further worsening. A disease-modifying drug, however, may indeed be efficacious in halting further degeneration or cleaning up cellular debris and not show any parallel effect on cognition.

Although it might be desired to use a disease modifier early in the course of illness or as a preventative measure, this might prove an unsuccessful strategy. The earlier into the course of illness one goes, the more obscure the diagnosis of that illness, the more heterogeneous and less impaired the target population is, the slower the clinical progression, the longer the trials have to be, and the safer the drug must be. Thus, using current ratings and outcomes trials would have to be longer and cognitive effects harder to discern. Another consideration is that any potential benefit of a disease-modifying drug given before the onset of dementia also would be offset by the risk of the drug in terms of adverse events during this pre-clinical or mild early phase of the illness.

Given the *caveats* discussed above, two clinical trials designs have been suggested for empirically demonstrating disease modification.[68-71] One is a randomized withdrawal design and the other a randomized start design.

In a randomized withdrawal design, patients are randomized to medication or placebo for the first part of the trial to establish the efficacy of treatment (Figure 2.2). In the next period, patients who had been randomly assigned to medication then receive double-blind placebo and the placebo patients continue on double-blind placebo. It is observed whether the formerly medicated patients (who must have improved relative to placebo-treated patients in the first period) continue to maintain their improvement compared to the ongoing placebo group, or whether their improvement during the first period regresses towards the placebo group. In the former case, an interpretation of disease modification might be made and in the latter case, a symptomatic effect is interpreted.

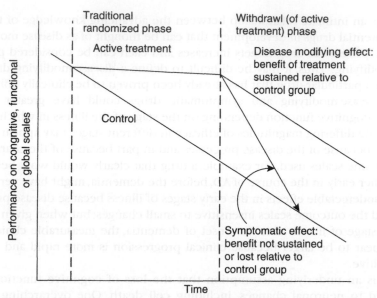

Figure 2.2   Diagram of a randomized withdrawal design. Subjects are randomized to active drug or placebo in the first Phase. During the second Phase (dotted vertical line) they are placed on placebo in the randomized withdrawal design. Benefits attributable to the active drug in the first Phase are maintained in the second Phase (the lines remain apart) if the drug modifies the underlying disease but not if the effect is symptomatic. Adapted from [68–70].

The randomized delayed start design requires first randomizing patients to drug or placebo in a parallel group fashion in order to demonstrate the efficacy of the drug as in the randomized withdrawal design (Figure 2.3). Then, in the second period, patients who originally received placebo receive double-blindly the active drug. If there is improvement in the placebo group towards the continuing active drug group, then that would be interpreted as a symptomatic effect, whereas if the originally randomized placebo group does not catch up with the originally active drug, if the effect seems parallel with the treated group, then it is considered that the active drug has a disease-modifying effect.

Despite their conceptual clarity, both trials designs would be very difficult to carry out in practice. Sample sizes would have to be large in order to both enhance the likelihood of efficacy in the first phase and to compensate for dropouts. There would have to be a sufficiently long duration of observation, an appropriate outcome rating, and methods for controlling dropouts would need to be addressed as dropouts may be most likely early in the trials and after initiating active medication.

An *ad hoc* European group under the auspices of the European AD Consortium (EADC) considered the potential for disease-modifying trials and recommended the following: (1) that patients with early, mild, or moderate AD would be appropriate for disease-modifying trials and not patients with MCI; (2) that disease modification is a long-term effect and trials necessarily should be parallel grouped and placebo controlled; and (3) that 18-month trial durations was the appropriate tradeoff between

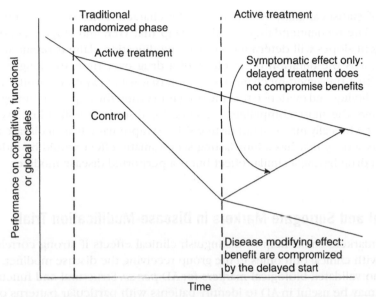

Figure 2.3 Diagram of a randomized delayed start design. Subjects are randomized to active drug or placebo in the first Phase. During the second Phase (second dotted line) subjects are placed on active drug in the randomized start design. Benefits attributable to the active drug in the first Phase are maintained in the second Phase (the lines remain apart) if the drug modifies the underlying disease but not if the effect is symptomatic. Adapted from [68–70].

allowing sufficient time for a clinical effect and to minimize threats to the validity of the trial due to high dropouts or economic costs.[68]

This group was vague and arbitrary on the outcomes to be used, hence reflecting the state of the field. They recommended that a "clinically relevant" endpoint should be defined at the beginning, without stating what it should be. They felt that such clinically relevant endpoints should involve multiple domains as discussed above and that composite measures of outcome might be appropriate. Rather surprisingly, they stated that the as yet unspecified outcome should show a reduction in the rate of progression from 30% to 50% with the active drug compared to placebo. More work needs to be done here to develop such a measure if this is thought desirable.

Other recommendations from this group include the use of statistical analyses that might address whether the clinical course over 18 months is different between the drug and placebo groups. These analyses might therefore include the use of generalized estimating equations (GEE) and slope analyses in which the differing slopes of decline of patients on medication or placebo are compared. Such approaches may be limited, however, not only by the heterogeneity of decline among patients entered into the trial, but also by practical clinical trials factors such as frequency of the measurement of the outcome, dropouts, the need to impute missing values, and the linearity of the changes in the outcome scales. Moreover, in such studies, the scales that have been used were designed to show symptomatic effects and are not different.

The difficulty with setting standards is that the issues with many recommendations are not fully worked through prior to the making the recommendations. For example, methods of statistical analysis depend on the characteristics of the sample and the outcomes. The recommendations of this group that GEE and slope analysis be used and divergent slopes will determine a disease-modification claim is premature.

In sum, it is the duration of an effect of a drug over time, the longer the better, coupled with a presumed mechanism of action that some experts consider potentially disease-modifying, and evidence that the drug is exerting the expected biological effect, that becomes the most compelling evidence for disease modification, even though such a trial technically may still not distinguish a symptomatic from a disease-modifying effect. Thus, a drug that has a long-lasting symptomatic effect would be indistinguishable from a drug having a similar effect but is a purported disease modifier.

Biological and Surrogate Markers in Disease-Modification Trials

Biological markers could help to distinguish clinical effects if strong correlations are observed with clinical outcomes in the group receiving the disease modifier. Currently, there are no validated biological markers for AD *per se*. Structural and functional neuroimaging may be useful in AD to identify patients with particular patterns of cerebral atrophy, glucose metabolism, β-amyloid peptide deposition, and brain volumes.

It is important to distinguish biological markers and surrogate markers. The former are assessments that are meant to reflect the presence, severity, or activity of a disease. A number of biomarkers are being investigated in AD and dementia. These include volumetric MRI, glucose uptake positron emission tomography scanning (PET), specific PET ligands, as well as blood and CSF measurements relating to elements of oxidation, tau proteins, and amyloid metabolism. Biomarkers to greater or lesser extents relate to the disease such that there is a difference in biomarker measurements between the people who have the illness and people who do not. A biomarker might also be an indication of severity of the pathology of the disease.

Thus in this context, relatively small hippocampal volumes are associated with AD, correlate with severity of cognitive impairment, and predict clinical progression of cognitive impairment. Pittsburgh imaging compound (PIB) is a ligand to β-amyloid peptide that indexes plaque density and thus one aspect of β-amyloid pathology in AD. However, it may not be a robust indicator of clinical progression of the illness as plaque density does not strongly correlate with severity of cognitive impairment.

A surrogate marker is different from a biomarker in that the former is meant to be a stand-in (i.e., a surrogate) for a clinical effect or primary outcome in a trial.[72] A surrogate marker has the properties of a "test" and in principle could be used in clinical trials in place of the primary clinical outcome. Thus, a surrogate marker is useful to the extent that it fully predicts and is more efficient than the outcome it is replacing. In this case a validated surrogate marker needs to be easier to use, more efficient, or "better" than the cognitive test it is replacing.

A surrogate marker does not have to be fully validated and fully replace a primary clinical outcome, however. The 1997 FDA Modernization Act[73] allows a drug to be approved for marketing if the drug has an effect on a surrogate marker that is reasonably likely to predict clinical benefit. Operationalizing "reasonably likely to predict" becomes a challenge, however.

Surrogate markers become important in the development of drugs that might have an effect on disease progression. A drug that may have an effect on a proposed surrogate marker or even an actual direct effect on the underlying pathology of the disease, but does not show clinical effects, is a drug that does not have an effect on a surrogate marker (but does have an effect on a biological marker). Whereas a biological marker may be only correlationally linked and related to the pathology, there has to be a clinicopathologic understanding of the relationship between the surrogate marker and the clinical outcome.

It has also been considered that the effect of a drug on a surrogate marker in the presence of a clinical effect should be taken as evidence that a drug is disease-modifying. From a practical point of view, this suggests that a surrogate marker should only be used when it is impractical to assess the clinical outcome. One attraction of a potential surrogate marker for dementia is that it is perceived as more precise, easier, or more straightforward to obtain. Thus, for example, an assay of a surrogate marker in CSF would be perceived as more desirable than cognitive testing. This example illustrates how the development and use of surrogate markers in neurodegenerative disease is so difficult.

In order to use a biomarker in clinical trials as the evidence for disease modification, the biomarker would have to be strongly linked both to the pathophysiologic progression of the illness and to the expected clinical outcome. Under these considerations, it would have to be assessed how strongly the biomarker predicts clinical outcomes, and it would need to be shown that the drug both affects the biological marker as well as the underlying pathology of the illness. Moreover, the effect of the drug on the marker needs to be interpreted as clinically meaningful and strongly linked to a clinical outcome.

Statistical Considerations

Statistical approaches to the evaluation of treatments intended to slow a gradual decline in patients with AD are complex. The use of slope analyses or GEE as primary analytic methods for regulatory agency recommended outcomes such as the ADAS-cog or the CDR has certain limitations. First, sponsors argue that slope analysis will allow the inference of a disease-modifying effect of a drug if the slopes of the rate of change of the outcomes are significantly divergent.

Issues here, however, involve the fact that rates of change on the ADAS-cog and other instruments may not be linear in AD, that outcomes from dropouts or non-compliers are not missing completely at random, and slope analysis depends in large part on the number and intervals of the repeated measurements of the outcome used to estimate the slope. The extent to which a decline in the ADAS-cog may be linear also may depend on the severity of patients at baseline.

Some forms of an adaptive trial design might be considered in very long trials that use slope analysis if it emerges that the rate of decline is less than expected. Such an adaptive design may allow for the inclusion of additional patients or patients who are more or less severe than those originally intended to be in the study. The study designs of the current 18-month clinical trials cannot distinguish between effects on AD symptoms from effect on progression of the underlying illness even if a GEE or slope analysis shows divergence.

Prevention Trials

Prevention trials[74,75] can be divided into primary and secondary prevention trials. Primary prevention trials would use subjects who do not have the illness. Secondary prevention trials would include patients with early signs and symptoms of cognitive impairment or AD and before diagnosis, but who still do not have the illness. The border area of trials between primary and secondary prevention is the planned inclusion of patients who do not have signs but may have one or several risk factors for AD and questionable or non-specific symptoms such as memory complaints.

In effect sample selection for these trials are enriched samples, primary prevention trials and are intended to increase the expected rate of onset of AD in the trials and thus decrease the sample sizes required. Examples of such "at risk" factors include older age, family history of AD, APOE4 genotype, cardiovascular disease, and memory complaints.

Part of the rationale for prevention trials is that drugs might have particular therapeutic actions during a critical preclinical period of AD, i.e., during the early development of AD brain pathology, that they would not exert after the illness manifested itself. Prevention trials, with or without enrichment, however, require relatively large sample sizes, ranging between 2500 and 20,000 when the outcome is dementia because the incidences of cognitive worsening or dementia onset are fairly low in these groups. Moreover, sample sizes for prevention trials are generally based on the expectations for incidence of dementia in the overall population. Yet, individuals who volunteer for clinical studies are likely to be healthier than the general population and may be less likely to develop dementia.

Two prevention trials, that of naproxen (Naprelan®/Naprosyn®) and celecoxib (Celebrex®) and of hormone replacement therapy, that used time to onset of AD or MCI as endpoints yielded significant outcomes, but were in favor of placebo. Contemplation of the these trial results however led to the critique of the underlying assumptions of the trials, for example, that women over 65 years of age would benefit from the initiation of estrogen replacement when the epidemiology suggested younger women would; and to the criticism that because the onset of AD was occurring within 5 years of starting medications that the patients already had the pathology of AD and that any effect was not so much an advancing of the illness (the opposite of delaying) but rather an uncovering of the cognitive symptoms earlier (essentially a symptomatic effect). Primary prevention trials probably need to involve much younger patients, and hence would have to be larger and longer in order to accommodate the very low event rates.

Examples of primary prevention trials include those that were primarily designed to assess cognitive impairment and AD and those in which the incidence of dementia was a secondary outcome or add-on project (Table 2.8). Notably, the prevention trials with anti-inflammatories, equine estrogens, and *Ginkgo biloba* were undertaken in the face of negative placebo-controlled trials of 6-month to 1-year durations in patients with mild to moderate AD. In most of these trials a time-to-AD component was added

Table 2.8 Characteristics of selected placebo-controlled primary prevention trials[a,b]

Study name/drug/sponsor	Criteria/ enrichment	Number enrolled/follow-up/outcomes	Status
ADAPT/Naproxen, celecoxib/ NIA[76]	First-degree relatives with AD, age ≥70 years,	$N \approx 2528$; 5–7 years Incidence of AD, cognitive decline	Trial stopped early because of potential NSAID toxicity; increased risk for AD with both treatments
GEM/Ginkgo biloba extract/ NICAM with Schwabe Pharma support[77]	Asymptomatic, 60% or MCI, 40% age ≥75 years	$N \approx 3072$; 8.5 years Incident dementia, rate of cognitive decline, cardiovascular outcomes	Ongoing
GUIDAGE/Ginkgo biloba extract/ EU with Ipsen Pharma support[78]	Memory complaints, age >70 years	$N \approx 2630$; 4 years Incident dementia	Ongoing
Physicians' Health Study-II/ Vitamin E, folic acid, beta-carotene/NIH[79]	Asymptomatic, age >65 years	$N \approx 10\,000$; 9 years Telephone cognitive testing (add-on study)	Ongoing
Heart Protection Study/Vitamins E, C, beta-carotene and simvastatin/MRC[80]	Asymptomatic with cardiovascular risk factors, age 40–80 years	$N \approx 20{,}536$; 5 years Telephone Interview for Cognitive Status (TICS) and incident dementia (add-on)	No differences with either vitamins or simvastatin
PREADVISE/Selenium, vitamin E/NIH[81]	Asymptomatic men, age ≥60 years	$N \approx 10{,}400$; 12 years Dementia onset, cognitive tests (add-on)	Ongoing, expected completion 2013
HERS/Estrogen and medroxyprogesterone[82]	Asymptomatic women, mean age 67	$N \approx 1060$; 4.2 years Cognitive tests (add-on)	One test improved
Women's Health Initiative Memory Study/Estrogen and medroxyprogesterone[83]	Women without dementia, ages 65–80 years	$N \approx 4532$; 4–5 years Incident dementia and MCI, cognitive scores (add-on)	Increased risks for MCI/dementia; worse cognitive scores with hormone therapy
Women's Health Initiative Memory Study Estrogen alone/NIH[84]		$N \approx 2497$; 4–5 years	

Abbreviations: MCI, mild cognitive impairment; AD, Alzheimer's disease.
[a]Modified from Green and DeKosky[85] and from Schneider.[86]
[b]Most have enriched sample selection. The last five were add-ons to larger trials.

on to a trial designed to assess the effect of the drugs on other medical conditions (e.g., cardiovascular disease, prostate disease, cancer, osteoporosis). The determination of time-to-AD dementia or MCI is problematic, however, as it is on a continuum and subject to some judgment.

The prevention of dropouts or patients lost to follow-up is a more important issue with longer term trials than it is in shorter trials. Since dropouts occur non-randomly, as a result of medication side effects, lack of efficacy, worsening clinical condition, intercurrent illnesses, and loss of interest, among other reasons, they will very much affect the validity of any outcomes. Imputing outcomes of missing patients are not satisfactory statistical compensation. Therefore, it is important in longer term studies to work on ways of retaining subjects. The larger the trial, the more sites and countries involved the greater the importance of preventing patients from becoming lost to follow-up.

Choosing participants for long-term clinical trials in order to minimize dropouts results in tradeoffs such as choosing a medically healthier population, better educated, and younger patients. Thus, the expected statistical power of the study to see a significant difference would be diminished as the incidence of the endpoint would decrease. Trials that require a proxy informant have the increased risk for losing the patient if the proxy drops out. The trials burdens on proxies or study partners accumulate as they do with the patients. Requirements for frequent clinic visits may decrease recruitment and follow-up. Methods need to be developed for following up patients and could include remote assessments by telephone or internet.

Drugs for prevention studies have to be perceived as relatively safe, at least safe enough for patients who will not develop dementia. Some of the barriers to implementing prevention trials aside from their obvious length involve being able to recruit and maintain subjects in the trial, providing informed consent that may change over time, disclosing risk factors, including the fact that a patient may be chosen because of an enhanced risk for developing AD, using appropriate tools and the appropriate definitions of endpoints.

Assuming that a sponsor would develop a drug using a prevention trial as the Phase III pivotal trial and that the trial was statistically significant in favor of the drug, a regulatory consideration would involve whether a single trial can be accepted as pivotal, whether or not simply because it is a single and very large trial, it may not be subject to bias, and whether or not results are internally consistent.

An important point in considering prevention trials is whether they have to be done at all as a requirement for drug approval. Would it be better to develop the drug for shorter term effects for marketing and then use the marketed drug in longer term prevention trials?

Concluding Remarks

If new drugs are developed using the current "standard" paradigms, then the potential for effective drugs to not be recognized as effective would be great and effective treatments would less likely be found. The clinical expression of AD needs to be recognized earlier than the dementia. Sample selection and relevant outcomes for mild AD are important; simply making the trials longer or using different statistical techniques will not adequately address effectiveness, nor would this gain a disease-modification claim. Longer trials that demonstrate significant improvements in cognition and function, however, will be recognized as having symptomatic effects over the course of the trial, and many consumers will interpret a long-term effect as the same as disease-modifying. Prevention trials may be impractical for drug development and might be better employed in Phase IV post-registration studies. Trials using times to certain endpoints or milestones as indicators of efficacy, including prevention trials, need to be re-visited for the appropriateness of the chosen endpoints and their intimate involvement with the illness process.

SECTION 3: CONDUCT OF CLINICAL TRIALS, DRUG DEVELOPMENT, AND GCP

This section overviews the conduct of clinical trials, and GCP from the point of view that perceptions of GCP may impair study conduct and international drug development. It reviews some of what is involved in conducting clinical trials of cognitive enhancers, including the sites, staffing, sample selection, samples of convenience, that may lead only to the potential to demonstrate internal validity but not external validity, outcome measures applied to multi-site trials and internationally, the issues of randomization and blinding, the practical distinctions between Phase II and III trials in this area, and safety assessment.

Perception that GCP May Impair Study Conduct and Drug Development

Clinical trials in general are intended to conform to the International Conference on Harmonization (ICH); Guidance on General Considerations for Clinical Trials, Nonclinical Safety Studies for the Conduct of Human Clinical Trials for Pharmaceuticals, and GCP: Consolidated Guidance.[v] These guidelines have been updated regularly. ICH guidance complements FDA GCP regulations[vi] set requirements for a minimum level of trial quality.

GCP guidelines seek to raise the standard of trials conduct and are implemented to ensure that all phases of clinical trials are properly designed, carried out and documented. They are also intended to ensure proper ethical and safety considerations are carried out when administering experimental drugs and biologics in human subjects. According to the ICH guidelines, GCP "...is an international ethical and scientific quality standard for designing, conducting, recording and reporting trials that involve the participation of human subjects. Compliance with this standard provides public assurance that the rights, safety and well-being of trial subjects are protected, consistent with the principles that have their origin in the Declaration of Helsinki, and that the clinical trial data are credible."[vii] Although mandated by regulators they do not address issues of skill and expertise for dementia trials.

---

[v] 62 Fed. Reg. 66113, December 17, 1997; 62 Fed. Reg. 62922, November 25, 1997; 62 Fed. Reg. 25692, May 9, 1997.
[vi] Title 21 Code of Federal Regulations Part 312 and other parts.
[vii] Guideline for good clinical practice. ICH harmonised tripartite guideline, E6(R1), 1996, p. 1.

Some issues that will be addressed below include the prevailing thought that very large sample sizes are needed in both Phase II as well as Phase III in order to assess efficacy, and that the more economical and faster and approach would be the larger trials; the current US clinical trials infrastructure involves individual or groups of private and university sites of variable quality and ability to recruit and accurately evaluate patients; a current trend is to use more sites with the expectation of fewer patients per site; and as sites from different countries are combined in the same study, issues of consistency of diagnosis and precision of outcomes given in different languages emerge.

Conducting Clinical Trials of Cognitive Enhancers

Practical Distinctions Between Phase II and III Trials

A blurring of distinctions between Phase II and III trials characterizes the AD drug development process with the major distinction being sample size.[viii] A large part of this may have been due to historical reasons that tacrine, the first marketed drug indicated for AD, was previously marketed and used clinically prior to its development program for AD so that dosage ranges and formulations were largely known and *ad hoc* studies suggested efficacy at certain doses. Thus, the drug could more easily and quickly be used in trials that could be viewed as either Phase II or III. Both tacrine and donepezil were approved on the basis of a 12-week trial and a 6-month trial, and there was little to distinguish the 12-week, dose-ranging trials from Phase II dose-ranging or proof of concept trials. Subsequently, 4-, 6-month Phase III rivastigmine trials were launched, including both dose-ranging and adjustable dosing trials on the basis of one 12-week Phase II trial. Thus, there is a history in AD drug development of either doing minimal Phase II work or combining Phase II with Phase III. This may be due to perceptions that that efficacy of AD drugs cannot be determined in short-term, 3-month trials (although they were with tacrine and donepezil) so that they would not be informative for making development decisions.

More recent drugs – mainly being developed for disease modification – tend to rely on only one Phase II trial, in effect a "proof of concept study," sometimes as long as 12–18 months, before launching large Phase III trials. These trials, however, generally did not yield an efficacy signal or one was found only after *post hoc* analyses.

The blurring of distinctions between Phase II and III includes the use of the same relatively restrictive diagnostic criteria, that both Phase II and III may do dose finding, that the duration of the trial and the clinical outcomes are often the same. A consequence of skimping in Phase II development is that less is known about the

---

[viii] Phases of development may be summarized briefly: Phase I – initial administration to humans, pharmacokinetics and pharmacodynamics, and early measurement of biological and/or clinical activity; Phase II – the exploration of efficacy, involving patients selected by clearly defined criteria, close monitoring of clinical trials, dosage determination, and evaluation of efficacy; Phase III – pivotal trials that provide confirmation of therapeutic efficacy and safety, further define dose response, and explore the use in wider patient samples. See also McEvoy and Freudenreich, Issues in the design and conductance of clinical trials, in Volume 1, Psychiatric Disorders for further discussion of changes in clinical development phases.

drug at the end of Phase III, and the outcomes of Phase III determine the future of the drugs.

Thus, currently, among the Phase III trials listed in Table 2.7:

1. Xaliproden (Sanofi-Aventis) apparently did not achieve its Phase III objectives in two trials involving a total of approximately 2400 patients, yet the company will continue its development based on differences in hippocampal volume in subsets of patients from these trials.
2. Tramiprosate (Neurochem) was entered into two Phase III trials of approximately 1000 patients each as well, after a non-informative Phase II trial; and its development was stopped after the first Phase III trial was acknowledged to not have been significant.
3. Tarenflurbil (R-flurbiprofen/Flurizan®) was entered into two Phase III trials of approximately 1684 and 841 patients, each based on one Phase II trial that was overall not significant but showed salutary effects in the higher dose and more mildly impaired patient subgroups.
4. Four Phase III trials were launched for bapineuzumab (AAB-001, Elan) before the single 18-month long Phase II trial of 240 patients was completed.

These programs may have been done because of a prevailing thought that very large sample sizes would be needed in both Phase II as well as Phase III in order to assess efficacy, and that the more economical and faster and approach would be the larger trials sooner. This may or may not be the case however, and may actually be an artifact of sample selection and outcomes choice. The consequences of these development choices may lead both to disappointment and more uncertainty.

Clinical Trials Infrastructure

The current US clinical trials infrastructure involves individual or groups of private and university sites of variable quality and ability to recruit and accurately evaluate patients, and several competing private and academic contract research organizations (CROs).[ix] The latter are often divisions of large healthcare corporations, whose performance measures primarily involve costs and recruitment rates, without further considerations of quality. The CROs establish preferred provider agreements with large pharmaceutical companies and bid against other CROs on trials contracts from smaller companies.

Each new clinical trial requires a new contract, choice of sites, recruitment effort, and monitoring, and leads to considerable uncertainty about most aspects of a trial. Company medical directors may have to use the CROs approved by their purchasing departments. The CROs often choose the sites, sometimes in collaboration with the sponsor, based on closely held criteria that are often not fully rational or on faulty metrics and economics.

At any time, the staff at any of the academic or private sites, CROs, or drug companies may be inexperienced in dementia trials or trials in general, especially considering

[ix] See also McEvoy and Freudenreich, Issues in the design and conductance of clinical trials, in Volume 1, Psychiatric Disorders for further discussion on the clinical research industry.

the ebb of flow of clinical trials contracts and the impermanence of clinical trial workers and research assistants. The CROs, clinical sites, and drug companies compete mainly on the basis of cost and not quality. Although the federally mandated GCP regulations (Title 21 Code of Federal Regulations Part 312 and other parts) set requirements for a minimum level of trial quality, they do not address issues of skill and expertise for dementia trials.

Western Europe, Canada, Australia/New Zealand are roughly similar. There are some collaborative clinical trials consortia such as the ADCS, the European AD Consortium (http://eadc.alzheimer-europe.or), the UK Dementias and Neurodegenerative Diseases Research Network (http://www.dendron.org.uk/index.html), Consortium of Canadian Centres for Clinical Cognitive Research (http://www.c5r.ca). These more specialized groups still have limited capacity to undertake trials considering the large number of patients and sites needed for the many future trials. Indeed, the characteristic that they share cross-nationally is that they are academic sites doing various kinds of research and each site may not have access to sufficient patients or have clinical trials as a priority. Many countries elsewhere have more rudimentary dementia trials experiences.

Within and beyond North America and Europe, many clinics may be experienced in evaluating dementia patients but possibly not in ways similar to Western Europe, and often have no clinical trials experiences or GCP expertise. This poses obvious problems.

Site Selection

Clinical trials for dementia drugs have expanded internationally in recent years, both in order to be more representative, and for a sponsor to be better positioned to market medications internationally, and because it has been increasingly more challenging to enroll patients for cognitive impairment trials in North America and the European Union. Site selection, however, has affected the intrinsic design of Phase II and III trials. The numbers of sites per trial has increased rather remarkably from approximately 20–30 sites for 400–600 patient trials in the early 1990s to over 130 sites for current longer term trials involving 600–1600 patients. Therefore, the trend is to use more sites with the expectation of fewer patients per site.

Many sites have limited or no experience prior to the trials; many sites recruit only one or two patients over the trial. There become wide imbalances in patients recruited per site. Moreover, as sites from different countries are combined in the same study, issues of consistency of diagnosis and precision of outcomes given in different languages emerge.

Skills of the Sites and Personnel

The skills of clinical sites vary and often are not controlled for in the current infrastructure. For example, the cognitive raters in US sites vary greatly in training from being research technicians to PhD level clinical psychologists. In France, by comparison, cognitive raters must be neuropsychologists and have at least a master's degree in psychology. The CIBIC+ was designed and intended for experienced clinicians, mainly physicians and psychologists to administer, yet in the US technicians often administer it.

Moreover, because of staff changes and availability over the length of trials the same raters often are not available to do pre- and post-treatment assessments on the same patients. The meaning of change of the CIBIC+ differs in some trials from an assessment of overall change in a trial, to a more specific change in cognition. Implications of this have yet to be appreciated but certainly stand to lessen the ability to compare results from different trials, although the CIBIC+ was intended merely to obtain an experienced clinician's judgment of change as a test of clinically meaningful change.

Although the sponsors recognize the need and are putting more effort into training, at least at investigator's meetings, the thoroughness and effectiveness of such training has not been systematically evaluated. In fact, other companies and CROs compete to provide such training and this is considered proprietary information. Most trials managers do not continue training throughout the course of recruitment. Training is especially important for the cognitive testing and its need is not lessened by the use of computerized testing.

Monitoring

GCP requires that each stage of the clinical trial be monitored not only to ensure proper adherence to protocol, but also prevent, or to detect fraud such as falsified data, enrollment of ineligible patients, or indeed enrollment of fictional patients. Ethical compliance such as enrolment of well-informed patients participating in the trial with written consent is mandatory. Also GCP requires that the certification and other credentials of researchers are adequately confirmed. As trials become more multi-national, the due diligence of proper and consistent monitoring becomes more difficult.

Safety and Adverse Events

Safety assessments for cognitively enhancing drugs should be no different than with other drugs in development and are based on FDA and ICH guidelines. Total clinical experience must include data on a large and representative group of patients,[x] it should be considered that long-term safety may be different in the various subtypes of dementia. Specific guidelines include a minimum of 1000 patients exposed for several weeks to relevant dose-range and a minimum of 300 patients exposed to doses above the median for 6 months to a year.

Adverse events should be assessed in relationship to treatment duration, dosage duration, and clinical characteristics of the patients. Safety and tolerability are relative concepts however. Adverse events and risks in patients with early cognitive impairment or with conditions that progress slowly have to be considered differently from patients with more severe or rapidly progressive illness.

Psychiatric and neurological and cardiovascular adverse events should be particularly noted, as well as the effects of withdrawal of drugs in clinical trials. For example,

[x] See ICH Harmonised Tripartite Guideline E1. The extent of population exposure to assess clinical safety for drugs intended for long-term treatment of non-life-threatening conditions http://www.ich.org/LOB/media/MEDIA435.pdf

confusion, disorientation, extrapyramidal symptoms, gait disorders, seizures, cerebrovascular events, delusions, hallucinations, aggression, agitation and other behavioral
abnormalities, orthostatic hypotension, cardiac arrhythmias should be particularly
noted. Specific claims in this respect, improvement of neuro-behavioral abnormalities,
have to be based on specific studies.

Studies on morbidity and mortality are not required before marketing approval.
However, effects on mortality should be monitored on a long-term basis. This can be
done post-marketing by implementing a risk minimization or risk management plan.

Methodological issues
Patient Selection
The potential and actual confound of inadequate patient selection has been discussed
above. Issues pertaining not only to the heterogeneity of the dementias and their
presumed causes, but even to the actual definition of levels of AD such as what is
actually meant by "mild" and "moderate" AD; notwithstanding the use of MMSE that
was originally conceived as a clinical screening instrument to identify and stratify
patients are yet to be resolved. Further potential confounds such as the use of advertising for patients, type of residence and support potential patient–volunteers enjoy
make it appear that they are recruited largely on the basis of convenience that is,
patient–volunteers that clinical sites *can* recruit, rather than the patient–volunteers
who *need* to be recruited. Difficulty in recruitment has subsequently led to expansion
of trials worldwide, an expansion that brings with it associated confounds of language,
culture, class and education.

Outcome Measures Applied to Multi-site Trials and Internationally
The currently used outcomes in Phase II to IV trials were invented and originally validated in the United States and Canada. They are of course language and culturally
based. With respect to cognition, although certainly the cognitive processes that are
assessed are not culture dependent, the way they are assessed may be subject to such
differences. Global assessments depend on the investigators expectations and valuing
of clinically significant change, and may differ among cultures and economic levels.
ADLs are particularly culturally related.

The internationalization of trials leads to the conduct of trials and the recruiting of sites and patients from many different cultures and using different languages.
The mandates of some companies are to broaden the participation of countries and
regions, to essentially "internationalize" clinical drug development programs. Although
many development programs will concentrate their trials sites in North America and
Western Europe, others are recruiting sites representing countries throughout the
world. Current Phase II and III trials may involve from 100 to over 200 sites and over a
dozen languages.

Cognitive outcomes in AD trials are particularly language dependent, relying on
wordlist-learning, naming objects, language comprehension, and expression. Moreover,
they and ADLs are also culturally, educationally, and socioeconomically dependent.
Equivalent cognitive forms are used in many trials but it is not clear that these forms

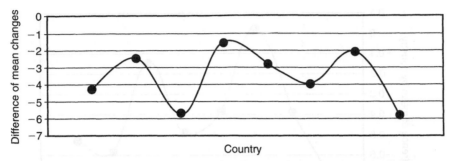

Figure 2.4 ADAS-cog difference of mean changes by country from galantamine trial GAL-INT-1, including 7 European countries and Canada. Negative sign favors galantamine over placebo. From Galantamine New Drug Application 21-169 FDA statistical review, table 2.7.1.

are equivalent across languages. Cognitive tests are subject to administration and scoring errors as well and these errors however small, and if systematic, may affect outcomes.

ADAS-cog scores most likely vary greatly among countries, likely due to the fact that the test itself has limited precision and may not be precisely enough equivalent across languages and cultures. Differences between language versions includes objects for naming and items for verbal memory, the imagery of the words/objects used, and the number of versions or lists. Some inter-European studies suggest that the differences between different country versions of the ADAS-cog can be reduced and harmonized by adjusting, adapting, and harmonizing the various versions of the ADAS-cog.[87]

The FDA in evaluating a New Drug Application for galantamine demonstrated the ranges of country to country variations on the ADAS-cog and CIBIC+ (FDA Center for Drug Evaluation Research Approval Package for: Application Number 21-169 Statistical Review, http://www.fda.gov/cder/foi/nda/2001/21-169Reminylstatr.pdf). Figure 2.4 shows the variations in mean differences in ADAS-cog scores between the marketed cholinesterase inhibitor, galantamine and placebo across several countries. Although this Phase III pivotal trial showed over significant effects for galantamine, the mean ADAS-cog differences ranged from about −1.5 to −6 among countries.

Similarly, CIBIC+ scores vary by country with drug-placebo differences ranging from 0 to −0.7 (Figure 2.5). The latter might be considered counter-intuitive since the CIBIC+ is basically an overall judgment of change performed by a clinician and might have been expected not to show such variation. As can be seen, a comparison between the mean effects of the ADAS-cog and the CIBIC+ by country do not necessarily correlate with each other.

No information is available on the ADL outcomes from this trial, nor is information generally made available from other propriety trials. Clearly, such disclosure would help in planning future clinical trials.

Randomization and Blinding

Maintaining the methodological quality of Phase II and III trials is a challenge with CNS drugs in general and with AD drugs in particular. Poor enrollment among sites,

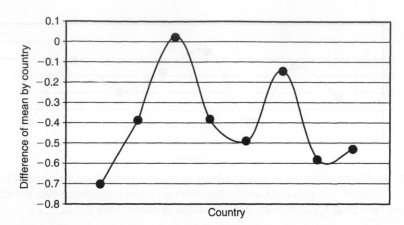

Figure 2.5   CIBIC+ difference of mean changes by country from galantamine trial GAL-INT-1, including 7 European countries avd Canada. Negative sign favors galantamine over placebo. From Galantamine New Drug Application 21-169 FDA statistical review, table 2.7.2.

imbalances among sites in multicenter trials, concomitant usage of cholinesterase inhibitors and adverse events are among the factors that threaten the trial and the blinding of treatments. There appear to be differences among countries as well as among sites.

Trials that are too small often do not achieve balanced randomization and important characteristics may be differentially represented among treatment groups; and unfortunately statistical modelling or adjustments cannot correct these imbalances. Randomization in blocks and by sites is one effort to achieve balance.

Randomization schemes with constrains or minimization on certain characteristics may help in smaller studies (e.g., balancing APOE genotype status or baseline severity).

CONCLUSIONS AND FUTURE DIRECTIONS

The diagnosis of AD is general and based on clinical phenotype. A number of genetic variants of the clinical expression of AD can be described and more will be identified in the future. APOE allele variant is one example. Phenotypic and genetic variants might show differential clinical courses and responses to medications. The course of AD is clinically heterogeneous and this has greater impact on sample selection and the assessment of outcomes in trials than can be appreciated.

Biomarkers have more particular potential for a neurodegeneration model but need further research. The currently discussed potential biomarkers will change over the course of the illness and their utility for drug development remains to be determined. It is uncertain the extent to which they can serve as surrogate markers of outcomes.

The assessment of memory is important to document in early drug development. This may be a variance to a disease-modification model.

Disease-modification drugs should show symptomatic, cognitive effects if in fact they counteract β-amyloid or affect β-amyloid oligimer synaptic effects or synaptic plasticity. Some 18-month-long trials purport to model AD as a progressive neurodegenerative process but considering that modeling is based on cognitive impairment clinical effects in these longer trials are likely to be interpreted as symptomatic. In drug development for dementia and other cognitive impairment disorders, a cognition model should be used where advantageous cognitive outcomes are essential.

The FDA and EMEA standards for efficacy, safety and marketing approval of drugs for dementia are fairly minimal and general, and constitute low thresholds to approval rather than high barriers. Yet, regulatory authorities and their advisors are at risk for "overspecifying" required trials designs and outcomes based on dementia and cognition models that may not apply to the drug in development or that are clinically relevant. For regulators a definition of clinical meaning or relevance is more related ADLs and health economics than to the overall illness.

Because so many patients are taking cholinesterase inhibitors drugs as a standard of medical care there is the need to perform well-designed, long-term trials with currently marketed drugs, to assess better how effective these drugs really are over the long term in order to estimate any effect with new drugs.

Methods for translating pre-clinical outcomes assessments to clinical development are needed. Current drug development in this area shows little connection to the preclinical models. Finally, a major barrier to the advancement of clinical development of drugs for cognitive impairment is that development methods have been treated as proprietary and there has been an absence of cooperation in sharing trials data among sponsors. This leads to the potential to repeat previous mistakes and does not encourage progress

ACKNOWLEDGMENTS

NIH grant P50 AG 05142, the University of Southern California Alzheimer's Disease Research Center (ADRC), and the State of California Alzheimer's Research and Clinical Center, and the Alzheimer's Association (United States).

REFERENCES

1. McKhann, G., Drachman, D., Folstein, M., Katzman, R., Price, D., and Stadlan, E.M. (1984). Clinical diagnosis of Alzheimer's disease: Report of the NINCDS-ADRDA Work Group under the auspices of Department of Health and Human Services Task Force on Alzheimer's Disease. *Neurology*, 34:939–944.
2. American Psychiatric Association. (2000). *Diagnostic and Statistical Manual of Mental Disorders DSM-IV-TR.*. American Psychiatric Press, Washington, DC.
3. Petersen, R.C., Smith, G.E., Waring, S.C., Ivnik, R.J., Tangalos, E.G. *et al.* (1999). Mild cognitive impairment: Clinical characterization and outcome. *Arch Neurol*, 56:303–308.
4. Morris, J.C., Storandt, M., Miller, J.P., McKeel, D.W., Prince, J.L. *et al.* (2001). Mild cognitive impairment represents early-stage Alzheimer disease. *Arch Neurol*, 58:397–405.
5. Dubois, B., Feldman, H.H., Jacova, C., Dekosky, S.T., Barberger-Gateau, P., Cummings, J. *et al.* (2007). Research criteria for the diagnosis of Alzheimer's disease: Revising the NINCDS-ADRDA criteria. *Lancet Neurology*, 6(8):734–746.

6. Chui, H.C., Victoroff, J.I., Margolin, D., Jagust, W., Shankle, R., and Katzman, R. (1992). Criteria for the diagnosis of ischemic vascular dementia proposed by the State of California Alzheimer's Disease Diagnostic and Treatment Centers (see comments). *Neurology*, 42(3 Pt 1):473–480.

7. Roman, G.C., Tatemichi, T.K., Erkinjuntti, T., Cummings, J.L., Masdeu, J.C., Garcia, J.H. *et al.* (1993). Vascular dementia: Diagnostic criteria for research studies. Report of the NINDS-AIREN International Workshop. *Neurology*, 43(2):250–260.

8. McKeith, I.G., Galasko, D., Kosaka, K., Perry, E.K., Dickson, D.W., Hansen, L.A. *et al.* (1996). Consensus guidelines for the clinical and pathologic diagnosis of dementia with Lewy bodies (DLB): Report of the consortium on DLB international workshop. *Neurology*, 47(5):1113–1124.

9. Emre, M., Aarsland, D., Brown, R. *et al.* (2007). Clinical diagnostic criteria for dementia associated with Parkinson's disease. *Mov Disord*, 22(12):1689–1707.

10. Crook, T.H., Bartus, R.T., Ferris, S.H. *et al.* (1986). Age-associated memory impairment: proposed diagnostic criteria and measures of clinical change – Report of a National Institute of Mental Health workgroup. *Dev Neuropsych*, 2:261–276.

11. Petersen, R.C., Smith, G.E., Ivnik, R.J., Tangalos, E.G., Schaid, D.J., Thibodeau, S.N. *et al.* (1995). Apolipoprotein E status as a predictor of the development of Alzheimer's disease in memory-impaired individuals. *JAMA*, 26; 273(16):1274–1278.

12. Visser, P.J., Scheltens, P., and Verhey, F.R. (2005). Do MCI criteria in drug trials accurately identify subjects with predementia Alzheimer's disease?. *J Neurol Neurosurg Psychiatr*, 76:1348–1354.

13. Petersen, R.C., Stevens, J.C., Ganguli, M. *et al.* (2001). Practice parameter: Early detection of dementia: Mild cognitive impairment (an evidence-based review). Report of the Quality Standards Subcommittee of the American Academy of Neurology. *Neurology*, 56:1133–1142.

14. Larrieu, S., Letenneur, L., Orgogozo, J.M., Fabrigoule, C., Amieva, H., Le Carret, N. *et al.* (2002). Incidence and outcome of mild cognitive impairment in a population-based prospective cohort. *Neurology*, 59(10):1594–1599.

15. Visser, P.J. And Brodaty, H. (2006). MCI is not a clinically useful concept. *Int Psychogeriatr*, 18:402–409.

16. United States Prescribing Information for Exelon http://www.pharma.us.novartis.com/product/pi/pdf/exelon.pdf

17. Kavirajan, H. And Schneider, L.S. (2007). The efficacy and adverse effects of cholinesterase inhibitors and memantine in vascular dementia: A systematic review and meta-analysis of controlled trials. *Lancet Neurol*, 6:782–792. Online doi:10.1016/S1474-4422(07)70195-3

18. McKeith, I.G., Dickson, D.W., Lowe, J., Emre, M., O'Brien, J.T., Feldman, H. *et al.* (2005 Dec 27). Diagnosis and management of dementia with Lewy bodies: Third report of the DLB Consortium. *Neurology*, 65(12):1863–1872.

19. McKeith, I., Teodoro Del Ser, T., PierFranco Spano, P., Murat Emre, M., Wesnes, K., Anand, R., Cicin-Sain, A., Ferrara, R., and Spiegel, R. (2000). Efficacy of rivastigmine in dementia with Lewy bodies: A randomised, double-blind, placebo-controlled international study. *Lancet*, 356:2031–2036.

20. Folstein, M.F., Folstein, S.E., and McHugh, P.R. (1975). "Mini-mental state". A practical method for grading the cognitive state of patients for the clinician. *J Psychiatr Res*, 12(3):189–198.

21. Rosen, W.G., Terry, R.D., Fuld, P.A., Katzman, R., and Peck, A. (1980). Pathological verification of ischemic score in differentiation of dementias. *Ann Neurol*, 7(5):486–488.

22. Mohr, E., Feldman, H., and Gauthier, S. (1995). Canadian guidelines for the development of antidementia therapies: A conceptual summary. *Can J Neurol Sci*, 22(1):62–71.

23. FDA Psychopharmacological Drugs Advisory Committee (2000). Development of Drugs for Psychiatric Disturbances Associated with Alzheimer's Disease and other Dementias. March 9, 2000. http://www.fda.gov/ohrms/dockets/ac/00/minutes/3590m.htm

24. National Institute for Clinical and Healthcare Excellence (NICE) (2006). Donepezil, galantamine, rivastigmine (review) and memantine for the treatment of Alzheimer's disease (amended) November 2006 (amended September 2007) http://guidance.nice.org.uk/TA111/guidance/pdf/English

25. Schneider, L.S. (2006). The post-modern world of Alzheimer's disease trials: How much is an ADAS-cog point worth in Central London? *Int J Ger Psychiatr*, 21(1):9–13.

26. Rosen, W.G., Mohs, R.C., and Davis, K.L. (1984). A new rating scale for Alzheimer's disease. *Am J Psychiatr*, 141:1356–1364.

27. Mohs, R.C., Knopman, D., Petersen, R.C., Ferris, S.H., Ernesto, C., Grundman, M. *et al.* (1997). Development of cognitive instruments for use in clinical trials of antidementia drugs: Additions to the Alzheimer's Disease Assessment Scale (ADAS) that broaden its scope. *Alzheimer Dis Assoc Disord*, 11(Suppl 2):S13–S21.

28. Petersen, R.C., Thomas, R.G., Grundman, M., Bennett, D., Doody, R., Ferris, S. *et al.* (2005 Jun 9). Vitamin E and donepezil for the treatment of mild cognitive impairment (see comment). *New Engl J Med*, 352(23):2379–2388.

29. Kertesz, A. And Mohs, R.C. (1999). Cognition. In Gauthier, S. (ed.), *Clinical Diagnosis and Management of Alzheimer's Disease*, Second ed. Martin Dunitz, Ltd., London, pp. 179–196.

30. Saxton, J., McGonigle-Gibson, K.L., Swihart, A.A., Miller, V.J., and Boller, F. (1990). Assessment of the severely impaired patient: Description and validation of a new neuropsychological test battery. *Psychological Assessment: A Journal of Consulting and Clinical Psychology*, 2:298–303.

31. Schmitt, F.A., Ashford, W., Ernesto, C., Saxton, J., Schneider, L.S., Clark, C.M., Ferris, S.H., Mackel, J.A., Schafer, K., Thal, L.J., and the Alzheimer's Disease Cooperative Study (1997). The severe impairment battery: Concurrent validity and the assessment of longitudinal change in Alzheimer's disease. *Alzheimer Dis Assoc Disord*, 11(suppl 2): S51–S56.

32. Gelinas, I., Gauthier, L., McIntyre, M., and Gauthier, S. (1999). Development of a functional measure for persons with Alzheimer's disease: The disability assessment for dementia. *Am J Occup Ther*, 53(5):471–481.

33. Feldman, H., Sauter, A., Donald, A., Gelinas, I., Gauthier, S., Torfs, K. *et al.* (2001). The disability assessment for dementia scale: A 12-month study of functional ability in mild to moderate severity Alzheimer disease. *Alzheimer Dis Assoc Disord*, 15(2):89–95.

34. Galasko, D., Bennett, D., Sano, M., Ernesto, C., Thomas, R., Grundman, M., and Ferris, S. (1997). An inventory to assess activities of daily living for clinical trials in Alzheimer's disease. The Alzheimer's Disease Cooperative Study. *Alzheimer Dis Assoc Disord*, 11(Suppl 2):S33–S39.

35. Schneider, L.S. (1996). An overview of rating scales used in dementia research. *Alzheimer Insights*, 2(3):1–7.

36. Schneider, L.S. (2001 Aug). Assessing outcomes in Alzheimer's disease. *Alzheimer Dis Assoc Disord*, 15(S):S8–S18.

37. Blessed, G., Tomlinson, B.E., and Roth, M. (1988). Blessed-Roth Dementia Scale (DS). *Psychopharmacology Bulletin*, 24(4):705–708.

38. DeJong, R., Osterlund, O.W., and Roy, G.W. (1989). Measurement of quality-of-life changes in patients with Alzheimer's disease. *Clin Therapeut*, 11(4):545–554.

39. Bentham, P., Gray, R., Sellwood, E., and Raftery, J. (1999). Effectiveness of rivastigmine in Alzheimer's disease. Improvements in functional ability remain unestablished. *BMJ*, 319(7210):640–641.

40. Teunisse, S., Derix, M.M., and van Crevel, H. (1991). Assessing the severity of dementia. Patient and caregiver. *Arch Neurol*, 48(3):274–277.

41. Burns, A., Rossor, M., Hecker, J., Gauthier, S., Petit, H., Moller, H.J. *et al.* (1999). The effects of donepezil in Alzheimer's disease-results from a multinational trial. *Dement Geriatr Cognit Disord*, 10(3):237–244.

42. Gelinas, I. And Auer, S. (1996). Functional autonomy. In: Gautheir, S. (ed.), *Clinical Diagnosis and Management of Alzheimer's Disease*. Martin Dunitz Ltd, London.

43. Guy, W. (1976). Clinical Global Impressions (CGI). In Guy, W. (ed.), *ECDEU Assessment Manual for Psychopharmacology*. US Department of Health and Human Services, Public Health Service, Alcohol Drug Abuse and Mental Health Administration, NIMH Psychopharmacology Research Branch, Rockville, MD, pp. 218–222.

44. Morris, J.C. (1993). The Clinical Dementia Rating (CDR): Current version and scoring rules. *Neurology*, 43(11):2412–2414.

45. Reisberg., B., Ferris, S.H., de Leon, M.J., and Crook, T. (1982). The global deterioration scale (GDS): An instrument for the assessment of primary degenerative dementia (PDD). *Am J Psychiatr*, 139:1136–1139.

46. Forstl, H., Burns, A., Levy, R., Cairns, N., Luthert, P., and Lantos, P. (1992). Neurologic signs in Alzheimer's disease. Results of a prospective clinical and neuropathologic study. *Arch Neurol*, 49(10):1038–1042.

47. Leber, P. (1990). Guidelines for the Clinical Evaluation of Antidementia Drugs (First Draft). November 8, unpublished.

48. Schneider, L.S., Olin, J.T., Doody, R.S., Clark, C.M., Morris, J.C., Reisberg, B. *et al.* (1997). Validity and reliability of the Alzheimer's Disease Cooperative Study-Clinical Global Impression of Change. The Alzheimer's Disease Cooperative Study. *Alzheimer Dis Assoc Disord*, 11(Suppl 2):S22–S32.

49. Olin, J.T., Schneider, L.S., Doody, R.S., Clark, C.M., Ferris, S.H., Morris, J.C. *et al.* (1996). Clinical evaluation of global change in Alzheimer's disease: Identifying consensus. *J Geriatr Psychiatr Neurol*, 9(4):176–180.

50. Leber, P. (2002). Criteria used by Drug Regulatory Authorities. In Qizilbash, N., Schneider, L., Chui, H., *Evidence-based Dementia Practice*. Blackwell Science Ltd, Oxford, pp. 376–387.

51. European Medicines Agency (2007). Committee for Medicinal Products for Human Use, Guideline on medicinal products for the treatment of Alzheimer's disease and other dementias, London, July 19, 2007 Doc. Ref. CPMP/EWP/553/95 Rev. 1 (Draft)

52. European Medicines Agency (1997). Committee for Proprietary Medicinal Products (CPMP) note for guidance on medicinal products in the treatment of Alzheimer's disease. http://www.emea.europa.eu/pdfs/human/ewp/055395en.pdf

53. European Medicines Agency (2006). EMEA/CHMP/EWP Workshop: slowing the progression of neurodegenerative diseases: Medicinal Products (MP) Clinical Development, London, October 2, 2006, Doc. Ref. EMEA/512562/2006 (http://www.emea.europa.eu)

54. Schneider, L.S. (2008). The prevention therapeutics of dementia. Alzheimer Dement 4(1):5122–5130.

55. Doody, R.S., Stevens, J.C., Beck, C. *et al.* (2001). Practice parameter: Management of dementia (an evidence-based review). Report of the Quality Standards Subcommittee of the American Academy of Neurology (see comment). *Neurology*, 56(9):1154–1166.

56. Waldemar, G., Dubois, B., Emre, M. *et al.* (2007). Recommendations for the diagnosis and management of Alzheimer's disease and other disorders associated with dementia: EFNS guideline. *Eur J Neurol*, 14:e1–e26.

57. Tariot, P.N., Farlow, M.R., Grossberg, G.T., Graham, S.M., McDonald, S., and Gergel, I. (2004). Memantine Study Group. Memantine treatment in patients with moderate to severe Alzheimer disease already receiving donepezil: A randomized controlled trial. *JAMA*, 291(3):317–324.

58. Courtney, C., Farrell, D., Gray, A. *et al.* (2004 Jun 26). Long-term donepezil treatment in 565 patients with Alzheimer's disease (AD2000): Randomised double-blind trial. *Lancet*, 363(9427):2105–2115.

59. Reisberg, B., Doody, R., Stoffler, A., Schmitt, F., Ferris, S., Mobius, H.J. *et al.* (2003). Memantine in moderate-to-severe Alzheimer's disease (see comment). *New Engl J Med*, 348(14):1333–1341.

60. Winblad, B. And Portis, N. (1999). Memantine in severe dementia: Results of the M-Best Study. *Int J Geriatr Psych*, 14:135–146.

61. Harrison, J., Minassian, S.L., Jenkins, L., Black, R.S., Koller, M., and Grundman, M. (2007). A neuropsychological test battery for use in Alzheimer's disease clinical trials. *Arch Neurol*, 64(9):1323–1329.

62. Sano, M., Ernesto, C., Klauber, M.R., Schafer, K., Woodbury, P., Thomas, R., Grundman, M., Growdon, J., Cotman, C.W., Pfeiffer, E., Schneider, L., and Thal, L. (1997). A controlled trial of selegiline, α-tocopherol or both as treatment for Alzheimer's disease. *New Engl J Med*, 336:1216–1222.

63. Petersen, R.C., Thomas, R.G., Grundman, M., Bennett, D., Doody, R., Ferris, S. *et al.* (2005 Jun 9). Vitamin E and donepezil for the treatment of mild cognitive impairment (see comment). *New Engl J Med*, 352(23):2379–2388.

64. Feldman, H.H., Ferris, S., Winblad, B., Sfikas, N., Mancione, L., He, Y. *et al.* (2007). Effect of rivastigmine on delay to diagnosis of Alzheimer's disease from mild cognitive impairment: The InDDEx study (see comment). *Lancet Neurol*, 6(6):501–512.

65. Johnson & Johnson Pharmaceutical Research & Development. GAL-INT-11 trial synopsis. (May 20, 2005; http://www.clinicalstudyresults.org/documents/company-study_96_1.pdf); kJohnson & Johnson Pharmaceutical Research & Development. GAL-INT-18 trial synopsis (May 20, 2005; http://www.clinicalstudyresults.org/documents/company-study_96_2.pdf)

66. Raschetti, R., Albanese, E., Vanacore, N., and MAggini, M. (2007). Cholinesterase inhibitors in mild cognitive impairment: A systematic review of randomized trials. *PLoS Med*, 4(11): 0001–00011.

67. Vellas, B., Andrieu, S., Sampaio, C., and Wilcock, G. (2007). Disease-modifying trials in Alzheimer's disease: A European task force consensus. *Lancet Neurol*, 6:56–62.

68. Qizilbash, N. And Schneider, L.S. (2002). Dementia trials for cognitive symptoms and modification of prognosis: Past, present and future. In: Qizilbash, N., Schneider, L.S., Chui, H., Tariot, P., Brodaty, H., Kaye, J., and Erkinjuntti, T. (eds.), *Evidence-based Dementia Practice*. Blackwell Publishing, Oxford, UK, pp. 405–417.

69. Qizilbash, N. (2002). Introduction to specific therapies for cognitive symptoms or modifying disease prognosis. In Qizilbash, N., Schneider, L.S., Chui, H., Tariot, P., Brodaty, H., Kaye, J., and Erkinjuntti, T. (eds.), *Evidence-based Dementia Practice*. Blackwell Publishing, Oxford, UK, pp. 461–466.

70. Leber, P. (1996). Observations and suggestions on antidementia drug development. *Alzheimer Dis Assoc Disord*, 10(S1):31–35.

71. Mani, R.B. (2004). The evaluation of disease modifying therapies in Alzheimer's disease: A regulatory viewpoint. *Stat Med*, 23:305–314.

72. Katz, R. (2004). Biomarkers and surrogate markers: An FDA perspective. *NeuroRx*, 1(2):189–195.

73. Food and Drug Administration Modernization Act Section 506b http://www.fda.gov/cder/guidance/105-115.htm

74. Mohs, R.C., Kawas, C., and Carillo, M.C. (2006). Optimal design of clinical trials for drugs designed to slow the course of Alzheimer's disease. *Alzheimer Dement*, 2(3):131–139.

75. Thal, L.J., Carta, A., Doody, R., Leber, P., Mohs, R., Schneider, L., Shimohama, S., and Silber, C. (1997). Prevention protocols for Alzheimer's disease: Position paper from the International Working Group on Harmonization of Dementia Drug Guidelines. *Alzheimer Dis Assoc Disord*, 11(suppl 3):46–49.

76. ADAPT Research Group. (2007). Naproxen and celecoxib do not prevent AD in early results from a randomized controlled trial. *Neurology*, 68:1800–1808.

77. DeKosky, S.T., Fitzpatrick, A., and Ives, D.G. (2006). Ginkgo Evaluation of Memory (GEM) Study: Design and baseline data of a randomized trial of *Ginkgo biloba* extract in prevention of dementia. *Contemp Clin Trials*, 27:238–253.

78. Vellas, B., Andrieu, S., Ousset, P.J., Ouzid, M., Mathiex-Fortunet, H., for the GuidAge Study G (2006). The GuidAge study: Methodological issues. A 5-year double-blind randomized trial of the efficacy of EGb 761(R) for prevention of Alzheimer disease in patients over 70 with a memory complaint. *Neurology*, 67:S6–S11.

79. Christen, W.G., Gaziano, J.M., and Hennekens, C.H. (2000). Design of Physicians' Health Study II – a randomized trial of beta-carotene, vitamins E and C, and multivitamins, in prevention of cancer, cardiovascular disease, and eye disease, and review of results of completed trials (abstract). A*nn Epidemiol*, 10(2):125–134. http://phs.bwh.harvard.edu/phs2.htm

80. Group HPSC. (2002). MRC/BHF Heart Protection Study of cholesterol lowering with simvastatin in 20,536 high-risk individuals: A randomised placebo-controlled trial (comment). *Lancet*, 360:7–22.

81. Runyons, C.R., Schmitt, F.A., and Caban-Holt, A. (2005). Antioxidants for the prevention of dementia: Overview of the PREADVISE trial. *Alzheimers Dement*, 1(1):S74.

82. Grady, D., Yaffe, K., Kristof, M., Lin, F., Richards, C., and Barrett-Connor, E. (2002). Effect of postmenopausal hormone therapy on cognitive function: The Heart and Estrogen/progestin Replacement Study. *Am J Med*, 113:543–548.

83. Shumaker, S.A., Legault, C., Rapp, S.R., Thal, L., Wallace, R.B., Ockene, J.K. *et al.* (2003). Estrogen plus progestin and the incidence of dementia and mild cognitive impairment in postmenopausal women: The Women's Health Initiative Memory Study: A randomized controlled trial. *JAMA*, 289(20):2651–2662.

84. Shumaker, S.A., Legault, C., Kuller, L., Rapp, S.R., Thal, L., Lane, D.S. *et al.* (2004). Conjugated equine estrogens and incidence of probable dementia and mild cognitive impairment in postmenopausal women: Women's Health Initiative Memory Study. *JAMA*, 291(24):2947–2958.

85. Green, R.C. And DeKosky, S.T. (2006). Primary prevention trials in Alzheimer's disease. *Neurology*, 67:S2–S5.

86. Schneider, L.S. (1998). Designing Phase III trials of antidementia drugs with a view toward pharmaco economic considerations. In Wimo, A., Jonsson, B., Karlsson, G., and Winblad, B. (eds.), *Health Economics of Dementia*. John Wiley & Sons, Oxford, pp. 451–464.

87. Verhey, F.R., Houx, P., Van Lang, N. *et al.* (1998). Cross-national comparison and validation of the Alzheimer's Disease Assessment Scale: Results from the European Harmonization Project for Instruments in Dementia (EUROHARPID). *Int J Geriatr Psychiatr*, 19:41–50.

88. Fleisher, A.S., Sun, S., Taylor, C., Ward, C.P., Gamst, A.C., Petersen, R.C., Jack Jr, C.R., Aisen, P.S., and Thal, L.J. (2008 Jan 15). Volumetric MRI vs clinical predictors of Alzheimer disease in mild cognitive impairment. *Neurology*, 70(3):191–199.

CHAPTER 3

Molecular and Cellular Mechanisms of Learning Disabilities: A Focus on Neurofibromatosis Type I

Carrie Shilyansky[1], Weidong Li[1], M. Acosta[2], Y. Elgersma[3], F. Hannan[4], M. Hardt[5], K. Hunter-Schaedle[6], L.C. Krab[3], E. Legius[7], B. Wiltgen[1] and Alcino J Silva[1]

[1]Department of Neurobiology, University of California, Los Angeles
[2]Department of Neurology, Children's National Medical Center, Washington DC
[3]Neuroscience Institute, Erasmus University, Rotterdam
[4]Cell Biology and Anatomy Department, New York Medical College, New York
[5]Department of Psychology and Clinical Neuroscience Laboratory, University of California, Los Angeles
[6]Children's Tumor Foundation, New Jersey
[7]Department of Human Genetics, Catholic University of Leuven, Leuven

Animal and Translational Models for CNS Drug Discovery,
Vol. 2 of 3: Neurological Disorders
Robert McArthur and Franco Borsini (eds), Academic Press, 2008

INTRODUCTION

Learning disabilities (LD) affect approximately 15% of the US population, but currently there are no generally effective therapies for this class of cognitive disorders. To address this problem, we have initially focused on Neurofibromatosis type I (NF1), a single gene disorder associated with learning disabilities. Previous studies showed that mice with a heterozygous null mutation of the NF1 gene have behavioral deficits related to the cognitive phenotype of NF1 patients. Studies of these mice showed increased Ras/MAPK signaling in the hippocampus and prefrontal cortex which results in the upregulation of GABA release underlying the spatial, attention and working memory deficits of the mutants. Statins can be used to decrease the isoprenylation and therefore the activity of Ras. Recent results demonstrate that a short treatment with statins, which is ineffective in controls, can reverse the increases in Ras-MAPK signaling, the synaptic plasticity, attention, and spatial learning deficits of the Nf1 mutant mice. To test whether statins can also reverse the neurological and cognitive deficits associated with NF1 in patients, we have initiated a series of collaborative pilot clinical studies in children and adults with NF1. These studies will not only have an impact on our understanding of cognitive deficits associated with NF1, it will also serve as a case study for how to investigate and treat learning disabilities.

Introduction to learning disabilities

Learning disability is a class of neurological disorders affecting approximately 15% of the US population. The diagnosis of learning disability is broad; it reflects difficulties in learning of specific academic skills in subjects with otherwise normal cognition. Learning disabilities differ from mental retardation or learning problems caused primarily by visual, auditory, or motor handicaps. Unlike these other disorders, learning disabilities are characterized by specific impairments restricted to certain domains of mental function. Therefore, individuals with learning disabilities have multiple areas of strengths, but their academic performance is confounded by significant weaknesses in certain skill sets.

The simplest definition of a learning disorder is a discrepancy between tests of intellectual capability and actual achievement.[1] Intellectual capability is typically quantified with IQ tests like the Wechsler scales (WISC-IV, WAIS-III) or the Stanford Binet (SB-IV). These tests provide reliable measures that are standardized across specific age groups.[2] Academic achievement is also determined using standardized tests that assess performance level in multiple academic areas (e.g., Woodcock-Johnson (WJ-III)[2] or WIAT.[3] Learning disability is diagnosed when performance in tests of achievement is significantly below predictions based on IQ score.

Beyond this general definition of learning disability, several systems attempt to categorize the disorder into subtypes. The DSM-IV places learning disabilities into three major categories: reading disorder, mathematical disorder, and disorders of written expression.[1,4] These categories are determined by the specific set of cognitive abilities that are impaired in an individual. In addition to these categories, the DSM-IV also recognizes non-verbal learning disorders and learning disorder not otherwise specified. These latter categories represent learning disabilities which cause a pattern of weaknesses that do not fall neatly into one of the first three DSM-IV categories of learning disability.[5] The DSM-IV categories are also considered distinct from other developmental disorders such as motor skills disorders and communication disorders.

Other diagnostic systems are based on specific descriptions of the skills that are most impaired by the learning disability; For example, dyslexia (reading disorder), dysgraphia (writing disorder), dyscalculia (problems with arithmetic and math), dyspraxia (motor coordination).[4] Attention deficit disorder often occurs in individuals with learning disorder, but is considered a separate, co-morbid diagnosis.

In addition, the etiology of learning disabilities is multivariate, making the problem even more complex. In some genetic or neurological conditions, specific learning problems are part of the phenomenology associated with the diagnosis. However, in other diagnosis a non-specific impairment defines the associated learning disability. In practice, definitions regarding impairments in learning are complex and require a careful evaluation of the cognitive profile of the affected individual, including the performance area that is impacted (e.g., difficulties in visuospatial organization could result in deficits in mathematical abilities and in phonological decoding required for reading). A careful assessment can provide a better overview of the profile of strengths and difficulties and allow the clinician to understand a changing pattern of individual performance in response to increasing demands from the environment.

Careful description of the impairments of individuals with learning disability is important, because it allows appropriate intervention and support to be implemented. Parents and school teachers would be able to make accommodations according to the weaknesses of an individual. Such an individualized program allows learning to be less dependent on weaker cognitive abilities, and the individual can use their strengths to bypass potential deficits. These support-based interventions improve the achievement of an individual with learning disabilities. However, they require a lifelong, intensive commitment from an individual with learning disability as well as their parents and teachers. Further, the effectiveness of the intervention depends on the accuracy and completeness with which the learning disability subtype is diagnosed and strengths and weaknesses of the student are described. The diagnostic criteria described above identify patterns of learning problems, but may not capture the entire clinical picture. It is unclear whether diagnostic criteria reflect fundamental differences in underlying neuronal mechanisms. A better understanding of the neuronal mechanisms that are impaired in learning disability disorders could lead to more accurate diagnosis and the development of more effective treatments.

NF1 AND LEARNING DISABILITIES

The causes for learning disabilities are multivariate. However, several neurological diseases of known etiology have learning disability as a prominent symptom. NF1 is one such disease. NF1 is diagnosed by the presence of a combination of symptoms in multiple organ systems. As a model of learning disabilities, NF1 provides an important advantage as it is caused by mutations to a single known gene. Importantly, it is associated with a very high frequency of learning disabilities (30–80%) and a low frequency of mental retardation (6–8% compared with 4% in the general population).

This wide range of estimated learning disability is due in part to studies using differing definitions of a learning disorder, as well as use of small groups without appropriate controls.[6,7] It is important to note that patients with NF1 do not show pronounced deficits on IQ tests and other neuropsychological measures sensitive to overall cognitive impairment.[8] Although specific, learning disabilities and cognitive impairments in patients with NF1 do limit their academic and social gains, sometimes quite severely.

In NF1 patients, impairments greater than predicted based on IQ are seen in four main cognitive areas: visuospatial function, executive function and planning, attention, and reading/vocabulary.[9] NF1 has been historically associated with deficits in visuospatial skills. Several studies have found consistent deficits in the Judgment of Line Orientation (JLO) test in this patient population. However, JLO requires more than just visuospatial skills. Recent studies have demonstrated that the pattern of learning and cognitive deficits in patients with NF1 is more complex than those detected by JLO, and that it includes visuospatial organization, motor abilities, and social skills. Most notably, NF1 is associated with robust deficits in tests of visuospatial functioning and impaired performance in spatial learning tests.[7,8] Also, patients with NF1 demonstrate deficits in organizational skills and planning. Further, they have notable social problems, related to impairments in attention and perception of social cues.[6,7]

In addition, NF1 patients demonstrate language-based learning problems. Patients with NF1 have deficits in expressive and receptive language, vocabulary, visual naming, and phonologic awareness. In fact, reading and spelling are repeatedly found to be impaired more severely than predicted by IQ in NF1.[9] Consistent with these impairments in language-based learning, NF1 patients show poorer academic achievement in reading and writing, compared to their unaffected siblings. However, in NF1 patients, there appears to be no discrepancy between verbal IQ and performance IQ.[6] Hence, performance-related impairments and motor coordination problems are also common in NF1.

The pattern of learning disabilities seen in NF1, as it is the case with other disorders, does not fall cleanly into one of the DSM-IV defined categories. Instead, the occurrence of multiple types of learning problems suggests that NF1 impairs a fundamental learning process.

NF1 AND ADHD

In addition to learning disabilities, deficits in other behavioral and cognitive domains can limit academic and social achievement in patients with NF1. This has been highlighted by studies showing that up to 40% of children with NF1, who were identified as academic underachievers, were nevertheless normal on neuropsychological tests for learning disabilities.[8] In such cases, underachievement may be caused by deficits in attention, planning, and organization skills,[7-9] which are consistently seen in NF1 patients.

There is a high co-morbidity between NF1 and attention deficit disorder. Studies have reported incidence rates of 30–50% of attention deficits in NF1 populations,[9-11] an occurrence three times more frequent than that observed in unaffected siblings.[9] Attention deficit in NF1 has been found at early ages and persists throughout adulthood. The inattentive subtype of ADHD is most frequently present in NF1 patients, followed by the combined subtype.[9] The effects of attention deficit in children with NF1 are quite broad, and they may affect both academic and social learning. Children with NF1 tend to have social problems and appear socially awkward and withdrawn, in comparison to their siblings and to children with other chronic, life-threatening illnesses.[12] Parents commonly complain that their children with NF1 are unable to engage in successful peer relationships.[8] Some evidence suggests that social deficits are related to poor interpersonal skills, which may occur as a result of decreased attention to social cues. When social skills are assessed using the Social Skills Rating System, children with ADHD and NF1 have the poorest outcomes compared to children with NF1 alone or with NF1 and learning disabilities.[12,13] Among the many symptoms associated with NF1, co-morbid attention deficit disorder in NF1 is increasingly recognized as having dramatic and important effects on quality of life for affected individuals.[i]

OTHER NF1 PHENOTYPES

Aside from the cognitive and behavioral phenotypes, NF1 is associated with a myriad of symptoms affecting multiple organ systems, including tumors, bone changes, and cardiovascular problems. The *NF1* gene codes for a tumor suppressor and therefore, loss of the wild-type *NF1* allele in a variety of cell types results in tumor formation.[14] Benign nervous system tumors such as neurofibromas and gliomas are frequent in NF1. Some other tumors associated with NF1 are pheochromocytomas, gastrointestinal stromal tumors, non-ossifying fibromas of bone, and glomus tumors of the finger tips. Malignancies seen at increased frequency in NF1 include peripheral nerve sheath tumors, glioblastoma multiforme, rhabdomyosarcoma, and juvenile myelomonocytic leukemia.[15] Abnormalities of melanocyte proliferation are virtually always present and result in café-au-lait spots, skin fold freckling, and iris hamartomas (Lisch nodules).[16]

The skeletal phenotype in NF1 is characterized by mild short stature, osteopenia, and pectus excavatum. In some patients a local bone dysplasia can result in severe scoliosis, sphenoid bone dysplasia, or pseudarthrosis.[17]*NF1* mutations also affect the cardiovascular and cerebrovascular system resulting in an increased frequency of congenital pulmonic valve stenosis, essential hypertension, renal artery stenosis, and cerebrovascular malformations.[18,19] Several growth, cardiovascular, cognitive, cutaneous, and facial characteristics of NF1 are similar to other conditions resulting from genetic abnormalities in the RAS-MAPKinase pathway such as LEOPARD syndrome (*PTPN11*), Noonan syndrome (*PTPN11, KRAS*), Cardio-facio-cutaneous syndrome (*BRAF, KRAS*), and Costello syndrome (*HRAS*). These conditions have been grouped under the name of "neuro-cardio-facial-cutaneous" (NCFC) syndromes.[20]

Neurofibromin, the protein product of the *NF1* gene, is a negative regulator of an important signal transduction pathway (RAS-MAP kinase pathway). The central role of this pathway in cellular function is reflected in the many different clinical problems

---

[i] For further discussion of learning disabilities, please refer to Tannock *et al.*, Perspectives on ADHD: An integrative assessment of the use of animal models for developing novel therapeutic agents and Bartz *et al.*, Preclinical animal models of autistic spectrum disorders (ASD) in Volume 1, Psychiatric Disorders.

that can be seen in individuals with NF1. Animal models of NF1 have provided extensive insight into the mechanisms by which changes in this pathway result in the clinical manifestations of NF1.

MODEL STUDIES OF NF1: DROSOPHILA AND MICE

Animal models of NF1-related learning disorders offer many advantages, including rapid testing of learning and memory behaviors in genetically well-defined organisms, with rigorous experimental controls. In addition to its effects on Ras, NF1 also controls adenylyl cyclase (AC) activity in both fruit flies and mammals.[21-23] A novel growth factor stimulated AC pathway that requires both NF1 and Ras has been recently identified in flies.[23] There are also at least two separate neurotransmitter activated G-protein dependent AC pathways in flies that are controlled by NF1.[23] NF1 acting via Gsα and the Rutabaga AC is required for olfactory learning in flies,[24] while the NF1/Ras pathway is necessary for long-term memory in flies.[25] Strikingly, separate domains of the NF1 protein control each pathway since the GAP domain alone is sufficient for long-term memory, while the C-terminal portion is essential for learning.[25] The fruit fly long-term memory task is equivalent to the mouse spatial learning task, since both require multiple rounds of training and are dependent on protein synthesis.[26,27] Both the Ras and the AC pathways are important for hippocampal-dependent spatial learning in mice.[28] Further, studies of spatial learning defects in *Nf1* heterozygous mice (*Nf1*±) show that pharmacologic or genetic manipulation of the Ras pathway can rescue learning in these mice.[29-32] Currently available therapeutics such as lovastatin, a cholesterol lowering agent, decrease Ras activity, and fully rescue the spatial learning defect in *Nf1*± mice.[32] The current statin clinical trials for learning disabilities associated with NF1 were directly stimulated by these most recent findings in mice.[32] Thus, animal models of NF1 have had a central role in therapeutic development for NF1.

ANATOMICAL CORRELATES OF LEARNING DISABILITIES AND COGNITIVE SYMPTOMS IN NF1

Converging evidence from both human and animal studies implicates the hippocampal, prefrontal, and cerebellar systems in the learning disabilities and cognitive problems associated with NF1. Learning and remembering new facts and general information about the world requires the hippocampus and surrounding medial temporal cortex.[33,34] Spatial learning tasks are known to depend on the hippocampus.[35,36] Damage to the hippocampus produces profound amnesia for spatial information and difficulties navigating through space. Also, patients with damage to this area often have considerable difficulty learning and retrieving new vocabulary words.[37] Although considerably milder than patients with lesions, the pattern of deficits in NF1 suggests that hippocampal-dependent domains are affected, such as spatial processing as well as reading comprehension and vocabulary learning in school. Learning disabilities associated with NF1, therefore, may be better understood by considering how NF1 affects hippocampus function, physiology, and ability to process information.

Data from human studies suggests that the prefrontal cortex also plays a critical role in many of the cognitive processes affected in NF1. Symptoms seen in NF1, such as increased impulsiveness, attention deficit, and difficulties with planning and behavioral organization, are commonly seen in syndromes involving prefrontal dysfunction.

Finally, NF1 patients display symptoms suggestive of cerebellar dysfunction. NF1 is associated with a variety of fine and gross motor function impairments, including problems with fine motor coordination, hypotonia and problems with balance and gait.[38-41] Half of the NF1 children seen at the Sophia's children hospital/Erasmus MC is scored "clumsy" on physical examination by a pediatric neurologist and almost 60% of these patients require physiotherapy.[42] There are several candidate brain regions that could play a role in the motor deficits in NF1, such as the premotor- and association areas, the primary motor cortex, the basal ganglia, and different sub-regions of the cerebellum.[43] The cerebellum is of special interest in NF1, since this region is critically involved in fine motor control. Although NF1 patients are not clearly ataxic, NF1-related hypotonia and clumsiness can very well arise from dysfunction of the vermis and/or intermediate zone of the cerebellum.[43] Moreover, the cerebellum is one of the predominant sites for NF1-related hyperintensities visible on T2-weighted MRI, which have been implicated in fine-motor problems.[44] To understand how NF1 affects hippocampal, prefrontal, and cerebellar circuits it is critical to understand how this protein modulates molecular and physiological function in these structures.

MOLECULAR MECHANISMS UNDERLYING THE COGNITIVE DEFICITS IN NF1

Studies in the mouse model of NF1 have revealed how changes in the NF1/ras pathway cause behavioral learning deficits associated with the disease. The NF1 mouse model (*Nf1* ± mouse) shows behavioral phenotypes in several cognitive domains affected by NF1 in patients. These phenotypes include impairments in spatial learning,[29] attention,[32] and possibly behavioral planning. Spatial learning and memory in mice requires experience-dependent plasticity in the hippocampus. During learning, synapses in the hippocampus undergo long-term potentiation (LTP), a persistent, activity-dependent increase in synaptic strength. *Nf1* ± mice have impaired hippocampal LTP, which very likely causes their spatial learning impairments in behavioral tasks. LTP deficits in the *Nf1* ± mice are caused by an abnormally high level of activity of the RAS/MAP Kinase pathway. The Nf1 gene product, neurofibromin, is a negative regulator of the ras signaling pathway.[45,46] Therefore, loss of neurofibromin function in NF1 leads to increased ras signaling.[32] LTP deficits can be rescued in the *Nf1* ± mice by manipulations which normalize the level of ras activity. These same manipulations also rescue behavioral impairments in spatial learning.[32,47]

Behavioral data from the *Nf1* ± mouse model also suggests that ras-dependent prefrontal dysfunction contributes to impairments in attention and planning. *Nf1* ± mice show impairments in behavioral tests of attention and planning which depend on prefrontal cortex. For example, the NF1 mouse shows impairments in the lateralized reaction time task, a test of visuospatial attention[32] developed from a task that is sensitive to lesions and manipulations of prefrontal function in humans.[48-50] Performance deficits of the $Nf1\pm$ mice in this task are also ras dependent, similarly to the spatial learning impairments,[32] since these deficits can be rescued by manipulations that decrease ras activity. Therefore, the $Nf1\pm$ mouse model demonstrates that both learning and attention deficits in NF1 are caused by increased ras activity.

Increased ras levels in the $Nf1\pm$ mouse cause an abnormal increase in inhibitory activity in the hippocampus.[47] This high level of inhibition disrupts activity-dependent plasticity in the hippocampus, causing the spatial learning impairments in the $Nf1\pm$ mice. Ras-dependent increases in activity of inhibitory networks may also occur in other brain areas where increased RAS activity is seen in NF1. This includes the prefrontal cortex, where increased RAS activity was shown in the $Nf1\pm$ mouse, and where balanced inhibition is thought to be critical for function. This may also be expected to include the cerebellum. Purkinje cells, which are the sole output of the cerebellar cortex, are GABA-ergic neurons, and among the highest neurofibromin expressing cells in the brain.[51,52] In prefrontal cortex and cerebellum, ras-dependent increases in inhibition offer a compelling potential mechanism by which NF1 deletion can disrupt the physiological function of these structures to cause multiple cognitive symptoms of NF1 such as attention, planning, and motor coordination impairments.

REVERSING THE MOLECULAR, PHYSIOLOGICAL AND COGNITIVE DEFICITS OF NF1 WITH STATINS

As stated above, the key pathophysiologic mechanism underlying multiple NF1 symptoms in both humans[53,54] and mice[47,55-57] is Nf1-dependent Ras/MAPK activity. Data from the mouse model of NF1 clearly place increased ras activity as central to cognitive symptoms of NF1 such as attention and learning deficits.[32,47] Therefore, therapeutic interventions designed to inhibit p21Ras function have been proposed as treatments for NF1.[58] Post-translational isoprenylation is required for the membrane localization and function of p21Ras, and isoprenylation provides a potential target for NF1 pharmacotherapy.[59] Indeed, pharmacologic inhibitors of farnesyltransferase downregulate p21Ras activity and can rescue physiological and spatial learning deficits associated with $Nf1\pm$ mice.[47] It is unknown, however, whether any of these inhibitors have the *in vivo* pharmacokinetics, biodistribution, and safety profile required for the long-term treatment of cognitive dysfunction in NF1.[60] Fortunately, other pharmacologic agents with better-established safety profiles, such as the statins, are also able to regulate p21Ras isoprenylation. Isoprenyl groups are synthesized during an intermediate step in cholesterol synthesis. Statins, cholesterol lowering agents widely prescribed to treat hyperlipidemia,[61] inhibit cholesterol synthesis by irreversibly blocking the rate-limiting enzyme in this process (HMG-CoA reductase). In this manner, statins are able to decrease the availability of isoprenyl groups and thus lower p21Ras isoprenylation.[62,63]

Lovastatin, a statin which passes the blood–brain barrier, was shown to inhibit the enhanced p21Ras-MAPK activity in the cortex and hippocampus of $Nf1\pm$ mice[32] at doses that do not seem to affect controls. In preclinical experiments using the mouse model of NF1, lovastatin was found to effectively reverse molecular, physiological, and behavioral impairments. Even a short 4-day treatment with lovastatin in adult

Nf1 ± mice normalized Ras activity and LTP at hippocampal synapses. Lovastatin treatment also rescued behavioral impairments, reversing both spatial learning and attention deficits.[32] These results, taken together with the fact that lovastatin is a widely prescribed drug that is known to be well-tolerated even in long-term treatments, make lovastatin a viable potential treatment option for cognitive deficits associated with NF1 in humans. These preclinical findings have spurred multi-center clinical trials examining the safety and efficacy of lovastatin treatment for cognitive symptoms in the NF1 patient population. This represents the first scientifically based pharmacological treatment for learning disabilities. Positive results could foment tests of this and perhaps other pharmacologic agents in other learning disabilities.

As with NF1, the evolving richness of the genetics and pharmacology of memory could be used to identify the molecular, cellular, systems, and cognitive mechanisms underlying learning disabilities. This would mark a paradigm shift for helping the 6% of children in public schools currently receiving help for their learning disabilities (about 2.8 million in 2002 in the USA alone).[64]

MEASURING EFFICACY IN STATIN CLINICAL TRIALS

In clinical trials designed to assess the effect of statins on cognition, it is of pivotal importance to use a carefully designed battery of tasks. These tasks should be sensitive, quantitative and have high test–retest reliability. These tasks should also address robust, core features and underlying mechanisms of the cognitive symptoms seen in patients. Also, it is important to include tests that closely reflect the cognitive domains that have already been shown to be responsive to statins in mice. Clinical trials designed in this way could provide sensitive and clearly interpretable results. In this design, disease mechanisms described in the NF1 mouse model guide the choice of both the therapeutic being tested (lovastatin) and the clinical endpoints being used to measure drug efficacy. Two experimental tests that can contribute to the available test battery are working memory and motor learning tests, both of which are developed to assess specific impairments that are found in NF1 patients and studied in animal models.

Prefrontal cortex dysfunction is thought to contribute to many of the cognitive symptoms seen in NF1 patients. Importantly, preclinical studies showed that lovastatin rescued prefrontal RAS/MAPK dysfunction, as well as deficits in attention in *Nf1* ± mice.[32] Therefore, clinical trials could utilize tasks, such as working memory tasks, which are known to require prefrontal function and have been shown to be sensitive to prefrontal impairment in other disease states.[65,66] Performance in specific working memory tasks reflects prefrontal cortex engagement and function.[67] A battery of such working memory tasks has been designed to isolate two distinct facets of working memory, maintenance and manipulation. Working memory maintenance can be tested by asking subjects to mentally maintain the spatial location of several items (1–7) in memory over a short time. Manipulation of information in working memory can be tested by asking subjects to mentally flip the spatial items over a horizontal line. Such tasks should be paired with an equivalent verbal task to explore whether any observed deficit is specific to spatial encoding. By changing the number of items presented, these tasks allow working memory load to be parametrically varied, ensuring that even minor behavioral deficit can be detected.[65-67]

This battery of tasks isolates specific processes of working memory, while retaining the sensitivity to reveal small changes in working memory ability associated with drug treatment. In a clinical trial, the sensitivity of these measures is critical given that the drug dose being tested may not have been optimized and so treatment-related improvements may be relatively small. Such working memory tests can be included in a clinical trial as one measure of the efficacy of lovastatin in improving prefrontal-related cognitive symptoms in NF1.

Since motor skills are impaired in NF1 patients, adding a parameter of motor functioning is important when assessing the effect of statins in NF1. In addition to tests for fine motor skills, such as the Beery Visual Motor Integration test, functional integrity, and plasticity in the brain areas involved in motor skills can be assessed by testing adaptation of motor skills (i.e., motor learning).

One motor learning test that could be applied to this purpose is the prism adaptation test, a quantitative, easy and quick way to measure the adaptation of eye–hand movements to visual displacement of the environment by prism glasses. Prism adaptation is thought to be dependent not only on plasticity in the anterior and caudal posterior lobe of the cerebellar cortex, but also on plasticity in various other motor areas.[68,69] Since prism adaptation can be rapidly learned, well-quantified and is not sensitive to a placebo or test–retest effect it is ideal measures to include in the assessment of drugs that potentially improve brain function.

THE ROLE OF PATIENT ORGANIZATIONS IN STUDIES OF LEARNING DISABILITIES

The child with NF1 is at risk for physically devastating and potentially life-threatening neurological tumors, bone deformities, and an array of other complications. It is unpredictable if and when these might appear, and there are still no effective NF1 drugs. For many parents, however, one of the first (and for many, the most distressful) issues they confront after NF1 diagnosis is being told their child may "struggle in school". Again unpredictable, this may range from mild to severe. Fortunately, there are organizations such as the Children's Tumor Foundation and NF Inc. that offer support networks and information, such as the location of NF clinics and the medical resources patients need. These networks of support are a very important and effective way to organize and empower patients, and to provide the support they need in dealing with the significant life-changing problems associated with NF1. Patient organizations are also having an increasingly active role in all aspects of research and development. They are an important source of motivation and inspiration for scientists working in the area. They often provide much needed pilot resources that allow laboratories to venture into a particular area of research, and they facilitate the process of translating basic laboratory findings into clinical trials. Patient organizations have also had important roles in lobbying governmental organizations and obtaining the required support for research. In this respect, these organizations can also have a critical role in facilitating the complex process of drug development and implementation of new treatments.

It is critical that patient organizations are active participants in the complex, tortuous and often lengthy process of developing treatments for disorders as complex as learning disabilities. NF1 is a wonderful example of how the involvement and commitment of families of affected individuals can have an enormous impact on research and development.

FINDINGS FROM STUDIES OF NF1: IMPLICATION TO LEARNING DISABILITIES

Most learning disabilities have no known etiology or treatment and they can impact every aspect of an individual's life. The emerging biology of learning and memory – which spans molecular, cellular, systems, and behavioral findings – promises to revolutionize the study and treatment of learning disabilities. These studies have uncovered a number of molecular, cellular, and systems mechanisms that could account for the cognitive profiles observed in learning-disabled patients. Specific ion channels, neurotransmitters, receptor complexes, signal transduction mechanisms, transcription factors, and genes, have become part of the fast evolving molecular puzzle of memory.[70] Furthermore, environmental influences add complexity to this tantalizing puzzle. It is very likely that genes primarily responsible for one learning disability may also contribute to natural variation of the phenotype in another learning disability. Additionally, genes that affect any one aspect of a learning disability may also have an impact on other phenotypes associated with the disability, or could even contribute or exacerbate other neurological or psychiatric disorders.

There is a considerable amount of insight into the molecular mechanisms disrupted by NF1 mutations and these have been instrumental in unraveling both the cause of the disorder and in developing treatments. Furthermore, studies of the NF1 learning and memory deficits have revealed the involvement of mechanisms previously uncovered in more general studies of learning and memory. Thus, the emerging biology of learning and memory is useful in understanding the underlying causes of learning disabilities, and the study of these disorders also promises to be broadly relevant to other learning disabilities and to our understanding of normal learning and memory.

GENETIC AND PHARMACOLOGICAL MANIPULATIONS THAT ENHANCE LEARNING AND MEMORY: AN ALTERNATIVE STRATEGY

Current understanding of the neurobiology of learning can also be used to devise strategies for cognitive enhancement which would not require identification of underlying disease causing mechanisms. This approach is important since the majority of learning-disabled individuals are not part of clearly identified groups, and their disorders do not have known etiologies. Such general enhancement strategies may be valuable not only for learning disabilities but also in other disorders associated with cognitive dysfunction, particularly those of heterogeneous or undefined etiology. For example, genetic analysis has shown that schizophrenia[71] and depression[72] are heterogeneous conditions, each caused by the cumulative effects of numerous mutations and many incompletely understood developmental and environmental factors. In such cases, as in many learning disability subcategories, it is unclear which single mechanism or molecular pathway should be targeted for pharmacotherapy. Thus, in developing therapeutics for such disorders, it is worthwhile to consider strategies to improve cognitive function which could be used irrespective of detailed knowledge of the underlying pathophysiology. It is important to note that the FDA has already approved a number of drugs that are thought to enhance cognitive function, including donepezil (Aricept®), rivastigmine tartrate (Exelon®), galantamine HBr (Razadyne®), memantine (Namenda®), and modafinil (Provigil®).[73] These and other compounds could be tested for their usefulness in treating learning disabilities.

Molecular and cellular studies into cognitive enhancements may identify additional targets for therapeutics aimed at potentiating learning processes to compensate for the disruptive effects of disease causing mutations. Enhancing the strength of induction of learning processes may compensate for downstream deficits. Alternatively, enhancing the sensitivity of the final molecular events in synaptic plasticity and learning may be able to compensate for disease-related impairments in induction.

Currently, there is considerable evidence for animal models with dramatic cognitive enhancements.[28] In several of these animal models, genetic and pharmacological manipulations that enhance induction of LTP also facilitate behavioral learning and memory.[28] The over-expression of genes known to be required for LTP induction can result in enhancements in LTP and learning. For example, activation and opening of the NMDA receptor (NMDAR) is a critical initial step in the induction of LTP. The transgenic over-expression of the NMDAR subunit 2B enhances the opening time of the NMDAR. Such transgenic mice show enhancements in LTP and several forms of behavioral learning.[74] Further, the mutation of negative regulators of LTP induction can also lead to learning enhancements. The nociceptin receptor normally acts as a negative regulator of LTP induction. Mice carrying inactivating mutations of nociceptin show increased hippocampal LTP as well as improved spatial learning and memory.[75]

Learning enhancements are also seen in mice with genetic manipulations of downstream effectors of LTP. Tissue plasminogen activator (TPA) is an extracellular protease that is thought to be involved in synaptic remodeling triggered by plasticity and learning. Such synaptic remodeling is thought to maintain learning in a neuronal network. Transgenic over-expression of TPA enhances LTP expression and behavioral learning.[76] In contrast, a null mutation of this gene impairs these two phenomena.[77] Thus, molecules such as TPA may modulate the downstream processes involved in expression and maintenance of synaptic plasticity. Such molecules may represent a potential molecular target which can enhance the ability of even impaired learning processes to become effectively encoded.

The list of known memory-enhancing mutations is by no means limited to the examples presented. Other genetic manipulations which enhanced LTP and learning targeted pre-synaptic Growth Associated Protein 43,[78] adenylyl cyclase,[79] telencephalon-specific cell adhesion molecule,[80] calcineurin, Rim 1 (a ras effector), and forebrain H-ras^{G12V}.[81] Finding common molecular, cellular, and systems changes underlying the learning and memory enhancements in this diverse collection of mutants may be especially informative for developing future approaches to identifying novel therapeutics for learning disabilities.

REFERENCES

1. Kronenberger, W.G. and Dunn, D.W. (2003). Learning disorders. *Neurol Clin*, 21(4):941–952.
2. Palumbo, D. and Lynch, P.A. (2006). Psychological testing in adolescent medicine. *Adolesc Med Clin*, 17(1):147–164.
3. Wechsler, D. (ed.) (2001). *Wechsler Individual Achievement Test*, 2nd edition. The Psychological Corporation, San Antonio, TX.
4. Kelly, D.P. (2004). Chapter 29: Neurodevelopmental dysfunction in the school-aged child. In Behrman (ed.) *Nelson Textbook of Pediatrics*, 17th edition. Saunders, An Imprint of Elsevier.
5. Tramontana, M.G. (2006). Section 5, Chapter 38: Disorders usually presenting in middle childhood (6–11 years) or adolescence (12–18 years). In Michael, P.T.L., Ebert, H. and N. Barry (eds.), *Current Diagnosis and Treatment in Psychiatry*.
6. North, K.N. *et al.* (1997). Cognitive function and academic performance in neurofibromatosis. 1: consensus statement from the NF1 Cognitive Disorders Task Force. *Neurology*, 48(4):1121–1127.
7. North, K. (2000). Neurofibromatosis type 1. *Am J Med Genet*, 97(2):119–127.
8. Kayl, A.E. and Moore, B.D. (2000). 3rd, Behavioral phenotype of neurofibromatosis, type 1. *Ment Retard Dev Disabil Res Rev*, 6(2):117–124.
9. Hyman, S.L., Shores, A., and North, K.N. (2005). The nature and frequency of cognitive deficits in children with neurofibromatosis type 1. *Neurology*, 65(7):1037–1044.
10. Mautner, V.F. *et al.* (2002). Treatment of ADHD in neurofibromatosis type 1. *Dev Med Child Neurol*, 44(3):164–170.
11. Hofman, K.J. *et al.* (1994). Neurofibromatosis type 1: The cognitive phenotype. *J Pediatr*, 124(4):S1–S8.
12. Barton, B. and North, K. (2004). Social skills of children with neurofibromatosis type 1. *Dev Med Child Neurol*, 46(8):553–563.
13. Barton, B. and North, K. (2007). The self-concept of children and adolescents with neurofibromatosis type 1. *Child Care Health Dev*, 33(4):401–408.
14. Legius, E. *et al.* (1993). Somatic deletion of the neurofibromatosis type 1 gene in a neurofibrosarcoma supports a tumour suppressor gene hypothesis. *Nat Genet*, 3(2):122–126.
15. Arun, D. and Gutmann, D.H. (2004). Recent advances in neurofibromatosis type 1. *Curr Opin Neurol*, 17(2):101–105.
16. De Schepper, S. *et al.* (2005). Pigment cell-related manifestations in neurofibromatosis type 1: An overview. *Pigment Cell Res*, 18(1):13–24.
17. Wu, X. *et al.* (2006). Neurofibromin plays a critical role in modulating osteoblast differentiation of mesenchymal stem/progenitor cells. *Hum Mol Genet*, 15(19):2837–2845.
18. Friedman, J.M. *et al.* (2002). Cardiovascular disease in neurofibromatosis 1: Report of the NF1 Cardiovascular Task Force. *Genet Med*, 4(3):105–111.
19. Rosser, T.L., Vezina, G., and Packer, R.J. (2005). Cerebrovascular abnormalities in a population of children with neurofibromatosis type 1. *Neurology*, 64(3):553–555.
20. Bentires-Alj, M., Kontaridis, M.I., and Neel, B.G. (2006). Stops along the RAS pathway in human genetic disease. *Nat Med*, 12(3):283–285.
21. Tong, J. *et al.* (2002). Neurofibromin regulates G protein-stimulated adenylyl cyclase activity. *Nat Neurosci*, 5(2):95–96.
22. Dasgupta, B., Dugan, L.L., and Gutmann, D.H. (2003). The neurofibromatosis 1 gene product neurofibromin regulates pituitary adenylate cyclase-activating polypeptide-mediated signaling in astrocytes. *J Neurosci*, 23(26):8949–8954.
23. Hannan, F. *et al.* (2006). Effect of neurofibromatosis type I mutations on a novel pathway for adenylyl cyclase activation requiring neurofibromin and Ras. *Hum Mol Genet*, 15(7):1087–1098.

24. Guo, H.F. *et al.* (2000). A neurofibromatosis-1-regulated pathway is required for learning in Drosophila. *Nature*, 403(6772):895–898.
25. Ho, I.S. *et al.* (2007). Distinct functional domains of neurofibromatosis type 1 regulate immediate versus long-term memory formation. *J Neurosci*, 27(25):6852–6857.
26. Meiri, N. and Rosenblum, K. (1998). Lateral ventricle injection of the protein synthesis inhibitor anisomycin impairs long-term memory in a spatial memory task. *Brain Res*, 789(1):48–55.
27. Tully, T. *et al.* (1994). Genetic dissection of consolidated memory in Drosophila. *Cell*, 79(1):35–47.
28. Silva, A.J. (2003). Molecular and cellular cognitive studies of the role of synaptic plasticity in memory. *J Neurobiol*, 54(1):224–237.
29. Silva, A.J. *et al.* (1997). A mouse model for the learning and memory deficits associated with neurofibromatosis type I. *Nat Genet*, 15(3):281–284.
30. Costa, R.M. *et al.* (2001). Learning deficits, but normal development and tumor predisposition, in mice lacking exon 23a of Nf1. *Nat Genet*, 27(4):399–405.
31. Costa, R.M. and Silva, A.J. (2002). Molecular and cellular mechanisms underlying the cognitive deficits associated with neurofibromatosis 1. *J Child Neurol*, 17(8):622–626. discussion 627-9, 646-51
32. Li, W. *et al.* (2005). The HMG-CoA reductase inhibitor lovastatin reverses the learning and attention deficits in a mouse model of neurofibromatosis type 1. *Curr Biol*, 15(21):1961–1967.
33. Bayley, P.J. and Squire, L.R. (2005). Failure to acquire new semantic knowledge in patients with large medial temporal lobe lesions. *Hippocampus*, 15(2):273–280.
34. Schmolck, H. *et al.* (2002). Semantic knowledge in patient H.M. and other patients with bilateral medial and lateral temporal lobe lesions. *Hippocampus*, 12(4):520–533.
35. Burgess, N., Maguire, E.A., and O'Keefe, J. (2002). The human hippocampus and spatial and episodic memory. *Neuron*, 35(4):625–641.
36. Squire, L.R., Stark, C.E., and Clark, R.E. (2004). The medial temporal lobe. *Annu Rev Neurosci*, 27:279–306.
37. Verfaellie, M., Koseff, P., and Alexander, M.P. (2000). Acquisition of novel semantic information in amnesia: Effects of lesion location. *Neuropsychologia*, 38(4):484–492.
38. North, K. *et al.* (1994). Specific learning disability in children with neurofibromatosis type 1: Significance of MRI abnormalities. *Neurology*, 44(5):878–883.
39. Chapman, C.A. *et al.* (1996). Neurobehavioral profiles of children with neurofibromatosis 1 referred for learning disabilities are sex-specific. *Am J Med Genet*, 67(2):127–132.
40. Brewer, V.R., Moore, B.D., 3rd, and Hiscock, M. (1997). Learning disability subtypes in children with neurofibromatosis. *J Learn Disabil*, 30(5):521–533.
41. Korf, B.R. (2002). Clinical features and pathobiology of neurofibromatosis 1. *J Child Neurol*, 17(8):573–577. discussion 602-4, 646-51
42. Cnossen, M.H. *et al.* (1998). A prospective 10 year follow up study of patients with neurofibromatosis type 1. *Arch Dis Child*, 78(5):408–412.
43. Gazzaniga, M.S., Irvy, R., and Mangun, G.R. (1998). *Cognitive Neuroscience - The Biology of the Mind*. W.W. Norton & Company, Chapter 10.
44. Feldmann, R. *et al.* (2003). Neurofibromatosis type 1: Motor and cognitive function and T2-weighted MRI hyperintensities. *Neurology*, 61(12):1725–1728.
45. Xu, G.F. *et al.* (1990). The catalytic domain of the neurofibromatosis type 1 gene product stimulates ras GTPase and complements ira mutants of S. cerevisiae. *Cell*, 63(4):835–841.
46. Ballester, R. *et al.* (1990). The NF1 locus encodes a protein functionally related to mammalian GAP and yeast IRA proteins. *Cell*, 63(4):851–859.

47. Costa, R.M. *et al.* (2002). Mechanism for the learning deficits in a mouse model of neurofibromatosis type 1. *Nature*, 415(6871):526-530.

48. Maddux, J.M. *et al.* (2007). Dissociation of attention in learning and action: Effects of lesions of the amygdala central nucleus, medial prefrontal cortex, and posterior parietal cortex. *Behav Neurosci*, 121(1):63-79.

49. Fletcher, P.J. *et al.* (2007). A sensitizing regimen of amphetamine impairs visual attention in the 5-choice serial reaction time test: reversal by a d1 receptor agonist injected into the medial prefrontal cortex. *Neuropsychopharmacology*, 32(5):1122-1132.

50. Christakou, A., Robbins, T.W., and Everitt, B.J. (2005). Prolonged neglect following unilateral disruption of a prefrontal cortical-dorsal striatal system. *Eur J Neurosci*, 21(3):782-792.

51. Nordlund, M.L. *et al.* (1995). Neurofibromin expression and astrogliosis in neurofibromatosis (type 1) brains. *J Neuropathol Exp Neurol*, 54(4):588-600.

52. Gutmann, D.H. *et al.* (1995). Expression of the neurofibromatosis 1 (NF1) isoforms in developing and adult rat tissues. *Cell Growth Differ*, 6(3):315-323.

53. Basu, T.N. *et al.* (1992). Aberrant regulation of ras proteins in malignant tumour cells from type 1 neurofibromatosis patients. *Nature*, 356(6371):713-715.

54. DeClue, J.E. *et al.* (1992). Abnormal regulation of mammalian p21ras contributes to malignant tumor growth in von Recklinghausen (type 1) neurofibromatosis. *Cell*, 69(2):265-273.

55. Costa, R.M. *et al.* (2001). Learning deficits, but normal development and tumor predisposition, in mice lacking exon 23a of Nf1. *Nat Genet*, 27(4):399-405.

56. Brannan, C.I. *et al.* (1994). Targeted disruption of the neurofibromatosis type-1 gene leads to developmental abnormalities in heart and various neural crest-derived tissues. *Genes Dev*, 8(9):1019-1029.

57. Jacks, T. *et al.* (1994). Tumour predisposition in mice heterozygous for a targeted mutation in Nf1. *Nat Genet*, 7(3):353-361.

58. Weiss, B., Bollag, G., and Shannon, K. (1999). Hyperactive Ras as a therapeutic target in neurofibromatosis type 1. *Am J Med Genet*, 89(1):14-22.

59. Yan, N. *et al.* (1995). Farnesyltransferase inhibitors block the neurofibromatosis type I (NF1) malignant phenotype. *Cancer Res*, 55(16):3569-3575.

60. Mazieres, J., Pradines, A., and Favre, G. (2004). Perspectives on farnesyl transferase inhibitors in cancer therapy. *Cancer Lett*, 206(2):159-167.

61. Corvol, J.C. *et al.* (2003). Differential effects of lipid-lowering therapies on stroke prevention: A meta-analysis of randomized trials. *Arch Intern Med*, 163(6):669-676.

62. Mendola, C.E. and Backer, J.M. (1990). Lovastatin blocks N-ras oncogene-induced neuronal differentiation. *Cell Growth Differ*, 1(10):499-502.

63. Sebti, S.M., Tkalcevic, G.T., and Jani, J.P. (1991). Lovastatin, a cholesterol biosynthesis inhibitor, inhibits the growth of human H-ras oncogene transformed cells in nude mice. *Cancer Commun*, 3(5):141-147.

64. NCLD. *LD basics and fast facts*. 2002 cited; Available from: http://ncld.org/info/index.cfm.

65. Cannon, T.D. *et al.* (2005). Dorsolateral prefrontal cortex activity during maintenance and manipulation of information in working memory in patients with schizophrenia. *Arch Gen Psychiatry*, 62(10):1071-1080.

66. Karlsgodt, K.H. *et al.* (2007). The relationship between performance and fMRI signal during working memory in patients with schizophrenia, unaffected co-twins, and control subjects. *Schizophr Res*, 89(1-3):191-197.

67. Glahn, D.C. *et al.* (2002). Maintenance and manipulation in spatial working memory: Dissociations in the prefrontal cortex. *Neuroimage*, 17(1):201-213.

68. Baizer, J.S., Kralj-Hans, I., and Glickstein, M. (1999). Cerebellar lesions and prism adaptation in macaque monkeys. *J Neurophysiol*, 81(4):1960-1965.

69. Pisella, L. *et al.* (2005). Ipsidirectional impairment of prism adaptation after unilateral lesion of anterior cerebellum. *Neurology*, 65(1):150–152.

70. Weeber, E.J. and Sweatt, J.D. (2002). Molecular neurobiology of human cognition. *Neuron*, 33(6):845–848.

71. Harrison, P.J. and Weinberger, D.R. (2005). Schizophrenia genes, gene expression, and neuropathology: On the matter of their convergence. *Mol Psychiatry*, 10(1):40–68. image 5

72. Lesch, K.P. (2004). Gene-environment interaction and the genetics of depression. *J Psychiatry Neurosci*, 29(3):174–184.

73. Mehlman, M.J. (2004). Cognition-enhancing drugs. *Milbank Q*, 82(3):483–506. table of contents

74. Tang, Y.P. *et al.* (1999). Genetic enhancement of learning and memory in mice. *Nature*, 401(6748):63–69.

75. Manabe, T. *et al.* (1998). Facilitation of long-term potentiation and memory in mice lacking nociceptin receptors. *Nature*, 394(6693):577–581.

76. Madani, R. *et al.* (1999). Enhanced hippocampal long-term potentiation and learning by increased neuronal expression of tissue-type plasminogen activator in transgenic mice. *EMBO J.*, 18(11):3007–3012.

77. Huang, Y.Y. *et al.* (1996). Mice lacking the gene encoding tissue-type plasminogen activator show a selective interference with late-phase long-term potentiation in both Schaffer collateral and mossy fiber pathways. *Proc Natl Acad Sci USA*, 93(16):8699–8704.

78. Routtenberg, A. *et al.* (2000). Enhanced learning after genetic overexpression of a brain growth protein. *Proc Natl Acad Sci USA*, 97(13):7657–7662.

79. Wang, H. *et al.* (2004). Overexpression of type-1 adenylyl cyclase in mouse forebrain enhances recognition memory and LTP. *Nat Neurosci*, 7(6):635–642.

80. Nakamura, K. *et al.* (2001). Enhancement of hippocampal LTP, reference memory and sensorimotor gating in mutant mice lacking a telencephalon-specific cell adhesion molecule. *Eur J Neurosci*, 13(1):179–189.

81. Kushner, S.A. *et al.* (2005). Modulation of presynaptic plasticity and learning by the H-ras/extracellular signal-regulated kinase/synapsin I signaling pathway. *J Neurosci*, 25(42):9721–9734.

Development, Optimization and Use of Preclinical Behavioral Models to Maximize the Productivity of Drug Discovery for Alzheimer's Disease

Mark D. Lindner[1], Robert A. McArthur[1], Sam A. Deadwyler[2], Robert E. Hampson[2], and Pierre N. Tariot[3]

[1]McArthur and Associates GmbH, Basel, Switzerland
[2]Department of Physiology and Pharmacology, Wake Forest University School of Medicine, Medical Center Boulevard, Winston Salem, NC, USA
[3]Memory Disorders Center, Banner Alzheimer's Institute, Phoenix, AZ, USA

Animal and Translational Models for CNS Drug Discovery,
Vol. 2 of 3: Neurological Disorders
Robert McArthur and Franco Borsini (eds), Academic Press, 2008

INTRODUCTION

In the United States alone 2–4 million people have Alzheimer's disease (AD), at a cost of more than $100 billion per year, and as the population ages, it is expected that the size of this patient population and associated costs will increase 3–4 times over by the year 2050 (for review,[1]). In addition to the costs of the disease to society, considerable public and private resources have also been devoted to study and develop new therapeutics for AD, which is characterized by molecular and neuropathological features, and a clinical phenotype that includes loss of cognitive function – especially memory, loss of overall functional capacity, and erosion of personality.

Currently available treatments for AD provide only modest symptomatic relief, they do not stop disease progression, and despite government initiatives and a concerted effort from the pharmaceutical industry and academia to produce drugs that are more efficacious for the treatment of this disorder, some have argued that many of the treatments under development are not very innovative and may not be any more effective than existing treatments.[2] Furthermore, even after 12–15 years of research, at a total cost of 0.8–1.6 billion US dollars,[3-7] the final results of Phase III trials often show that potential new treatments are not effective. In fact, despite evidence of potential efficacy in the preclinical models, lack of efficacy is the single biggest reason why drugs fail in clinical trials.[8-11] The acknowledged limitations of existing pharmacological treatments for AD, combined with the lack of progress in discovering and developing new drugs, the apparent lack of predictive validity of the preclinical models, the lack of creativity and innovation and other inefficiencies in the system, all contribute to a growing sense of urgency among all stakeholders, including patients and investors, who are beginning to demand that the field find more effective and efficient ways to develop novel treatments for AD.

The objective of this chapter is to examine how preclinical behavioral models can be developed, validated, and used, in order to maximize their predictive validity and improve the productivity of the drug discovery process. It is written from the perspective of translational research, which involves interactions between scientists in academia and the biotech/pharmaceutical industry, working together with clinical scientists, to identify and validate the most appropriate models and endpoints in animals and humans, by which efficacy can be predicted and confirmed. It is our belief that such a collaborative, integrated, translational approach, is both useful and necessary in order to be able to predict more accurately which treatments will ultimately prove to be truly effective, based on the results of preclinical models and early clinical trials.

AD: CLINICAL PRESENTATION

Virtually every aspect of a person's life is affected by AD, but with considerable variability in the pattern of its effects from one individual to another. Despite the heterogeneity of the effects of AD within and across individuals, it is possible to categorize them using three overlapping and somewhat arbitrary conceptual domains (see Table 4.1): cognition, daily functioning, and potential neuropsychiatric issues. Cognitive deficits are usually evident early on and include: impairments in learning and memory, attention, language in all of its aspects (speaking, understanding speech, reading, and writing), naming or object recognition, orientation to space and time, visuospatial function, praxis, and executive function (the ability to respond to information in the environment and execute a logical plan). Initially, cognitive impairment leads to the loss of complex (or instrumental) functions, but as the disease progresses, more basic functional abilities are also ultimately affected. There is also a nearly 100% lifetime risk of significant psychopathological features at some point in the illness.[12]

Table 4.1 Conceptual domains affected in AD

Cognitive functions
Memory, attention, language, orientation, visuospatial function, praxis, executive function

Daily functioning
Instrumental: Driving, finances, work, shopping, cooking, household management, communication
Basic: Dressing, hygiene, toileting, feeding, ambulation

Neuropsychiatric issues
Apathy, anxiety, depression, psychosis, agitation

TARGETS AND COMPOUNDS IN THE CLINIC: FAILED, APPROVED, AND UNDER DEVELOPMENT

Although there are a number of different components of AD-related pathology, classical "symptomatic" treatment approaches and preclinical paradigms have typically addressed only a limited part of the entire phenotype, primarily improving cognition or ameliorating cognitive decline. "Disease-modifying" treatments, on the other hand, focus on slowing or arresting the underlying disease processes, which would presumably be more effective at attenuating deficits across all of the functional domains. Any of the AD-related cognitive, functional, and psychiatric deficits could at least be attenuated by either "symptomatic" or "disease-modifying" therapies, but for the purposes of this chapter, we will focus on models and treatments for the dementia and cognitive components of the disease.

The "symptomatic" treatment of AD was driven initially by the cholinergic hypothesis of AD, which integrates the clinical and basic research observations that (a) changes in brain cholinergic parameters such as acetylcholinesterase (AChE) or choline acetyltransferase (ChAT) activity is reduced in AD patients, (b) pharmacological antagonists or lesions of the cholinergic systems of the brain lead to amnesia in both humans and animals, and (c) that AChE inhibitors (AChEIs) such as tacrine (Cognex®) or donepezil (Aricept®) can ameliorate cognitive decline in patients with AD.[13,14] Indeed, AChEIs have become the pharmacological "gold standards" of AD treatment by which clinical efficacy of novel compounds are judged. However, relief of cognitive impairment by AChEIs is modest, on average, and cognitive and functional decline continue despite ongoing therapy.[15] The introduction of memantine, a glutameric NMDA receptor antagonist,[16] has augmented the pharmacological armamentarium, but there is still a need for additional treatment options to preserve or improve cognitive function, as well as to derail the neurodegenerative process.

Just as the cholinergic hypothesis has provided a productive theoretical framework for the discovery and development of symptomatic treatments for AD, the amyloid cascade hypothesis has served an equivalent role for several pharmacological and biological disease-modifying approaches to the neurodegenerative aspects of this disease.[17,18] Faulty processing of the amyloid precursor protein (APP), leading to the production and accumulation of amyloid products such as $A\beta_{42}$ and soluble oligomeric species in the brain, followed by the development of amyloid plaques, is one of the neurological hallmarks of AD.[19,20] Considerable effort has been devoted to understanding the mechanisms by which faulty APP processing occurs, and how novel treatments could be developed to intervene at this point of the disease,[21-23] with the expectation that the neurodegenerative process might be arrested by early inhibition of amyloid production. As a corollary of this therapeutic approach are attempts to reduce the existing amyloid burden in Alzheimer's patients' brains through the disruption of amyloid plaques and the clearance of amyloid pharmacologically, or through recruitment of natural immune systems and antibody-mediated amyloid clearance.[24,25] Of particular note have been the anti-amyloid immunization trials initiated by Elan.[26,27] Despite the appearance of meningoencephalitis in a number of patients,[28,29] this approach is still being actively pursued.[30]

In addition to the presence of amyloid deposits in the Alzheimer's brain, this disease is also characterized by the presence of neurofibrillary tangles that are thought to result in part from hyperphosphorylation of tau protein, leading to insoluble paired helical filaments and unstable microtubule formation in neurons, and eventual loss of neuronal function.[31] These observations and others have led to the formation of the Tau hypothesis of AD and other axonal transport neurodegenerative diseases.[32,33] Notwithstanding the emphasis that has been placed on amyloid for the past 10–15 years, it is clear that renewed interest in tau is lending new impetus to this therapeutic approach;[34] although it should be stated that the actual relationship of either amyloid or hyperphosphorylated tau and subsequent neurotoxicity and cognitive decline, has yet to be fully understood.

Since the introduction of the first cholinergic treatment of AD, tacrine, there have been many drug candidates introduced as potential symptomatic treatments for AD which have failed, or whose development has been curtailed or abandoned. This attrition can best be described by the data illustrated in Figure 4.1, which is a compendium of drugs that have reached clinical development for AD and/or cognition (Phase I, II, or III), or which have subsequently been discontinued.[35,36] There are five drugs presently registered and accepted in the US, EU, or Japan for the symptomatic treatment of AD, and their dates of introduction are: tacrine (Cognex®) 1993; donepezil (Aricept®) 1996; rivastigmine (Exelon®) 2000; galantamine (initially Reminyl, then renamed Razadyne®) 2001; and memantine (Nameda®) 2003. Nootropics such as nicergoline (Sermion®), piracetam (Nootropil®), and aniracetam (Draganon®, registered in Japan in 1993) have been used extensively in the EU and Japan for the treatment of AD.[37] Indeed, Nootropil® was one of the first pharmacological treatments available for AD, but the mechanism of action of the nootropics and even whether they were truly efficacious was never completely clear,[38] leading to their delisting. Nootropil® and Draganon®, for example, were removed from the Japanese market in 1998 and 2000, respectively. Consequently, these drugs have not been included in our analysis.

We have identified 172 compounds that have been listed in various databases as potential therapeutics for AD and/or cognition since the introduction of Cognex®.[i] Of these, 48% have reached at least Phase I of clinical development and have subsequently been discontinued (Figure 4.1(a)), but 52% of the identified compounds are still in clinical development; 16%, 27%, and 9% in Phase I, II and III, respectively. These investigational drugs are sorted by drug class in Figure 4.1(b), which shows the shift away from the development of the nootropic class of drugs, whose mechanism of action is not very well defined and of equivocal clinical efficacy,[39] and the emphasis still placed on the discovery and development of compounds working through a cholinergic mechanism of action, targeting either the inhibition of AChE, or cholinergic receptor subtypes such as the muscarinic M_1 receptor, for example, Sabcomeline,[40] or

[i] The authors acknowledge the collaboration of Sarah Vogel and Dr. Rudy Schreiber from Roche Palo Alto, LLC, in compiling this table of compounds. Published sources[35-37] and the Investigational Drugs Database (IDdb – http://scientific.thomson.com/products/iddb/) were consulted during the compilation of this table. Compounds-in-the-pipeline analyses are useful to obtain a snapshot of the competition and observe trends in drug development. However, they are limited in the sense that the information is only as good as the number and quality of the databases consulted. Some compounds may be listed for many years with no work being done on them, for example, or discontinued or reactivated without notice. Consequently, these types of analyses should be interpreted with a certain amount of caution.

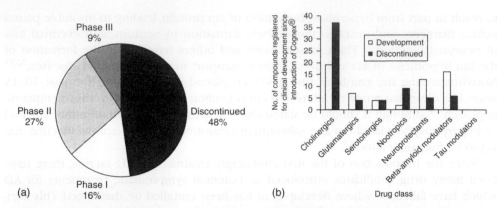

Figure 4.1   Compounds that reached clinical development as potential pharmacotherapies for cognitive impairments in AD since the introduction of Cognex®, divided according to (a) stage of development, and (b) by drug class.

nicotinic β4 receptors, for example, SIB-1553A[41] despite the high failure rate of compounds in this class.

Many of the cholinergic compounds underwent extensive preclinical evaluation and demonstrated potential efficacy in rodent and non-human primate (NHP) tests and models of cognition, but were discontinued nevertheless (Table 4.2). These include 12 AChEIs, 12 muscarinic receptor agonists, and 3 nicotinic receptor agonists. Similarly, of the 11 compounds working through a glutamatergic mechanism of action, 4 have been discontinued, perhaps most noteworthy of these has been the partial agonist at the glycine-B regulatory site on the NMDA receptor, D-cycloserine.[42] Despite positive effects in animals, D-cycloserine has shown equivocal results in clinical trials for AD, which may or may not be related to dose.[43,44]

Nicotinic ligands are currently receiving great interest as potential treatments for AD,[45,46] and many of these compounds have even been tested for efficacy in NHPs,[47] but the effectiveness of these compounds in clinical trials for the symptomatic treatment of AD is still to be demonstrated. Among the front runners, ABT-418[48] was discontinued apparently because of lack of oral bioavailability (http://www.adi-sinsight. com/), and SIB-1553A[41] was discontinued for unknown reasons. ABT-089[49] was last reported to be in Phase II clinical development for the treatment of ADHD in 2006, but this compound is no longer listed in the Abbott pipeline (http://www.abbott. com). SIB-1508,[50] for the treatment of the cognitive effects of Parkinson's disease or AD, was licensed to Lilly, and they were co-developing this compound with Meiji Seika in Japan, but this compound is no longer listed in either the Lilly (http://www.lilly. com) or the Meiji Seika (http://www.meiji.co.jp/en/index.html) pipelines. The fact that ABT-089 and SIB-1508 are no longer listed in the pipeline suggests that they may have been discontinued.

Among muscarinic compounds, Sabcomeline improved acquisition and reversal learning of a visual object discrimination task in marmosets,[40] and other muscarinic compounds previously in clinical development with positive NHP cognitive results include: Civimeline or AF-102B,[51,52] WAY-132983,[53] Xanomeline,[54] Milameline or

Table 4.2 The numbers of compounds that reached clinical development as potential pharmacotherapies for cognitive impairments in AD since the introduction of Cognex®, divided according to drug class, proposed mechanism of action and stage of development

Class	Sub-class	Development	Discontinued
Cholinergics		19	37
	AChEI	8	12
	Muscarinics	2	12
	Nicotinics	5	3
	Modulators	4	10
Glutamatergics		7	4
	NMDA	4	3
	AMPA	3	1
Serotonergics		7	4
	$5\text{-}HT_{1a}$	4	0
	$5\text{-}HT_{3/4}$	2	4
	$5\text{-}HT_6$	1	0
Nootropics		2	9
Neuroprotectants		13	5
	Anti inflammatories	10	3
	Anti oxidants	2	2
	Phosphodiesterase inhibitors	1	0
β-amyloid modulators		16	6
	Synthesis inhibitors	5	2
	Aggregation inhibitors	9	3
	Vaccines	2	1
Tau modulators		0	0
Others[a]		31	29

[a]Compounds with other mechanisms of action, including catecholaminergic, histaminergic, GABAergic, growth factor stimulants, compounds affecting lipid metabolism and ion channel modulators. Some compounds are listed with more than one proposed mechanism of action (see also Table 4.3).

CI-979/RU 3592,[55] and Talsaclidine.[56] Interestingly, the cognitive-enhancing effects of Milameline by itself in the primate were not very robust but synergized with those of tacrine.[57] The weak effect of Talsaclidine in the clinic[58] was confirmed *post hoc* in the primate, and while Xanomeline was originally targeted for the improvement of cognitive impairments in schizophrenia,[59] it was also claimed to be effective in clinical trials for AD.[60] Toxicological concerns have been addressed in both rodent and NHP testing through careful separation of cognitive-enhancing and cholinergic-stimulating doses,[53,56] but robust efficacy has not yet been demonstrated for this class of compounds in the clinic.

While lack of efficacy is the single biggest reason why drugs fail in clinical trials,[8-11] toxicity, poor pharmacodynamics, and changes in development strategy by the sponsoring company also account for many discontinuations.[ii] For example, a poor safety profile and low bioavailability of the first generation of muscarinics has generally been cited as the reason why further development of this class of compounds was discontinued.[62] As another example, the US Food and Drug Administration (FDA) put Cortex Pharmaceuticals' clinical trials of its AMPA modulator, CX717, on hold because it produced histopathological changes in animals. These concerns were addressed by Cortex and the compound is presently back in clinical trials. Cortex's Ampalex (CX516), on the other hand, was discontinued because of its poor bioavailability, but experience with this drug served to improve the design of subsequent drugs. Strategic re-positioning of compounds such as Sibia's SIB-1553A, following the acquisition of Sibia by Merck & Co. in 1999, might account for the abandonment of this compound.

DRUG DISCOVERY STRATEGIES: PROVEN, TESTED, AND HYPOTHETICAL

Examples of some of the different treatment strategies for AD are shown in Table 4.3. It is important to note that some that have failed thus far (e.g., anti-inflammatory agents) may yet show efficacy. At present, the most viable treatment strategies target neurotransmitter dysfunctions. Counteracting the misprocessing of Aβ is theoretically attractive and has spurred the development of secretase inhibitors as well as active and passive immunization techniques, but it remains to be seen if these approaches will be safe, tolerable, and effective. It appears that clearance of deposited amyloid by immunization may be possible, but with uncertain clinical benefit, in some cases causing fatal immune reactions.[28,63] Nevertheless, *post hoc* analyses of the cognitive abilities of surviving subjects suggests that this treatment may improve cognition.[64]

The potential relationship between plaque and tangle pathology may indicate shared intracellular signaling pathways, which may be important in the development of effective treatments. Other therapeutic targets are suggested by known or inferred physiological disturbances, ranging from impaired stress responses to abnormal neuro-inflammation. There are significant differences in the design of clinical trials between strategies developed primarily for treatment of clinically evident disease (e.g., AChEIs), for prevention (e.g., anti-inflammatories and hormones), or both (e.g., anti-oxidants and anti-excitotoxic agents). Most of the disease-modifying pathways will be assessed in clinical trials that examine treatment effects on the underlying disease-related mechanisms, as opposed to only assessing their immediate effects on the existing signs and symptoms of AD. This clinical trial design will entail studies that begin treatment earlier in the disease process, including persons at risk for AD but clinically normal. Some of these studies have already been initiated.

[ii] The reader is invited to consult a review by McArthur and Borsini,[61] which discusses this apparent discontinuity between positive results in animal models and subsequent abandonment of novel drugs, using depression as an example.

Table 4.3 Selected therapeutic strategies for treatment of AD (adapted from[335])

Strategy	Proven, tested, or hypothetical therapy
Anti-amyloid	Secretase inhibitors[a] Immunotherapy[a]
Normalizing tau phosphorylation	Kinase inhibitors[a]
Cholinergic	Cholinesterase inhibitors[c]
Glutamatergic	Memantine[c] AMPA receptor modulators[a] Vitamin E[b]
Antioxidant	Selegiline[b] *Ginkgo biloba* extracts[b]
Anti-inflammatory	NSAIDs[d] Prednisone[d]
Hormonal	Nerve growth factor[b] Estrogen[b]
Reduction of other risk factors	Statins[b] Vitamins B$_6$ and B$_{12}$, folate[b]
Agents used in possible combinations	Memantine Cholinesterase inhibitors Vitamin E *Ginkgo biloba* extracts Selegiline

[a]*In early development for AD treatment and/or prevention.*
[b]*Possibly beneficial for AD treatment and/or prevention based on epidemiology, small clinical studies and/or variable results, but of unproven efficacy.*
[c]*Beneficial for AD treatment based on large, consistent clinical trial results.*
[d]*Shown to be ineffective.*

CLINICAL TRIALS OF TREATMENTS FOR AD: HOW IS EFFICACY ESTABLISHED?

In general terms, Phase I studies typically address safety and tolerability across a range of doses of the agent, often addressing pharmacodynamic and pharmacokinetic issues as well. Although frequently conducted in non-diseased humans, this is not always the case. Phase II studies also examine safety and tolerability, but begin to explore the impact of treatments on measures of efficacy in patients, while larger, Phase III trials are the ultimate and final test of efficacy and safety for FDA approval.[iii] The FDA adopted pragmatic criteria for Phase III trials with potentially approvable "anti-dementia"

[iii] Please refer to McEvoy and Freundenreich, Issues in the design and conductance of clinical trials, Volume 1, Psychiatric Disorders, for a comprehensive discussion of clinical trial designs for behavioral disorders.

therapies,[65] which require that patients meet criteria for a specific dementia such as AD, for example, using either DSM-IV-TR or National Institute of Neurological and Communicative Disorders and Stroke–Alzheimer's Disease and Related Disorders Association (NINCDS–ADRDA) Work Group Criteria;[66] and that appropriate efficacy instruments be used in at least two positive trials. The agent must show efficacy relative to placebo treatment in improving memory or retarding its deterioration, and must show a meaningful impact on global clinical outcomes or functional impairment. Despite the frequency and morbidity of non-cognitive behavioral changes, they are not a target for regulatory approval at this time.

Phase II and III clinical trials of anti-dementia drugs are typically conducted in patients with either mild to moderate AD, or moderate to severe AD. Trials with mild to moderate AD patients rely on the Alzheimer's Disease Assessment Scale – cognitive subscale (ADAS-Cog)[67] which assesses word recall, naming, commands, constructional and ideational praxis, orientation, language, and recall of test instructions. Trials in moderate to severe AD often use the Severe Impairment Battery (SIB)[67] as the cognitive outcome. The majority of trials also incorporate a Clinical Global Impression of Change (CGIC) as the "global" clinical measure.[69] Some have used a functional measure instead, such as the Alzheimer's Disease Cooperative Study – Activities of Daily Living (ADCS-ADL) Scale, to assess aspects of daily functioning.[70]

CRITICAL ROLE OF BEHAVIORAL MODELS AND ENDPOINTS

Clearly, AD is a disorder of concern because of its effects on high-level cognitive and behavioral functions, such as attention, learning and memory, the ability to interact appropriately with others in work and social settings,[66] and the ability to live independently and care for oneself. Regulatory agencies such as the FDA recognize the importance of cognitive and other behavioral functions and require that novel treatments demonstrate therapeutic effects on measures of these cognitive and other behavioral functions. In fact, FDA approval of efficacy is based exclusively on whether treatments affect cognitive and other behavioral measures. The core cognitive and behavioral functions relevant to the disease can be assessed in preclinical models, and despite the present emphasis on biomarkers,[71,72] [iv] it is important to recall Claude Bernard's observation that measures of simpler, more reductionist phenomena, cannot fully capture all aspects of more complex phenomena.[73] In order to maximize the predictive validity of preclinical assessments, novel treatments should be evaluated with preclinical models that measure treatment effects at the same level of complexity as required to assess therapeutic potential in clinical trials.

This point is supported by a considerable amount of empirical research across a wide range of disorders. For example, it is faster, easier and cheaper to show effects

[iv] Please refer to Tannock *et al.*, Towards a biological understanding of ADHD and the discovery of novel therapeutic approaches, in Volume 1, Psychiatric Disorders, for further discussion regarding biomarkers in behavioral disorders.

of cancer treatments on tumor size, instead of treatment-related reductions in mortality rates,[74] or to show treatment-related reductions in blood pressure instead of reductions in the number of strokes in a treatment group, relative to a placebo-control group.[75-77] However, these biomarkers and surrogate endpoints usually only measure treatment effects on the disease target and detect potentially therapeutic effects. It is difficult to find biomarkers that are highly correlated with a treatment's overall effects because treatments often have non-specific and adverse effects, independent of their effects on the disease process, which can off-set whatever beneficial, therapeutic effects they may have.[75,76,78] For that reason, biomarkers usually suggest that treatments are effective, even when they actually have no effect or may even be harmful, increasing morbidity and mortality (Table 4.4).

Validation of a surrogate endpoint typically requires analyses of numerous randomized, controlled trials,[71] and even after a surrogate marker has been validated for treatments with one mechanism of action, it may not be valid for use with treatments that have different mechanisms of action. For example, low-dose diuretics reduce blood pressure in hypertensive patients, which reduces rates of death, heart attack and stroke, but calcium channel blockers that also lower blood pressure may actually be associated with an increased risk for myocardial infarction ([76]; for review see[79])

Although biomarkers are not adequate substitutes for primary endpoints, when combined with behavioral and other primary endpoints, biomarkers can add considerable value to the research, beyond the use of behavioral and other primary endpoints alone, by helping to validate the clinical relevance of the target and the mechanism of action and therapeutic potential of the prospective treatment. For example, AD was initially characterized histopathologically by Alois Alzheimer – who identified plaques and tangles in the brain of one of his patients 100 years ago. It was assumed that they played a critical, probably primary role in the etiology of the disease. This assumption holds even today where a definite diagnosis of AD cannot be confirmed unless dense plaques and tangles are seen at autopsy,[66,80,81] even though a causal relationship between plaques and tangles and the degree of neurodegeneration and dementia has still not been established. In fact, more and more studies have raised questions about the primary role that amyloid plaques were initially believed to play in the etiology of AD. For example, clinical studies have shown that levels of total Aβ are not closely related to neuronal loss, number of neurofibrillary tangles, or duration or severity of dementia in AD patients.[82,83] At autopsy, 22–50% of demented patients with probable AD have Aβ levels that are not high enough to confirm a diagnosis of definite AD,[84,85] while up to 50% of non-demented subjects have sufficient levels of amyloid plaques to meet the neuropathological criteria for a diagnosis of AD.[86-88] In one prospective study, there were no differences in mental performance between groups that met the neuropathological criteria for a diagnosis of AD and those that did not.[89,90] Only in these studies that measured both primary endpoints such as dementia severity, together with biological measures of the degree of pathology, has it been possible to determine that AD may be mediated by soluble forms of Aβ more than the Aβ that has aggregated into insoluble plaques. Such studies have recently shown that levels of soluble Aβ are elevated early in AD, and they are more closely correlated with measures of disease severity (e.g., age at death and reductions in synaptic density), than measures of insoluble Aβ.[91,92]

Table 4.4 Lack of correlation between treatment effects on biomarkers and primary endpoints across a wide range of clinical disorders

Indication	Treatment mechanisms	Biomarkers	Primary endpoints
Cardiovascular disease[336–343]	PDE inhibitor, β_1 selective partial agonist, various anti-arrhythmic and cholesterol lowering agents	Maximum exercise HR and systolic BP, maintenance of sinus rhythm, reduced arrhythmias, reduced cholesterol	No change or up to 3X Increased heart attacks and overall mortalities
Cancer[344]	Thymidylate synthase inhibitor	Reduced tumor size	No change in mortality rate
AIDS[345–347]	Immune system facilitators	Increased CD-4 lymphocyte levels	Unreliable reductions in mortalities
	Anti-bacterial agents	Reduced bacterial loads	Increased mortality rates
Diabetes[348]	Increased hepatic and peripheral insulin sensitivity and reduced insulin resistance	Reduced levels of fasting glucose and glycated hemoglobin	Increased heart attacks and possibly increased mortalities
Osteoporosis[349]	Fluoride treatment	Increased bone mass	Increased bone fractures
Chronic granulomatous disease[79,350 a]	Interferon-gamma to increase macrophage production of superoxides	No increase in macrophage production of superoxide	Decrease in serious infections

[a]*Biomarkers usually suggest that treatments are effective even when they are not, but sometimes they suggest that treatments are ineffective when they are actually effective.*

HISTORICAL ORIGINS OF ANIMAL MODELS OF COGNITIVE PROCESSES

It has long been the goal of animal experimentation in the cognitive sciences to discover processes that are critical for learning and memory in one or more brain regions,[93–96] and much of our understanding of cognitive brain function stems from the use of such models; historically traceable through many-celled organisms[97] to NHPs.[98] Notwithstanding the early hopes that cognitive disorders such as AD could be regarded as a cholinergic equivalent to Parkinson's disease, and that the treatment of AD could be effected by replacement therapy, it was soon evident that deficits in cognition were not going to be solved by identification of a single brain-related neurological event such as nigro-striatal degeneration. Rather, it became clear through the pioneering work of Olton,[94] Squire,[99] Mishkin,[98] Morris,[100] and many others, that memory was a multifaceted process and that different memories were derived from different brain regions (neocortex, hippocampus, amygdala, and striatum). In addition, it was determined that different types of cellular and biochemical mechanisms might be involved for the duration of those memories (i.e., long-term versus short-term) within a structure. Cognitive deficits in humans do not occur through any single neurological "event." Instead, combinations of different processes, operating simultaneously, in parallel, give rise to different *cognitive functions*. With advancements in the areas of human brain imaging and increased understanding of the underlying neural events that produce those imaged changes, it may be possible to identify specific biochemical and cellular targets directly, without the use of animal models, but until then, most of our understanding of cognitive processes will continue to come from investigating cognitive and behavioral functions in animals.

CLINICALLY RELEVANT COGNITIVE DEFICITS IN AD

Spatial Memory and Spatial Mapping

Memory for locations in space is primarily the province of the hippocampus and related structures.[101] Richard Morris was the first to demonstrate this conclusively with the development of the water maze task for rodents.[100] Damage to the hippocampus in rodents is nearly always associated with deficits in acquiring spatial memory, as well as deficits encoding spatial position,[102] and this finding has been extended to some types of tasks in NHPs.[103] There is no question that memory of spatial relations, and spatial orientation using landmarks in the environment, is disrupted in AD, and that this type of memory impairment produces a major demand on patient care. Animal models confirm that spatial mapping and navigation are severely impaired after damage to the hippocampus and related structures, such as the subiculum, entorhinal, and perirhinal cortex.[104-106] The importance of hippocampal and related structures for spatial memory and navigation in man is supported by evidence in humans that medial temporal lobe structures are selectively activated during tasks involving navigation and spatial memory.[107,108]

Episodic and Recognition Memory

Memory for particular details related to a given context or circumstance has been demonstrated in animals, from rats to monkeys.[98,109-112] In man, this type of memory has been called declarative, syntactical, and most recently, episodic. In the latter instance, memory for particular incidences (i.e., episodes) requires recall of a number of factors that can be probed easily in humans, but is more difficult to demonstrate in lower species. Conclusions drawn from such studies require qualification because of the lack of a generalized paradigm that can be shown to require the same neural processes related to "episodic" recall in all forms of the tasks that are employed. One form is recognition memory, usually demonstrated in delay type tasks requiring identification of a stimulus or physical object amongst a group of different elements after an initial exposure to the object or stimulus. Animal models of recognition memory include memory for odors,[113] tactile sensations,[114] and con-specifics,[115] which apply to several types of memory deficits in AD.

Global Functional Deficits

Clinicians assess global functional abilities in interviews with the patient and their primary caregiver by asking about their cognitive abilities, overall abilities, and social and daily functioning. These assessments can include questions about functions that are not usually considered cognitive in nature, such as bathing, dressing, eating, and walking, and compounds must demonstrate significant effects on these measures of global functional abilities in order to be approved by the FDA.[69,70] What is noticeably lacking in animal models are measures of these types of global functional deficits.[116-118] Most preclinical efforts have focused on developing models of specific cognitive deficits, care is often taken to determine if the behavioral effects being studied can be attributed to non-cognitive factors, and if so, the results are often seen as not interpretable or irrelevant for AD. Given the importance of global functional abilities in AD patients and clinical trials, it might be important to develop measures of similar functional abilities in preclinical models. These might include measures of spontaneous activity levels, motor function, grooming, and feeding. Aged rats and mice do seem to show global functional decline, and a range of behaviors could be used to assess the therapeutic potential of novel treatments on global functional deficits, in aged and impaired rodents and primates.

ANIMAL MODELS USED TO ASSESS DRUG CANDIDATES FOR IMPAIRED COGNITION IN AD

Just as there are no models of global dysfunction, there are also no models available that fully capture all aspects of AD pathology. Nevertheless, a number of models have been developed to study different aspects of the pathology, such as models of the dysfunction of the cholinergic systems, models of hippocampal degeneration, models of deficits related to amyloid, etc. These models have been used to assess the effects of potential treatments on different components of the disease.[v]

---

[v] Historically, there has been a good deal of confusion regarding the terms "models" and "tests or procedures" used in behavioral research. The interested reader is invited to consult the following sources for a more detailed discussion of the subject,[119,120] as well as Steckler *et al.*, Developing novel anxiolytics: Improving preclinical detection and clinical assessment, and, Wagner *et al.*, Huntington Disease, in this volume for further discussion regarding "models" or procedures. We concur with Steckler and colleagues' definition that a model attempts to recapitulate the pathophysiology and produce the symptoms of the disorder through experimental manipulations, while tests or procedures are used to measure and confirm that the experimental manipulations did in fact produce the same signs, symptoms and behaviors that are characteristic of the disorder.

Pharmacological Models

Models of cognition in the rodent have been examined using pharmacological interventions to disrupt neurotransmitter systems suspected to be involved in memory. Blockade of cholinergic transmission with scopolamine is historically one of the first pharmacological agents used in memory research,[121] and remains one of the main pharmacological models in preclinical and clinical use today. Other agents such as benzodiazepines also show selective effects on suspected memory processes,[122] but they are not usually used either in preclinical or clinical drug discovery and development. Behavioral screens are widely employed to assess compounds that might reverse these drug-induced deficits. However, the interpretation of these "reversal" studies is subject to pharmacological interactions, and they have to be assessed for such potential actions. The most useful applications of these pharmacological models of memory disruption are those that can be reversed by receptor-specific agonists of the normal transmitter system, after disruption has been demonstrated.[123] Any suspected memory-facilitative agent can then be compared to the agonist, to reverse the pharmacological blockade of the normal transmitter system. However, such demonstrations usually require extensive dose effect analyses to rule out non-specific effects and drug interactions. For example, abnormal glutamatergic transmission in AD has been particularly difficult to model because of the pronounced locomotor effects of glutamate antagonists.[124] Nevertheless, pharmacologically induced glutamatergic deficits are used to model impaired cognition processes in schizophrenia.[125][vi]

Lesions

Models based on the mechanical, electrical, or chemical ablation of selected brain areas or neurotransmitter pathways were among the first established in neuroscience research to study brain anatomy and function.[126,127] Lesions of ascending cholinergic pathways from the septum to the hippocampus, or from the nucleus basalis to the cortex,[128] provided much of the initial evidence supporting the cholinergic hypothesis of AD. Lesion techniques are still being used today to dissect components of memory-related circuits in the brain[129] and to examine non-cholinergic contributions to learning and memory.[130] However, these models have largely been superseded because of extra, non-specific damage that is produced, and the difficulty of attenuating or reversing lesion-induced deficits.[131,132]

Neurogenesis

Recent studies have examined the potential for neurogenesis to replace neurons lost to AD.[133] Studies involving neurogenesis in appropriate brain areas such as the dentate gyrus[134-136] suggest that some "reversal" of the deficit is possible, provided that the lesion technique does not result in total ablation of the dentate gyrus (i.e., using doses of neurotoxins and axotomy procedures that leave some remaining neurons). While many of the causative factors in age-related decline in neurogenesis are unclear, there

---

[vi] Please refer to Jones *et al.*, Animal and translational models of schizophrenia, in this volume.

is a clear reduction in neurogenesis with age in animal models that parallels the reduction in regenerative potential in human AD patients. Animal models of AD involving neurogenesis are now proceeding on multiple fronts: (a) using inhibition of neurogenesis as a model of age-related cognitive decline;[137-139] (b) focusing on whether neurotrophic factors that promote neurogenesis can alleviate AD;[140,141] (c) examining the role of neuroprotective or anti-inflammatory actions (e.g., steroids) in neurogenesis for alleviating AD;[133,142-144] and (d) determining whether stem cell therapy – specifically with respect to restoring neurogenic properties – has potential as a therapeutic agent for AD.[145-147]

Aged Animals

AD is an age-related disorder, and in addition to the loss of neuroplasticity and neurogenesis mentioned above, aged rats exhibit AD-related pathologies such as brain atrophy, especially in the hippocampus,[148] and dysfunction of cholinergic neurons in the hippocampus and basal forebrain.[149,150] Aged animals are also an attractive animal model of AD because there are considerable individual differences in cognitive functions among aged animals, and these individual differences are correlated with neurobiological changes relevant to AD.[149-152] For example, it has been reported that aged rats show loss of neurogenesis that is related to their cognitive abilities[153], but see[154]. The aged unimpaired animals make excellent controls, and it should be noted that cognitive deficits among impaired aged rats can exceed 4 standard deviations from the mean of the unimpaired aged rats.[155,156] Among clinical populations, cognitive deficits of 1–2 standard deviations from normal age-matched controls are classified as age-associated memory impairment and mild cognitive impairment (MCI), and deficits of 2–4 standard deviations from normal age-matched controls are classified as demented.[157,158] In contrast to the subtle deficits seen in many transgenic mouse models of AD, the magnitude of the cognitive deficits in impaired aged rats are comparable to the severe cognitive deficits seen in demented patients. Aged rodents do not normally exhibit plaques and tangles or significant neurodegeneration; however, other species such as the lemur (*Microcebus murinus*,[159]), the domestic cat,[160] and the beagle dog,[161] but see[162] do develop age-associated plaques and have been used as animal models of AD.

Genetic

Transgenic animals – typically mice, although there are a few transgenic rat models – provide the opportunity to study specific phenomena associated with AD, such as loss of specific neurotransmitters or receptors (cholinergic) and presence or absence of protein (synapsin, amyloid, etc.). Mutant strains can be produced with the genetic manipulations present from birth – however, this produces concerns regarding potential abnormal development. Inducible transgenes – in which the genes are activated at specific developmental stages or at maturity, provide a better model for studying systems affected by AD. Limitations still exist in producing the desired mutations or limiting them to specific brain areas or neuron types. One possible solution to this limitation is the use of viral vectors. Genes can be targeted to specific brain areas via viruses with an affinity for the hippocampus, amygdala, basal ganglia, and etc. Once the virus attaches to target cells and injects the custom gene product – the gene is expressed only by the target cells. Viral vector-mediated neurodegeneration has been used to induce a model of Parkinson's disease in monkeys,[163,164] and a Huntington's disease model in rats,[165] as well as to provide a potential therapy.[166] This technique has recently been used to create a model of AD in rats via induction of amyloid protein,[167,168] and therapeutic applications are likely to follow.[169]

A number of transgenic mouse models of AD have been produced, and while they may provide the best face validity for evaluating new drug treatments for AD, they do not reproduce all of the pathological features of the disease, and the behavioral and cognitive deficits they exhibit are often subtle, which is not consistent with the magnitude of deficits seen in AD patients. For example, the Tg_{2576} APP transgenic mouse originally developed by Hsiao and her colleagues,[170] has been used extensively in neurobiological research on the role of amyloid and the development of drugs for AD. In some studies, no significant deficits in performance of cognitive tasks were detected. In one study, the mice were tested in six cognitively based tasks (i.e., Y-maze, visible platform, Morris water maze, circular platform, passive avoidance, and active avoidance) through 19 months, and the results revealed that Tg+ mice only exhibited statistically significant deficits in the Y-maze and visible platform tasks.[171] Other attempts to develop tests that should be especially sensitive have also failed to detect significant deficits in these mice. For example, AD-related pathology is especially prevalent in the olfactory bulbs of AD patients,[172] and robust olfactory deficits occur very early in the disease.[173-176] Given the high levels of amyloid in Tg_{2576} mice, especially in their olfactory bulbs, it was expected that these mice would have olfactory deficits. One of the authors (RMcA) carried out a complex GO-NO GO olfactory discrimination study in aged (>11 months) Tg+, Tg− Tg_{2576} mice, including age-matched background control (C57Bl/6SJL$_{F1}$) mice.[177] The mice were trained to go to the back of an operant conditioning chamber and place their nose in a small hole which activated an air pump that delivered one of two odors. If one odor was presented (S+) the mouse had to return to the front of the operant chamber and press a lever 10 times in order to earn a sweet saccharine reward. If the other odor was presented (S−), the mouse had to refrain from pressing the lever in order to receive a reward. Once the mice learned this task, the two odors were reversed, that is, the odor that was initially paired with pressing the lever now required the mouse to withhold its response. The data shown in Figure 4.2(a) indicate that both Tg+ (Subject 15725) and Tg− (Subject 20487) Tg_{2576} mice were capable of reaching choice accuracies of 70 to 80% correct, and they were both impaired when compared to their C57Bl/6SJL$_{F1}$ background control (Subject 21926). Reversing this discrimination, in other words suppressing their learned response to the odor that signaled "press the lever for reward" and pressing the lever in response to the odor that previously signaled "do not press the lever for reward," was more difficult (Figure 4.2(b)). Nevertheless, both the Tg+ and the background control mouse were capable of this reversal. Interestingly, the Tg− mouse was unable to do so. Thus, the ability to learn this task was transgene-independent as well as amyloid load-independent, as indicated by the histological examination of the brains of these representative animals (Figure 4.2(c)).

In some cases, special procedures have been developed that successfully tease out statistically significant effects in transgenic models of AD. For example, an elaborate

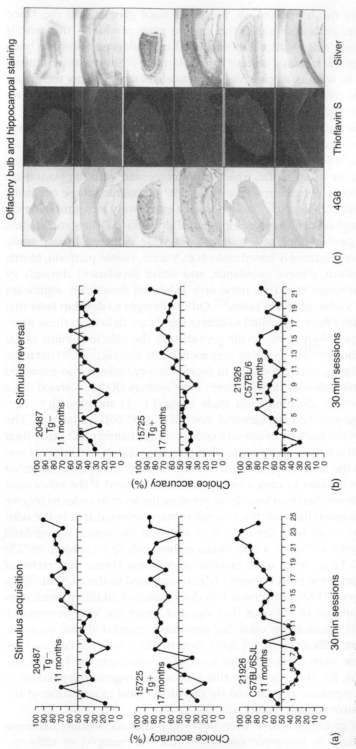

Figure 4.2 Rates of learning to discriminate odors and then to reverse that discrimination in a GO-NO GO odor discrimination task in representative aged (>11 months) Tg$_{2576}$ Tg+, Tg−, and C57BL/6SJF$_1$ mice. (a) stimulus acquisition, (b) stimulus reversal, and (c) olfactory bulb and hippocampal staining. The figures illustrate the increase in choice accuracy (% correct discriminations) in learning to press or not press a lever for food, depending on which of 2 odors (cinnamon or peppermint) were presented (a), and the subsequent reversal of that behavior (b) in an odor discrimination task by representative aged Tg−, Tg+, and C57BL/6SJF1 background good discriminating mice over 25–30 min training sessions. Fifty percent represents chance levels of responding. The levels of amyloid deposition and neurodegeneration of these mice were assessed (c) through examination of olfactory bulb (upper sections) and hippocampal formation (lower sections) stained with 4G8 (plaque formation), thioflavin S (dense plaque formation), or silver staining (neuritic processes). The authors acknowledge the contribution made by S. Franklin, J. Oostveen, and A. Buhl (ex. Pharmacia and Upjohn, Kalamazoo MI) and of A. Goodwin to this study.

variation of the standard MWM was used to demonstrate water maze deficits in the PDAPP mouse[178] (see details of procedure in section on Radial Arm and Water Mazes). Until then, the PDAPP model had been questioned as a model of AD because profound cognitive deficits had not been detected reliably in these mice, despite extensive amyloid deposition in brain areas such as the hippocampus and cortex (cf.,[179]). While there were no differences between Tg+ and Tg− PDAPP transgenic mice in finding the visible platform, or in swim speeds, an age-independent difference in the number of trials needed to reach criterion locating a single platform was observed. PDAPP transgenic mice, regardless of age, required more trials to learn the location of a submerged platform. However, an age-dependent impairment in ability to learn two or more locations was evident. Young (6–9 months) PDAPP transgenic mice learned faster than middle-aged (13–15 month old) and aged (18–21 month old) mice. In terms of learning capacity, both Tg− and Tg+ learned fewer locations in 10 days than the non-transgenic controls, but the Tg+ transgenic mice were most impaired. While there does not appear to be a significant difference in either training to criterion or learning capacity between middle-aged and aged PDAPP transgenic mice, a significant negative correlation with amyloid plaque burden was observed. A water version of the radial arm maze has also been used to detect cognitive deficits in transgenic mice with mutations in presenilin-1 APP (APP(670, 671)[180], and to show amelioration of these impairments through Aβ immunization.[181] Recently, a triple transgenic mouse model has been developed which reportedly produces plaques and tangles and behavioral deficits,[182–184] but additional research must be conducted to fully characterize and validate this new model.

PROCEDURES USED TO ASSESS COGNITION IN ANIMALS

Passive and Active Avoidance

Avoidance tasks require an animal to recognize a cue or context associated with an aversive stimulus and avoid the stimulus either by moving much slower than before the aversive event or freezing and not moving at all (passive avoidance), or actively performing a different behavior (active avoidance). An example of passive avoidance is the "step-down" paradigm where the animal is placed on an elevated platform next to a shock-grid, such that the animal receives a foot-shock when it steps down from the platform onto the grid. When next placed on the platform, the rat or mouse passively avoids the shock by remaining on the platform for a much longer period of time before stepping down, indicating recollection of the aversive experience. Active avoidance tasks employ operant conditioning, and require that the animal perform behaviors that avoid the aversive stimulus (e.g., pressing a lever to prevent shock or exiting the shock chamber in a shuttle box). Passive avoidance reflects classical conditioning within the context of the step-down paradigm, where latency to respond is increased due to the recollection that foot-shock was previously delivered after stepping onto a floor consisting of metal rods.[185,186] Much of what we know about memory, including enhancement, consolidation, and retrieval, comes from earlier studies with these paradigms, and many drugs were shown to facilitate performance in these active and passive avoidance tasks.[187] More recently, these paradigms have been used to explore the role of steroids in avoidance memory, and the involvement of arousal as an important feature in encoding memory.[188]

Conditioned Fear

Fear conditioning is often conducted as a type of avoidance task in which the cue associated with the aversive stimulus is the environmental context. The fear conditioning task used extensively by Fanselow *et al.*[189] consists of a two-compartment operant box. One compartment is covered and dark, the other open and lighted. Rodents are nocturnal, so their natural preference is to spend more time in the dark chamber. However, entry into that chamber is accompanied by a foot-shock. The animal will avoid getting the shock by actively avoiding the darkened half of the chamber. Note that the conditioned cue for the aversive stimulus is the environmental context of the darkened chamber. Other contextual cues can be used – and the animal will avoid them even when no shock is present. Conditioned fear can also be conducted by measuring the amount of time the animal spends freezing in a box (i.e., the context) where it previously received a shock. Freezing is a natural, species-specific defensive behavior in rodents, and can easily and automatically be quantified using image analysis equipment. Such tasks test episodic memory (specific event plus context) as well as the rapid consolidation to reference memory – often requiring only a single association between context and shock to produce lasting memory. The brain areas involved in avoidance behaviors are primarily the amygdala and basal ganglia. The hippocampus is invoked primarily in associating the cue or context with the aversive stimulus. Thus, deficits in avoidance behavior do not necessarily suggest cognitive deficits, but can result from alterations in sensory responses to the aversive stimulus, or to changes in perception of the "emotional content" of the environment.[188,190,191] Fear conditioning tasks are quickly learned, since many responses (particularly passive "freezing") to the aversive stimulus, *per se*, do not have to be learned; only the association of cue or context with the stimulus must be learned.

Novel Object or Social Recognition

Object recognition, often termed "novel" object recognition, is a task in which the animal must make a response based on recognition of an object. Novel object recognition in rodents refers to some form of selection or preference for a novel physical object that has been added to a previously explored environment.[192] For example, in a familiar environment, rats will spend more time sniffing, rearing, and climbing on novel objects than familiar ones. The task is quickly acquired, often requiring only 3–5 testing sessions to establish baseline performance. Object recognition tasks where experimenters measure the time an animal spends examining different physical features in an environment differ from discrimination tasks in which the animal must displace a physical feature that covers a food well.[193] Early lesion studies indicated hippocampal involvement in object recognition,[194-197] but more recent studies downplay the role of the hippocampus.[192] C-fos activation indicates that it is the perirhinal cortex that is primarily responsible for object recognition memory.[198,199] Interpretation of the results of novel object experiments is complicated by the fact that the behavior can be affected by changes in activity levels and anything that makes what should be a familiar environment appear unfamiliar. For example, if an animal has reference memory deficits, or if an otherwise familiar room is filled with a new odor, a familiar environment may seem unfamiliar.[192]

Delayed Matching and Non-Matching to Sample

Operant tasks first require that an animal associate an instrumental response with a reward that reinforces that behavior – for example, pressing a lever produces a small amount of food or water, which reinforces lever pressing. A series of instrumental responses can then be chained together, as in the delayed-match-to-sample (DMTS) or delayed-non-match-to-sample (DNMTS). For example, with rats, a single lever is presented. When the animal presses the lever, a cue light comes on indicating that the next appropriate response is a nosepoke into the food bin. Once the nosepoke is performed, two levers are presented. When the animal then presses the appropriate lever, the reinforcement is given.[128,200-202] Incorrect responses are not reinforced. Instead, a lights-out timeout is presented. Operant tasks can require extensive training (weeks or even months) depending on whether a delay is instituted in the task. Cognitive functions tested using operant responding are attention, procedural memory (learning the "rules" of the task), reference memory, and in the case of tasks incorporating a delay – working memory. Performance in these tasks can be affected by the use of non-cognitive, mediating strategies. For example, rats may learn to stand in front of the correct lever until it is extended. Additional procedures can be included to limit the use of such mediating strategies, such as training the rat to wait with its nose in a food bin at the back of the cage so that it cannot simply stand in front of the correct lever, but detailed assessments of performance must still be conducted in order to rule out the effects of potential confounding factors.[203]

Radial Arm and Water Mazes

Maze tasks incorporate many features of both object recognition and operant responding. The classic eight-arm radial maze requires animals to visit each arm without revisiting any given arm, until every arm has been entered.[204-206] The delay form of the task introduces a delay after four arms have been entered. The animal is removed from the maze, the delay elapses (1, 4, or 24 h), and then the animal is placed back in the maze and must enter the other four arms without re-entering any of the arms visited before the delay. There are several variants of the maze task which test different cognitive processes. The floor or walls of the different arms can be covered with different smells or textures – making it a cued-recognition task. There may be no proximal (-intramaze) cues, only distal (environmental or extramaze) cues – making it a spatial memory task.[100] Variations such as "T" or "Y" mazes allow introduction of alternation or even DMTS/DNMTS to test working memory.

The water maze was developed by Morris[100] as a method in which spatial navigation and memory could be assessed without using food or water deprivation as a primary motivator. This procedure is probably the most common for testing compounds with cognitive-enhancing potential. Morris' original procedure uses a pool of milky, opaque water in which the animal must swim to a location to find a hidden platform and climb out of the water. The animal is aided in this navigational task by extra- and/or intra-maze visual stimuli with which the animal can orient itself and the target platform in space. The task is learned quickly, with a noticeable improvement in performance each day. Criterion performance is often reached in 4–10 testing days, with 2–4 trials per day. The rapid learning of maze tasks allows testing of two different memory systems. Day-to-day acquisition of the task measures consolidation into reference memory, while within-day acquisition (and delayed match or non-match) measures working memory.[207,208] The Morris water maze (MWM) procedure is also used to measure the retention of the spatial memory of the submerged platform through the use of "probe" trials in which the platform is removed. The proportion of time spent swimming in the quadrant in which the platform was originally placed is taken as a measure of memory retention. There are variations of the MWM procedure including placing the submerged platform in different quadrants of the pool and measuring the rate at which the animal learns the new position and ignores the original placement of the submerged platform.

Recently, Morris and his colleagues have described a variant of the typical place navigation task for use with transgenic mice.[209] Mice are required to undergo a series of water maze tasks over time. Initially, the mice are required to swim to a visible platform for 5 days. This task helps evaluate the sensorimotor abilities of the mice. Once this initial training is achieved, the mice are then trained in a standard place navigation task of swimming to a submerged platform in a fixed location. The number of trials and/or daily sessions is not fixed, but training proceeds at a rate of up to eight daily trials until the mouse can find the submerged platform within 20 s for three consecutive trials. Once this criterion is reached the location of the platform is changed and the mouse is required to ignore the previous location and learn a new one, re-training to criterion in up to five different locations. Another variant of this procedure measures the total number of different locations that the mouse can learn to criterion in a 10-day period. This procedure has been used to tease out deficits in the PDAPP mouse that were difficult to detect with the standard MWM procedure (see previous discussion in section on Genetic Models).

Set Shifting

Set shifting tasks are used to assess executive functions, which include the ability to monitor, regulate, and change previously learned strategies if they are no longer effective. For example, in the Wisconsin Card Sorting Task,[210] cards are selected or sorted according to simple rules. Subjects may need to learn to sort the cards based on their color, but after a few choices, the rules are changed and the subject must learn to switch to a different strategy, such as sorting the cards based on the number of objects on the cards. This task is very sensitive to deficits in executive function in AD patients because they can learn any single rule, but they have difficulty realizing that previously successful strategies are no longer effective. They tend to perseverate, making choices based on strategies that are no longer effective, despite receiving feedback after each choice. A version of the Wisconsin Card Sorting Task has been developed for use in NHPs,[211,212] and a number of simple versions of this test have been developed for rodents.[213,214] In one version of the task, a rat learns to dig in bowls for a food reward. The bowls have different odors and different materials in them. First, the rat learns to dig in the bowl based on the type of material in the bowl (e.g., glass beads or wood shavings), but after learning this strategy, it must learn to switch, to pick the bowl based on the odor (e.g., nutmeg or thyme). The difficulty of the task is increased because the critical strategic changes occur on "extra-dimensional" cues. In other words, after learning to find food rewards based on the texture of the digging materials, the rat is not just learning to respond to a different texture, it must learn to respond to completely different types of cues, such as odors.

ROLE OF BEHAVIORAL MODELS IN DRUG DISCOVERY FOR AD

Primary Screening

In the past, before the molecular revolution and the advent of target-based discovery processes, preclinical behavioral models played a critical role in the initial screening of compounds. Very simple, fairly high-throughput behavioral models and tests, such as acute electroconvulsive shock-induced amnesia and step-down passive avoidance were used to screen compounds,[215-217] and compounds were initially tested in these relatively time-consuming and labor-intensive behavioral tests, sometimes on a trial and error basis, until therapeutic potential was detected. Then, testing continued on a relatively large number of compounds in order to optimize the molecular structure – a process known as defining the structure activity relationship (SAR).[vii]

Target Validation and Proof of Concept

In the last 10–15 years, tremendous progress has been made in a number of areas relevant to drug discovery and development. For example, gene sequencing machines were developed, the human genome project was completed, and gene expression profiling techniques became available that simultaneously determine the gene expression pattern of the entire genome. At the same time, compound libraries have grown in size and chemical diversity, and automated assay procedures have been developed that allow hundreds of thousands of compounds to be quickly tested for binding and/or functional effects on the target. X-ray crystallography and computer automated 3-dimensional modeling technologies have also been developed to facilitate the design

---

[vii] For further discussion of the role of animal models in various stages of drug discovery, please refer to Bartz *et al.*, Preclinical animal models of Autistic Spectrum Disorders (ASD), in Volume 1, Psychiatric Disorders; Heidbreder, Impulse and reward deficit disorders: drug discovery and development; Markou *et al.*, Contribution of animal models and preclinical human studies to medication development for nicotine dependence; Wilding *et al.*, Anti-obesity drugs: from animal models to clinical efficacy, in Volume 3 Reward Deficit Disorders.

of compounds that precisely fit the binding site. These scientific and technological advances have led to target-based drug discovery in which a molecular target related to a disease is selected at the beginning of a drug discovery project, and hits can be quickly identified and optimized using *in vitro* assays and measures of the pharmacokinetic and pharmacodynamic properties of the compound. Advancement of compounds with potential for treating cognitive deficits can now be based on proof of concept studies with only a few development candidates, using more sophisticated, complex, clinically relevant and appropriate models and behavioral tasks. For example, it is now easier to justify the use of expensive, aged, cognitively impaired rats and transgenic mice, and tasks that can require fairly extensive training such as acquisition and retention of spatial maps, delayed matching, or set-shifting, in order to target the most clinically relevant and specific biological mechanisms and cognitive functions.[viii]

Final Preclinical Testing in NHPs

Since behavioral responses can be more easily identified and assessed by the nature of the stimulus presentations, displays, response and reinforcement devices employed with NHPs, less inference is required to define the cognitive processes being assessed experimentally than in rodent studies. Cognitive tasks can be refined to approximate similar processes in humans, once it is determined that monkeys are using the same strategies and principles to solve the tasks.[218-220] Other advantages of testing in NHPs are that effective dose, bioavailability, and time course of action can be estimated for human applications with more certainty than in rodents. Finally, as an infrequently used but nonetheless important option, it is possible to equate drug action in humans using brain imaging correlates of the task.[221]

Because of the relative cost incurred, NHP studies typically include fewer and much smaller groups, relative to rodent experiments and clinical trials, which means that fewer treatments and/or conditions can be examined and there is less statistical power, and testing of compounds in NHPs (rhesus macaque, cynomologus, vervet, and spider monkeys) is usually relegated to the final step, prior to testing in humans. Furthermore, these animals live longer and tend to be used to test several different types of drugs during their lifetime. Although occasionally used for drug discovery,[50,222,223] lesion-induced models of impaired cognition in NHPs are usually used when studying the neurobiology of cognitive processes.[211,224-227] In drug discovery, the use of NHPs usually relies on pharmacologically induced cognitive deficits, using compounds such as scopolamine,[228-230] or glutamate receptor antagonists.[231,232] As previously mentioned, these pharmacologically induced deficit models are subject to potential drug interactions, which can confound the results, and given the mechanism of action of the therapeutic agents, appropriate antagonists are not always available.

[viii] For further discussion regarding the demands placed upon behavioral pharmacologists developing and working with animal models of behavioral disorders within the context of pharmaceutical drug discovery environments, please refer to Bartz *et al.*, Preclinical animal models of Autistic Spectrum Disorders (ASD), in Volume 1, Psychiatric Disorders.

Late-stage drug discovery for AD has also relied on age-related cognitive deficits in NHPs[233-235] to examine the cognitive enhancing potential of novel compounds, based on the assumption that memory impairments in aged subjects are similar in nature to those in Alzheimer's patients. The therapeutic potential of novel compounds has also been assessed using NHPs with cognitive deficits due to sleep deprivation, or fatigue (such as in tests of sustained attention), and etc.[221] However, just as with rodent studies, the possibility that non-specific performance variables may be affecting the results needs to be considered with these models of cognitive deficits before attributing the drug action to cognition.

SUGGESTED PROCEDURES TO ASSESS POTENTIAL EFFICACY USING DONEPEZIL AS AN EXAMPLE

A review of the data with donepezil might help to illustrate how preclinical assessments can be conducted to maximize predictive validity. Donepezil was approved in 1996 after consistently producing statistically significant effects in AD patients in numerous, large, well-controlled clinical trials. Donepezil has a wide therapeutic index and now captures more than 80% of the market for dementia-related cognitive deficits, with annual sales of approximately 1.0 billion US dollars. A recent review of well-controlled clinical trials[236] showed that the largest effects of donepezil, were seen in patients treated with a high dose (10 mg/day) for an extended period of time (24 weeks)[237]. Unfortunately, even this maximum improvement leaves AD patients more like non-treated AD patients than normal controls. To illustrate this point, the means and standard deviations of ADAS-Cog scores for non-demented controls and AD patients treated with donepezil or placebo were estimated from several studies,[238-244] as illustrated in Figure 4.3. The mean changes in ADAS-Cog scores following donepezil treatment indicate a relatively small improvement compared to AD patients treated with placebo. Even the largest effects of donepezil leave AD patients much closer to non-treated AD patients than to non-demented age-matched controls, and the standard deviations almost completely overlap between the two groups, as shown in the figure on the left. Only with large samples, such as those typically used in clinical trials shown in the figure on the right, is the standard error of the means small enough so that the the effects of donepezil can be reliably detected.

Review Publications in the Literature

When assessing the therapeutic potential of any novel target, it is important, of course, to begin by examining what has been published. A survey of the literature was conducted to identify publications that assessed the potential efficacy of donepezil in preclinical models (Table 4.5). While donepezil has produced therapeutic effects in preclinical studies, there were fewer preclinical studies demonstrating the therapeutic potential of donepezil than might be expected, given its length of time on the market, market share and gross sales. On the other hand, the limited number of preclinical studies demonstrating efficacy with donepezil is consistent with the very small effects produced in AD patients.

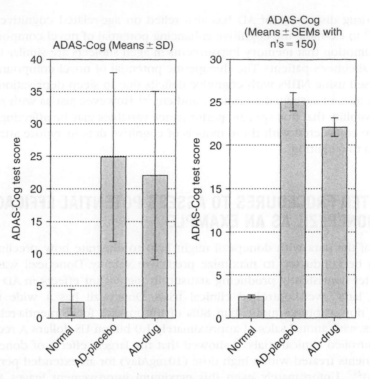

Figure 4.3 Examination of the variability associated with changes in ADAS-Cog scores of normal aged-matched controls, and AD patients treated with donepezil or placebo. Means and standard deviations of ADAS-Cog scores in non-demented controls and AD patients treated with donepezil or placebo were estimated from several studies.[238–244]

In addition to the small number of studies that demonstrated potential efficacy, many of these studies reported a narrow range of therapeutic doses, and the effective doses varied from one study to another. For example, inverted U-shaped dose–response curves were seen in animals with scopolamine-induced deficits in the radial arm maze: therapeutic effects were detected only at 0.25 or 0.30 mg/kg, and there were no beneficial effects of donepezil at slightly lower doses (0.18–0.30 mg/kg) or at slightly higher doses of 0.5–0.60 mg/kg i.p.[245,246] Inverted U-shaped functions in other studies were shifted to a completely different range. AF64A-lesioned rats in a radial arm maze were improved at 1.0 and 2.0 mg/kg, but there was no effect of donepezil at 0.6 or 3.0 mg/kg.[247] Scopolamine-induced deficits on measures of working memory in a radial arm maze task in rats were also attenuated by donepezil at 0.7 mg/kg, but there was no effect at 0.5 mg/kg, and the effects at 1.0 mg/kg were significant but smaller than at 0.7 mg/kg.[248]

Behavioral effects also varied from one study to the next. For example, in an operant DMTS task in rats, 1.0 mg/kg (but not 0.1 or 0.3 mg/kg) attenuated deficits produced by scopolamine with delays of 4, 8, and 16 s in one study,[249] but in another DMTS study, 1.0 mg/kg attenuated scopolamine-induced deficits, but only

Table 4.5 Preclinical experiments of the potential for donepezil to attenuate cognitive deficits

Behavioral test	Publication	Deficit	Significant doses	Non-significant doses
Passive avoidance	Carey et al.[255]	No deficit, normal young rats	0.01, 0.1, 1.0 mg/kg, PO (all doses equally effective)	
	Smith et al.[351]	No deficit, normal young rats	0.0003 mg/kg, SC	0.003, 0.03, 3.0 µg/kg
	Tokita et al.[352]	Scopolamine 1.0 mg/kg, IP	1.0 mg/kg, IP	0.032, 0.1, 0.32, 3.2 mg/kg, IP
	Yamaguchi et al.[353]	Scopolamine 2.0 mg/kg IP	0.1 mg/kg PO	0.01, 1.0, 10.0 mg/kg PO
	Sato et al.[354]	ICV DCG-IV (mGluR II agonist)-induced deficits	1.0 mg/kg SC	0.1, 0.5 mg/kg SC
	Sato et al.[354]	ICV LY341495 (mGluR II antagonist)-induced deficits	1.0 mg/kg SC	0.1, 0.5 mg/kg SC
	Tokita et al.[352]	NbM lesions	0.32, 3.2 mg/kg, IP	0.032, 0.1, 1.0 mg/kg, IP
	Ogura et al.[254]	NbM lesions	0.125, 0.25, 0.5, 1.0 mg/kg, PO	
	Suzuki et al.[355]	Cycloheximide 150 mg/kg, SC	0.3 and 1.0 mg/kg, PO	0.03, 0.1 mg/kg, PO
	Suzuki et al.[355]	Hemicholinium-3 0.3 µg, ICV	3.0 and 10.0 mg/kg, PO	0.3 and 1.0 mg/kg, PO
	Tokita et al.[352]	Aged, 24–26 months aged rats	No improvement	0.032, 0.32, 3.2 mg/kg, IP
Contextual and cued fear conditioning	Dong et al.[356]	9–10 months Tg$_{2576}$ Aβ+ mice	0.3 mg/kg SC	0.1, 1.0 mg/kg SC
Lick suppression	Dawson and Iverson[251]	Scopolamine 0.6 mg/kg, SC	0.1 and 0.6 mg/kg, SC	1.0 mg/kg, SC

(continued)

Table 4.5 (Continued)

Behavioral test	Publication	Deficit	Significant doses	Non-significant doses
T-maze continuous alternation	Spowart-Manning and van der Staay[357]	No deficit, normal young mice	0.3, 1.0, 3.0 mg/kg PO	
	Spowart-Manning and van der Staay[357]	Scopolamine 1.0 mg/kg, IP	3.0 mg/kg PO	
	Bontempi[358]	Scopolamine 1.2 mg/kg SC	0.9, 2.7 mg/kg SC	0.45, 5.5, 8.2 SC
	Bontempi[358]	24–26 months aged mice	0.18 mg/kg SC	0.046, 0.091, 0.36, 0.73 mg/kg SC
5-Choice serial reaction-time test	Kirkby et al.[359]	Scopolamine 0.075 mg/kg, SC	1.0/kg, IP	
	Balducci et al.[360]	Cholinergic AMPA lesions of the NbM	1.0/kg IP	0.5 mg/kg IP
Novel object recognition	Luine et al.[361]	Ovariectomized female rats	1.0 mg/kg/day SC	
	Pirckaerts et al.[362]	Normal rats with 24 h delay	1.0 mg/kg PO	0.1, 0.3 mg/kg
Water T-maze spatial learning and reversal	Dong et al.[356]	9–10 months Tg$_{2576}$ Aβ+ mice	0.3, 1.0 mg/kg SC	0.1/kg SC
Delayed (non-) matching to sample	Higgins et al.[250]	Scopolamine 0.06 mg/kg, SC	1.0 mg/kg, IP and 3.0 mg/kg, PO	
	Kirkby et al.[359]	Scopolamine 0.075 mg/kg, SC	1.0 mg/kg, IP	0.1 and 0.3 mg/kg, IP
	Poorheidari et al.[249]	Scopolamine 0.1 mg/kg, SC	1.0 mg/kg, SC	
	Dawson and Iversen[251]	Scopolamine 0.4 mg/kg, IP	0.1, 0.3, 1.0 mg/kg, IP	0.1 and 0.3 mg/kg, SC
	Carey et al.[255]	Normal young monkeys	0.3 and 1.0 mg/kg, PO	
	Higgins et al.[250]	Perforant path lesions	No improvement	1.0 and 3.0 mg/kg, PO

(*continued*)

Table 4.5 (Continued)

Behavioral test	Publication	Deficit	Significant doses	Non-significant doses
	Higgins *et al.*[250]	Transient cerebral ischemia	No improvement	1.0 mg/kg, IP
	Bontempi[358]	24–26 months aged mice	0.091, 0.36 mg/kg SC	0.046, 0.18, 0.73 mg/kg SC
Radial arm maze	Wang and Tang[246]	Scopolamine 0.15 mg/kg, IP	0.3, 0.6, and 0.9 mg/kg, PO	0.15 and 1.2 mg/kg, PO
	Cheng, Ren and Tang[248]	Scopolamine 0.20 mg/kg, IP	0.5, 0.7, 1.0 mg/kg, PO	0.3 mg/kg, PO
	Braida *et al.*[245]	Scopolamine 0.25 mg/kg, SC	0.25 mg/kg, PO	0.125, 0.18, 0.5 mg/kg, PO
	Ogura *et al.*[254]	Scopolamine 0.5 mg/kg	0.5 mg/kg, PO	0.25 mg/kg
	Yamaguchi *et al.*[353]	Scopolamine 0.5 mg/kg IP	10.0 mg/kg PO	0.01, 0.1, 1.0 mg/kg PO
	Cheng and Tang[247]	AF64A-lesioned rats	1.0 and 2.0 mg/kg, PO	0.6, 3.0 mg/kg, PO
Spatial cone field orientation	Van der Staay[363]	Scopolamine 0.5 mg/kg IP	No improvement	0.1, 0.3, 1.0 mg/kg IP
Morris water maze	Van der Staay[364]	Young normal rats	No improvement	0.3, 1.0, 3.0 mg/kg PO
	Rogers and Hagan[365]	4 and 7 day delay for forgetting	No improvement	0.3, 1.0 mg/kg, PO
	Chen *et al.*[366]	Scopolamine in acquisition and retention (0.4 and 1.5 mg/kg, respectively)	0.1, 0.3, 1.0 mg/kg, IP	
	Ogura *et al.*[254]	Medial septal lesions	0.5 mg/kg, PO	2.0 mg/kg, IP ($p = 0.055$)
	Xu *et al.*[367]	4-vessel occlusion/ischemia	0.3, 1.0 mg/kg	0.1 mg/kg
	Van Dam *et al.*[368]	4 months APP23 mice	0.3, 0.6 mg/kg/day IP	
	Abe *et al.*[369]	24–25 months rats	0.25, 0.50 mg/kg PO	1.0 mg/kg POO

Table 4.6 Potential efficacy of donepezil in preclinical cognition models

Deficit	No. positive experiments	No. negative experiments
Scopolamine	16	1
NbM lesions	3	0
Transgenic mice	3	0
Aging	3	1
Normal animals, delay	4	2
mGlurR2 antagonist	2	0
Cycloheximide	1	0
Hemicholinium-3	1	0
AF64A	1	0
Perforant path lesions	0	1
Transient cerebral ischemia	0	1

Donepezil was primarily reported to be efficacious in models of specific cholinergic deficits, such as scopolamine-induced deficits and lesions of cholinergic cell bodies (NbM).

at intermediate delays of 8 and 16 seconds, not at the shorter or longer delays.[250] In yet another DMTS study, all doses of donepezil (0.1, 0.3, and 1.0 mg/kg) attenuated scopolamine-induced deficits, but the improvement was only evident at the shorter delays (1, 2, and 4 s.). At the longer delays donepezil tended to impair performance at all doses used.[251]

With respect to deficit models, a number of studies failed to detect any therapeutic effects of donepezil. For example, chronic treatment with donepezil failed to improve age-related deficits in the MWM,[252] donepezil failed to improve performance in rats with perforant path lesions or transient cerebral ischemia,[250] and it failed to improve retention in the MWM in young normal rats at 0.3 or 1.0 mg/kg.[253] As might be expected given the mechanism of action of AChEIs, therapeutic effects of donepezil were most often reported in animals with cholinergic deficits, such as those produced with the anti-cholinergic scopolamine or lesion of the cholinergic cell bodies in the nucleus basalis (Table 4.6), and the magnitude of the effects were largest in simple conditioning tasks (Table 4.7). For example, donepezil improved performance in a passive avoidance task in NBM-lesioned rats equally well at all doses tested, from 0.125–1.0 mg/kg,[254] and donepezil reversed scopolamine-induced deficits in a passive avoidance task at all doses tested, across a log-scale dose-range from 0.01–1.0 mg/kg.[255]

Table 4.7 Potential efficacy of donepezil in preclinical tests of cognitive function

Behavioral function	Test	No. positive[a]	No. negative
Spatial mapping	Morris water maze	5	2 (normal forgetting)
	Spatial cone field orientation	0	1
Working memory	Radial arm maze	6	0
	Delayed (non-) matching to sample	6	2 (lesion models)
	T-maze spatial alternation	5	0
	Novel object recognition	2	0
Attention	Serial choice reaction-time	1	0
Classical conditioning	Passive avoidance and fear conditioning	12	1 (age)

[a] *Number of experiments that demonstrated potential efficacy with donepezil.*

Determine if Potential Efficacy can be Replicated in Rodents

In order to assess the reliability of the efficacious effects of donepezil reported in these publications in rodents, one of the authors (MDL), tested donepezil in rats. Since the efficacious effects of donepezil were most often detected in models of specific cholinergic deficits, such as with scopolamine-induced deficits, replication studies were conducted with scopolamine-induced deficits, using a range of behavioral tests.[256] Even when tested against selective, scopolamine-induced cholinergic deficits, the effects of the AChEI, donepezil, were very small in the most clinically relevant tests of higher cognitive functions, such as the MWM, the RAM, and DNMTS tests of spatial mapping and working memory, accounting for only about 1% of the variance in the data, which is comparable to the magnitude of the effects of donepezil seen in AD patients (Table 4.8).

Determine if Potential Efficacy can be Replicated in NHPs

In addition to replicating studies conducted in rodents, if therapeutic effects of a novel compound have been reported in NHPs, then replication studies should be conducted in NHPs as well. Buccafusco titrated both task difficulty and individual doses of donepezil,[257] as well as other cholinergic compounds such as physostigmine[258] and nicotine,[259] to demonstrate therapeutic effects in NHPs, in a DMTS task. Titration procedures were used in order to avoid floor and ceiling effects, to reduce variability between subjects, and to bring performance into a range most likely to detect therapeutic effects. These procedures are used with NHPs and in humans; especially aged

Table 4.8 Effect size between scopolamine and scopolamine + donepezil treatment groups

Behavioral function	Test	Effect size ω^2	Power[a]
Spatial mapping	Cumulative error in MWM	~0.2	6%
Working memory	RAM entries until first error and DNMTS % correct	~0.6	15%
Classical conditioning	Fear conditioning	6.2	45%
Attention	5-CSRTT % correct	10.0	60%
Psychomotor function	DNMTS no. trials completed and 5-CSRTT % omissions	18.7 and 49.4	98%

ω^2 = % of variance. Small effect = 1%, medium effect = 6%, large effect = 14%.[370]
[a]Power is the probability that the largest effect in this group would be detected as statistically significant with n's = 20 (from Ref. [256]).

and demented subjects,[233,258,260-262] and when testing compounds for AD in NHP.[263-265] For example, instead of imposing fixed levels of delay (e.g., 5, 10, 20, 40 s between sample response and presentation of the choice stimuli), monkeys may be tested prior to drug administration to determine the level of delay necessary for them to maintain a standard zero delay level of accuracy (85-100%), short delay (75-85%), intermediate or medium delay (65-74%) and long delay (55-64%). This procedural modification was described by Paule and colleagues,[264] and is used by Buccafusco and his colleagues in all their studies.[266] After adjusting task difficulty, animals are also often tested using a range of doses of a particular compound, and the "best dose" is identified for each individual animal.[ix] Animals are then tested again using both the task difficulty and dose that are most likely to detect therapeutic effects.

In order to determine the reliability of the efficacious effects previously reported for donepezil in NHPs, one of the present authors (RMcA) explored the therapeutic potential of donepezil and other cholinergic compounds using similar task difficulty and individual dose titration procedures, in order to maximize the probability of detecting therapeutic effects. First, young (5 years of age) and aged (approximately 25 years old) male rhesus monkeys were trained either on a delayed color matching paradigm,[259] illustrated in Figure 4.4(a), or a touch-screen paired associates paradigm,[267,268] illustrated in Figure 4.4(b). This study compared the accuracy of making a correct choice in a task whose complexity, or "memory load" was increased by prolonging the delay between a stimulus presentation and choice phase (delayed color matching), or by holding the delay constant at 5 s and increasing the number of paired associates and spatial locations made to the original cue (visuospatial paired associates).

[ix] Please refer to[266] or[260] for more detailed discussions of the "best dose" strategy.

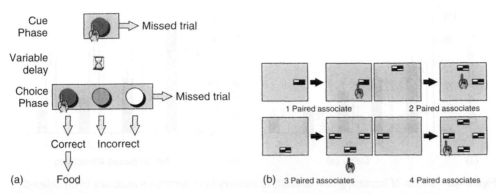

Figure 4.4 Illustration of two common matching paradigms used with primates in cognitive research, (a) delayed color matching paradigm,[259,267] one of three color cues are presented initially by illuminating a stimulus light. The subject is required to respond to this cue by touching the illuminated button within a user-defined time. The cue light then turns off, and after a variable delay of up to 12s, a row of three buttons will turn on with three colored lights. Correctly matching the cue color by pressing the button illuminated with that color produces a food reward. Incorrect responses of pressing a button illuminated with a different color, or failure to respond within a predetermined time produces a 10s time-out period followed by the next trial. (b) Visuospatial paired associates paradigm,[268] a complex geometrical stimulus is presented initially at semi-random positions on a computer-controlled touch-screen. A monkey that has been trained previously to respond to stimuli appearing on this touch-screen by touching the stimulus with its finger/hand is required to touch the stimulus causing it to disappear for a user-defined time period. At the end of this period, the stimulus re-appears in one or more positions on the touch-screen. The monkey must remember the original position of the stimulus and touch the stimulus in that position before being rewarded with a food pellet. The complexity of the task can be manipulated by increasing the number of paired associates with which the subject is presented. (The authors acknowledge the excellent technical assistance provided by Mr. Robert Cole of Pharmacia and Upjohn, who carried out the daily training and testing of these monkeys.)

The data illustrated in Figure 4.5 indicate that regardless of the method used, there was a very clear effect of task difficulty (i.e., the greater the memory load the less accurate the monkeys were). However, there were differences between these procedures with respect to the effects of age. No effect of age was noted in the monkeys responding to delayed color matching (Figure 4.5(a)), but there was a very clear effect of age, which interacted significantly with task difficulty, in monkeys responding to paired associates (Figure 4.5(b)). Although it had been used for this purpose in another laboratory,[269] in the present study the delayed color matching paradigm did not detect age-related changes in cognitive ability in rhesus monkeys. In contrast, the results indicated that the touch-screen paired associates paradigm was sensitive to differences in choice accuracy due not only to task difficulty, but also to age, which more strongly supported the validity of this task.[258] Therefore, the effects of donepezil, physostigmine, and nicotine were examined by increasing the number of paired associates that the monkey had to remember in order to make a correct response (Figure 4.6).

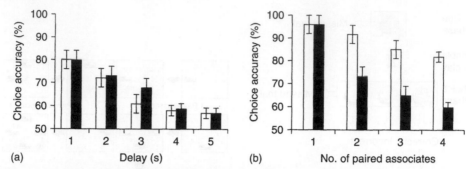

Figure 4.5 Effects of increasing task difficulty or memory load, on choice accuracy in (a) delayed color matching paradigm in young and aged rhesus monkeys, reduction of choice accuracy on the delayed color matching task by increasing the delay between stimulus presentation and choice in young (□ <7 years) or aged (■ >25 years) rhesus monkeys. A significant delay-dependant decrease in delayed color matching was observed, but no age-related impairment. (b) Visuospatial paired associates paradigm in young and aged rhesus monkeys, reduction of choice accuracy on the paired associates task by increasing the number of visuospatial paired associates to be remembered young (□ <7 years) or aged (■ >25 years) rhesus monkeys. Significant delay- and age-dependant decreases in paired associate responding were observed with a significant age by paired associates interaction. (The authors acknowledge the excellent technical assistance provided by Mr. Robert Cole of Pharmacia and Upjohn, who carried out the daily training and testing of these monkeys.)

Various doses of each compound were tested initially in young and aged rhesus monkeys. While there were significant effects of task difficulty and age on choice accuracy in paired associates learning, none of the cholinergic compounds showed any dose related or other therapeutic effect on choice accuracy in either the young or aged monkeys. Consequently, each monkey's choice accuracy was examined *post hoc*, in order to identify the dose of each compound that produced the best improvement in responding. The paired associate studies were repeated using the best dose of each compound for each subject (Figure 4.7).

While task difficulty and age effects were still observed, neither donepezil, nicotine, nor physostigmine altered choice accuracy significantly, even when administered at the "best dose" for each monkey (Figure 4.7). These data illustrate that, despite the titration of dose and task difficulty to maximize the probability of achieving a positive result, these methodological manipulations did not guarantee a positive outcome for donepezil or other cholinergic compounds.

Evaluate Potential Efficacy Based on Thorough Analysis of all the Evidence

Robust effects of donepezil had been reported in the MWM, RAM and DNMTS in rodents, and in DMTS in NHP, but those results were not reliable enough to be reproduced. Replication studies verified that donepezil attenuates scopolamine-induced effects on psychomotor function, and reproduced the efficacious effects previously reported with tests of attention and simple conditioning in rodents. Those findings

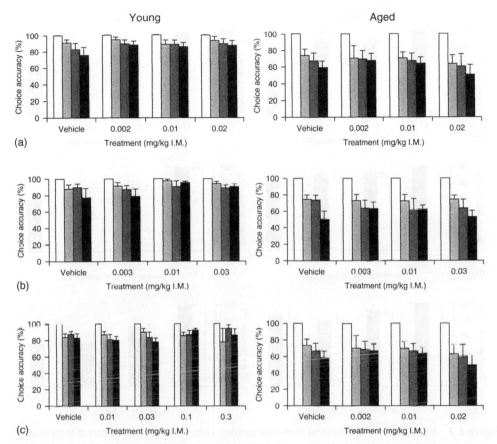

Figure 4.6   Paired associates learning in rhesus monkeys after intramuscular (I.M.) administration of three doses of either (a) nicotine, (b) physostigmine, or (c) donepezil. The data refer to the choice accuracy (%) of ☐ 1, ▨ 2, ▧ 3 or ■ 4 paired associates in young (6–7 years of age) and aged (25–30 years of age) monkeys.

suggest that while compounds may produce fairly robust effects in less clinically relevant behavioral tests, the use of more clinically relevant tests, in this case tests of higher-level cognitive functions, most accurately reflect the effects treatments will have in AD patients.[256] By examining the pattern of the results, both in terms of the magnitude and reliability of the effects, as well as the clinical relevance of the different models and behavioral tests, preclinical assessments can be conducted in a way that optimizes their predictive validity.

TRANSLATIONAL INITIATIVES IN AD

This section will address in more detail how preclinical, behavioral assessments of potential efficacy can be optimized in order to maximize their predictive validity and the productivity of drug discovery and development.

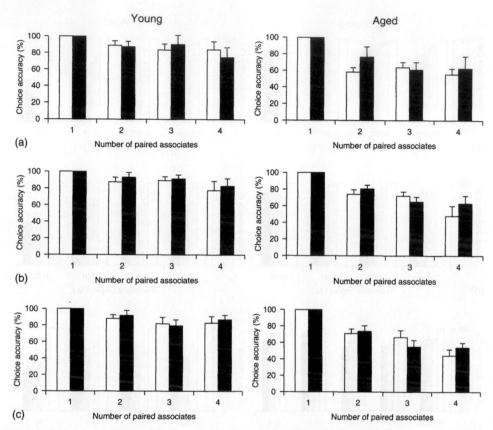

Figure 4.7 Paired associates learning in rhesus monkeys after I.M. administration of individual best doses of either (a) nicotine, (b) physostigmine, or (c) donepezil. The data refer to the choice accuracy (%) of ☐ vehicle or ■ "best dose" in young (6–7 years of age) and aged (25–30 years of age) monkeys.

Explore Non-Cholinergic Targets and Models without AChEIs as Positive Control

Some have assumed that the procedures used to develop the current "gold standard" AChEIs, such as reversing scopolamine-induced deficits, should continue to be used to develop novel treatments. However, as reviewed in the previous section, the small number of preclinical studies that detected efficacious effects with donepezil, the narrow range of effective doses and the lack of consistency between studies with respect to which doses were effective, the fact that efficacious effects were primarily detected only in models with specific cholinergic deficits, and the fact that donepezil only produced very small and inconsistent effects in the most clinically relevant tests of higher cognitive functions, all suggest that donepezil cannot be used as a reliable positive control. Likewise, the therapeutic potential of novel, non-cholinergic compounds may not be detected in people or animals with selective cholinergic deficits such as those produced by administering scopolamine, so those procedures should not be required for the assessment or validation of novel treatments, either in preclinical models or in early clinical trials with healthy human volunteers.

Optimize Clinical Relevance of Models and Behavioral Tests

In order to improve their predictive validity, models and behavioral tests should be selected based on their clinical relevance. In the past, models and behavioral tests were often selected largely based on their expediency: on their ability to demonstrate therapeutic potential for the compounds being tested, and the speed at which those compounds could be screened. Even now, many compounds continue to be advanced into the clinic based on data from models and behavioral tests that are able to detect the most robust therapeutic effects. For example, AChEIs were tested primarily in models of specific cholinergic deficits (Table 4.6), and behavioral tests of simple, one-trial conditioning (e.g., passive avoidance and fear conditioning, Table 4.7). Cholinergic dysfunction is only one component of AD-related pathology, and testing AChEIs in models specific to their mechanism of action tends to overestimate their therapeutic potential. Likewise, it may be easier to attenuate deficits in simple tests of cognitive function, and relying on these results may also overestimate the therapeutic potential of novel treatments (Table 4.8).

High-level cognitive functions are most severely affected in demented patients, and more appropriate preclinical tests of these functions are available. These include the MWM[270] test of spatial orientation and the acquisition and retention of spatial maps, the RAM,[271,272] and DMTS/DMNTS[128,273,274] tests of working memory, and the 5-CSRT test of attention.[275,276] With respect to models, specific cholinergic deficits are still relevant for development of AChEIs and compounds with cholinergic mechanisms, but in the absence of an effective standard, other potential targets and mechanisms can be assessed by examining the magnitude and pattern of cognitive and behavioral deficits they produce. For example, amyloid transgenic mice have been developed, and while they do exhibit cognitive deficits, the magnitude and pattern of those deficits suggest that β-amyloid alone may not account for the severe dementia seen in clinical patients. In addition to assessing the clinical relevance of the target, models of target-specific deficits can also be used to assess the therapeutic potential of treatments aimed at that target.

Develop and Validate Clinically Relevant Behavioral Tests

Model and behavioral test development in neurological and psychiatric disorders has traditionally been a "feed backwards" process in which preclinical investigators have taken their cue from the clinic as to what disorder-relevant factors and/or symptoms need to be produced in animals, and how those disorders will be measured. However, there is at least one example in the AD field that is unique in that procedures to measure changes in human cognitive processing have been developed in animals and subsequently adapted for use in humans.[x] As discussed in the section on historical origins

---

[x] Please refer to Large *et al.*, Developing therapeutics for bipolar disorder: from animal models to the clinic, in Volume 1, Psychiatric Disorders, for another example of attempts to translate methods used in animal testing back up to humans.

of animal models of cognitive processes, the procedures developed in the primate work by preclinical investigators such as Mishkin,[98] Squire,[99] and Goldman-Rakic[277] not only have been fundamental for the study of the neurobiology of cognition in animal species, but also in humans. Robbins and his colleagues realized very early that the use of non-verbal and cultural context-free visual stimuli in primates could be adapted to study similar cognitive processes in humans. Consequently the Cambridge Neuropsychological Test Automated Battery (CANTAB) was developed using geometrical shapes and colors presented on touch-sensitive screens that could be used in both NHPs and human subjects.[278,279]

The CANTAB test battery has undergone extensive validation in normal and abnormal humans. In order to determine normative values in middle-aged to elderly populations, a factor analysis of the various CANTAB subtests was carried out, initially in 787 subjects from 55 to 88 years of age,[280] and later followed up in another 341 normal volunteers from 21 to 79 years of age,[281] and normative data in normal human volunteers covering a much wider age span has recently been reported by De Luca and her colleagues.[282] These studies indicated that performance in various CANTAB subtests could distinguish among different cognitive functions. Thus, subtests such as paired associates learning, DMTS and pattern recognition are related to general learning and memory and speed of responding, while executive functions and visual perception are more related to subtests such as spatial working memory, tower of London and intra- and extra-dimensional (ID/ED) set-shifting.

One of the advantages of the CANTAB testing battery is that both the stimuli and test procedures are identical, or very similar, in both the human and primate versions. This has helped to make more direct comparisons between subjects and species. The strategy of comparing response patterns in the various CANTAB subtests of NHPs lesioned in specific brain areas with those of human subjects who have undergone surgical or disease-related lesions in homologous areas, has helped to strengthen the mapping of function to brain area; particularly impaired function. Patients with frontal lobectomies, but not with temporal lobe or amygdalo-hippocampectomy excisions, for example, have great difficulty with extra-dimensional set-shifting when tested on instruments such as the Wisconsin Card sort,[283] or on the CANTAB ID/ED subtest.[284] Similar extra-dimensional set-shifting deficits have been observed in prefrontal cortex-lesioned marmosets.[212] CANTAB subtests have detected early signs of cognitive impairment in asymptomatic HIV-infected subjects;[285] impairments that can be modeled and assessed in SIV-infected primates.[286] Furthermore, modified CANTAB-like subtests have been used successfully with brain imaging techniques in both humans[261,287-290] and in NHPs.[291]

Despite the considerable investment required in setting up a primate unit and then training NHPs on the various subtests such as DMTS and paired associates learning,[230,268,292] CANTAB methodology is attracting the attention of the pharmaceutical industry for use in both drug discovery[293] and clinical development. Part of this interest has been generated by the relationship between paired associates learning and rates of progression in AD. Fowler and colleagues[294,295] first indicated the utility of the CANTAB paired associates learning subtest to identify patients with questionable Alzheimer's dementia from those of probable AD, and compared their response patterns to subjects with Parkinson's disease or depressed subjects. At early stages of dementia, when patients begin to have difficulties remembering and start consulting their physicians, it can be difficult to distinguish between subjects with "benign forget-fulness" and those with AD that are beginning to exhibit its symptoms. It was observed that at initial testing, those subjects with questionable dementia tended to commit a similar number of paired associates errors (>30) as those diagnosed with probable AD, by NINCDS–ADRDA criteria, and within 12–24 months they were re-classified as AD. Those who had scored less than 30 errors were no more likely to develop AD than elderly controls within the same time period. Interestingly, there are no major differences in blood-oxygen-level-dependent responses in occipitoparietal regions measured by fMRI between elderly controls and subjects with mild AD.[261] The authors suggest that AD subjects have a "greater recruitment of the same brain regions as age-matched controls as a means of compensating for neuropathology and associated cognitive impairment in Alzheimer disease".[296]

Several implications can be drawn from these studies. First, the studies show the utility of a battery of computerized, non-verbal, culture-free behavioral testing procedures that can be used in both human and NHPs. This battery of tests can be used to follow subjects over time, and repeated computerized testing with paired associates learning can be used as a more objective measure of disease progression to monitor not only the effects of potential symptomatic, but also disease-modifying therapics in AD. This latter approach has already shown promise in the clinical development of the combined AChEI and βAPP modifier phenserine.[297,298] This compound showed significant positive results in the CANTAB paired associates test during a double-blind, placebo-controlled Phase II AD trial.[299] Unfortunately, these promising results were not confirmed in an extended Phase III trial, but the results suggested that drug exposures were too low, and if a new formulation can be developed that will allow higher exposure levels, this target and mechanism may be examined again.

Combine Behavioral/Functional with Molecular/Biological Measures

As discussed in the section reviewing assessments of donepezil, the absence of a reliable standard or positive control to validate new models and targets and to assess novel compounds adds an additional layer of complexity to an already daunting task. However, the power and predictive validity of preclinical assessments can be enhanced by combining behavioral measures with additional measures of the mechanisms that mediate the cognitive functions of interest. These additional measures are most valuable if they are collected concurrently with the behavioral data, especially in a well-characterized behavioral task. For example, two of the authors (SAD and REH) have demonstrated electrophysiological correlates of behavior in rodents and primates performing well-characterized working memory tasks.[218,300] Using these techniques, it has been possible to identify neural activity patterns and even specific brain regions involved in cognitive decisions[218,301-304] during different stages of a spatial DNMTS task that assesses working memory.[203,305] The results of these studies suggest that different cognitive processes are mediated by different brain areas, and that the cognitive basis for behavioral success in performing the DNMTS task in these studies could not have been ascertained in the absence of electrophysiological recording (cf., [306,307]).

A similar series of experiments were conducted with ampakines, positive allosteric modulators of AMPA receptors that enhance depolarization of neurons and ultimately enhance NMDA receptor-mediated activation of neurons.[308-310] These studies demonstrated that disruption of cognitive processing was alleviated by CX717 mentioned above, as evidenced by[1] recovery of performance on a multi-object DMTS task by monkeys, and[2] concomitant reversal of disruptive influences of brain imaging correlates that characterized successful performance of the task *in the same monkeys during the same testing sessions.*[221] In that study, measurement of brain metabolic markers (local cerebral glucose utilization) of DMTS task correlates provided a means of identifying which brain regions (i.e., medial temporal lobe, prefrontal cortex, and striatum) were engaged while monkeys performed the task; permitting determination of the functional significance of those brain regions when performance of the task was disrupted by sleep deprivation. Once characterized in this context it was possible to determine whether a drug (CX717): (a) alleviated the behavioral effects of sleep deprivation, and (b) did so by reversing the alterations in brain metabolic *correlates of task performance* resulting from sleep deprivation.

The internal consistency afforded by such testing is a valuable tool in ruling out several factors that often plague extrapolation of drug testing in animals to humans. The likelihood that brain correlates of successful task performance would be differentially altered from the behavioral measures of those same events is very low, and therefore both measures together provide the means to: [1] determine the efficacy of the drug on performance and [2] determine whether the drug is affecting a process critical for that performance. A dissociation of the two implies a false positive outcome due to non-specific drug actions, a circumstance that can lead to a false prediction of efficacy in humans if the corresponding functional brain correlates are not available.

As mentioned above, in some cases it is possible to identify constituents of memory tasks in animals that can be translated more directly to humans. Although this is more difficult with cognitive variables, current methods may allow this type of assessment in the future and could result in limiting the number of instances in which positive effects in animal studies are not related to success in the clinic. Figure 4.8 shows the results of a study in which DMTS task difficulty was categorized with respect to performance accuracy in terms of trial-to-trial variation in difficulty or "cognitive load," a variable that has been repeatedly used in human studies of cognitive performance.[311-315] DMTS trials with more complex parameters (i.e., increased duration of delay and number of objects to choose from) ranked routinely and systematically lower in performance accuracy across animals than trials with shorter delays and fewer objects. The graph in Figure 4.8(c) shows that trials characterized in this manner had performance levels appropriately above and below the continuum of difficulty demarcated by the mean across all trials presented in normal sessions (All). Using PET scans of uptake of 18Flourodoxhyglucose (FDG) as an indication of local brain cerebral glucose metabolism during the task,[221] it was possible to distinguish areas that were engaged on high versus low cognitive load trials. By comparing isolated sessions in which only one type of trial was presented with those in which both types (high and low load) were presented together, it was determined that the brain regions

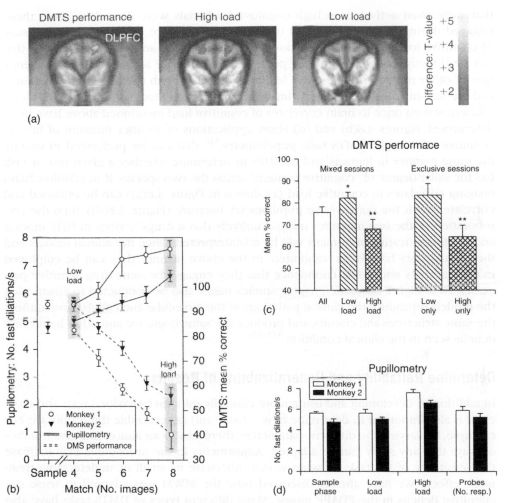

Figure 4.8 A translational model for cognitive load using NHPs. Measures of cognitive load in NHPs performing a DMTS task (a) SPM statistical maps of local cerebral glucose metabolic rate (CMRglc) from PET scans of 18Fluorodeoxyglucose uptake in prefrontal (DLPFC) brain region while monkeys performed DMTS task. Colored voxels superimposed on MRI images reflect the degree to which different brain areas were activated on high versus low cognitive load trials. (b) Comparison of pupillometry and DMTS performance (right axis) across different types of DMTS trials that range from low to high cognitive load. Pupillary dilation frequency increases (left axis) and DMTS performance declines along the same dimension of DMTS task complexity. (c) Mean DMTS task performance during imaging sessions above in which only high or low cognitive load trials were presented. Performance was the same as when those same trials were presented randomly in normal sessions. (d) Pupillometric measures of cognitive load in same two monkeys shown in (b). Mean (± SEM) number of rapid (fast) pupillary dilations increased under conditions of high cognitive workload. Frequency of rapid pupil dilations was not different from the single image sample phase for low load trials. Probe: presentation of 6–8 images as on high cognitive load trials presented independently without response contingency. This type of analysis also demonstrated that performance on high cognitive load trials was the primary factor that was facilitated by the ampakine CX717.[221] (The authors acknowledge and greatly appreciate the combined efforts and expertise of Dr. Linda Porrino, Mack Miller, and Kathryn Gill.)

that were most activated on high cognitive load trials were dissociable from those engaged during low cognitive load trials (images in Figure 4.8(a)). Using a measure of cognitive load can provide additional insight into drug action in NHP studies that can be directly assessed in human preclinical imaging. In addition, the implementation of other measures of cognitive load that correlate with the same brain measures and are non-invasive and easier to implement in human studies can serve as a more efficient screen once its brain correlates of cognitive load mentioned above have been determined. Figures 4.8(b) and (d) show applications of another measure of human cognitive load to the DMTS task, pupillometry,[316] that can be performed in exactly the same manner in humans and in NHPs to determine whether a given test or task has the same degree of "cognitive content" across the two species. If, in addition, brain imaging correlates of cognitive load (as shown in Figure 4.8(a)) can be obtained and correlated with the non-invasive pupillometry measure (Figure 4.8(d)), then the corroboration of the two measures make it unlikely that a drugs' actions in NHP models and in clinical testing in humans will be misinterpreted. Once the animal models and the human tests have been "calibrated" in the above manner, they can be employed in clinical trials with some confidence that they engage the same drug sensitive processes. New high-T magnetic imaging studies might also be conducted to ensure that the models reproduce the clinical pathology at the molecular and cellular levels, affect the same structures and circuits, and produce the same cognitive and other behavioral deficits seen in the clinical condition.[317-321]

Determine Reliability and Generalizability of Results

In addition to developing and using more clinically relevant behavioral tests and models, it is also important to determine how reliable and generalizable the results are. For example, by varying the different parameters, there can be an almost limitless number of ways that any study can be adapted. Adjustments in the procedures may increase the sensitivity of the task for what would otherwise be small or undetectable treatment effects. We have already discussed how the MWM was adapted to tease out cognitive deficits in the PDAPP mouse. Many different types of DMTS tasks have also evolved over the last 30–40 years, and current technology provides very different implementations than were used previously.[218,221] DMTS tasks in NHPs can include discrimination between as few as two lights on a console across a 30 s delay,[269,322] matching faces or other objects displayed across longer (>120 s) delays,[323,324] or performing a well-characterized touch-screen task that is also performed by humans.[192,325] It is important to consider whether all these different versions of the task measure similar cognitive processes, and whether they are differentially sensitive to non-cognitive factors, which could produce differences in their predictive validity.

It is also important to consider how reliable the results are from one experiment to another, even when using the same procedures. Using donepezil as an example of how to assess the therapeutic potential of novel compounds, it is clear that therapeutic effects reported in the literature are not always replicated, which emphasizes the importance of conducting replication studies. Failure to replicate results can be attributed to methodological differences, but if therapeutic effects are detected only with specific parameters and procedures, this suggests that the effects may not be generalizable to clinical populations, and/or that the effects might be attributed to some non-specific effect.

Consider Potential Non-Specific, Non-Cognitive Confounds

In addition, it is important to be very cautious in the interpretation of the apparent cognitive deficits displayed by the animals, and the changes in behavior induced by the drug treatment employed. It is important to consider and explore the possibility that non-specific, non-cognitive factors might be affecting the results. For example, the Tg_{2576} mouse overexpresses amyloid, but also carries other mutations that can conceivably affect behavior and cognition. Because of the C57Bl/6SJL background on which they were bred, Tg_{2576} mice have a 25% probability of inherited retinal degeneration.[326] This mutation has also been found in three other transgenic lines (APPsw, P301L, APPsw + P301L[327]). The Tg_{2576} mouse is also prone to seizures and to death during early development.[328] Not only could these genetic abnormalities contribute directly to behavioral effects, but they could also affect the behavioral results indirectly. For example, male Tg_{2576} mice are very aggressive, and as a consequence, they are housed individually rather than in groups. Since social isolation is a stressor that induces anxious-like behaviors in mice (cf.,[329]), the housing conditions required with these mice could confound their performance in tests of cognitive function.

As with any test of cognitive function, the dependent variable is an indirect measure of a psychological construct. Therefore, investigators must constantly guard against simplistic assumptions and overgeneralizations when interpreting their results. For example, aged rats and mice suffer loss of visual acuity, and it is usually assumed that, since the MWM is dependent on visual–spatial cues, the most severely impaired aged animals may simply suffer from loss of visual acuity. However, studies with blind young rats has shown that these animals still perform fairly well, despite being completely blind, perhaps because they are using a strategy of "looping" around the pool.[330] Even if impaired aged rats were completely blind, that would not account for the severity of their deficits in the MWM. Nevertheless, aged rats do lose visual acuity, and a treatment that improved vision might improve their performance in the MWM. Aged rats also do not thermoregulate as well as young animals, and after being placed in and out of the water during their daily trials, they become hypothermic.[331] Warming the aged rats to maintain normothermia between trials improved their performance, suggesting that part of their age-related deficits was a result of hypothermic amnesia. Again, improvements in MWM performance due to a treatment that helps the aged animals maintain normothermia could incorrectly be interpreted as evidence that the treatment is a cognitive enhancer. Experimenters should never accept evidence of therapeutic potential at face value, but should constantly be on guard, considering the possibility that their results might be affected by non-specific confounds, and should explore these possibilities so that they can be ruled out.

Increase Communication and Collaborations

Differences between the procedures used in preclinical and clinical assessments of potential efficacy may also contribute to the lack of success in developing effective novel treatments for AD. For example, preclinical scientists are able and even expected to conduct their studies using experimental manipulations and invasive sampling procedures that are not acceptable for clinical investigators. To satisfy reviewers as part of the peer review process required for publication, preclinical scientists must include specific control measures, address questions about the potential mechanism of action, the pharmacological specificity and functional significance of the treatment; procedures that are sometimes difficult or even impossible to include in clinical trials. In addition, sometimes preclinical scientists do not design their preclinical studies to be consistent with the way these compounds will be assessed in the clinic because they are simply unaware of FDA regulations, requirements and restrictions, which can make it impossible to design clinical studies using precisely the same procedures used in the preclinical studies. Clinical protocols are also sometimes developed without sufficient input or communication with the preclinical investigators who may have years of experience with the compound. The result is that clinical trials may be conducted in ways that were never examined in prior studies with animal models, or in ways that the preclinical investigators, based on their experience, would predict is unlikely to be successful. If not properly designed, clinical trials can fail to detect efficacy for a treatment that is actually effective, which may account for some of the discrepancies between results with preclinical models and clinical trials.

Improve Experimental and Decision-Making Processes

In clinical trials, the hopes, beliefs, and expectations – together referred to as the biases of the patients and investigators, can affect the results, usually to exaggerate the therapeutic effects of the treatment being evaluated. Partly for that reason, procedures intended to reduce or limit the effects of experimenter bias have been mandated by the FDA. The effects of experimenter bias are at least as robust and consistent in experiments with animals as in clinical trials;[332,333] however, preclinical proof of concept studies rarely control for potential bias.[333] The predictive validity of preclinical assessments of potential efficacy would be improved by using the same procedures that have proven so effective to control for bias in clinical trials. For example, protocols should be finalized and approved before starting the experiment, and the protocol should define the most relevant, primary endpoints, exclusion criteria, and analytical procedures, and all procedures used to conceal treatment allocation and limit bias should be reported (for review, see[333]). In addition to using more rigorous controls within individual experiments, the management and decision-making processes in drug discovery could also be improved. Top-down decision-making dominated by market analyses and the inappropriate application of a manufacturing ethos from non-scientist, non-technical executive managers who have little training or appreciation for the scientific method and the complexities of scientific research, the use of high quotas and mandated results, as well as other inefficiencies common in the large bureaucracies that have emerged within pharmaceutical companies, all contribute to the declining levels of productivity in drug discovery that have been evident since the 1970s (for review, see[333,334]).

SUMMARY AND CONSENSUS STATEMENT

The predictive validity of preclinical assessments of potential efficacy could be improved by using the best procedures that are already available. For example, assessments should be based on a pattern analysis of all the data generated, positive and negative, with special attention devoted to the clinical relevance of the models and measures, the magnitude, reliability and generalizability of the results, and taking care to consider and rule out artefacts due to non-specific effects. Additional advancements and improvements to the models, behavioral assessment procedures and decision-making processes can also be made, beyond what is already available, which will further improve the predictive validity of the models. For example, efforts should continue to develop a model that exhibits the full array of AD-related pathology, including the pattern and severity of behavioral/functional deficits, perhaps with special consideration for measures of the global, functional deficits often measured in clinical trials. No model or preclinical assessment procedure has perfect predictive validity, but high levels of productivity are not dependent on perfect predictive validity. By using the best procedures available today, continuing to optimize those procedures and developing better models and behavioral tests, preclinical assessments of potential efficacy can be performed in a way that will reduce the rate of clinical failures due to lack of efficacy and increase the return on investment in drug discovery.

REFERENCES

1. Rice, D.P., Fillit, H.M., Max, W., Knopman, D.S., Lloyd, J.R., and Duttagupta, S. (2001). Prevalence, costs, and treatment of Alzheimer's disease and related dementia: A managed care perspective. *Am J Manag Care*, 7(8):809–818.
2. Barbui, C., Cipriani, A., Lintas, C., Bertele, V., and Garattini, S. (2007). CNS drugs approved by the centralised European procedure: true innovation or dangerous stagnation? *Psychopharmacology (Berl)*, 190(2):265–268.
3. Dickson, M. and Gagnon, J.P. (2004). The cost of new drug discovery and development. *Discov Med*, 4(22):172–179.
4. Tollman, P., Philippe, G., Altshuler, J., Flanagan, A., and Steiner, M. (2001). *A revolution in R&D: How genomics and genetics are transforming the biopharmaceutical industry*. The Boston Consulting Group, Boston, MA.
5. DiMasi, J.A., Hansen, R.W., and Grabowski, H.G. (2003). The price of innovation: New estimates of drug development costs. *J Health Econ*, 22(2):151–185.
6. Gilbert, J., Henske, P., and Singh, A. (2003). Rebuilding big pharma's business model. *In Vivo: The Business and Medicine Report*, 21(10):1–10.
7. DiMasi, J.A. (1995). Trends in drug development costs, times, and risks. *Drug Inform J*, 29:375–384.
8. Kennedy, T. (1997). Managing the drug discovery/development interface. *Drug Discov Today*, 2:436–444.

9. DiMasi, J.A. (2001). Risks in new drug development: Approval success rates for investigational drugs. *Clin Pharmacol Ther*, 69(5):297-307.

10. Prentis, R.A., Lis, Y., and Walker, S.R. (1988). Pharmaceutical innovation by the seven UK-owned pharmaceutical companies (1964-1985). *Br J Clin Pharmacol*, 25(3):387-396.

11. Schuster, D., Laggner, C., and Langer, T. (2005). Why drugs fail – A study on side effects in new chemical entities. *Curr Pharm Des*, 11(27):3545-3559.

12. Lyketsos, C.G., Steinberg, M., Tschanz, J.T., Norton, M.C., Steffens, D.C., and Breitner, J.C. (2000). Mental and behavioral disturbances in dementia: Findings from the Cache County Study on Memory in Aging. *Am J Psychiatr*, 157(5):708-714.

13. Bartus, R.T., Dean, R.L., III., Beer, B., and Lippa, A.S. (1982). The cholinergic hypothesis of geriatric memory dysfunction. *Science*, 217(4558):408-414.

14. Bartus, R.T. and Emerich, D.F. (1999). Cholinergic markers in Alzheimer disease. *JAMA*, 282(23):2208-2209.

15. Lahiri, D.K. and Farlow, M.R. (2003). Review: Cholinesterase inhibitors have a modest effect on neuropsychiatric and functional outcomes in Alzheimer's disease. *Evid Based Ment Health*, 6(3):94.

16. Peskind, E.R., Potkin, S.G., Pomara, N., Ott, B.R., Graham, S.M., Olin, J.T. *et al.* (2006). Memantine treatment in mild to moderate Alzheimer's disease: A 24-week randomized, controlled trial. *Am J Geriatr Psychiatr*, 14:704-715.

17. Hardy, J. (2006). Alzheimer's disease: The amyloid cascade hypothesis: An update and reappraisal. *J Alzheimers Dis*, 9(3 Suppl):151-153.

18. Hardy, J.A. and Higgins, G.A. (1992). Alzheimer's disease: The amyloid cascade hypothesis. *Science*, 256(5054):184-185.

19. Selkoe, D.J., Yamazaki, T., Citron, M., Podlisny, M.B., Koo, E.H., Teplow, D.B. *et al.* (1996). The role of APP processing and trafficking pathways in the formation of amyloid beta-protein. *Ann N Y Acad Sci*, 777:57-64.

20. Gong, Y., Chang, L., Viola, K.L., Lacor, P.N., Lambert, M.P., Finch, C.E. *et al.* (2003). Alzheimer's disease-affected brain: Presence of oligomeric Aβ ligands (ADDLs) suggests a molecular basis for reversible memory loss. *Proc Natl Acad Sci USA*, 100(18):10417-10422.

21. Hardy, J. and Selkoe, D.J. (2002). The amyloid hypothesis of Alzheimer's disease: Progress and problems on the road to therapeutics. *Science*, 297(5580):353-356.

22. Felsenstein, K.M. (2000). Aβ modulation: The next generation of AD therapeutics. *Ann N Y Acad Sci*, 920(1):269-273.

23. Lahiri, D.K., Farlow, M.R., Sambamurti, K., Greig, N.H., Giacobini, E., and Schneider, L.S. (2003). A critical analysis of new molecular targets and strategies for drug development in Alzheimer's disease. *Curr Drug Targets*, 4(2):97-112.

24. Aisen, P.S. (2005). The development of anti-amyloid therapy for Alzheimer's disease: From secretase modulators to polymerisation inhibitors. *CNS Drugs*, 19(12):989-996.

25. Wang, Y.J., Zhou, H.D., and Zhou, X.F. (2006). Clearance of amyloid-beta in Alzheimer's disease: Progress, problems and perspectives. *Drug Discov Today*, 11(19-20):931-938.

26. Nicoll, J.A., Wilkinson, D., Holmes, C., Steart, P., Markham, H., and Weller, R.O. (2003). Neuropathology of human Alzheimer disease after immunization with amyloid-beta peptide: A case report. *Nat Med*, 9(4):448-452.

27. Schenk, D.B., Seubert, P., Lieberburg, I., and Wallace, J. (2000). Beta-peptide immunization: A possible new treatment for Alzheimer disease. *Arch Neurol*, 57(7):934-936.

28. Gilman, S., Koller, M., Black, R.S., Jenkins, L., Griffith, S.G., Fox, N.C. *et al.* (2005). Clinical effects of Aβ immunization (AN1792) in patients with AD in an interrupted trial. *Neurology*, 64(9):1553-1562.

29. Orgogozo, J.M., Gilman, S., Dartigues, J.F., Laurent, B., Puel, M., Kirby, L.C. *et al.* (2003). Subacute meningoencephalitis in a subset of patients with AD after Abeta42 immunization. *Neurology*, 61(1):46-54.

30. Schenk, D.B., Seubert, P., Grundman, M., and Black, R. (2005). Aβ immunotherapy: Lessons learned for potential treatment of Alzheimer's disease. *Neurodegener Dis*, 2(5):255–260.

31. Lee, V.M. (1996). Regulation of tau phosphorylation in Alzheimer's disease. *Ann N Y Acad Sci*, 777:107–113.

32. Lee, V.M. (1995). Disruption of the cytoskeleton in Alzheimer's disease. *Curr Opin Neurobiol*, 5(5):663–668.

33. Trojanowski, J.Q. and Lee, V.M.Y. (2005). The Alzheimer's brain: Finding out what's broken tells us how to fix it. *Am J Pathol*, 167(5):1183–1188.

34. Lee, V.M. and Trojanowski, J.Q. (2006). Progress from Alzheimer's tangles to pathological tau points towards more effective therapies now. *J Alzheimers Dis*, 9(3 Suppl):257–262.

35. Kwon, M.O. and Herrling, P. (2006). List of drugs in development for neurodegenerative diseases. Update June 2006. *Neurodegener Dis*, 3(3):148–186.

36. Melnikova, I. (2007). Therapies for Alzheimer's disease. *Nat Rev Drug Discov*, 6(5):341–342.

37. Roses, A.D. and Pangalos, M.N. (2003). Drug development and Alzheimer disease. *Am J Geriatr Psychiatr*, 11(2):123–130.

38. Lopez Arrieta, J.M. (2002). Role of meta-analysis of clinical trials for Alzheimer's disease. *Drug Dev Res*, 56(3):401–411.

39. Gualtieri, F., Manetti, D., Romanelli, M.N., and Ghelardini, C. (2002). Design and study of piracetam-like nootropics, controversial members of the problematic class of cognition-enhancing drugs. *Curr Pharm Des*, 8(2):125–138.

40. Harries, M.H., Samson, N.A., and Cilia, J. (1998). A.J. Hunter. The profile of sabcomeline (SB-202026), a functionally selective M1 receptor partial agonist, in the marmoset, *Br J Pharmacol*, 124(2):409–415.

41. Bontempi, B., Whelan, K.T., Risbrough, V.B., Rao, T.S., Buccafusco, J.J., Lloyd, G.K. *et al.* (2001). SIB-1553A, (+/−)-4-[[2-(1-methyl-2-pyrrolidinyl)ethyl]thio]phenol hydrochloride, a subtype-selective ligand for nicotinic acetylcholine receptors with putative cognitive-enhancing properties: Effects on working and reference memory performances in aged rodents and nonhuman primates. *J Pharmacol Exp Ther*, 299(1):297–306.

42. Hood, W.F., Compton, R.P., and Monahan, J.B. (1989). D-cycloserine: A ligand for the *N*-methyl-D-aspartate coupled glycine receptor has partial agonist characteristics. *Neurosci Lett*, 98(1):91–95.

43. Randolph, C., Roberts, J.W., Tierney, M.C., Bravi, D., Mouradian, M.M., and Chase, T.N. (1994). D-cycloserine treatment of Alzheimer disease. *Alzheimer Dis Assoc Disord*, 8(3):198–205.

44. Tsai, G.E., Falk, W.E., Gunther, J., and Coyle, J.T. (1999). Improved cognition in Alzheimer's disease with short-term D-cycloserine treatment. *Am J Psychiatr*, 156(3):467–469.

45. Mazurov, A., Hauser, T., and Miller, C.H. (2006). Selective alpha7 nicotinic acetylcholine receptor ligands. *Curr Med Chem*, 13(13):1567–1584.

46. Oddo, S. and LaFerla, F.M. (2006). The role of nicotinic acetylcholine receptors in Alzheimer's disease. *J Physiol Paris*, 99(2–3):172–179.

47. Buccafusco, J.J., Letchworth, S.R., Bencherif, M., and Lippiello, P.M. (2005). Long-lasting cognitive improvement with nicotinic receptor agonists: mechanisms of pharmacokinetic-pharmacodynamic discordance. *Trends Pharmacol Sci*, 26(7):352–360.

48. Anderson, D.J., Williams, M., Pauly, J.R., Raszkiewicz, J.L., Campbell, J.E., Rotert, G. *et al.* (1995). Characterization of [3H]ABT-418: A novel cholinergic channel ligand. *J Pharmacol Exp Ther*, 273(3):1434–1441.

49. Rueter, L.E., Anderson, D.J., Briggs, C.A., Donnelly-Roberts, D.L., Gintant, G.A., Gopalakrishnan, M. *et al.* (2004). ABT-089: Pharmacological properties of a neuronal nicotinic acetylcholine receptor agonist for the potential treatment of cognitive disorders. *CNS Drug Rev*, 10(2):167–182.

50. Schneider, J.S., Tinker, J.P., Van, V.M., Menzaghi, F., and Lloyd, G.K. (1999). Nicotinic acetylcholine receptor agonist SIB-1508Y improves cognitive functioning in chronic low-dose MPTP-treated monkeys. *J Pharmacol Exp Ther*, 290:731–739.

51. O'Neill, J., Fitten, L.J., Siembieda, D.W., Crawford, K.C., Halgren, E., Fisher, A. *et al.* (1999). Divided attention-enhancing effects of AF102B and THA in aging monkeys. *Psychopharmacology (Berl)*, 143(2):123–130.

52. O'Neill, J., Siembieda, D.W., Crawford, K.C., Halgren, E., Fisher, A., and Fitten, L.J. (2003). Reduction in distractibility with AF102B and THA in the macaque. *Pharmacol Biochem Behav*, 76(2):301–306.

53. Bartolomeo, A.C., Morris, H., Buccafusco, J.J., Kille, N., Rosenzweig-Lipson, S., Husbands, M.G. *et al.* (2000). The preclinical pharmacological profile of WAY-132983, a potent M1 preferring agonist. *J Pharmacol Exp Ther*, 292(2):584–596.

54. Andersen, M.B., Fink-Jensen, A., Peacock, L., Gerlach, J., Bymaster, F., Lundbaek, J.A. *et al.* (2003). The muscarinic M1/M4 receptor agonist xanomeline exhibits antipsychotic-like activity in *Cebus apella* monkeys. *Neuropsychopharmacology*, 28(6):1168–1175.

55. Schwarz, R.D., Callahan, M.J., Coughenour, L.L., Dickerson, M.R., Kinsora, J.J., and Lipinski W.J. *et al.* (1999). Milameline (CI-979/RU35926): A muscarinic receptor agonist with cognition-activating properties: Biochemical and in vivo characterization. *J Pharmacol Exp Ther*, 291(2):812–822.

56. Terry, A.V., Jr., Buccafusco, J.J., Borsini, F., and Leusch, A. (2002). Memory-related task performance by aged rhesus monkeys administered the muscarinic M(1)-preferring agonist, talsaclidine. *Psychopharmacology (Berl)*, 162(3):292–300.

57. Callahan, M.J. (1999). Combining tacrine with milameline reverses a scopolamine-induced impairment of continuous performance in rhesus monkeys. *Psychopharmacology (Berl)*, 144(3):234–238.

58. Weinrich, M., Ceci, A., Ensinger, H.A., Gaida, W., Mendla, K.D., Osugi, T. *et al.* (2002). Talsaclidine (W2014 FU), a muscarinic M1 receptor agonist for the treatment of Alzheimer's disease. *Drug Dev Res*, 56:321–334.

59. Mirza, N.R., Peters, D., and Sparks, R.G. (2003). Xanomeline and the antipsychotic potential of muscarinic receptor subtype selective agonists. *CNS Drug Rev*, 9(2):159–186.

60. Bodick, N.C., Offen, W.W., Levey, A.I., Cutler, N.R., Gauthier, S.G., Satlin, A. *et al.* (1997). Effects of xanomeline, a selective muscarinic receptor agonist, on cognitive function and behavioral symptoms in Alzheimer disease. *Arch Neurol*, 54(4):465–473.

61. McArthur, R. and Borsini, F. (2006). Animal models of depression in drug discovery: A historical perspective. *Pharmacol Biochem Behav*, 84(3):436–452.

62. Fisher, A., Pittel, Z., Haring, R., Bar-Ner, N., Kliger-Spatz, M., and Natan, N. *et al.* (2003). M1 muscarinic agonists can modulate some of the hallmarks in Alzheimer's disease: Implications in future therapy. *J Mol Neurosci*, 20(3):349–356.

63. Orgogozo, J.M. (2006). Vaccination treatment of AD, *Alzheimer's Dementia 2*, S94.

64. Hock, C., Konietzko, U., Streffer, J.R., Tracy, J., Signorell, A., Muller-Tillmanns, B. *et al.* (2003). Antibodies against beta-amyloid slow cognitive decline in Alzheimer's disease. *Neuron*, 38(4):547–554.

65. Leber, P. (2002). Not in our methods, but in our ignorance. *Arch Gen Psychiatr*, 59(3):279–280.

66. McKhann, G., Drachman, D., Folstein, M., Katzman, R., Price, D., and Stadlan, E.M. (1984). Clinical diagnosis of Alzheimer's disease: Report of the NINCDS-ADRDA work group under the auspices of department of health and human services task force on Alzheimer's disease. *Neurology*, 34:939–944.

67. Mohs, R.C., Knopman, D., Petersen, R.C., Ferris, S.H., Ernesto, C., Grundman, M. *et al.* (1997). Development of cognitive instruments for use in clinical trials of antidementia drugs: Additions to the Alzheimer's Disease Assessment Scale that broaden its scope. The Alzheimer's Disease Cooperative Study. *Alzheimer Dis Assoc Disord*, 11(Suppl 2): S13–S21.

68. Schmitt, F.A., Ashford, W., Ernesto, C., Saxton, J., Schneider, L.S., Clark, C.M. *et al.* (1997). The severe impairment battery: Concurrent validity and the assessment of longitudinal change in Alzheimer's disease. The Alzheimer's Disease Cooperative Study. *Alzheimer Dis Assoc Disord*, 11(Suppl 2):S51–S56.

69. Schneider, L.S., Olin, J.T., Doody, R.S., Clark, C.M., Morris, J.C., Reisberg, B. *et al.* (1997). Validity and reliability of the Alzheimer's Disease Cooperative Study-Clinical Global Impression of Change. The Alzheimer's Disease Cooperative Study. *Alzheimer Dis. Assoc. Disord.*, 11(Suppl. 2):S22–S32.

70. Galasko, D., Bennett, D., Sano, M., Ernesto, C., Thomas, R., Grundman, M. *et al.* (1997). An inventory to assess activities of daily living for clinical trials in Alzheimer's disease. The Alzheimer's Disease Cooperative Study. *Alzheimer Dis Assoc Disord*, 11(Suppl. 2):S33–S39.

71. Katz, R. (2004). Biomarkers and surrogate markers: An FDA perspective. *NeuroRx*, 1(2):189–195.

72. Thal, L.J., Kantarci, K., Reiman, E.M., Klunk, W.E., Weiner, M.W., Zetterberg, H. *et al.* (2006). The role of biomarkers in clinical trials for Alzheimer disease. *Alzheimer Dis Assoc Disord*, 20(1):6–15.

73. Bernard, C. (1865). *An Introduction to the Study of Experimental Medicine*. Dover Publications Inc., New York.

74. Friedman, L.M., Furberg, C.D., and DeMets, D.L. (1998). *Fundamentals of Clinical Trials*, 3rd ed. Springer, New York.

75. Fleming, T.R. (2000). Surrogate end points in cardiovascular disease trials. *Am Heart J*, 139(4):S193–S196.

76. Temple, R.J. (1995). A regulatory authority's opinion about surrogate endpoints. In Nimmo, W.S. and Tucker, G.T. (eds.), *Clinical Measurement in Drug Evaluation*. John Wiley & Sons, New York.

77. Prentice, R.L. (1989). Surrogate endpoints in clinical trials: Definition and operational criteria. *Stat Med*, 8(4):431–440.

78. Lindner, M.D., Plone, M.A., Francis, J.M., and Cain, C.K. (1999). Chronic morphine reduces pain-related disability in a rodent model of chronic, inflammatory pain. *Exp Clin Psychopharmacol*, 7(3):187–197.

79. Fleming, T.R. and DeMets, D.L. (1996). Surrogate end points in clinical trials: Are we being misled? *Ann Intern Med*, 125(7):605–613.

80. Small, D.H. and Cappai, R. (2006). Alois Alzheimer and Alzheimer's disease: A centennial perspective. *J Neurochem*, 99(3):708–710.

81. Khachaturian, Z.S. (1985). Diagnosis of Alzheimer's disease. *Arch Neurol* (42):1097–1105.

82. Gomezisla, T., Hollister, R., West, H., Mui, S., Growdon, J.H., Petersen, R.C. *et al.* (1997). Neuronal loss correlates with but exceeds neurofibrillary tangles in Alzheimer's disease. *Ann Neurol*, 41(1):17–24.

83. Arriagada, P.V., Growdon, J.H., Hedley-Whyte, E.T., and Hyman, B.T. (1992). Neurofibrillary tangles but not senile plaques parallel duration and severity of Alzheimer's disease. *Neurology*, 42(3 Pt 1):631–639.

84. Crystal, H.A., Dickson, D., Davies, P., Masur, D., Grober, E., and Lipton, R.B. (2000). The relative frequency of "dementia of unknown etiology" increases with age and is nearly 50% in nonagenarians. *Arch Neurol*, 57(5):713–719.

85. Petrovitch, H., White, L.R., Ross, G.W., Steinhorn, S.C., Li, C.Y., Masaki, K.H. *et al.* (2001). Accuracy of clinical criteria for AD in the Honolulu-Asia Aging Study, a population-based study. *Neurology*, 57(2):226–234.

86. Crystal, H., Dickson, D., Fuld, P., Masur, D., Scott, R., Mehler, M. *et al.* (1988). Clinico-pathologic studies in dementia: Nondemented subjects with pathologically confirmed Alzheimer's disease. *Neurology*, 38(11):1682–1687.

87. Dickson, D.W., Crystal, H.A., Mattiace, L.A., Masur, D.M., Blau, A.D., Davies, P. *et al.* (1992). Identification of normal and pathological aging in prospectively studied nondemented elderly humans. *Neurobiol Aging*, 13(1):179–189.

88. Geddes, J.W., Tekirian, T.L., Soultanian, N.S., Ashford, J.W., Davis, D.G., and Markesbery, W.R. (1997). Comparison of neuropathologic criteria for the diagnosis of Alzheimer's disease. *Neurobiol Aging*, 18(4 Suppl):S99–S105.

89. Schmitt, F.A., Davis, D.G., Wekstein, D.R., Smith, C.D., Ashford, J.W., and Markesbery, W.R. (2000). "Preclinical" AD revisited: Neuropathology of cognitively normal older adults. *Neurology*, 55(3):370–376.

90. Davis, D.G., Schmitt, F.A., Wekstein, D.R., and Markesbery, W.R. (1999). Alzheimer neuropathologic alterations in aged cognitively normal subjects. *J Neuropathol Exp Neurol*, 58(4):376–388.

91. McLean, C.A., Cherny, R.A., Fraser, F.W., Fuller, S.J., Smith, M.J., Beyreuther, K. *et al.* (1999). Soluble pool of Abeta amyloid as a determinant of severity of neurodegeneration in Alzheimer's disease. *Ann Neurol*, 46(6):860–866.

92. Lue, L.F., Kuo, Y.M., Roher, A.E., Brachova, L., Shen, Y., Sue, L. *et al.* (1999). Soluble amyloid beta peptide concentration as a predictor of synaptic change in Alzheimer's disease. *Am J Pathol*, 155(3):853–862.

93. Thompson, R.F. (2005). In search of memory traces. *Annu Rev Psychol*, 56:1–23.

94. Olton, D.S. (1989). Mnemonic functions of the hippocampus: Past, present and future. In Squire, L.R. and Lindenlaub, E. (eds.), *The Biology of Memory*. F.D. Schattauer Verlag, New York, NY, pp. 427–440.

95. Ledoux, J. (2003). The emotional brain, fear, and the amygdale. *Cell Mol Neurobiol*, 23:727–738.

96. Morris, R.G. and Rugg, M.D. (2004). Messing about in memory. *Nat. Neurosci.*, 7:1171–1173.

97. Kandel, E.R. (2001). The molecular biology of memory storage: A dialogue between genes and synapses. *Science*, 294:1030–1038.

98. Mishkin, M., Vargha-Khadem, F., and Gadian, D.G. (1998). Amnesia and the organization of the hippocampal system. *Hippocampus*, 8:212–216.

99. Squire, L.R. and Zola-Morgan, S.M. (1988). Memory: Brain systems and behavior. *TINS*, 11:170–175.

100. Morris, R. (1984). Developments of a water-maze procedure for studying spatial learning in the rat. *J Neurosci Methods*, 11:47–60.

101. O'Keefe, J. and Nadel, L. (1978). *The Hippocampus as a Cognitive Map*. Oxford University Press, Oxford.

102. Jarrard, L.E. (1991). On the neural bases of the spatial mapping system: Hippocampus vs. hippocampal formation. *Hippocampus*, 1:236–239.

103. Suzuki, W.A. and Amaral, D.G. (2004). Functional neuroanatomy of the medial temporal lobe memory system. *Cortex*, 40:220–222.

104. Witter, M.P. and Moser, E.I. (2006). Spatial representation and the architecture of the entorhinal cortex. *Trends Neurosci*, 29:671–678.

105. Leutgeb, S., Leutgeb, J.K., Moser, M.B., and Moser, E.I. (2005). Place cells, spatial maps and the population code for memory. *Curr Opin Neurobiol*, 15:738–746.

106. Eichenbaum, H. (2000). A cortical-hippocampal system for declarative memory. *Nat Rev Neurosci*, 1:41–50.

107. Spiers, H.J., Burgess, N., Maguire, E.A., Baxendale, S.A., Hartley, T., Thompson, P.J. *et al.* (2001). Unilateral temporal lobectomy patients show lateralized topographical and episodic memory deficits in a virtual town. *Brain*, 124:2476–2489.

108. Maguire, E.A., Frith, C.D., Burgess, N., Donnett, J.G., and O'Keefe, J. (1998). Knowing where things are parahippocampal involvement in encoding object locations in virtual large-scale space. *J Cogn Neurosci*, 10:61–76.

109. Suzuki, W.A. (2003). Declarative versus episodic: Two theories put to the test. *Neuron*, 38:5-7.
110. Squire, L.R. and Zola, S.M. (1998). Episodic memory, semantic memory, and amnesia. *Hippocampus*, 8:205-211.
111. Rolls, E.T., Xiang, J., and Franco, L. (2005). Object, space, and object-space representations in the primate hippocampus. *J Neurophysiol*, 94:833-844.
112. Gaffan, D. (1991). Spatial organization of episodic memory. *Hippocampus*, 1:262-264.
113. Fortin, N.J., Wright, S.P., and Eichenbaum, H. (2004). Recollection-like memory retrieval in rats is dependent on the hippocampus. *Nature*, 431:188-191.
114. Malkova, L., Mishkin, M., and Bachevalier, J. (1995). Long-term effects of selective neonatal temporal lobe lesions on learning and memory in monkeys. *Behav Neurosci*, 109(2):212-226.
115. Petrulis, A., Alvarez, P., and Eichenbaum, H. (2005). Neural correlates of social odor recognition and the representation of individual distinctive social odors within entorhinal cortex and ventral subiculum. *Neuroscience*, 130:259-274.
116. Kolb, B. (2005). Neurological Models. In Whishaw, I.Q. and Kolb, B. (eds.), *The Behavior of the laboratory Rat*. Oxford University Press, New York, pp. 449-461.
117. Bartus, R.T., Flicker, C., Dean, R.L., Pontecorvo, M., Figuciredo, J.C., and Fisher, S.K. (1985). Selective memory loss following nucleus basalis lesions: Long term behavioral recovery despite persistent cholinergic deficiencies. *Pharmacol Biochem Behav*, 23:125-135.
118. Whishaw, I.Q. (1989). Dissociating performance and learning deficits on spatial navigation tasks in rats subjected to cholinergic muscarinic blockade. *Brain Res Bull*, 23:347-358.
119. Geyer, M.A. and Markou, A. (1995). Animal models of psychiatric disorders. In Bloom, F.E. and Kupfer, D.J. (eds.), *Psychopharmacology, The Fourth Generation of Progress*. Raven Press, New York, pp. 787-798.
120. Willner, P. (1994). *Behavioural Models in Psychopharmacology: Theoretical, Industrial and Clinical Perspectives*. Cambridge University Press, Cambridge.
121. Berger, B.D. and Stein, L. (1969). An analysis of the learning deficits produced by scopolamine. *Psychopharmacologia*, 14(4):271-283.
122. Patel, S. and Tariot, P.N. (1991). Pharmacologic models of Alzheimer's disease. *Psychiatr Clin North Am*, 14(2):287-308.
123. Preston, G.C., Ward, C., Lines, C.R., Poppleton, P., Haigh, J.R., and Traub, M. (1989). Scopolamine and benzodiazepine models of dementia: Cross-reversals by Ro 15-1788 and physostigmine. *Psychopharmacology (Berl)*, 98(4):487-494.
124. Wozniak, D.F., Olney, J.W., Kettinger, L., III., Price, M., and Miller, J.P. (1990). Behavioral effects of MK-801 in the rat. *Psychopharmacology (Berl)*, 101(1):47-56.
125. Jentsch, J.D. and Roth, R.H. (1999). The neuropsychopharmacology of phencyclidine: From NMDA receptor hypofunction to the dopamine hypothesis of schizophrenia. *Neuropsychopharmacology*, 20(3):201-225.
126. Higgins, G.A. and Lashley, K.S. (1950). In search of the engram. *Society of Experimental Biology Symposium No. 4: Physiological Mechanisms in Animal Behavior*. Cambridge University Press, Cambridge. pp. 287-313.
127. Sperry, R.W. (1961). Cerebral control and behavior. *Science*, 133:1749-1757.
128. Dunnett, S.B. (1985). Comparative effects of cholinergic drugs and lesions of nucleus basalis or fimbria-fornix on delayed matching in rats. *Psychopharmacology*, 87:357-363.
129. Kirkby, D.L. (1998). Characterization of perforant path lesions in rodent models of memory and attention. *Eur J Neurosci*, 10(3):823-838.
130. Myhrer, T. (1993). Animal models of Alzheimer's disease: Glutamatergic denervation as an alternative approach to cholinergic denervation. *Neurosci Biobehav Rev*, 17(2): 195-202.
131. Jarrard, L.E. (1993). On the role of the hippocampus in learning and memory in the rat. *Behav Neural Biol*, 60(1):9-26.

132. Galani, R., Obis, S., Coutureau, E., Jarrard, L., and Cassel, J.C. (2002). A comparison of the effects of fimbria-fornix, hippocampal, or entorhinal cortex lesions on spatial reference and working memory in rats: Short versus long postsurgical recovery period. *Neurobiol Learn Mem*, 77:1–16.

133. Brinton, R.D. and Wang, J.M. (2006). Therapeutic potential of neurogenesis for prevention and recovery from Alzheimer's disease: Allopregnanolone as a proof of concept neurogenic agent. *Curr Alzheimer Res*, 3:185–190.

134. Melvin, N.R., Spanswick, S.C., Lehmann, H., and Sutherland, R.J. (2007). Differential neurogenesis in the adult rat dentate gyrus: An identifiable zone that consistently lacks neurogenesis. *Eur J Neurosci*, 25(4):1023–1029.

135. Frielingsdorf, H., Simpson, D.R., Thal, L.J., and Pizzo, D.P. (2007). Nerve growth factor promotes survival of new neurons in the adult hippocampus. *Neurobiol Dis*, 26:47–55.

136. Lagace, D.C., Noonan, M.A., and Eisch, A.J. (2007). Hippocampal neurogenesis: A matter of survival. *Am J Psychiatr*, 164:205.

137. Elder, G.A., De, G.R., and Gama Sosa, M.A. (2006). Research update: Neurogenesis in adult brain and neuropsychiatric disorders. *Mt. Sinai J Med*, 73:931–940.

138. Chevallier, N.L., Soriano, S., Kang, D.E., Masliah, E., Hu, G., and Koo, E.H. (2005). Perturbed neurogenesis in the adult hippocampus associated with presenilin-1 A246E mutation. *Am J Pathol*, 167:151–159.

139. Haughey, N.J., Nath, A., Chan, S.L., Borchard, A.C., Rao, M.S., and Mattson, M.P. (2002). Disruption of neurogenesis by amyloid beta-peptide, and perturbed neural progenitor cell homeostasis, in models of Alzheimer's disease. *J Neurochem*, 83:1509–1524.

140. Kelleher-Andersson, J. (2006). Discovery of neurogenic, Alzheimer's disease therapeutics. *Curr Alzheimer Res*, 3:55–62.

141. Gouras, G. and Fillit, H. (2006). Neurogenesis as a therapeutic strategy for cognitive aging and Alzheimer's disease. *Curr Alzheimer Res*, 3:3.

142. Becker, M., Lavie, V., and Solomon, B. (2007). Stimulation of endogenous neurogenesis by anti-EFRH immunization in a transgenic mouse model of Alzheimer's disease. *Proc Natl Acad Sci USA*, 104:1691–1696.

143. Rosenberg, P.B. (2005). Clinical aspects of inflammation in Alzheimer's disease. *Int Rev Psychiatr*, 17:503–514.

144. Mattson, M.P., Duan, W., Wan, R., and Guo, Z. (2004). Prophylactic activation of neuroprotective stress response pathways by dietary and behavioral manipulations. *NeuroRx*, 1:111–116.

145. Sugaya, K., Alvarez, A., Marutle, A., Kwak, Y.D., and Choumkina, E. (2006). Stem cell strategies for Alzheimer's disease therapy. *Panminerva Med*, 48:87–96.

146. Limke, T.L. and Rao, M.S. (2003). Neural stem cell therapy in the aging brain: pitfalls and possibilities. *J Hematother Stem Cell Res*, 12:615–623.

147. Shors, T.J. (2003). Can new neurons replace memories lost? *Sci Aging Knowledge Environ*, 2003(49): Pe35. (http://sageke.sciencemag.org/cgi/content/full/2003/49/pe35)

148. Rapp, P.R., Stack, E.C., and Gallagher, M. (1999). Morphometric studies of the aged hippocampus: I. Volumetric analysis in behaviorally characterized rats. *J Comp Neurol*, 403(4):459–470.

149. Sugaya, K., Greene, R., Personett, D., Robbins, M., Kent, C., Bryan, D. *et al.* (1998). Septohippocampal cholinergic and neurotrophin markers in age-induced cognitive decline. *Neurobiol Aging*, 19(4):351–361.

150. Smith, T.D., Adams, M.M., Gallagher, M., Morrison, J.H., and Rapp, P.R. (2000). Circuit-specific alterations in hippocampal synaptophysin immunoreactivity predict spatial learning impairment in aged rats. *J Neurosci*, 20(17):6587–6593.

151. Baxter, M.G. and Gallagher, M. (1996). Neurobiological substrates of behavioral decline: Models and data analytic strategies for individual differences in aging. *Neurobiol Aging*, 17(3):491–495.
152. Fischer, W., Chen, K.S., Gage, F.H., and Bjorklund, A. (1992). Progressive decline in spatial learning and integrity of forebrain cholinergic neurons in rats during aging. *Neurobiol Aging*, 13:9–23.
153. Drapeau, E., Mayo, W., Aurousseau, C., Le, M.M., Piazza, P.V., and Abrous, D.N. (2003). Spatial memory performances of aged rats in the water maze predict levels of hippocampal neurogenesis. *Proc Natl Acad Sci USA*, 100(24):14385–14390.
154. Bizon, J.L., Lee, H.J., and Gallagher, M. (2004). Neurogenesis in a rat model of age-related cognitive decline. *Aging Cell*, 3(4):227–234.
155. Lindner, M.D. (1997). Reliability, distribution, and validity of age-related cognitive deficits in the Morris water maze. *Neurobiol Learn Memory*, 68(3):203–220.
156. Lindner, M.D., Hogan, J.B., Krause, R.G., Machet, F., Bourin, C., Hodges, D.B., Jr. *et al.* (2006). Soluble Aβ and cognitive function in aged F-344 rats and Tg2576 mice. *Behav Brain Res*, 173(1):62–75.
157. Grundman, M., Petersen, R.C., Ferris, S.H., Thomas, R.G., Aisen, P.S., Bennett, D.A. *et al.* (2004). Mild cognitive impairment can be distinguished from Alzheimer disease and normal aging for clinical trials. *Arch Neurol*, 61(1):59–66.
158. Pillon, B., Dubois, B., Ploska, A., and Agid, Y. (1991). Severity and specificity of cognitive impairment in Alzheimer's, Huntington's, and Parkinson's diseases and progressive supranuclear palsy. *Neurology*, 41:634–643.
159. Bons, N., Rieger, F., Prudhomme, D., Fisher, A., and Krause, K.H. (2006). *Microcebus murinus*. A useful primate model for human cerebral aging and Alzheimer's disease?. *Genes Brain Behav*, 5(2):120–130.
160. Head, E., Moffat, K., Das, P., Sarsoza, F., Poon, W.W., Landsberg, G. *et al.* (2005). Beta-amyloid deposition and tau phosphorylation in clinically characterized aged cats. *Neurobiol Aging*, 26(5):749–763.
161. Head, E., Barrett, E.G., Murphy, M.P., Das, P., Nistor, M., Sarsoza, F. *et al.* (2006). Immunization with fibrillar Abeta(1–42) in young and aged canines: Antibody generation and characteristics, and effects on CSF and brain Abeta. *Vaccine*, 24(15):2824–2834.
162. Ball, M.J., MacGregor, J., Fyfe, I.M., Rapoport, S.I., and London, E.D. (1983). Paucity of morphological changes in the brains of ageing beagle dogs: Further evidence that Alzheimer lesions are unique for primate central nervous system. *Neurobiol Aging*, 4(2):127–131.
163. Kirik, D. and Bjorklund, A. (2003). Modeling CNS neurodegeneration by overexpression of disease-causing proteins using viral vectors. *Trends Neurosci*, 26:386–392.
164. Kirik, D., Annett, L.E., Burger, C., Muzyczka, N., Mandel, R.J., and Bjorklund, A. (2003). Nigrostriatal alpha-synucleinopathy induced by viral vector-mediated overexpression of human alpha-synuclein: a new primate model of Parkinson's disease. *Proc Natl Acad Sci USA*, 100:2884–2889.
165. de Almeida, L.P., Ross, C.A., Zala, D., Aebischer, P., and Deglon, N. (2002). Lentiviral-mediated delivery of mutant huntingtin in the striatum of rats induces a selective neuropathology modulated by polyglutamine repeat size, huntingtin expression levels, and protein length. *J Neurosci*, 22:3473–3483.
166. Carlsson, T., Bjorklund, T., and Kirik, D. (2006). Restoration of the striatal dopamine synthesis for Parkinson's disease: Viral vector-mediated enzyme replacement strategy. *Curr Gene Ther*, 7:109–120.
167. Mouri, A., Noda, Y., Hara, H., Mizoguchi, H., Tabira, T., and Nabeshima, T. (2007). Oral vaccination with a viral vector containing Aβ cDNA attenuates age-related Aβ accumulation

and memory deficits without causing inflammation in a mouse Alzheimer model. *FASEB J*, 21(9):2135-2148.

168. Gong, Y., Meyer, E.M., Meyers, C.A., Klein, R.L., King, M.A., and Hughes, J.A. (2006). Memory-related deficits following selective hippocampal expression of Swedish mutation amyloid precursor protein in the rat. *Exp Neurol*, 200(2):371-377.

169. Wong, L.F., Goodhead, L., Prat, C., Mitrophanous, K.A., Kingsman, S.M., and Mazarakis, N.D. (2006). Lentivirus-mediated gene transfer to the central nervous system: Therapeutic and research applications. *Hum Gene Ther*, 17:1-9.

170. Hsiao, K., Chapman, P., Nilsen, S., Eckman, C., Harigaya, Y., Younkin, S. *et al.* (1996). Correlative memory deficits, Abeta elevation, and amyloid plaques in transgenic mice. *Science*, 274(5284):99-102.

171. King, D.L. and Arendash, G.W. (2002). Behavioral characterization of the Tg2576 transgenic model of Alzheimer's disease through 19 months. *Physiol Behav*, 75(5):627-642.

172. Esiri, M.M. and Wilcock, G.K. (1984). The olfactory bulbs in Alzheimer's disease. *J Neurol Neurosurg Psychiatr*, 47(1):56-60.

173. Devanand, D.P., Michaels-Marston, K.S., Liu, X., Pelton, G.H., Padilla, M., Marder, K. *et al.* (2000). Olfactory deficits in patients with mild cognitive impairment predict Alzheimer's disease at follow-up. *Am J Psychiatr*, 157(9):1399-1405.

174. Doty, R.L., Reyes, P.F., and Gregor, T. (1987). Presence of both odor identification and detection deficits in Alzheimer's disease. *Brain Res Bull*, 18(5):597-600.

175. Morgan, C.D., Nordin, S., and Murphy, C. (1995). Odor identification as an early marker for Alzheimer's disease: Impact of lexical functioning and detection sensitivity. *J Clin Exp Neuropsychol*, 17(5):793-803.

176. Murphy, C., Gilmore, M.M., Seery, C.S., Salmon, D.P., and Lasker, B.R. (1990). Olfactory thresholds are associated with degree of dementia in Alzheimer's disease. *Neurobiol Aging*, 11(4):465-469.

177. McArthur, R.A., Franklin, S.F., Goodwin, A., Oostveen, J., and Buhl, A.E. (2000). APP-overexpressing transgenic mice (Tg$_{2576}$) are not impaired in the acquisition of an olfactory discrimination, *30th Annual Meeting Society for Neuroscience*, New Orleans, November 4-9.

178. Games, D., Adams, D., Alessandrini, R., Barbour, R., Berthelette, P., Blackwell, C. *et al.* (1995). Alzheimer-type neuropathology in transgenic mice overexpressing V717F beta-amyloid precursor protein. *Nature*, 373(6514):523-527.

179. Dodart, J.C., Meziane, H., Mathis, C., Bales, K.R., Paul, S.M., and Ungerer, A. (1999). Behavioral disturbances in transgenic mice overexpressing the V717F beta-amyloid precursor protein. *Behav Neurosci*, 113(5):982-990.

180. Arendash, G.W., King, D.L., Gordon, M.N., Morgan, D., Hatcher, J.M., Hope, C.E. *et al.* (2001). Progressive, age-related behavioral impairments in transgenic mice carrying both mutant amyloid precursor protein and presenilin-1 transgenes. *Brain Res*, 891(1-2):42-53.

181. Arendash, G.W., Gordon, M.N., Diamond, D.M., Austin, L.A., Hatcher, J.M., Jantzen, P. *et al.* (2001). Behavioral assessment of Alzheimer's transgenic mice following long-term Abeta vaccination: task specificity and correlations between Abeta deposition and spatial memory. *DNA Cell Biol*, 20(11):737-744.

182. Oddo, S., Caccamo, A., Shepherd, J.D., Murphy, M.P., Golde, T.E., Kayed, R. *et al.* (2003). Triple-transgenic model of Alzheimer's disease with plaques and tangles: intracellular Aβ and synaptic dysfunction. *Neuron*, 39(3):409-421.

183. Oddo, S., Caccamo, A., Kitazawa, M., Tseng, B.P., and LaFerla, F.M. (2003). Amyloid deposition precedes tangle formation in a triple transgenic model of Alzheimer's disease. *Neurobiol Aging*, 24(8):1063-1070.

184. Billings, L.M., Oddo, S., Green, K.N., McGaugh, J.L., and LaFerla, F.M. (2005). Intraneuronal Aβ causes the onset of early Alzheimer's disease-related cognitive deficits in transgenic mice. *Neuron*, 45(5):675–688.
185. Decker, M.W. and McGaugh, J.L. (1989). Effects of concurrent manipulations of cholinergic and noradrenergic function on learning and retention in mice. *Brain Res*, 477(1–2):29–37.
186. Jensen, R.A., Martinez, J.L., Jr., Vasquez, B.J., and McGaugh, J.L. (1979). Benzodiazepines alter acquisition and retention of an inhibitory avoidance response in mice. *Psychopharmacology (Berl)*, 64:125–126.
187. McGaugh, J.L. and Cahill, L. (1997). Interaction of neuromodulatory systems in modulating memory storage. *Behav Brain Res*, 83(1–2):31–38.
188. Cahill, L. and McGaugh, J.L. (1998). Mechanisms of emotional arousal and lasting declarative memory. *Trends Neurosci*, 21:294–299.
189. Tinsley, M.R. and Fanselow, M.S. (2005). Fear. In Whishaw, I.Q. and Kolb, B. (eds.), *The Behavior of the Laboratory Rat*. Oxford University Press, New York, pp. 410–421.
190. Rau, V., DeCola, J.P., and Fanselow, M.S. (2005). Stress-induced enhancement of fear learning: An animal model of posttraumatic stress disorder. *Neurosci Biobehav Rev*, 29:1207–1223.
191. Mayer, E.A. and Fanselow, M.S. (2003). Dissecting the components of the central response to stress. *Nat Neurosci*, 6:1011–1012.
192. Mumby, D.G. (2005). Object Recognition. In Whishaw, I.Q. and Kolb, B. (eds.), *The Behavior of the Laboratory Rat*. Oxford University Press, New York, pp. 383–391.
193. Hughes, R.N. (1997). Intrinsic exploration in animals: Motives and measurement. *Behavioural Processes*, 41:213–226.
194. Mumby, D.G. (2001). Perspectives on object-recognition memory following hippocampal damage: Lessons from studies in rats. *Behav Brain Res*, 127(1–2):159–181.
195. Bussey, T.J., Duck, J., Muir, J.L., and Aggleton, J.P. (2000). Distinct patterns of behavioural impairments resulting from fornix transection or neurotoxic lesions of the perirhinal and postrhinal cortices in the rat. *Behav Brain Res*, 111(1–2):187–202.
196. Jackson-Smith, P., Kesner, R.P., and Chiba, A.A. (1993). Continuous recognition of spatial and nonspatial stimuli in hippocampal-lesioned rats. *Behav Neural Biol*, 59(2):107–119.
197. Ainge, J.A., Heron-Maxwell, C., Theofilas, P., Wright, P., de, H.L., and Wood, E.R. (2006). The role of the hippocampus in object recognition in rats: Examination of the influence of task parameters and lesion size. *Behav Brain Res*, 167(1):183–195.
198. Aggleton, J.P. and Brown, M.W. (1999). Episodic memory, amnesia, and the hippocampal-anterior thalamic axis. *Behav Brain Sci*, 22(3):425–444.
199. Brown, M.W. and Aggleton, J.P. (2001). Recognition memory: What are the roles of the perirhinal cortex and hippocampus? *Nat Rev Neurosci*, 2:51–61.
200. Dunnett, S.B. (1989). Comparison of short-term memory deficits in animal models of aging using an operant delayed response task in rats. In Squire, L.R. and Lindenlaub, E. (eds.), *The Biology of Memory*. F.K. Schattauer Verlag, New York, NY, pp. 581–603.
201. Hampson, R.E., Heyser, C.J., and Deadwyler, S.A. (1993). Hippocampal cell firing correlates of delayed-match-to-sample performance in the rat. *Behav Neurosci*, 107(5):715–739.
202. Deadwyler, S.A., Bunn, T., and Hampson, R.E. (1996). Hippocampal ensemble activity during spatial delayed-nonmatch-to-sample performance in rats. *J Neurosci*, 16:354–372.
203. Deadwyler, S.A. and Hampson, R.E. (2004). Differential but complementary mnemonic functions of the hippocampus and subiculum. *Neuron*, 42:465–476.
204. Olton, D.S., Becker, J.T., and Handelmann, G.E. (1979). Hippocampus, space, and memory. *Behav Brain Sci*, 2:313–365.
205. Wible, C.G., Findling, R.L., Shapiro, M., Lang, E.J., Crane, S., and Olton, D.S. (1986). Mnemonic correlates of unit activity in the hippocampus. *Brain Res*, 399(1):97–110.

206. Zeldin, R.K. and Olton, D.S. (1986). Rats acquire spatial learning sets. *J Exp Psychol Anim Behav Process*, 12:412–419.

207. Morris, R.G., Hagan, J.J., and Rawlins, J.N. (1986). Allocentric spatial learning by hippocampectomised rats: A further test of the spatial mapping and working memory theories of hippocampal function. *Q J Exp Psychol [B]*, 38:365–395.

208. Morris, R.G. (1991). Distinctive computations and relevant associative processes: Hippocampal role in processing, retrieval, but not storage of allocentric spatial memory. *Hippocampus*, 1:287–290.

209. Chen, G., Chen, K.S., Knox, J., Inglis, J., Bernard, A., Martin, S.J. *et al.* (2000). A learning deficit related to age and beta-amyloid plaques in a mouse model of Alzheimer's disease. *Nature*, 408(6815):975–979.

210. Paolo, A.M., Axelrod, B.N., Troster, A.I., Blackwell, K.T., and Koller, W.C. (1996). Utility of a Wisconsin Card Sorting Test short form in persons with Alzheimer's and Parkinson's disease. *J Clin Exp Neuropsychol*, 18(6):892–897.

211. Dias, R., Robbins, T.W., and Roberts, A.C. (1996). Primate analogue of the Wisconsin Card Sorting Test: Effects of excitotoxic lesions of the prefrontal cortex in the marmoset. *Behav Neurosci*, 110(5):872–886.

212. Dias, R., Robbins, T.W., and Roberts, A.C. (1996). Dissociation in prefrontal cortex of affective and attentional shifts. *Nature*, 380(6569):69–72.

213. Stefani, M.R., Groth, K., and Moghaddam, B. (2003). Glutamate receptors in the rat medial prefrontal cortex regulate set-shifting ability. *Behav Neurosci*, 117(4):728–737.

214. Birrell, J.M. and Brown, V.J. (2000). Medial frontal cortex mediates perceptual attentional set shifting in the rat. *J Neurosci*, 20(11):4320–4324.

215. Duncan, C.P. (1949). The retroactive effect of electroshock on learning. *J Comp Physiol Psychol*, 42:32–44.

216. Jarvik, M.E. and Kopp, R. (1967). An improved one-trial passive avoidance learning situation. *Psychol Rep*, 21:221–224.

217. Luttges, M.W. and McGaugh, J.L. (1967). Permanence of retrograde amnesia produced by electroconvulsive shock. *Science*, 156:408–410.

218. Hampson, R.E., Pons, T.P., Stanford, T.R., and Deadwyler, S.A. (2004). Categorization in the monkey hippocampus: A possible mechanism for encoding information into memory. *Proc Natl Acad Sci USA*, 101:3184–3189.

219. Freedman, D.J., Riesenhuber, M., Poggio, T., and Miller, E.K. (2003). A comparison of primate prefrontal and inferior temporal cortices during visual categorization. *J Neurosci*, 23:5235–5246.

220. Miller, E.K., Nieder, A., Freedman, D.J., and Wallis, J.D. (2003). Neural correlates of categories and concepts. *Curr Opin Neurobiol*, 13:198–203.

221. Porrino, L.J., Daunais, J.B., Rogers, G.A., Hampson, R.E., and Deadwyler, S.A. (2005). Facilitation of task performance and removal of the effects of sleep deprivation by an ampakine (CX717) in nonhuman primates. *PLoS Biol*, 3:e299.

222. Aigner, T.G., Mitchell, S.J., Aggleton, J.P., DeLong, M.R., Struble, R.G., Price, D.L. *et al.* (1987). Effects of scopolamine and physostigmine on recognition memory in monkeys with ibotenic-acid lesions of the nucleus basalis of Meynert. *Psychopharmacology (Berl)*, 92(3):292–300.

223. Fournier, J., Steinberg, R., Gauthier, T., Keane, P.E., Guzzi, U., Coude, F.X. *et al.* (1993). Protective effects of SR 57746A in central and peripheral models of neurodegenerative disorders in rodents and primates. *Neuroscience*, 55(3):629–641.

224. Easton, A., Ridley, R.M., Baker, H.F., and Gaffan, D. (2002). Unilateral lesions of the cholinergic basal forebrain and fornix in one hemisphere and inferior temporal cortex in the opposite hemisphere produce severe learning impairments in rhesus monkeys. *Cereb Cortex*, 12(7):729–736.

225. Ridley, R.M., Gribble, S., Clark, B., Baker, H.F., and Fine, A. (1992). Restoration of learning ability in fornix-transected monkeys after fetal basal forebrain but not fetal hippocampal tissue transplantation. *Neuroscience*, 48(4):779–792.

226. Roberts, A.C., Robbins, T.W., Everitt, B.J., Jones, G.H., Sirkia, T.E., Wilkinson, J. *et al.* (1990). The effects of excitotoxic lesions of the basal forebrain on the acquisition, retention and serial reversal of visual discriminations in marmosets. *Neuroscience*, 34(2):311–329.

227. Zola-Morgan, S. and Squire, L.R. (1986). Memory impairment in monkeys following lesions limited to the hippocampus. *Behav Neurosci*, 100(2):155–160.

228. Aigner, T.G. and Mishkin, M. (1986). The effects of physostigmine and scopolamine on recognition memory in monkeys. *Behav Neural Biol*, 45(1):81–87.

229. Rupniak, N.M., Field, M.J., Samson, N.A., Steventon, M.J., and Iversen, S.D. (1990). Direct comparison of cognitive facilitation by physostigmine and tetrahydroaminoacridine in two primate models. *Neurobiol Aging*, 11(6):609–613.

230. Taffe, M.A., Weed, M.R., and Gold, L.H. (1999). Scopolamine alters rhesus monkey performance on a novel neuropsychological test battery. *Brain Res Cogn Brain Res*, 8(3):203–212.

231. Harder, J.A., Aboobaker, A.A., Hodgetts, T.C., and Ridley, R.M. (1998). Learning impairments induced by glutamate blockade using dizocilpine (MK-801) in monkeys. *Br J Pharmacol*, 125(5):1013–1018.

232. Rupniak, N.M., Duchnowski, M., Tye, S.J., Cook, G., and Iversen, S.D. (1992). Failure of D-cycloserine to reverse cognitive disruption induced by scopolamine or phencyclidine in primates. *Life Sci*, 50(25):1959–1962.

233. Bartus, R.T. (1979 Nov 30). Physostigmine and recent memory: Effects in young and aged nonhuman primates. *Science*, 206(4422):1087–1089.

234. Jackson, W.J., Buccafusco, J.J., Terry, A.V., Turk, D.J., and Rush, D.K. (1995). Velnacrine maleate improves delayed matching performance by aged monkeys. *Psychopharmacology (Berl)*, 119(4):391–398.

235. Prendergast, M.A., Terry, A.V., Jr., Jackson, W.J., Marsh, K.C., Decker, M.W., Arneric, S.P. *et al.* (1997). Improvement in accuracy of delayed recall in aged and non-aged, mature monkeys after intramuscular or transdermal administration of the CNS nicotinic receptor agonist ABT-418. *Psychopharmacology (Berl)*, 130(3):276–284.

236. Birks, J. and Harvey, R.J. (2006). Donepezil for dementia due to Alzheimer's disease. *Cochrane Database Syst Rev*(1). (CD001190)

237. Burns, A., Rossor, M., Hecker, J., Gauthier, S., Petit, H., Moller, H.J. *et al.* (1999). The effects of donepezil in Alzheimer's disease – Results from a multinational trial. *Dement Geriatr Cogn Disord*, 10(3):237–244.

238. Rogers, S.L. and Friedhoff, L.T. (1996). The efficacy and safety of donepezil in patients with Alzheimer's disease: Results of a US multicentre, randomized, double-blind, placebo-controlled trial, The Donepezil Study Group. *Dementia*, 7(6):293–303.

239. Matthews, H.P., Korbey, J., Wilkinson, D.G., and Rowden, J. (2000). Donepezil in Alzheimer's disease: Eighteen month results from Southampton Memory Clinic. *Int J Geriatr Psychiatr*, 15(8):713–720.

240. Rogers, S.L., Doody, R.S., Pratt, R.D., and Ieni, J.R. (2000). Long-term efficacy and safety of donepezil in the treatment of Alzheimer's disease: Final analysis of a US multicentre open-label study. *Eur Neuropsychopharmacol*, 10(3):195–203.

241. Rocca, P., Cocuzza, E., Marchiaro, L., and Bogetto, F. (2002). Donepezil in the treatment of Alzheimer's disease: Long-term efficacy and safety. *Prog Neuropsychopharmacol Biol Psychiatr*, 26(2):369–373.

242. Wilkinson, D.G., Passmore, A.P., Bullock, R., Hopker, S.W., Smith, R., Potocnik, F.C. *et al.* (2002). A multinational, randomised, 12-week, comparative study of donepezil and

rivastigmine in patients with mild to moderate Alzheimer's disease. *Int J Clin Pract*, 56(6):441–446.

243. Zec, R.F., Landreth, E.S., Vicari, S.K., Feldman, E., Belman, J., Andrise, A. *et al.* (1992). Alzheimer disease assessment scale: Useful for both early detection and staging of dementia of the Alzheimer type. *Alzheimer Dis Assoc Disord*, 6(2):89–102.

244. Rosen, W.G., Mohs, R.C., and Davis, K.L. (1984). A new rating scale for Alzheimer's disease. *Am J Psychiatr*, 141(11):1356–1364.

245. Braida, D., Paladini, E., Griffini, P., Lamperti, M., Maggi, A., and Sala, M. (1996). An inverted U-shaped curve for heptylphysostigmine on radial maze performance in rats: Comparison with other cholinesterase inhibitors. *Eur J Pharm*, 302(1–3):13–20.

246. Wang, T. and Tang, X.C. (1998). Reversal of scopolamine-induced deficits in radial maze performance by (-)-huperzine A: Comparison with E2020 and tacrine. *Eur J Pharm*, 349(2–3):137–142.

247. Cheng, D.H. and Tang, X.C. (1998). Comparative studies of huperzine A, E2020, and tacrine on behavior and cholinesterase activities. *Pharmacol Biochem Behav*, 60(2):377–386.

248. Cheng, D.H., Ren, H., and Tang, X.C. (1996). Huperzine A, a novel promising acetylcholinesterase inhibitor. *Neuroreport*, 8(1):97–101.

249. Poorheidari, G., Stanhope, K.J., and Pratt, J.A. (1998). Effects of the potassium channel blockers, apamin and 4-aminopyridine, on scopolamine-induced deficits in the delayed matching to position task in rats: A comparison with the cholinesterase inhibitor E2020. *Psychopharmacology (Berl)*, 135(3):242–255.

250. Higgins, G.A., Enderlin, M., Fimbel, R., Haman, M., Grottick, A.J., Soriano, M. *et al.* (2002). Donepezil reverses a mnemonic deficit produced by scopolamine but not by perforant path lesion or transient cerebral ischaemia. *Eur J Neurosci*, 15(11):1827–1840.

251. Dawson, G.R. and Iversen, S.D. (1993). The effects of novel cholinesterase inhibitors and selective muscarinic receptor agonists in tests of reference and working memory. *Behav Brain Res*, 57(2):143–153.

252. Barnes, C.A., Meltzer, J., Houston, F., Orr, G., McGann, K., and Wenk, G.L. (2000). Chronic treatment of old rats with donepezil or galantamine: Effects on memory, hippocampal plasticity and nicotinic receptors. *Neuroscience*, 99(1):17–23.

253. Rogers, D.C. and Hagan, J.J. (2001). 5-HT6 receptor antagonists enhance retention of a water maze task in the rat. *Psychopharmacology (Berl)*, 158(2):114–119.

254. Ogura, H., Kosasa, T., Kuriya, Y., and Yamanishi, Y. (2000). Donepezil, a centrally acting acetylcholinesterase inhibitor, alleviates learning deficits in hypocholinergic models in rats. *Meth Find Exp Clin Pharmacol*, 22(2):89–95.

255. Carey, G.J., Billard, W., Binch, H., III., Cohen-Williams, M., Crosby, G., Grzelak, M. *et al.* (2001). SCH 57790, a selective muscarinic M(2) receptor antagonist, releases acetylcholine and produces cognitive enhancement in laboratory animals. *Eur J Pharm*, 431(2):189–200.

256. Lindner, M.D., Hogan, J.B., Hodges, D.B., Jr., Orie, A.F., Chen, P., Corsa, J.A. *et al.* (2006). Donepezil primarily attenuates scopolamine-induced deficits in psychomotor function, with moderate effects on simple conditioning and attention, and small effects on working memory and spatial mapping. *Psychopharmacology (Berl)*, 188(4):629–640.

257. Buccafusco, J.J. and Terry, A.V. (2004). Donepezil-induced improvement in delayed matching accuracy by young and old rhesus monkeys. *J Mol Neurosci*, 24(1):85–91.

258. Bartus, R.T., Dean, R.L., and Beer, B. (1983). An evaluation of drugs for improving memory in aged monkeys: Implications for clinical trials in humans. *Psychopharmacol Bull*, 19(2):168–184.

259. Buccafusco, J.J. and Jackson, W.J. (1991). Beneficial effects of nicotine administered prior to a delayed matching-to-sample task in young and aged monkeys. *Neurobiol Aging*, 12(3):233–238.

260. Bartus, R.T. (2000). On neurodegenerative diseases, models, and treatment strategies: Lessons learned and lessons forgotten a generation following the cholinergic hypothesis. *Exp Neurol*, 163(2):495–529.

261. Gould, R.L., Brown, R.G., Owen, A.M., Bullmore, E.T., Williams, S.C., and Howard, R.J. (2005). Functional neuroanatomy of successful paired associate learning in Alzheimer's disease. *Am J Psychiatr*, 162(11):2049–2060.

262. Tariot, P.N., Farlow, M.R., Grossberg, G.T., Graham, S.M., McDonald, S., and Gergel, I. (2004). Memantine treatment in patients with moderate to severe Alzheimer disease already receiving donepezil: a randomized controlled trial. *JAMA*, 291(3):317–324.

263. Terry, A.V., Jr., Buccafusco, J.J., and Bartoszyk, G.D. (2005). Selective serotonin 5-HT2A receptor antagonist EMD 281014 improves delayed matching performance in young and aged rhesus monkeys. *Psychopharmacology (Berl)*, 179(4):725–732.

264. Paule, M.G., Bushnell, P.J., Maurissen, J.P., Wenger, G.R., Buccafusco, J.J., Chelonis, J.J. *et al.* (1998). Symposium overview: the use of delayed matching-to-sample procedures in studies of short-term memory in animals and humans. *Neurotoxicol Teratol*, 20(5):493–502.

265. Terry, A.V., Jr., Jackson, W.J., and Buccafusco, J.J. (1993). Effects of concomitant cholinergic and adrenergic stimulation on learning and memory performance by young and aged monkeys. *Cereb Cortex*, 3(4):304–312.

266. Buccafusco, J.J., Jackson, W.J., Stone, J.D., and Terry, A.V. (2003). Sex dimorphisms in the cognitive-enhancing action of the Alzheimer's drug donepezil in aged Rhesus monkeys. *Neuropharmacology*, 44(3):381–389.

267. Taffe, M.A., Weed, M.R., Gutierrez, T., Davis, S.A., and Gold, L.H. (2004). Modeling a task that is sensitive to dementia of the Alzheimer's type: Individual differences in acquisition of a visuospatial paired-associate learning task in rhesus monkeys. *Behav Brain Res*, 149(2):123–133.

268. Weed, M.R., Taffe, M.A., Polis, I., Roberts, A.C., Robbins, T.W., Koob, G.F. *et al.* (1999). Performance norms for a rhesus monkey neuropsychological testing battery: Acquisition and long-term performance. *Brain Res Cogn Brain Res*, 8(3):185–201.

269. Buccafusco, J.J., Terry, A.V., Jr., and Murdoch, P.B. (2002). A computer-assisted cognitive test battery for aged monkeys. *J Mol Neurosci*, 19:179–185.

270. Morris, R.G.M. (1981). Spatial localization does not require the presence of local cues. *Learn Motiv*, 12:239–260.

271. Jarrard, L.E. (1978). Selective hippocampal lesions: Differential effects on performance by rats of a spatial task with preoperative versus postoperative training. *J Comp Physiol Psychol*, 92(6):1119–1127.

272. Olton, D.S. and Papas, B.C. (1979). Spatial memory and hippocampal function. *Neuropsychologia*, 17:669–682.

273. Dunnett, S.B., Evenden, J.L., and Iversen, S.D. (1988). Delay-dependent short-term memory deficits in aged rats. *Psychopharmacology*, 96:174–180.

274. Dunnett, S.B. (1990). Role of prefrontal cortex and striatal output systems in short-term memory deficits associated with ageing, basal forebrain lesions, and cholinergic-rich grafts. *Can J Psychol*, 44(2):210–232.

275. Carli, M., Robbins, T.W., Evenden, J.L., and Everitt, B.J. (1983). Effects of lesions to ascending noradrenergic neurones on performance of a 5-choice serial reaction task in rats; implications for theories of dorsal noradrenergic bundle function based on selective attention and arousal. *Behav Brain Res*, 9(3):361–380.

276. Robbins, T.W. (2002). The 5-choice serial reaction time task: behavioural pharmacology and functional neurochemistry. *Psychopharmacology (Berl)*, 163(3–4):362–380.

277. Goldman-Rakic, P.S. (1996). The prefrontal landscape: implications of functional architecture for understanding human mentation and the central executive, *Philos Trans R Soc Lond B Biol Sci*. 351(1346): 1445–1453.

278. Fray, P.J., Robbins, T.W., and Sahakian, B.J. (1996). Neuropsychiatric applications of CANTAB. *Int J Geriatr Psychiatr*, 11:329–336.
279. Sahakian, B.J. (1990). Computerized assessment of neuropsychological function in Alzheimer's disease and Parkinson's disease. *Int J Geriatr Psychiatr*, 5:211–213.
280. Robbins, T.W., James, M., Owen, A.M., Sahakian, B.J., McInnes, L., and Rabbitt, P. (1994). Cambridge Neuropsychological Test Automated Battery (CANTAB): A factor analytic study of a large sample of normal elderly volunteers. *Dementia*, 5(5):266–281.
281. Robbins, T.W., James, M., Owen, A.M., Sahakian, B.J., Lawrence, A.D., McInnes, L. *et al.* (1998). A study of performance on tests from the CANTAB battery sensitive to frontal lobe dysfunction in a large sample of normal volunteers: Implications for theories of executive functioning and cognitive aging. Cambridge Neuropsychological Test Automated Battery. *J Int Neuropsychol Soc*, 4(5):474–490.
282. De Luca, C.R., Wood, S.J., Anderson, V., Buchanan, J.A., Proffitt, T.M., Mahony, K. *et al.* (2003). Normative data from the CANTAB. I: Development of executive function over the lifespan. *J Clin Exp Neuropsychol*, 25(2):242–254.
283. Martin, R.C., Sawrie, S.M., Gilliam, F.G., Palmer, C.A., Faught, E., Morawetz, R.B. *et al.* (2000). Wisconsin Card Sorting performance in patients with temporal lobe epilepsy: Clinical and neuroanatomical correlates. *Epilepsia*, 41(12):1626–1632.
284. Owen, A.M., Roberts, A.C., Polkey, C.E., Sahakian, B.J., and Robbins, T.W. (1991). Extra-dimensional versus intra-dimensional set shifting performance following frontal lobe excisions, temporal lobe excisions or amygdalo-hippocampectomy in man. *Neuropsychologia*, 29(10):993–1006.
285. Sahakian, B.J., Elliott, R., Low, N., Mehta, M., Clark, R.T., and Pozniak, A.L. (1995). Neuropsychological deficits in tests of executive function in asymptomatic and symptomatic HIV-1 seropositive men. *Psychol Med*, 25(6):1233–1246.
286. Weed, M.R., Gold, L.H., Polis, I., Koob, G.F., Fox, H.S., and Taffe, M.A. (2004). Impaired performance on a rhesus monkey neuropsychological testing battery following simian immunodeficiency virus infection. *AIDS Res Hum Retrovir*, 20(1):77–89.
287. Baker, S.C., Rogers, R.D., Owen, A.M., Frith, C.D., Dolan, R.J., Frackowiak, R.S. *et al.* (1996). Neural systems engaged by planning: A PET study of the Tower of London task. *Neuropsychologia*, 34(6):515–526.
288. Gould, R.L., Brown, R.G., Owen, A.M., ffytche, D.H., and Howard, R.J. (2003). fMRI BOLD response to increasing task difficulty during successful paired associates learning. *Neuroimage*, 20(2):1006–1019.
289. Stern, C.E., Owen, A.M., Tracey, I., Look, R.B., Rosen, B.R., and Petrides, M. (2000). Activity in ventrolateral and mid-dorsolateral prefrontal cortex during nonspatial visual working memory processing: Evidence from functional magnetic resonance imaging. *Neuroimage*, 11(5 Pt 1):392–399.
290. Reeves, S.J., Grasby, P.M., Howard, R.J., Bantick, R.A., Asselin, M.C., and Mehta, M.A. (2005 Oct 15). A positron emission tomography (PET) investigation of the role of striatal dopamine (D2) receptor availability in spatial cognition. *Neuroimage*, 28(1):216–226.
291. Pearce, P.C., Crofts, H.S., Muggleton, N.G., and Scott, E.A. (1998). Concurrent monitoring of EEG and performance in the common marmoset: A methodological approach. *Physiol Behav*, 63(4):591–599.
292. Spinelli, S., Pennanen, L., Dettling, A.C., Feldon, J., Higgins, G.A., and Pryce, C.R. (2004). Performance of the marmoset monkey on computerized tasks of attention and working memory. *Brain Res Cogn Brain Res*, 19(2):123–137.
293. Spinelli, S., Ballard, T., Gatti-McArthur, S., Richards, G.J., Kapps, M., Woltering, T. *et al.* (2005). Effects of the mGluR2/3 agonist LY354740 on computerized tasks of attention and working memory in marmoset monkeys. *Psychopharmacology (Berl)*, 179(1):292–302.

294. Fowler, K.S., Saling, M.M., Conway, E.L., Semple, J.M., and Louis, W.J. (1997). Computerized neuropsychological tests in the early detection of dementia: Prospective findings. *J Int Neuropsychol Soc*, 3(2):139–146.

295. Fowler, K.S., Saling, M.M., Conway, E.L., Semple, J.M., and Louis, W.J. (2002). Paired associate performance in the early detection of DAT. *J Int Neuropsychol Soc*, 8(1):58–71.

296. Gould, R.L., Arroyo, B., Brown, R.G., Owen, A.M., Bullmore, E.T., and Howard, R.J. (2006 Sep 26). Brain mechanisms of successful compensation during learning in Alzheimer disease. *Neurology*, 67(6):1011–1017.

297. Greig, N.H., Sambamurti, K., Yu, Q.S., Brossi, A., Bruinsma, G.B., and Lahiri, D.K. (2005). An overview of phenserine tartrate, a novel acetylcholinesterase inhibitor for the treatment of Alzheimer's disease. *Curr Alzheimer Res*, 2(3):281–290.

298. Shaw, K.T., Utsuki, T., Rogers, J., Yu, Q.S., Sambamurti, K., Brossi, A. *et al.* (2001). Phenserine regulates translation of beta-amyloid precursor protein mRNA by a putative inter-leukin-1 responsive element, a target for drug development. *Proc Natl Acad Sci USA*, 98(13):7605–7610.

299. Kirby, L.C., Baumel, B., Eisner, L.S., Safirstien, B.E., and Burford, R.G. (2002). The efficacy of phenserine tartrate following twelve (12) weeks of treatment in Alzheimer disease patients, *International Symposium on Advances in Alzheimer Therapy*, Geneva, Switzerland.

300. Hampson, R.E. and Deadwyler, S.A. (1994). Hippocampal representations of DMS/DNMS in the rat. *Behav Brain Sci*, 17:480–482.

301. Hampson, R.E. and Deadwyler, S.A. (1996). Ensemble codes involving hippocampal neurons are at risk during delayed performance tests. *Proc Natl Acad Sci USA*, 93:13487–13493.

302. Deadwyler, S.A. and Hampson, R.E. (1997). The significance of neural ensemble codes during behavior and cognition. In Cowan, W.M., Shooter, E.M., Stevens, C.F., and Thompson, R.F. (eds.), *Annual Review of Neuroscience*, Vol. 20. Annual Reviews, Inc., Palo Alto, CA, pp. 217–244.

303. Hampson, R.E., Simeral, J.D., and Deadwyler, S.A. (1999). Distribution of spatial and nonspatial information in dorsal hippocampus. *Nature*, 402:610–614.

304. Hampson, R.E., Simeral, J.D., and Deadwyler, S.A. (2001). What ensemble recordings reveal about functional hippocampal cell encoding. *Prog Brain Res*, 130:345–357.

305. Hampson, R.E. and Deadwyler, S.A. (2003). Temporal firing characteristics and the strategic role of subicular neurons in short-term memory. *Hippocampus*, 13:529–541.

306. Hampson, R.E., Rogers, G., Lynch, G., and Deadwyler, S.A. (1998). Facilitative effects of the ampakine CX516 on short-term memory in rats: Enhancement of delayed-nonmatch-to-sample performance. *J Neurosci*, 18:2740–2747.

307. Hampson, R.E., Rogers, G., Lynch, G., and Deadwyler, S.A. (1998). Facilitative effects of the ampakine CX516 on short-term memory in rats: Correlations with hippocampal ensemble activity. *J Neurosci*, 18:2748–2763.

308. Suppiramaniam, V., Bahr, B.A., Sinnarajah, S., Owens, K., Rogers, G., Yilma, S. *et al.* (2001). Member of the Ampakine class of memory enhancers prolongs the single channel open time of reconstituted AMPA receptors. *Synapse*, 40:154–158.

309. Arai, A.C., Kessler, M., Rogers, G., and Lynch, G. (2000). Effects of the potent ampakine CX614 on hippocampal and recombinant AMPA receptors: Interactions with cyclothiazide and GYKI 52466. *Mol Pharmacol*, 58:802–813.

310. Arai, A.C., Xia, Y.F., Rogers, G., Lynch, G., and Kessler, M. (2002). Benzamide-type AMPA receptor modulators form two subfamilies with distinct modes of action. *J Pharmacol Exp Ther*, 303:1075–1085.

311. Fukuda, K., Stern, J.A., Brown, T.B., and Russo, M.B. (2005). Cognition, blinks, eye-movements, and pupillary movements during performance of a running memory task. *Aviat Space Environ Med*, 76:C75–C85.

312. Van Gerven, P.W., Paas, F., Van Merrienboer, J.J., and Schmidt, H.G. (2004). Memory load and the cognitive pupillary response in aging. *Psychophysiology*, 41:167–174.

313. Granholm, E. and Steinhauer, S.R. (2004). Pupillometric measures of cognitive and emotional processes. *Int J Psychophysiol*, 52:1–6.

314. Granholm, E., Asarnow, R.F., Sarkin, A.J., and Dykes, K.L. (1996). Pupillary responses index cognitive resource limitations. *Psychophysiology*, 33:457–461.

315. Beatty, J. and Wagoner, B.L. (1978). Pupillometric signs of brain activation vary with level of cognitive processing. *Science*, 199:1216–1218.

316. Marshall, S.P. (2007). Identifying cognitive state from eye metrics. *Aviat Space Environ Med*, 78:B165–B175.

317. Delfino, M., Kalisch, R., Czisch, M., Larramendy, C., Ricatti, J., Taravini, I.R. *et al.* (2007). Mapping the effects of three dopamine agonists with different dyskinetogenic potential and receptor selectivity using pharmacological functional magnetic resonance imaging. *Neuropsychopharmacology*, 32(9):1911–1921.

318. Smirnakis, S.M., Brewer, A.A., Schmid, M.C., Tolias, A.S., Schuz, A., Augath, M. *et al.* (2005). Lack of long-term cortical reorganization after macaque retinal lesions. *Nature*, 435 (7040):300–307.

319. Zhao, F., Wang, P., and Kim, S.G. (2004). Cortical depth-dependent gradient-echo and spin-echo BOLD fMRI at 9.4T. *Magn Reson Med*, 51(3):518–524.

320. Poduslo, J.F., Wengenack, T.M., Curran, G.L., Wisniewski, T., Sigurdsson, E.M., Macura, S.I. *et al.* (2002). Molecular targeting of Alzheimer's amyloid plaques for contrast-enhanced magnetic resonance imaging. *Neurobiol Dis*, 11(2):315–329.

321. Fox, G.B., McGaraughty, S., and Luo, Y. (2006). Pharmacological and functional magnetic resonance imaging techniques in CNS drug discovery. *Expet Opin Drug Discov*, 1:211–224.

322. Elrod, K., Buccafusco, J.J., and Jackson, W.J. (1988). Nicotine enhances delayed matching-to-sample performance by primates. *Life Sci*, 43:277–287.

323. Rolls, E.T., Cahusac, P.M., Feigenbaum, J.D., and Miyashita, Y. (1993). Responses of single neurons in the hippocampus of the macaque related to recognition memory. *Exp Brain Res*, 93(2):299–306.

324. Tovee, M.J., Rolls, E.T., Treves, A., and Bellis, R.P. (1993). Information encoding and the responses of single neurons in the primate temporal visual cortex. *J Neurophysiol*, 70:640–654.

325. Morris, R.G.M., Evenden, J.L., Sahakian, B.J., and Robbins, T.W. (1987). Computer-aided assessment of dementia: Comparative studies of neuropsychological deficits in Alzheimer-type dementia and Parkinson's disease. In Stahl, S.M., Iversen, S.D., and Goodman, E.C. (eds.), *Cognitive Neuroschemistry*. Oxford University Press, Oxford, pp. 21–36.

326. Pittler, S.J. and Baehr, W. (1991). Identification of a nonsense mutation in the rod photoreceptor cGMP phosphodiesterase beta-subunit gene of the rd mouse. *Proc Natl Acad Sci USA*, 88(19):8322–8326.

327. Garcia, M.F., Gordon, M.N., Hutton, M., Lewis, J., McGowan, E., Dickey, C.A. *et al.* (2004). The retinal degeneration (rd) gene seriously impairs spatial cognitive performance in normal and Alzheimer's transgenic mice. *Neuroreport*, 15(1):73–77.

328. Hsiao, K., Borchelt, D.R. Sisodia, S. inventors, Johns Hopkins University RotUoM, assignee, (1999). Transgenic mice expressing APP-Swedish mutation develop progressive neurologic disease. *U.S. Patent Office patent US 5,877,399.*

329. Harris, J.C. (1989). Experimental animal modeling of depression and anxiety. *Psychiatr Clin North Am*, 12(4):815–836.

330. Lindner, M.D., Plone, M.A., Schallert, T., and Emerich, D.F. (1997). Blind rats are not profoundly impaired in the reference memory Morris water maze and cannot be clearly discriminated from rats with cognitive deficits in the cued platform task. *Brain Res Cogn Brain Res*, 5(4):329–333.

331. Lindner, M.D. and Gribkoff, V.K. (1991). Relationship between performance in the Morris water task, visual acuity, and thermoregulatory function in aged F-344 rats. *Behav Brain Res*, 45:45-55.

332. Rosenthal, R. (1966). *Experimenter Effects in Behavioral Research*. Appleton Century Crofts (Division of Meredith Publishing Co.), NY.

333. Lindner, M.D. (2007). Clinical attrition due to biased preclinical assessments of potential efficacy. *Pharmacol Ther*, 115(1):148-175.

334. Cuatrecasas, P. (2006). Drug discovery in jeopardy. *J Clin Invest*, 116(11):2837-2842.

335. Tariot, P.N. and Federoff, H.J. (2003). Current treatment for Alzheimer disease and future prospects. *Alzheimer Dis Assoc Disord*, 17(Suppl 4):S105-S113.

336. Packer, M., Carver, J.R., Rodeheffer, R.J., Ivanhoe, R.J., DiBianco, R., Zeldis, S.M. *et al.* (1991 Nov 21). Effect of oral milrinone on mortality in severe chronic heart failure, The PROMISE Study Research Group. *N Engl J Med*, 325(21):1468-1475.

337. The Cardiac Arrhythmia Suppression Trial (CAST) Investigators. (1989). Preliminary report: Effect of encainide and flecainide on mortality in a randomized trial of arrhythmia suppression after myocardial infarction. *N Engl J Med*, 321(6):406-412.

338. The Cardiac Arrhythmia Suppression Trial II Investigators. (1992). Effect of the antiarrhythmic agent moricizine on survival after myocardial infarction. *N Engl J Med*, 327(4):227-233.

339. The Xamoterol in Severe Heart Failure Study Group. (1990). Xamoterol in severe heart failure. *Lancet*, 336(8706):1-6.

340. Echt, D.S., Liebson, P.R., Mitchell, L.B., Peters, R.W., Obias-Manno, D., Barker, A.H. *et al.* (1991). Mortality and morbidity in patients receiving encainide, flecainide, or placebo. The Cardiac Arrhythmia Suppression Trial.. *N Engl J Med*, 324(12):781-788.

341. Coplen, S.E., Antman, E.M., Berlin, J.A., Hewitt, P., and Chalmers, T.C. (1990). Efficacy and safety of quinidine therapy for maintenance of sinus rhythm after cardioversion. A meta-analysis of randomized control trials. *Circulation*, 82(4):1106-1116.

342. Hine, L.K., Laird, N., Hewitt, P., and Chalmers, T.C. (1989). Meta-analytic evidence against prophylactic use of lidocaine in acute myocardial infarction. *Arch Intern Med*, 149(12):2694-2698.

343. Gordon, D.J. (1995). Cholesterol lowering and total mortality. In Rifkind, B.M. (ed.), *Lowering Cholesterol in High-Risk Individuals and Populations*. Marcel Dekker, Inc., New York, pp. 33-48.

344. Advanced Colorectal Cancer Meta-Analysis Project. (1992). Modulation of fluorouracil by leucovorin in patients with advanced colorectal cancer: Evidence in terms of response rate. *J Clin Oncol*, 10(6):896-903.

345. Fleming, T.R. (1994). Surrogate markers in AIDS and cancer trials. *Stat Med*, 13(13-14):1423-1435.

346. Fleming, T.R. (2005). Surrogate endpoints and FDA's accelerated approval process. *Health Aff (Millwood)*, 24(1):67-78.

347. Chaisson, R.E., Benson, C.A., Dube, M.P., Heifets, L.B., Korvick, J.A., Elkin, S. *et al.* (1994). Clarithromycin therapy for bacteremic Mycobacterium avium complex disease. A randomized, double-blind, dose-ranging study in patients with AIDS. AIDS Clinical Trials Group Protocol 157 Study Team. *Ann Intern Med*, 121(12):905-911.

348. Nissen, S.E. and Wolski, K. (2007). Effect of rosiglitazone on the risk of myocardial infarction and death from cardiovascular causes. *N Engl J Med*, 356(24):2457-2471.

349. Riggs, B.L., Hodgson, S.F., O'Fallon, W.M., Chao, E.Y., Wahner, H.W., Muhs, J.M. *et al.* (1990). Effect of fluoride treatment on the fracture rate in postmenopausal women with osteoporosis. *N Engl J Med*, 322(12):802-809.

350. The International Chronic Granulomatous Disease Cooperative Study Group. (1991). A controlled trial of interferon gamma to prevent infection in chronic granulomatous disease. *N Engl J Med*, 324(8):509–516.

351. Smith, R.D., Kistler, M.K., Cohen-Williams, M., and Coffin, V.L. (1996). Cholinergic improvement of a naturally-occurring memory deficit in the young rat. *Brain Res*, 707(1):13–21.

352. Tokita, K., Yamazaki, S., Yamazaki, M., Matsuoka, N., and Mutoh, S. (2002). Combination of a novel antidementia drug FK960 with donepezil synergistically improves memory deficits in rats. *Pharmacol Biochem Behav*, 73(3):511–519.

353. Yamaguchi, Y., Higashi, M., Matsuno, T., and Kawashima, S. (2001). Ameliorative effects of azaindolizinone derivative ZSET845 on scopolamine-induced deficits in passive avoidance and radial-arm maze learning in the rat. *Jpn J Pharmacol*, 87(3):240–244.

354. Sato, T., Tanaka, K., Ohnishi, Y., Irifune, M., and Nishikawa, T. (2003). Effect of donepezil on group II mGlu receptor agonist- or antagonist-induced amnesia on passive avoidance in mice. *Neural Plast*, 10(4):319–325.

355. Suzuki, M., Yamaguchi, T., Ozawa, Y., Ohyama, M., and Yamamoto, M. (1995). Effects of (−)-S-2, 8-dimethyl-3-methylene-1-oxa-8-azaspiro[4,5]decane L-tartrate monohydrate (YM796), a novel muscarinic agonist, on disturbance of passive avoidance learning behavior in drug-treated and senescence-accelerated mice. *J Pharmacol Exp Ther*, 275(2):728–736.

356. Dong, H., Csernansky, C.A., Martin, M.V., Bertchume, A., Vallera, D., and Csernansky, J.G. (2005). Acetylcholinesterase inhibitors ameliorate behavioral deficits in the Tg2576 mouse model of Alzheimer's disease. *Psychopharmacology (Berl)*, 181(1):145–152.

357. Spowart-Manning, L. and van der Staay, F.J. (2004). The T-maze continuous alternation task for assessing the effects of putative cognition enhancers in the mouse. *Behav Brain Res*, 151(1–2):37–46.

358. Bontempi, B., Whelan, K.T., Risbrough, V.B., Lloyd, G.K., and Menzaghi, F. (2003). Cognitive enhancing properties and tolerability of cholinergic agents in mice: A comparative study of nicotine, donepezil, and SIB-1553A, a subtype-selective ligand for nicotinic acetylcholine receptors. *Neuropsychopharmacology*, 28(7):1235–1246.

359. Kirkby, D.L., Jones, D.N., Barnes, J.C., and Higgins, G.A. (1996). Effects of anticholinesterase drugs tacrine and E2020, the 5-HT(3) antagonist ondansetron, and the H(3) antagonist thioperamide, in models of cognition and cholinergic function. *Behav Pharmacol*, 7(6):513–525.

360. Balducci, C., Nurra, M., Pietropoli, A., Samanin, R., and Carli, M. (2003). Reversal of visual attention dysfunction after AMPA lesions of the nucleus basalis magnocellularis (NBM) by the cholinesterase inhibitor donepezil and by a 5-HT1A receptor antagonist WAY 100635. *Psychopharmacology (Berl)*, 167(1):28–36.

361. Luine, V.N., Mohan, G., Tu, Z., and Efange, S.M. (2002). Chromaproline and Chromaperidine, nicotine agonists, and Donepezil, cholinesterase inhibitor, enhance performance of memory tasks in ovariectomized rats. *Pharmacol Biochem Behav*, 74(1):213–220.

362. Prickaerts, J., Sik, A., van der Staay, F.J., de Vente, J., and Blokland, A. (2005). Dissociable effects of acetylcholinesterase inhibitors and phosphodiesterase type 5 inhibitors on object recognition memory: Acquisition versus consolidation. *Psychopharmacology (Berl)*, 177(4):381–390.

363. van der Staay, F.J. and Bouger, P.C. (2005). Effects of the cholinesterase inhibitors donepezil and metrifonate on scopolamine-induced impairments in the spatial cone field orientation task in rats. *Behav Brain Res*, 156(1):1–10.

364. van der Staay, F.J., Hinz, V.C., and Schmidt, B.H. (1996). Effects of metrifonate, its transformation product dichlorvos, and other organophosphorus and reference cholinesterase inhibitors on Morris water escape behavior in young-adult rats. *J Pharmacol Exp Ther*, 278(2):697–708.

365. Hodges, H., Sowinski, P., Turner, J.J., and Fletcher, A. (1996). Comparison of the effects of the 5-HT3 receptor antagonists WAY-100579 and ondansetron on spatial learning in the water maze in rats with excitotoxic lesions of the forebrain cholinergic projection system. *Psychopharmacology (Berl)*, 125(2):146–161.

366. Chen, Z., Xu, A.J., Li, R., and Wei, E.Q. (2002). Reversal of scopolamine-induced spatial memory deficits in rats by TAK-1471. *Acta Pharmacol Sin*, 23(4):355–360.

367. Xu, A.J., Chen, Z., Yanai, K., Huang, Y.W., and Wei, E.Q. (2002). Effect of 3-[1-(phenylmethyl)-4-piperidinyl]-1-(2,3,4,5-tetrahydro-1H-1-benzazepin-8 -yl)-1-propanone fumarate, a novel acetylcholinesterase inhibitor, on spatial cognitive impairment induced by chronic cerebral hypoperfusion in rats. *Neurosci Lett*, 331(1):33–36.

368. Van, D.D., Abramowski, D., Staufenbiel, M., and De Deyn, P.P. (2005). Symptomatic effect of donepezil, rivastigmine, galantamine and memantine on cognitive deficits in the APP23 model. *Psychopharmacology (Berl)*, 180(1):177–190.

369. Abe, Y., Aoyagi, A., Hara, T., Abe, K., Yamazaki, R., Kumagae, Y. *et al.* (2003). Pharmacological characterization of RS-1259, an orally active dual inhibitor of acetylcholinesterase and serotonin transporter, in rodents: Possible treatment of Alzheimer's disease. *J Pharmacol Sci*, 93(1):95–105.

370. Cohen, J. (1988). *Statistical Power Analysis for the Behavioral Sciences*, 2 ed. Lawrence Erlbaum Associates, Inc., Hillsdale, New Jersey.

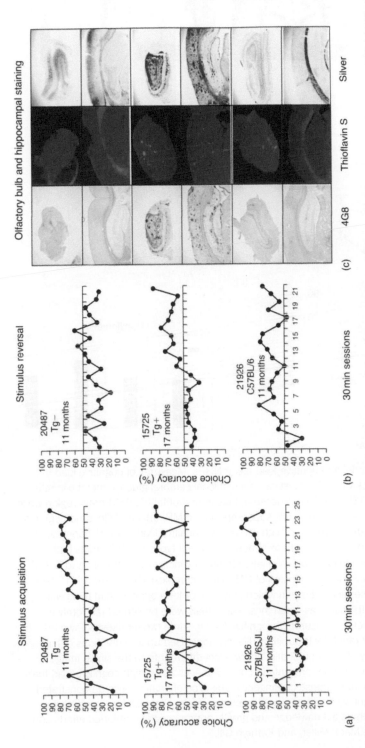

Figure 4.2 Rates of learning to discriminate odors and then to reverse that discrimination in a GO-NO GO odor discrimination task in representative aged (>11 months) Tg$_{2576}$ Tg+, Tg−, and C57BL/6SJ$_{F1}$ mice. (a) stimulus acquisition, (b) stimulus reversal, and (c) olfactory bulb and hippocampal staining. The figures illustrate the increase in choice accuracy (% correct discriminations) in learning to press or not press a lever for food, depending on which of 2 odors (cinnamon or peppermint) were presented (a), and the subsequent reversal of that behavior (b) in an odor discrimination task by representative aged Tg−, Tg+, and C57BL/6SJF1 background good discriminating mice over 25–30 min training sessions. Fifty percent represent chance levels of responding. The level of amyloid deposition and neurodegeneration of these mice were assessed (c) through examination of olfactory bulb (upper sections) and hippocampal formation (lower sections) stained with 4G8 (plaque formation), thioflavin S (dense plaque formation), or silver staining (neuritic processes). The authors acknowledge the contribution made by S. Franklin, J. Oostveen, and A. Buhl (ex. Pharmacia and Upjohn, Kalamazoo MI) and of A. Goodwin to this study.

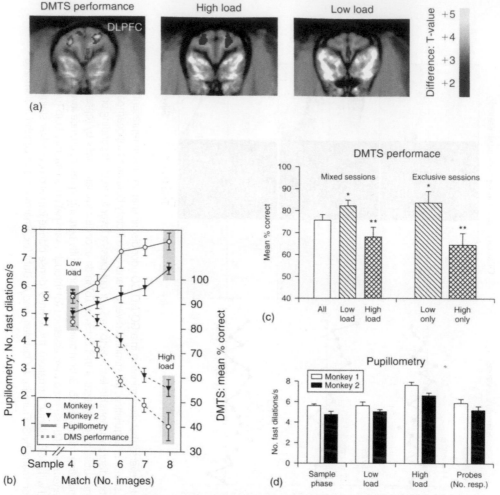

Figure 4.8 A translational model for cognitive load using NHPs. Measures of cognitive load in NHPs performing a DMTS task (a) SPM statistical maps of local cerebral glucose metabolic rate (CMRglc) from PET scans of 18Fluorodeoxyglucose uptake in prefrontal (DLPFC) brain region while monkeys performed DMTS task. Colored voxels superimposed on MRI images reflect the degree to which different brain areas were activated on high versus low cognitive load trials. (b) Comparison of pupillometry and DMTS performance (right axis) across different types of DMTS trials that range from low to high cognitive load. Pupillary dilation frequency increases (left axis) and DMTS performance declines along the same dimension of DMTS task complexity. (c) Mean DMTS task performance during imaging sessions above in which only high or low cognitive load trials were presented. Performance was the same as when those same trials were presented randomly in normal sessions. (d) Pupillometric measures of cognitive load in same two monkeys shown in (b). Mean (± SEM) number of rapid (fast) pupillary dilations increased under conditions of high cognitive workload. Frequency of rapid pupil dilations was not different from the single image sample phase for low load trials. Probe: presentation of 6–8 images as on high cognitive load trials presented independently without response contingency. This type of analysis also demonstrated that performance on high cognitive load trials was the primary factor that was facilitated by the ampakine CX717.[221] (The authors acknowledge and greatly appreciate the combined efforts and expertise of Dr. Linda Porrino, Mack Miller, and Kathryn Gill.)

CHAPTER 5

Animal Models of Parkinson's Disease to Aid Drug Discovery and Development

Kalpana M. Merchant[1], Marie-Françoise Chesselet[2], Shu-Ching Hu[3], and Stanley Fahn[3]

[1]Neuroscience Drug Discovery Research, Eli Lilly and Company, Indianapolis, IN, USA
[2]Department of Neurology, University of California, Los Angeles, CA, USA
[3]Department of Neurology, Columbia University Medical Center, New York, NY, USA

Animal and Translational Models for CNS Drug Discovery,
Vol. 2 of 3: Neurological Disorders
Robert McArthur and Franco Borsini (eds), Academic Press, 2008

INTRODUCTION

Parkinson's disease (PD) is the second most common, age-related progressive neurodegenerative disorder. World-wide, approximately 4.5 million people are thought to have been afflicted with PD in 2005 and this prevalence is projected to double by the year 2030 as the population ages.[1] Two recent events have impacted significantly the discovery and development approaches for novel therapeutics for PD: (a) the discovery of disease-causing mutations in multiple genes and (b) an emerging appreciation that the pathophysiology and associated symptoms of PD are more widespread than those resulting from the progressive loss of the nigrostriatal dopamine projections. Specifically, there has been an emergence of new animal models based on genetic etiology of familial PD and hence a renewed focus on using the new animal models to develop therapeutic strategies aimed at slowing the progression of the disease as well as treating non-motor symptoms of PD. This chapter aims to provide an overview of the current state of the PD research with a special emphasis on animal models that can help therapeutic discovery and development. Please note that the focus of this chapter is on animal models of disease pathophysiology and resultant symptoms and does not include a detailed discussion on models of dopaminergic drug-induced dyskinesias, although the latter is recognized as a major unmet medical need of the PD patients. We begin the chapter with a summary on the clinical syndrome and current therapies of PD. The objective is to set the context for the discussion to follow on commonly used animal models, their phenotypes and how they correlate/reproduce disease pathophysiology or specific symptoms of PD. The final section of this chapter will address the specific utility of animal models in drug discovery and development. Throughout the chapter, importance and attention will be paid to current challenges or gaps that hinder discovery and development of drugs addressing the unmet medical needs of PD patients. Additionally, some suggestions are offered on the utility of classical animal models as well as emerging models to address these gaps and facilitate development of therapeutic interventions.

BRIEF DESCRIPTION OF CLINICAL SYNDROME OF PD

In the 1817 monograph, "An Essay on the Shaking Palsy," James Parkinson described a disease characterized by tremor and impaired motility, which he named shaking palsy, to highlight these two motor symptoms.[2] As a plethora of other motor features were characterized and an expanding list of non-motor abnormalities recognized, the eponymous designation, PD, actually has illuminated better this multifaceted neurological disorder.

From the perspective of a movement disorder, PD has several motor features that are considered cardinal, in the sense that they are separate, distinct features common in this disease and their constellation increases the level of diagnostic certainty.[3] These cardinal symptoms are tremor, rigidity, bradykinesia, flexed posture, postural instability, and the freezing phenomenon. Those symptoms affecting the limbs tend to start unilaterally and stay asymmetrically more severe on the side of the onset even as the contralateral side becomes affected. The classic Parkinsonian tremor is a tremor-at-rest with a frequency between 4 and 6 Hz, and is most prominent in the distal regions such as the hand, foot and chin. Atypical tremors such as an action tremor can also occur in PD. Rigidity means increased muscle tone throughout the range of motion, and a ratchety quality that is called cogwheeling, also is detected frequently. Bradykinesia is defined as slowness, diminution or paucity of voluntary movements and the term akinesia refers to the same phenomenon with a more severe degree. Flexed posture affects the torso and limbs. Postural instability of PD is due to a loss of postural reflexes (righting reflex) and leads to a tendency to fall. Freezing describes an abrupt and transient cessation of motor activities, most commonly seen on gait initiation, turning and when reaching a destination, such as a chair in which to sit down. Neither of these cardinal symptoms nor a certain combination is omnipresent in PD. Nevertheless, several syndromic manifestations of PD emerge from the heterogeneity of symptoms, and are considered as subtypes of PD; for example, tremor-predominant, akinetic-rigid and postural-instability-gait-disorder subtypes of PD.[4,5] It is widely accepted that for a definite diagnosis of Parkinsonism, at least two of the cardinal signs must be present, with at least one being tremor-at-rest or bradykinesia.

Beyond the traditional boundary of a movement disorder, there is increasing awareness of non-motor symptoms of PD.[6] These include symptoms and signs that relate to functions of the cardiovascular, gastrointestinal, urinogenital, thermoregulatory, and pupillomotor systems and encompass virtually all levels of the neuraxis from the neural plexii innervating the heart, gut and pelvis to the hypothalamus and peripheral autonomic nervous system. Thus orthostatic hypotension and baroreflex failure, chronic constipation, and urinary urgency or incontinence are frequently present and can be disabling to patients. In addition, PD patients suffer from other non-motor symptoms such as depression, excessive daytime sleepiness, anosmia, cognitive deficits and REM sleep disorder. The non-motor symptoms of PD can compromise the patients' quality of life as greatly as the motor symptoms do. Certain non-motor symptoms clearly precede the motor symptoms in PD.[7,8] Therefore, recognition of these non-motor symptoms may facilitate an early diagnosis of PD, and thus can provide a timely window for neuroprotective interventions, which are considered more meaningful in an earlier phase of a progressive disease.[9] The development of non-motor and motor symptoms in the course of PD parallels the pathologic progression in which Lewy bodies and neurodegeneration first occur in the lower brain stem and olfactory bulb before it affects the substantia nigra, and eventually, other subcortical and cortical structures.[10]

The definite diagnosis of PD requires a histopathologic demonstration of selective neurodegeneration in the substantia nigra pars compacta and presence of the synuclein-containing Lewy bodies or neurites. Understandably, this level of diagnostic definitiveness is seldom achieved prior to an autopsy. Moreover, in at least one genetic form of PD, that caused by mutations in the *parkin* gene, Lewy bodies may be absent. Until reliable and practical biomarkers are available, PD will remain a disease for which the antemortem diagnosis relies exclusively on clinical observation. Therefore, limitations inherent to a clinical diagnosis of any disorder also exist in PD, namely the sensitivity and specificity of the clinical diagnosis as determined by the gold-standard pathologic diagnosis. Several clinical diagnostic criteria for PD have been proposed, for example, the UK PD Society Brain Bank and National Institute of Neurological Disorders and Strokes criteria.[11,12] The accuracy of these diagnostic criteria is estimated in the range between 76% and 92% based on several clinicopathologic studies.[13,14]

As a neurodegenerative disorder, PD progresses relentlessly. The progression is demonstrated pathologically by continuous neurodegeneration in the brain, and is reflected by clinical decline and changes on functional imaging. It is clear there is latency between the onset of neurodegeneration and clinical symptoms, and this presymptomatic period used to be considered protracted. With increasing sensitivity of clinical measures of motor and non-motor symptoms as well as functional imaging techniques, the estimate of the presymptomatic period continues to be reduced. Current estimates range between 3.1 and 6 years and correspond to about 33% loss of dopaminergic neurons in substantia nigra.[15,16] There is also increasing evidence that the progression of PD is non-linear and is more precipitous in the early phase of the disease.[16-18] These findings on the disease progression in presymptomatic and early phases indicate that neurodegeneration in PD is more active in the initial than in the advanced stage, and underpin the intense pursuit of effective neuroprotective treatment.

SYNOPSIS OF CURRENT TREATMENT OF PD

Treatment of any given progressive disease can be divided into two categories, symptomatic and disease-modifying. Symptomatic treatment remedies the symptoms but does not change the natural course of a disease. On the other hand, a disease-modifying treatment delays or reverses the progression of the disease, which is termed neuroprotective or neurorestorative, respectively. This dichotomy of symptomatic versus disease-modifying treatment, while conceptually distinct, does not preclude the possibility that a certain form of treatment can possess both properties.[i] Furthermore, although a purely disease-modifying treatment would exert its therapeutic effect directly on the pathogenesis but not on the symptoms of the disease, it should reduce the rate of deficits in symptoms as a consequence of delayed progression of the disease. Thus the benefit on symptoms is derived from a disease-modifying effect, and should not be considered as a direct symptomatic effect. Compared to a more immediate improvement in symptoms due to symptomatic or neurorestorative treatment, the pace of symptomatic improvement due to neuroprotective treatment will depend on the rate of progression of the disease and the degree of effectiveness of the therapeutic agent. In a chronic neurodegenerative condition such as PD, the observed symptomatic benefit of any neuroprotective therapy is expected to be delayed and gradual.

Based on available evidence, all currently established therapies of PD are considered symptomatic treatment, although some hold the promise of being disease-modifying as well.[19] There is a variety of medications effective for motor symptoms of PD[20] (Table 5.1). Pharmacologically, they are classified as dopamine precursor therapies (levodopa) with or without decarboxylase inhibitors (carbidopa, benserazide) and catechol-O-methyltransferase inhibitors (entacapone, tolcapone), dopamine receptor agonists (bromocriptine, pramipexole, ropinirole, apomorphine, cabergoline, lisuride, piribedil, rotigotine), monoamine oxidase (MAO) inhibitors (tranylcypromine, phenelzine, rasagiline), anticholinergics (biperiden, trihexiphenydil) and putative dopamine modulator (amantadine). Among them, levodopa (after being converted to dopamine) and dopamine receptor agonists act directly on dopaminergic

---

[i] For further discussion of symptomatic versus disease-modifying treatments, please refer to Lindner *et al.*, Development, optimization and use of preclinical behavioral models to maximize the productivity of drug discovery for Alzheimer's Disease, in this volume.

Table 5.1 PD treatments and product pipeline

Drug trade name	Generic name	Pharmacological mechanism	Intended use	Dosing route	Phase of development	Estimated launch
APPROVED DRUG PRODUCTS						
Dopamine precursor therapies						
Sinemet®, Madopar®	Levodopa/ carbidopa	Dopamine precursor/DDC inhibitor	Symptomatic for motor deficits	Oral	Approved	NA
Stalevo®	Entacapone/ levodopa/ carbidopa	COMT/dopamine precursor/DDC inhibitor	Symptomatic for motor deficits and motor complications	Oral	Approved	NA
Dopamine receptor agonists						
Parlodel®	Bromocriptine	D_2 receptor agonist	Symptomatic for motor deficits	Oral	Approved	NA
Permax®	Pergolide	D_2 receptor agonist	Symptomatic for motor deficits	Oral	Withdrawn in March 2007	NA
Apokyn®	Apmorphine	$D_1 + D_2$ receptor agonist	Symptomatic for motor deficits	Subcutaneous	Approved	NA
Requip®	Ropinrole	D_2 receptor agonists	Symptomatic for motor deficits	Oral	Approved	NA
Mirapex®/ Mirapexin®	Pramipexole	D_3 preferring, D_2 receptor agonist	Symptomatic for motor deficits	Oral	Approved	NA
Neupro®	Rotigotine	D_2 receptor agonist	Symptomatic for motor deficits	Transdermal	Approved	NA
MAO-B inhibitors						
Eldepryl®, Zelapar®	Selegiline	Irreversible MAO-B inhibitor	Symptomatic for motor deficits	Oral	Approved	NA

(continued)

Table 5.1 (Continued)

Drug trade name	Generic name	Pharmacological mechanism	Intended use	Dosing route	Phase of development	Estimated launch
Azilect®/Agilect®	Rasagiline	Irreversible MAO-B inhibitor	Symptomatic for motor deficits; disease-modifying efficacy being tested	Oral	Approved; Phase III for disease progression	NA; Results of efficacy on disease progression to be available in late 2008
Anticholinergic agents						
Artane®	Trihexyphenidyl	Antimuscarinic	Symptomatic for motor deficits	Oral	Approved	NA
Cogentin®	Benztropine	Antimuscarinic	Symptomatic for motor deficits	Oral	Approved	NA
Symmetrel®	Amantadine	Multiple mechanisms	Symptomatic for motor deficits and motor complications	Oral	Approved	NA
Others						
Exelon®		Acetylcholine esterase inhibitor	Symptomatic for cognitive deficits	Oral	Approved for PD-associated dementia	NA
INVESTIGATIONAL DRUGS (development recently halted after clinical trial results)						
	Liatermine	Recombinant GDNF	Disease-modifying	Intra-putamen	Phase II	Terminated
CEP 1347		Jnk inhibitor	Disease-modifying	Oral	Phase III	Terminated
TCH 346		Apoptosis inhibitor	Disease-modifying	Oral	Phase III	Terminated
INVESTIGATIONAL DRUGS (in development)						
Glutamate modulators						
E2007		AMPA receptor antagonist	L-DOPA induced dyskinesia		Phase III	2009

Code	Name	Mechanism	Indication	Route	Phase	Year
MRZ 2579	Neramexane	NMDA antagonist			Phase III	
LY 300164	Talampanel	AMPA receptor antagonist	L-DOPA induced dyskinesia		Phase II	
FP 0011		Glutamate release inhibitor			Phase II	
Adenosine receptor ligands						
KW 6002	Istradefylline	A$_{2A}$ antagonist	Symptomatic for motor deficits + disease modifying (has not been tested for effects on disease progression)	Oral	Pre-registration/Phase III	
SCH 63390		A$_2$ antagonist	Symptomatic for motor deficits + disease modifying	Oral	Phase III	
VR2006		A$_{2A}$ agonist	Symptomatic for motor deficits		Phase I	
Dopamine/Serotonin/Noradrenergic modulators						
SLV 308	Pardoprunox	Dopamine D$_2$ receptor partial agonist with 5-HT$_{1a}$ agonist activity	Symptomatic for motor deficits and co-morbid depression		Phase III	2010
EMD128130	Saritozan	D$_2$ receptor antagonist, 5-HT$_{1a}$ agonist	L-DOPA-induced dyskinesias	Oral	Phase III	
Sphera mine®		Dopamine secreting implants	Disease-modifying	implant	Phase IIb (fast-track status)	2008
ACP 103		5-HT$_{2A}$ inverse agonist	Symptomatic for motor deficits	Oral	Phase IIb	

(continued)

Table 5.1 (Continued)

Drug trade name	Generic name	Pharmacological mechanism	Intended use	Dosing route	Phase of development	Estimated launch
DAR 0100		D_1 receptor agonist	Symptomatic for motor deficits	Injectable	Phase II	
ACR 16		Dopamine normalizer	Symptomatic for motor deficits as add-on to dopamine agonists and L-DOPA; also for L-DOPA induced dyskinesias	Oral	Phase I	
JP 1730	Fipamezole	Adrenergic A_2 receptor antagonist	Symptomatic for L-DOPA-induced dyskinesias		Phase II	
Other miscellaneous mechanisms						
NW 1015	Safinamide	Na/Ca ion channel blocker + reversible MAO-B inhibitor	Symptomatic for motor deficits as add-on to dopamine agonists and L-DOPA	Oral	Phase III	
PD 02	Creatine	Antioxidant	Disease-modifying	Oral	Phase III	
	Ubidecarenone Coenzyme Q10		Disease-modifying			
GPI 1485		Neuroimmunophilin ligands	Disease-modifying		Phase II	Terminated
AEOL 10150		Antioxidant	Disease-modifying	Subcutaneous	Phase I	
AVE 1625		CB1 antagonist	Symptomatic		Phase I	
Gene therapy						
CERE 120		Neurturin gene therapy	Disease-modifying	Intra-putamen	Phase I	
NLX P101		Gene therapy	Disease-modifying		Phase I	

neurotransmission, and are more efficacious at providing symptomatic relief than other medications. Decarboxylase inhibitors and catechol-O-methyltransferase inhibitors have no intrinsic symptomatic effects, and are co-administered with levodopa to mitigate its peripheral complications or to prolong its action.

Levodopa, first introduced into clinical use in 1969,[21] still remains the most efficacious medication in treating PD. Combined with a decarboxylase inhibitor, levodopa is available in preparations of different pharmacokinetics. Not all motor symptoms of PD respond equally to levodopa. Rigidity and bradykinesia are most responsive, and tremor can respond fully, partially or not at all. Axial symptoms such as flexed posture, postural instability and freezing are usually less amenable to levodopa. Long-term exposure to levodopa is believed to cause or accelerate the occurrence of motor complications in PD.[22,23] Those motor complications of levodopa are involuntary movements called dyskinesias and fluctuations of motor improvement called wearing offs. Various temporal patterns of dyskinesias and wearing offs have been identified, including peak-dose dyskinesia, end-of-dose off, dyskinesia-improvement-dyskinesia (diphasic dyskinesias), sudden off, and off dystonia. When they are severe, levodopa-related motor complications become a major source of disability in patients with PD.

Next to levodopa in efficacy are the dopamine receptor agonists. Similar to levodopa, rigidity and bradykinesia are more responsive to dopamine receptor agonists than tremor or axial symptoms of PD. This class of drugs provides an alternative to levodopa when the symptoms of PD are mild in the early stage of the disease. However, as the disease progresses and the symptoms worsen, levodopa is needed inevitably for adequate symptomatic relief, although dopamine receptor agonists still remain an effective adjunct for reducing the wearing off phenomenon. Monotherapy with a dopamine receptor agonist rarely leads to dyskinesias; however, its addition may aggravate already existing levodopa-induced dyskinesias. Compared with levodopa, these agents have a higher propensity of inducing neuropsychiatric and sleep-related complications.

MAO inhibitors enhance dopaminergic neurotransmission by inhibiting degradation of dopamine. They can be separated into non-selective and type B-selective inhibitors according to their affinities for the type A and B isoforms of MAO, both expressed in the brain. Because the type A isoform is predominantly expressed in the gastrointestinal tract, use of non-selective MAO inhibitors requires adherence to a tyramine-free diet to prevent unwanted vasomotor complications caused by exogenous monoamines, the so-called "cheese effect." Such dietary restriction is usually not necessary for type B-selective MAO inhibitors, and therefore they are more convenient to use. Because levodopa can generate peripheral dopamine, non-selective MAO inhibitors should be avoided in the presence of levodopa therapy. Amantadine is another modulator of dopaminergic neurotransmission, enhancing release of dopamine from nerve terminals, but it also has anticholinergic and antiglutamatergic effects. Its symptomatic effect on the motor symptoms of PD is rapid in onset. Amantadine can be effective in reducing levodopa-induced dyskinesias, and is prescribed more often nowadays for its antidyskinetic effect. Anticholinergics also exert modest symptomatic effects on the motor symptoms of PD, but their use is less favored because of frequent adverse effects. In addition to medications for PD, surgeries targeting the basal ganglia have emerged as an effective modality in treating patients with refractory motor symptoms or levodopa-related motor complications in the last decade.[24,25] Because of its reversible nature, the implantation of deep brain stimulators has largely replaced the ablative procedures of thalamotomy and pallidotomy. The targets of deep brain stimulation to treat PD include the subthalamus, globus pallidus internus and thalamic ventrointermediate nucleus. Both subthalamic and pallidal stimulation are effective for a broader range of motor symptoms, whereas the effectiveness of thalamic stimulation is mainly confined to tremor.

UNMET MEDICAL NEEDS

Despite a growing armamentarium of options, there remain significant unmet medical needs in the treatment of PD. First and foremost is the void in disease-modifying therapies. Currently, all medical and surgical therapies for PD are deemed symptomatic. While symptomatic treatment is invaluable in improving functionality and quality of life, disease-modifying treatment for PD has been long desired for its curative merit. Hence, there is a need to develop markers of natural history of disease progression that may be used to assess therapeutic strategies that may alter that progression.

Although dopaminergic medications and deep brain stimulation are effective for certain motor symptoms of PD, they are less or not effective for other motor symptoms, such as flexed posture, postural instability and freezing. Similarly, most non-motor symptoms of PD do not respond to dopaminergic interventions, and their current treatment is typically derived from experience with similar symptoms in other disorders. These dopamine-unresponsive symptoms of PD deserve a place in the development of more specific treatment.

Levodopa-induced dyskinesias are another focus of effort in improving preventive or therapeutic strategies. Pulsatile dopaminergic stimulation due to intermittent administration of exogenous levodopa has been proposed to be a mechanism underlying levodopa-induced dyskinesias. Therefore, measures to deliver continuous instead of pulsatile dopaminergic stimulation are being investigated to determine if this approach would prevent or delay the onset of dyskinesias, although the rationale and efficacy of this approach are still debatable.[26] Medications with an intrinsic antidyskinetic property are also desirable in treating levodopa-induced dyskinesias once they occur.

In treatment of PD, a long-held and still unfolding controversy is the question whether dopaminergic medications could be neurotoxic, or to the contrary, be neuroprotective. Results from animal studies are often conflicting,[27-30] and those from clinical trials inconclusive.[18,31,32] As dopaminergic medications are the most frequently used ones in treating PD, there is a pressing need to clarify this uncertainty.

CLINICAL TRIALS OF TREATMENTS FOR PD

The concept of evidence-based medicine has permeated every aspect of clinical practice, and treatment of PD is no exception. All clinical trials in PD are subject to the reviewing algorithm of evidence-based medicine, which mirrors the requirements for approval of any therapeutics set by regulatory agencies like the US Food and Drug

Administration (FDA).[ii] Accordingly, guidelines, recommendations or reviews have been published by medical societies in the United States and Europe, and they outline the status of currently available treatment of PD.[33-35]

Pertinent to the therapeutic trials in PD is the way by which efficacy is determined. For clinical trials of symptomatic treatment, depending on the projected effects of interventions, the outcome is measured using clinical rating scales that assess different dimensions of symptoms in PD. Several rating scales are in wide use and are considered standards, including the Unified PD Rating Scale, Hoehn and Yahr Stage Scale, Schwab-England Activities of Daily Living Scale, Dopa Dyskinesia Severity Scale, Dyskinesia Activities of Daily Living Scale, and Parkinson's Psychosis Scale.[36] For those symptoms that can be measured and quantified electromechanically, biometric studies can supplement the clinical rating scales, for example, accelerometry for tremor. Most clinical trials of medications and surgeries for their symptomatic effects on PD are conducted in this fashion.

For clinical trials of disease-modifying treatment of PD, measuring outcome requires greater sophistication. The direct readout of the disease-modifying effect is, in theory, the change in the neurodegenerative process on serial pathological examinations, an impossible task in humans. Therefore, biomarkers of the progressive neurodegenerative process are required for clinical trials of disease-modifying treatment of PD,[37] and any proposed surrogate marker needs to be validated. Clinical outcomes, such as severity of symptoms on various clinical rating scales or time to a specific event like initiating symptomatic treatment, are convenient candidates for surrogate markers, although none of them have been validated pathologically. Therefore, clinical outcomes by themselves are not sufficient to get the regulatory approval for a new drug aimed at slowing disease progression. With regard to clinical markers, issues arise especially when the disease-modifying treatment being tested is known or suspected to possess also additional symptomatic benefits. In such a scenario, the perceived clinical benefit may be the summation of both symptomatic and disease-modifying effects. With a simple design of clinical trials, it is impossible to distinguish one from the other. The task of separating the disease-modifying effect from symptomatic effect demands more elaborate trial designs, and can be attempted in the following ways.

Theoretically, following an adequate washout period, the symptomatic effect is eliminated and the disease-modifying effect is exposed. However, there are limitations to this washout approach. For example, the patients may not be able to tolerate deprivation of the symptomatic effect, and as a consequence, the rate of dropout increases. The other *caveat* for this approach is the difficulty in determining the biological half-life of a drug and the adequacy of the length of the washout duration. For instance, levodopa is known to elicit both short- and long-duration responses, measured in hours and in days respectively.[38,39] Any given drug can carry similar dual responses. If the biological half-life is underestimated, it may result in an inadequate washout period, which in turn would lead to an apparent erroneous evidence of disease-modifying effect due to contamination by the symptomatic efficacy.[40]

[ii] See Code of Federal Regulations 2006; Title 21, Volume 5, Part 312: Investigational New Drug Application.

A delayed-start design, initially developed for Alzheimer's disease, is a methodology aimed at isolating the disease-modifying effect from symptomatic effect.[41,42] This approach consists of two-phases. The first phase of the study includes both active treatment (early-start group) and placebo (delayed-start group) arms. At the conclusion of the desired length of the first phase, the placebo arm from the first phase is switched to the active therapy while continuing to maintain the patients on the active therapy treatment arm during the second phase. Thus the clinical difference between the two arms in the first phase can be due solely to a symptomatic benefit and may be equivocal for a disease-modifying effect. However, differences in patient outcomes at the end of the second phase can be inferred to the disease-modifying effect of the active therapy. A MAO inhibitor, rasagiline, has been investigated in such a delayed-start design. The major criticism of a delayed-start design is that the second phase must be long enough to determine if the benefit in the delayed-start group would catch up to that obtained by the early-start group. In addition, disease-modifying effect from this type of clinical trial is revealed indirectly rather than directly.

In addition to clinical markers, neuroimaging markers of dopaminergic function have been used widely for PD. Besides their utility for a diagnostic application, they have the potential to distinguish between disease-modifying and symptomatic effects.[43] In clinical trials, commonly used imaging markers assess the state of nigrostriatal dopaminergic projections using functional imaging modalities of the positron emission tomography (PET) and single photon emission computed tomography (SPECT).[44] There are a number of radiotracers for nigrostriatal dopaminergic transmission, including the ones that measure various aspects of presynaptic dopamine functions such as [^{18}F]fluorodopa (measures the activity of L-aromatic acid decarboxylase, an enzyme that converts dopa to dopamine), [^{123}I]2β-carbomethoxy-3β-(4–iodophenyl)tropane (measures dopamine transporter function) and [^{11}C]dihydrotetrabenazine (measures the function of vesicular monoamine transporter, VMAT). Additionally there are radiotracers that assess postsynaptic dopamine D_2 receptors such as [^{11}C]raclopride and [^{123}I]iodobenzamide. Although these imaging techniques may provide quantitative information on the progression of PD, there are, unsolved issues regarding their use in clinical trials of disease-modifying agents. First, there are limited pathologic studies that validate the imaging markers for monitoring the progression of PD[45,46] and hence these markers are not acceptable as yet as surrogate markers of evidence of disease modification.[iii] Second, there are a small percentage of patients whose conditions meet the criteria of clinically definite PD, but

---

[iii] For further discussion regarding biomarkers and surrogate markers in behavioral disorders, please refer to Bartz et al., Preclinical animal models of Autistic Spectrum Disorders (ASD); Cryan et al., Developing more efficacious antidepressant medications: Improving and aligning preclinical detection and clinical assessment tools; Tannock et al., Towards a biological understanding of ADHD and the discovery of novel therapeutic approaches; Winsky et al., Drug discovery and development initiatives at the National Institute of Mental Health: From cell-based systems to proof of concept; Joel et al., Animal models of obsessive–compulsive disorder: From bench to bedside via endophenotypes and biomarkers; Large et al., Developing therapeutics for bipolar disorder: From animal models to the clinic, in Volume 1, Psychiatric Disorders; Lindner et al., Development, optimization and use of preclinical behavioral models to maximize the productivity of drug discovery for Alzheimer's Disease; Montes Translational Research in ALS; Wagner et al., Huntington Disease, in this volume; Dourish et al., Anti-obesity drugs: From animal models to clinical efficacy, in Volume 3, Reward Deficit Disorders.

have imaging scans without evidence of dopaminergic deficit (SWEDD). Inclusion of patients with SWEDD can negate an otherwise statistically significant result in several studies.[31,32] The clinical interpretation of SWEDD is not entirely settled.[47,48] Finally, there is the question whether the drug being tested in the clinical trial may interfere with the pharmacokinetics or pharmacodynamics of these radiotracers, and as a result, confound the interpretation.[44,49]

In testing disease-modifying treatment that clearly contains no immediate symptomatic effects; a simpler design in the methodology suffices. Biomarkers for progression of PD are nevertheless greatly desirable in these trials. For example, in a trial that involves an invasive surgical procedure, it may be difficult to have matched sham control or to have blinded clinical assessment. Use of biomarkers will be extremely useful to minimize the placebo effect, which may actually be higher in such trials.[50] The biomarkers also supplement the measurement of outcome with quantitative and objective data independent of clinical assessment, and therefore strengthen the validity of the results from the clinical trials. Finally, validated biomarkers can facilitate the approval of a new disease-modifying therapeutic intervention from regulatory authorities such as the FDA.

A key question arises from the discussion above: could animal models be developed to address the unmet medical needs and minimize challenges of clinical trials of disease-modifying treatment for PD? Indeed, animal models have played and will continue to play an indispensable bridge between the laboratory discoveries and clinical trials. The following section will provide a historical perspective on classical animal models that led to the discovery and development of currently marketed drugs as well as limitations of these models for assessment of therapeutics addressing unmet medical needs.

ANIMAL MODELS THAT LED TO THE DISCOVERY AND DEVELOPMENT OF CURRENTLY AVAILABLE DRUGS TO TREAT MOTORIC SYMPTOMS AND THEIR LIMITATIONS

Reserpine Model

Early animal models of PD can be traced back to the administration of reserpine in the 1950s.[51] This drug prevents uptake of dopamine into vesicles through the vesicular transporter, resulting in rapid destruction of dopamine in the cytoplasm by MAO, and a decrease in vesicular dopamine release. When administered to rats, reserpine causes a marked decrease in locomotion or induces "catalepsy." The discovery that this decrease in motor behavior is accompanied by a major decrease in the level of striatal dopamine, a finding similar to that in post-mortem brains from patients with PD, reinforced the suspicion that loss of nigrostriatal dopaminergic neurons was responsible for the major bradykinetic symptoms of PD. It is in the reserpine model that levodopa, the precursor of dopamine, was shown to improve dramatically motor symptoms, leading to the use of this drug to treat PD.[51] This example demonstrates the power of animal models of dopamine depletion to develop effective symptomatic treatments for PD.

6-Hydroxydopamine Model

A limitation of the reserpine model is the transient nature of the symptoms, and the lack of neurodegeneration, thus limiting the analogy between this model and the chronic, irreversible neurodegeneration of PD. A new model addressed these shortcomings using unilateral, stereotactic injections of the toxin, 6-hydroxydopamine, into the nigrostriatal pathway. The selectivity of 6-hydroxydopamine toxicity for catecholaminergic neurons is based on its specific uptake by both the dopaminergic and the noradrenergic transporters. Selectivity for dopaminergic versus noradrenergic neurons is achieved *in vivo* via pre-treatment with a blocker of the noradrenergic transporter, usually desipramine.[52] Upon uptake into the catecholamine neurons, 6-hydroxydopamine induces degeneration by oxidative stress and inhibition of mitochondrial complexes I and IV.[53,54] Infusion of 6-hydroxydopamine into the substantia nigra or medial forebrain bundle is used commonly to produce >90% loss of dopamine in the substantia nigra and the neostriatum via anterograde transport of the toxin. On the other hand, a partial lesion of the dopaminergic pathway is obtained by injection of the toxin into the neostriatum.[55] This procedure leads to retrograde degeneration of nigrostriatal neurons and is used often to induce lesions in mice. The time-courses of loss of dopamine cell bodies and terminals by anterograde versus retrograde degeneration vary considerably. Thus the striatal infusion of 6-hydroxydopamine is associated with a significantly protracted time course of loss of dopamine terminals and cell bodies than the nigral or medial forebrain bundle models.[56,57] Hence, the partial lesioned, striatal infusion model is preferred by some investigators for assessment of neuroprotective efficacy. Although it is possible technically to destroy nigrostriatal dopaminergic neurons bilaterally, this model is used rarely since it induces severe debility, which requires constant nursing and feeding of animals. This is an important limitation of this model because some experiments have clearly shown that bilateral versus unilateral lesions of the nigrostriatal dopaminergic system have different effects.[58] Another limitation is the need to perform stereotaxic surgery to inject the toxin. However, with good surgical techniques coupled with precautions to minimize oxidation of the toxin (addition of ascorbic acid and storage of the solution in cold, dark environment) the reproducibility of 6-hydroxydopamine-induced lesions is excellent.

Users of the unilateral 6-hydroxydopamine lesion models generally confirm the accuracy of the stereotaxic infusion and select animals that have the desired strength of lesions by assessing rotations induced by dopaminergic agonists.[54] Two agents are used typically to induce the rotational behavior: injection of amphetamine, a drug that releases dopamine from nigrostriatal terminals or apomorphine, a direct acting dopamine receptor agonist. Amphetamine challenge causes rotations toward the side of the lesion and is used for both the anterograde and retrograde lesion models. In contrast, apomorphine causes rotations contralateral to the side of the 6-hydroxydopamine infusion by stimulating the supersensitive postsynaptic dopaminergic receptors in the lesioned striatum.[54,59-61] Hence, apomorphine-induced rotations are significantly more robust in the anterograde lesion models, which typically produce >90% loss of striatal dopamine.

Numerous studies have validated the use of dopamine agonist-induced rotations as a surrogate indicator of the magnitude of dopamine depletion/survival while testing neuroprotective or neurorestorative activity of novel therapeutic agents. It should be noted, however, that improvement of this behavior is not proportional to the level of dopamine restoration, since only a small improvement in dopamine levels can lead to a major improvement in rotational response induced by the dopaminergic agonists. Another *caveat* is that repeated injections of the dopaminergic agonists can lead to supersensitivity, a possible confound in assessing the effects of neuroprotective treatments that require "before" and "after" tests of behavior. To address this concern a number of non-drug-induced behavioral tests have been developed to assess motor deficits induced by unilateral striatal dopamine depletion. These include the cylinder test, forced step test and step initiation test, in particular.[62-66] These tests can detect deficits after partial lesions[67] but need to be interpreted with caution.[68] The behavioral tests generally are based on the comparison between the paw on the side contralateral to the lesion (affected) to the paw ipsilateral to the lesion (non-affected). Although this is an acceptable practice for the behavioral tests, it should be stressed that unilateral brain lesions often have effects in the contralateral brain hemisphere.[52,69] Therefore, a sham-operated group should be always included as a control in biochemical or molecular studies to avoid erroneous conclusions.

The unilateral 6-hydroxydopamine model has been used widely to validate dopaminergic agonists that are now used in the symptomatic treatment of PD and led also to a better understanding of the pathophysiological changes induced in the basal ganglia as a result of dopamine depletion. It has been the model of choice to examine the beneficial effects of fetal or stem cells transplants into the striatum, and is commonly used to create models of L-dopa-induced dyskinesias.[70] Whether or not this model is suitable for assessing neuroprotective strategies is predicated on the assumption that the mechanism by which 6-hydroxydopamine induces cell death is similar to the mechanism of cell death in PD. This remains unknown and is being questioned as a result of recent failures of drugs to produce efficacy in patients despite the demonstration of neuroprotective efficacy in the 6-hydroxydopamine model.[iv]

MPTP Model

The next model that had a major impact on PD research is based on the use of the neurotoxin, 1-methyl-4-phenyl-1,2,3,6-tertahydropyridine (MPTP).[71-73] Its development followed the discovery that MPTP, a byproduct of heroin synthesis, can cause a loss of nigrostriatal dopaminergic neurons in humans and produce Parkinsonism that cannot be distinguished from the idiopathic disease.[74] The advantage of MPTP over 6-hydroxydopamine is that it can be administered systemically. In the brain, MPTP is metabolized first by the enzyme MAO-B to 1-methyl-4-phenyl-2, 3-dihydropyridium ($MPDP^+$), which undergoes deprotonation to generate the corresponding pyridium species, MPP^+. The specificity of systemic MPTP for dopaminergic lesions is based on the selective uptake of MPP^+, by dopaminergic neurons via the dopamine transporter. Peripheral injections of MPTP cause remarkably little cell death outside the mesencephalic dopaminergic cell groups, and within these groups, nigrostriatal neurons are more sensitive to the toxin than neurons of the ventral tegmental area.[71,75] A limitation of the MPTP model is that it cannot be reproduced effectively in rats[76] as a result of a greater sequestration of $MPP(^+)$ into vesicles via the vesicular monoamine transporter

---

[iv] See below in the section discussing the use of animal models for target identification and validation.

in the rat striatal dopamine terminals.[77] In mice, different strains have different sensitivity to the toxin due to differences in neostriatal MPP$^+$ concentration.[78] The most robust and reproducible results are obtained in male C57/Bl6 mice weighing at least 22 g.[79]

Several MPTP regimens have been described to achieve nigrostriatal cell loss in mice, each characterized by some unique biochemical and neuropathological features (cf.,[80]). Most regimens are acute or subacute. An example of a commonly used acute model pioneered by Przedborski and colleagues is the regimen of 4 injections of 20 mg/kg, ip, of MPTP, administered once every 2 h, which causes profound dopaminergic cell loss by 7 days.[72] In order to reproduce more faithfully the slow neurodegeneration occurring in PD, several groups have developed subacute or chronic regimens, in which 20–30 mg/kg of MPTP is administered daily or every other day for 5–30 days. Remarkably, a recently developed regimen using delivery of MPTP by Alzet minipump® seems to reproduce a host of features of PD, including proteasomal deficits and inclusion formation.[81] However, the reproducibility of this model in other laboratories remains to be established. Another variation in the mouse MPTP model requires co-administration of probenecid, to reduce the renal excretion of the toxin and shows an indication of α-synuclein aggregation due to lysosomal defects.[82] It is important to note that the different dosing regimens produce differential extent of cell death and may engage different mechanisms of cell death.[72,81,83,84-86] In general, the toxicity of MPTP is attributed to inhibition of mitochondrial complex I, III and IV as well as neuroinflammation.[87-89]

It should be noted that MPTP intoxication does not produce behavioral Parkinsonism in mice. Hence, the primary use of the MPTP mouse model is to test pharmacological or genetic manipulations that could reduce the size of MPTP-induced lesions with the goal of discovering neuroprotective therapies.[90] The test of neuroprotective efficacy is based on neurochemical and/or histological end-points.

As a result of the convenience of systemic treatment regimens, MPTP is the toxin of choice to induce nigrostriatal dopaminergic cell loss in non-human primates. Additionally, unlike the mouse, MPTP induces Parkinsonism in the non-human primates and a clinical scoring system has been established to monitor drug-induced amelioration of Parkinsonism. Again, several different dosing protocols have been developed and have their own champions.[91-95] The MPTP model in non-human primates has been undoubtedly critical for the development of new generations of dopaminergic agents, non-dopaminergic drugs and adjunct therapies such as COMT inhibitors for the treatment of PD.[96,97] In addition, this model has been instrumental in the development and pre-clinical validation of surgical treatments for PD, in particular deep brain stimulation of the subthalamic nucleus.[98,99] However, studies of functional and neurochemical recovery in the MPTP models have to be interpreted carefully because spontaneous amelioration can occur after MPTP administration.[100] Thus it is critical to validate a MPTP dosing regimen by studying the time course of dopamine neurodegeneration and demonstrating stability of the lesion.

Other Toxin-Based Models

The MPTP model inaugurated a wave of models based on the use of environmental toxins to kill dopaminergic neurons. Although MPTP itself is not present in the environment, its structure is similar to that of DDT, which has been widely used as an insecticide.[101] This chemical property, together with evidence from epidemiological studies described earlier, prompted the use of environmentally-relevant toxin to model PD in rodents. Two toxins have been more widely used to model PD: rotenone and paraquat.[102] Rotenone is mostly known as an inhibitor of mitochondrial complex I, although more complex effects have been described recently.[103-105] The rotenone model was introduced by Betarbet and colleagues and elicited a tremendous interest since for the first time, a peripherally administered inhibitor of mitochondrial function seemed to kill selectively nigrostriatal dopaminergic neurons without relying upon a selective uptake mechanism.[106] This raised the possibility that the dopamine-specific toxicity of rotenone was due to a selective vulnerability of the nigrostriatal dopaminergic neurons to mitochondrial dysfunction.[103] It soon became apparent, however, that direct inhibition of mitochondrial function may not be the sole or even primary mechanism of rotenone toxicity.[104,105] Furthermore, other limitations emerged. Individual animals (rats) show marked variations in their sensitivity to rotenone, leading to a wide range of lesion size and regional specificity in the same cohort of animals. For example, with the same dose of rotenone, some animals show no dopaminergic cell loss at all, a selective nigrostriatal cell loss, or toxicity to both the dopaminergic nigrostriatal neurons and their targets in the striatum.[107] This variability explains results of studies that challenged the selectivity of rotenone for dopaminergic neurons,[108,109] while others confirmed the specificity.[110,111] Importantly, the lack of consistent lesions is a major obstacle to the use of rotenone for the study of neuroprotective strategies. Another limitation is that rotenone has not been successfully used in mice due to species differences in metabolism.[112] Finally, rotenone itself is not linked to an increased risk of PD because it is rapidly degraded in the environment.[102] Despite these limitations, rotenone remains a very useful tool to explore the mechanisms by which toxins may cause the loss of nigrostriatal dopaminergic neurons.

In contrast to rotenone, the pesticide paraquat causes a remarkably reproducible loss of nigrostriatal dopaminergic neurons both in rats and in mice.[113-115] This loss, however, is limited to approximately 25–40% of nigrostriatal neurons based on stereological analyses of tyrosine-hydroxylase positive neuronal cell bodies in the substantia nigra pars compacta, with no or minimal loss of tyrosine-hydroxylase positive terminals and dopamine in the striatum, likely due to compensatory mechanisms. As a result of this modest neuronal loss, animals do not exhibit detectable behavioral deficits even when very sensitive tests are used.[114,115] Accordingly, this model is useful to explore mechanisms of dopaminergic cell death but not to assess symptomatic treatments. An additional use of paraquat has been to demonstrate increased vulnerability of dopaminergic neurons to the combined administrations of several environmental toxins. Specifically, animals exposed to the fungicide Maneb during development show an increase in neuronal loss after exposure to paraquat later in life,[116] although co-administration of both toxins does not have a synergistic effect.[113] Again, this model has been used primarily to explore neuropathological mechanisms rather than testing symptomatic therapies. Since the epidemiological evidence implicates paraquat and other environmental pesticides as risk factors in PD,[117] the paraquat-based models could provide useful tools also for testing potential neuroprotective therapies.

In addition to the toxins described above, local administration of the pro-inflammatory agent, lipopolysaccharide (LPS), in rats and mice has been used to induce nigrostriatal dopaminergic degeneration and to test the ability of anti-inflammatory agents to protect nigrostriatal neurons from inflammation-induced cell death.[118] Mention should be made also of toxin-induced dopaminergic cell loss in non-mammalian animal models, in particular the nematode worm and fruit-fly.[119-122] The use of these models in target identification is described below.

In summary, a number of neurotoxin models have been developed to induce dopaminergic neurodegeneration and Parkinsonism in rodents and non-human primates as well as model organisms. These models have been used to identify mechanisms by which the toxic agents cause dopamine cell loss *in vivo*.[102,123,124] Additionally, a number of genetic or pharmacological manipulations have shown neuroprotection in these models, latter often administered before the exposure.[125,126] Of these, the 6-OHDA rat model is commonly used to assess symptomatic efficacy and shows remarkable predictive validity.[v] On the other hand the MPTP, rotenone, paraquat and LPS models have been used to assess neuroprotective efficacy. The predictive validity of these toxin-induced animal models for neuroprotective efficacy remains questionable since it is unclear whether the mechanisms by which MPTP, paraquat and LPS cause cell death also operate in sporadic PD. This situation will be remedied only after the elucidation of the molecular etiology of dopamine neurodegeneration in sporadic PD. To this end, significant advances are being made as a result of identification of disease-causing mutations in several genes. The following sections summarize the emerging understanding of the etiopathology of PD, which has spurred new efforts in generation of genetic etiology-based animal models and their utility for development of novel therapeutic strategies for PD.

ETIOPATHOLOGY OF PD: GENETIC AND ENVIRONMENTAL FACTORS

PD is primarily a sporadic disease with a mean age of onset at 55 and a marked increase in incidence with aging thereafter. There are, however, exceptions to this common picture. Symptoms can appear earlier in life, sometimes before 50 years of age, which qualifies for "early onset PD." Furthermore, genetic inheritance plays a primary role in some rare familial forms of the disease. Only in the last decade, have there been extensive studies of the genetic etiology of PD, which have borne fruits. Until then, PD was not considered a genetic disorder. A significant contribution resulted from the tenacity of Roger Duvoisin in gathering DNA samples from a large Italian

---

[v] For further discussion of criteria of validity for models of behavioral disorders, please refer to Steckler *et al.*, Developing novel anxiolytics: Improving preclinical detection and clinical assessment; Joel *et al.*, Animal models of obsessive–compulsive disorder: From bench to bedside via endophenotypes and biomarkers, in Volume 1, Psychiatric Disorders; Lindner *et al.*, Development, optimization and use of preclinical behavioral models to maximize the productivity of drug discovery for Alzheimer's Disease in this volume; Koob, The role of animal models in reward deficit disorders: Views from academia; Markou *et al.*, Contribution of animal models and preclinical human studies to medication: Development for nicotine dependence, in Volume 3, Reward Deficits Disorders.

family, the Contursi kindred, which led to the identification of the first autosomal dominant PD-causing mutation, the A53T point mutation, in the *SNCA* gene encoding α-synuclein[127] Soon after, another point mutation, A30P, was found in different family.[128] More recently, an additional α-synuclein mutation, E46K, was discovered and importantly, duplications and triplications of the α-synuclein gene turned out to be sufficient to cause familial PD.[129-132]

The identification of mutations in α-synuclein was at the dawn of an incredibly fruitful era in PD research that continues to this day. Although point mutations in PD are exceedingly rare, their discovery led to the rapid identification of α-synuclein as a key pathological protein in sporadic PD. Soon after the publication of the Polymeropoulos paper,[127] Spillantini and colleagues published a short communication revealing that α-synuclein is a major component of the Lewy bodies.[133] These cytoplasmic inclusions are found in surviving nigrostriatal neurons, in many other neurons of the brain and peripheral nervous system, as well as the adrenal medulla.[10,134] The composition of the Lewy bodies had long eluded researchers and the presence of α-synuclein in these ubiquitinated inclusions immediately drew a connection between genetic and sporadic forms of the disease.

The rapidity of progress on understanding the pathophysiology of familial PD cases was related to a luck rarely encountered by human geneticists; α-synuclein had been identified previously as a vesicle-associated protein involved in song learning in birds and well characterized antibodies for this protein were already available.[135] Furthermore, a portion of α-synuclein protein had been identified as the non-amyloid component of amyloid plaques in Alzheimer's disease.[136] These tools and prior knowledge about the protein spurred a wealth of studies that soon established the ability of α-synuclein to form amyloid structures, and its toxicity *in vitro* as well as *in vivo* in *Drosophila*.[137,138] Furthermore, antibodies against α-synuclein led to the discovery of extensive α-synuclein pathology in PD brain and peripheral nervous system and to a new staging classification of the disease.[10] Finally, the finding of α-synuclein pathology in other neurodegenerative diseases that are distinct from PD led Trojanowski and colleagues to coin the term "synucleopathy," which linked PD with a host of different neurodegenerative illnesses that may share some common pathophysiological features.[139] Although the mechanistic contributions of α-synuclein to sporadic PD remain a matter of controversy, the discovery of PD-causing mutations in this protein, the major component of Lewy bodies, demonstrate the usefulness of the genetic approach in providing new clues for sporadic PD.

Soon after, mutations in a second gene, *parkin*, were identified as causative factors for recessive Parkinsonism. This discovery originally raised significant controversy because the family in which the first mutation was discovered presented with juvenile onset Parkinsonism that some neurologist were reluctant to call PD, especially because the brains of patients with *parkin* mutations did not contain Lewy bodies.[140] Skeptics, however, had to admit the role of *parkin* in PD pathophysiology when it became apparent that many different deletion and missense mutations in *parkin* gene cause familial forms of PD, and that these account for approximately 50% of early onset recessive Parkinsonism.[141,142] An important fallout of the discovery of mutations in parkin, an E3 ligase, is the implication that proteasomal dysfunction may play a role in PD. This hypothesis is strengthened by evidence from post-mortem human brain studies demonstrating decreases in proteasomal function in sporadic PD subjects.[143] A role for proteasomal dysfunction in PD is reinforced by the identification of mutations in the gene encoding an ubiquitin hydrolase, Ubiquitin C-terminal Hydrolase L-1 (UCHL-1) in two siblings with PD.[144,145] However, the lack of identification of additional families with UCHL-1 mutations has raised the question whether UCHL-1 mutations are pathogenic.

The next set of disease-causing mutations in familial forms of PD brought to the forefront a mechanism long suspected to cause sporadic PD: mitochondrial dysfunction. Mutations in PINK1 (PTEN-induced putative kinase-1), and DJ-1, two mitochondrial proteins whose physiologic functions have not been elucidated fully[146-149] cause recessive Parkinsonism, whose clinical presentation is similar to that caused by *parkin* mutations.

Although pointing to tantalizing putative mechanisms for neurodegeneration in PD, these mutations remain associated with unusual or very rare cases of PD, and some investigators continued to question their relevance for the vast majority of sporadic cases. This situation changed somewhat with the discovery of multiple missense mutations in a novel gene termed Leucine-rich Repeat Kinase 2 (LRRK2).[150,151] This gene encodes for a multi-domain protein that includes a kinase domain; however, the function and substrate for this kinase remain unclear. A case for LRRK2 in sporadic PD has been made because its mutations cause a disease that is indistinguishable from the common sporadic forms of PD, both clinically and, to some extent, pathologically.[152,153] Furthermore, mutations in LRRK2 are being detected in apparently sporadic, late onset cases of the disease.[154,155] Interestingly, one specific mutation, G2019S, shows high prevalence with frequencies ranging from >2% in the North American population to >10% in some isolated populations such as North African Arabs and Ashkenazi Jews.[155-157]

The list of PD-causing mutations is bound to increase since other PD-linked loci have been identified but the specific genes within these remain unknown. The very recent identification of a new potential disease-causing mutation in a lysosomal ATPase attests to this conjecture.[158] Researchers are taking advantage of these multiple genetic causes of PD to discover neuroprotective drugs. The allure of this approach should not make us forget that much remains to be learned from other risk factors for PD. Indeed, the role of genetic factors is not limited only to causal mutations that play a role in the rare familial forms of the disease. It is likely that many genetic risk factors are at play, although their contribution to late onset PD remains unclear.[159]

Genetic association studies can identify risk factors but are fraught with examples of lack of reproducibility of the results in multiple cohorts. This may be a sign of truly spurious results. Alternatively, it may indicate that the impact of genetic risk factors depends on other interactions with environmental conditions such as diet or other exposures. More extensive studies of gene and environment interactions are needed to resolve this issue (see below). A recent finding stands out because it has been reproduced in several independent studies so far. These studies have uncovered a higher prevalence of individuals who carry mutations known to cause Gaucher disease among patients with PD compared to controls.[160] Gaucher disease is a lysosomal storage disease caused by mutations in the gene encoding glucocerebrosidase. It is a recessive disease with heterozygous carriers appearing normal. In the most common form of the disease, Gaucher type 1, the onset in homozygous carriers of the mutation is in adulthood and the brain apparently is not affected. A few cases of Parkinsonism have been reported in Gaucher type 1 patients, but these are rare.[161,162] However, the Gaucher mutation is present in 10–30% of patients with PD, a marked increase compared to controls.[163] This association remains controversial, and it is not clear whether mechanisms triggered by the Gaucher mutation are involved in PD pathology. It is of interest, however, that recent work has implicated autophagy and age-related decrease in lysosomal function in PD.[164] Whether these findings will lead to new therapeutic approaches remains to be seen.

As indicated earlier, the impact of genetic risk factors could greatly depend on other conditions that may influence the risk of PD. Epidemiological studies have provided a strong case for environmental risk factors in PD. Since the seminal work of Andre Barbeau, it has been known that PD risk is higher in rural settings, especially in areas of industrialized agriculture and high pesticide use.[165,166] Specific agents have been implicated as PD risk factors, such as paraquat and maneb,[167] which has led to animal models of PD based on intoxication with these agents.[vi]

In summary, identification of etiopathological factors of PD such as genetic mutations in familial PD as well as genetic and environmental risk factors of sporadic PD offer a large range of possibilities to impact drug discovery. One immediate result of these breakthroughs can be seen in the generation genetic etiology-based cellular and animal models of the disease (see the following section), and for the discovery of new drug targets.[vii] Similarly, as discussed above, models of pesticide-induced dopaminergic toxicity have been used to assess mechanisms of dopamine neuronal degeneration or to assess neuroprotective activity. However, it should be stressed that the molecular etiology of sporadic PD remains to be elucidated. Hence, the relevance of these models to the pathophysiological mechanisms of sporadic forms of PD remains a matter of conjecture.

GENETIC ETIOLOGY-BASED MODELS; TRANSLATABILITY OF PHENOTYPES TO CLINICAL SYMPTOMS

Although toxin-based models of PD have been extremely useful for developing symptomatic treatments, both pharmacological and surgical, they suffer from two major limitations. First, as previously mentioned, the relevance of the mechanism of action of the toxins to PD etiopathology remains purely speculative. Second, they generally reproduce only the loss of nigrostriatal dopaminergic neurons, and not the broad pathology that characterizes PD.[10] The importance of this second limitation has been appreciated only recently. Patients, their care-takers and physicians have recognized that the spectrum of symptoms of PD goes beyond the motor deficits induced by the degeneration of the nigrostriatal dopamine pathway. The non-motor symptoms of PD include olfactory deficits, sleep disturbance, affective disorders (anxiety and

---

[vi] See above in the section discussing animal models that led to the discovery and development of currently available drugs for PD.

[vii] See below in the section discussing the use of animal models for target identification and validation.

depression), autonomic dysfunction and cognitive deficits. More importantly, these non-motor symptoms are generally resistant to levodopa and direct-acting dopamine receptor agonist treatments and represent a major unmet medical need. This is not surprising since pathological studies have revealed the existence of cell loss in extra-nigral regions of the brain, and the widespread presence of Lewy bodies in non-dopaminergic neurons.[10,168] These observations clearly point to a widespread systemic nature of PD pathophysiology, which is not recapitulated by toxin-based models. Hence, there is a critical need to develop and characterize animal models with better construct validity and also the ability to offer the means to test treatments for non-motor symptoms of PD.

Models based on Mendelian inheritance of disease-causing genetic mutations should, at least in part, alleviate some of these limitations. For one, broad expression of a PD-causing mutation in a mouse is likely to reproduce a broader range of symptoms/pathophysiology experienced by the patients carrying the same mutation. Second, a mouse expressing a disease-causing mutation is clearly a mechanistically relevant model to at least some form of the disease and hence has greater construct validity. Thus the molecular genetic studies have given rise to several transgenic mouse models of PD. There are two major classes of the genetic etiology-based mouse models of PD: those which over-express a transgene coding for a human mutant protein or those in which the mouse orthologue of the human gene was knocked out by homologous recombination. The former class of models has been generated for mutations which cause autosomal dominant PD and likely represent gain of function (e.g., α-synuclein transgenic mice). The second class represents loss of function mutations causing recessive PD (parkin, DJ-1 and PINK1 knockout mice).

Because mutations in α-synuclein were discovered first, mice over-expressing α-synuclein were the first to be generated and remain the most extensively studied to this day. Previous reviews provide a detailed description of the first generation of α-synuclein over-expressors.[169,170] Several points, however, need to be emphasized. Although it is often claimed that these models lack the pathological hallmark of PD (i.e., the loss of nigrostriatal dopaminergic neurons) one line of mice shows a progressive loss of tyrosine-hydroxylase positive neurons in the substantia nigra pars compacta starting at 9 months of age[171,172] as well as protesomal dysfunction upon aging.[173] This mouse expresses a double mutant α-synuclein under the tyrosine hydroxylase promoter. Thus, expression of PD-causing mutations of α-synuclein can reproduce the canonical loss of nigrostriatal dopaminergic neurons in mice. A limitation of this model, however, is that the promoter restricts expression of the mutation to catecholaminergic neurons, precluding the use of this mouse model to explore the extra-nigral PD pathology, except possibly in the locus coeruleus.

In contrast to mice expressing double-mutations in α-synuclein, mice expressing single mutant or the wild-type forms of the protein have not, so far, exhibited nigrostriatal cell loss.[115,169,174,175] An important *caveat*, however, is that few studies have been performed in aged mice. Experience from other mouse models of neurodegenerative diseases indicates that cell loss rarely occurs before 15–18 months of age.[176] Among the first reported lines of mice over-expressing human α-synuclein,[174] the line with the highest level of expression showed a decrease in tyrosine hydroxylase levels and tyrosine hydroxylase positive terminals in the striatum. Another line of mice has been reported to exhibit loss of dopamine in the striatum, although stereological analysis of dopaminergic cell bodies has not been reported. These mice express a truncated form of the protein, which may, like the double mutation, increase its pathogenicity.[177] An additional line of mice expressing a truncated form of α-synuclein exhibited a significant loss of nigrostriatal neurons, however, this deficit occurred early in development and did not mimic the progressive nature of PD.[178] Together, these data suggest that it may be necessary to increase the ability of α-synuclein to form pathogenic oligomers or fibrils to achieve nigrostriatal neuronal loss within the lifespan of a mouse. It is conceivable that in humans, environmental or aging factors contribute to the increased pathogenicity of wild-type forms of the protein.[179]

It is noteworthy also that different promoters lead to distinct sets of phenotypes in the α-synuclein transgenic mice. In particular, when expressed under the prion promoter, both wild type and mutant α-synuclein tend to cause cell death of motoneurons, a cell type not usually lost in PD.[180,181] Some lines using the Thy1 promoter have motoneuron pathology[182,183] while others do not.[175] The presence of spinal pathology, of course, precludes the study of PD-related behaviors but can be exploited to understand mechanisms of neuronal death caused by α-synuclein overexpression *in vivo*.

Since only few lines of mice have been reported to show a progressive loss of nigrostriatal terminals or cell bodies, the use of genetic mouse models of α-synuclein overexpression for neuroprotective studies has been limited. However, many lines exhibit behavioral deficits indicative of functional neuronal dysfunction.[170] This is a common observation in many rodent models of neurodegenerative diseases, and suggests that neuronal dysfunction may precede neuronal death in patients also. If true, this phenomenon could have significant implications for clinical trials of neuroprotective treatments in patients. This raises an interesting question: should one expect the behavioral deficits occurring in the absence of neurodegeneration in α-synuclein transgenic mice to be responsive to levodopa? Indeed symptoms that are due to neuronal dysfunction, but not associated with loss of dopamine neurons, may not be improved by dopaminergic agonists. On the contrary, as expected from observations that excess dopamine can be detrimental,[184] levodopa or dopaminergic agonists worsen symptoms in these mice.[185] Accordingly, the α-synuclein transgenic mice are not useful for developing or testing new symptomatic therapies, but could be useful to identify treatments that interfere with the initial pathological effects of the mutations that cause the neuronal dysfunction. To this end, early deficits in motor and non-motor behaviors in these mice provide useful measures for studies of neuroprotective agents. Indeed, another particularly novel use of these models is the exploration of extra-nigral pathology and symptoms. As indicated earlier, toxin-based models are not appropriate for this use since they only reproduce the loss of nigrostriatal dopaminergic neurons. In mice over-expressing α-synuclein under a broadly expressed promoter that does not cause motoneuron pathology (e.g., some of the lines using the Thy-1 promoter[175]), it should be possible to test the hypothesis that excess levels of α-synuclein in extra-nigral regions cause the non-motor symptoms of PD. This already has been achieved for olfactory dysfunction, a prevalent symptom of PD, which can often precede overt motor symptoms by many years.[186] Although these studies may not spur research in therapeutic drugs that may cure olfactory dysfunction, they strengthen the construct validity of the animal model. Additionally, olfactory dysfunction can be rigorously assessed non-invasively in the clinic,[187] and is being proposed as a biomarker of PD susceptibility. Therefore, it would be interesting to monitor olfaction in the α-synuclein mice during aging and assess correlations between olfactory deficits and other pathophysiologic outcomes in these mice. Preliminary data suggest that in addition to olfactory deficits, these mice show digestive and cardiovascular deficits, and increases in anxiety-related behaviors as they age.[viii] The extra-nigral, non-motor symptoms in this line of transgenic mice may be related to the high level of α-synuclein expression throughout the brain. Importantly, these mice show formation of proteinase K-resistant, α-synuclein immunoreactive aggregates in many regions, including the substantia nigra, locus coeruleus and olfactory bulb.[ix][115,175] Thus, it appears that in addition to the non-motor behavioral symptoms of PD, this model may be useful to understand the early pathophysiology induced by α-synuclein fibrillation or accumulation; however, it will not allow the assessment of neuroprotective therapies to prevent dopaminergic neurodegeneration.

In order to avoid the limitation of the lack of dopamine neuronal loss of most α-synuclein transgenic mouse lines (with the exception of that generated by Richfield and colleagues,[171] Kirik and colleagues generated a rat model using viral-mediated gene transduction of α-synuclein in the substantia nigra.[188] Unlike the genetically modified mouse models, the rat viral-mediated gene transfer model has significantly greater expression of human α-synuclein protein, which likely explains the death of nigral dopaminergic neurons and an accumulation of intraneuronal α-synuclein in these rats. Kirik and colleagues are pursuing currently the same method to generate a non-human primate model of α-synuclein pathophysiology, which would facilitate characterization of motor and non-motor behavioral symptoms and their correlation to neurochemical and histopathological abnormalities.

Mice deficient in *parkin*, DJ-1, or PINK1 have failed, so far, to reproduce the canonical loss of nigrostriatal dopaminergic neurons seen in PD. However, like the α-synuclein mice, some of these models show progressive behavioral anomalies, as well as biochemical and molecular changes that provide clues to possible pathogenic mechanisms of PD. For example, *parkin* knockout mice fail to show dopamine neuronal degeneration or extrapyramidal behavioral deficits[189,190] but appear to have a functional deficit in the nigrostriatal dopamine system.[191-193] In contrast to the null mutations, a recent study indicates that mice expressing the Q311X *parkin* mutation expressed using DAT-BAC do have nigral dopamine neuronal loss.[194] These data indicate that the pathophysiology of parkin mutations involves more complex mechanisms than the simple loss of function produced by knocking out the expression of the gene. Similarly, there are four distinct lines of DJ-1 knockout mice that have been characterized. Although none of these lines show nigral dopamine cell loss or α-synuclein-positive aggregates, they do show subtle locomotor deficits and alterations in dopamine neurotransmission, which are progressive in some cases.[195-198] On the other hand, a conditional RNAi-mediated silencing of PINK1 gene expression in a transgenic mouse model fails to show any PD-related phenotype.[199] This is in contrast to the *Drosophila* models in which knockout of the dPINK1 gene leads to dopamine neurodegeneration.[200]

---

viii Fleming and Chesselet, in preparation.
ix Hutson and Chesselet, in preparation.

A common feature of many genetically modified mouse lines was uncovered by studies assessing their sensitivity to the neurotoxin, MPTP. Thus overexpression of α-synuclein or loss of *parkin* and DJ-1 render the mice more susceptible to MPTP-induced nigrostriatal dopamine loss.[171,197,198] An important *caveat* of these results is that the DJ-1 mice show enhanced sensitivity to MPTP as a result of increases in DAT-mediated MPP^+ uptake whereas the α-synuclein and *parkin* mice may involve other mechanisms. Thus further studies of interactions between MPTP and *parkin* or MPTP and α-synuclein may shed light on the pathophysiology of the genetic etiological factors.

DIFFICULTIES IN PD RESEARCH

The discussion in the sections above may lead to the following major conclusions about the difficulties in PD research aimed at addressing the unmet medical need of PD patients:

a. A major unmet medical need is the lack of disease-modifying treatments of PD. The etiology and specific molecular mechanisms underlying the progressive pathology of sporadic PD of the disease remain unclear. This precludes the ability to generate animal models of PD pathophysiology that can enable evaluation of disease-modifying treatment or to identify druggable targets for disease-modifying therapy.

b. Although the neurotoxin-based animal models have been and will continue to be useful to develop symptomatic treatment strategies as well as those based on gene therapy and cell transplant, their predictive validity for assessment of disease-modifying therapies has come into question as a result of the failure of recent purportedly neuroprotective agents in clinical studies (see below).

c. The new genetic models provide an opportunity to identify or validate novel targets for PD or test novel drug candidate. However, their predictive validity for sporadic PD patient outcomes remains unknown. So far, only one direct link exists between mutations in a gene (α-synuclein) whose product is associated with a hallmark pathology (Lewy bodies) of PD.[10] However, it is still unclear whether aggregates of this protein are causative, protective or a mere epiphenomenon. For the other known mutations, a link with sporadic PD is only suggested by shared mechanisms between the effects of the mutation and pathological features of sporadic PD such as proteasomal or mitochondrial dysfunction.[123,201]

d. The pathology of PD is much more widespread and includes both peripheral and central neuraxis beyond the nigrostriatal dopamine system. Likely as a result, the current symptomatic therapies which augment dopaminergic neurotransmission do not adequately control non-dopamine-related symptoms. Animal models based on selective loss of dopamine neurons are not useful for studies of these so-called non-dopa responsive symptoms. Thus new animal models need to be characterized, as is being done for an α-synuclein transgenic mouse line[170] to assess their utility for the non-motor symptoms of PD.

Clinical development of drugs that may slow the progression of PD is hampered by lack of objective, validated biomarkers of disease progression.

The following section provides an overview of how animal models may be developed or used to address the difficulties listed above and facilitate discovery and development of new drugs.

UTILITY OF ANIMAL MODELS IN THE PROCESS OF DRUG DISCOVERY AND DEVELOPMENT

The probability of technical success for a new therapeutic agent aimed to address the unmet medical need for PD patients is linked critically to decisions driven on the basis of data from animal models employed throughout its discovery and development. Specifically, key decisions that can impact the probability of successfully developing a drug could be classified into the following four major categories: animal models used for (a) target identification and/or validation, (b) understanding target-specific pharmacology of the drug candidate, (c) assessment of efficacy predictive of clinical benefit and (d) discovery of a clinically translatable biomarker(s) to help set the dose range and/or assess efficacy in human clinical trials. It is noteworthy that for PD, a vast majority of the investigational agents and drugs currently in clinical practice listed in Table 5.1 used the 6-OHDA and MPTP mouse/monkey models to demonstrate efficacy of clinical relevance to PD patients. As discussed earlier, this is not surprising for the approved drugs since they primarily provide palliative treatment, for which the toxin-based models have served well to reproduce extrapyramidal motor deficits associated with loss of dopamine neurons. However, at issue is that these models continue to be the center piece of evaluation of disease-modifying efficacy of new investigational drugs as well as palliative treatment targeting non-dopaminergic mechanisms. The shortcoming of this approach is exemplified by the failure of three recent clinical trials to demonstrate efficacy of purportedly disease-modifying drugs that had demonstrated robust neuroprotective and/or neurorestorative efficacy in the MPTP and 6-OHDA models. Thus in randomized, controlled trials, the GAPDH inhibitor, TCH346,[202] the mixed lineage kinase inhibitor, CEP-1347,[203] and the neurotrophic factor, GDNF[204] did not show clinical benefit. The lack of clinical efficacy of the two putative anti-apoptotic compounds, TCH346 and CEP-1347, was unexpected in light of data showing significant dose-dependent neuroprotection in the mouse as well as monkey MPTP models and the rat 6-OHDA model.[205-207] These trial results have brought into question the animal models used to predict efficacious dose range and the predictive validity of these animal models for disease-modifying efficacy in the clinic. In contrast to CEP-1347 and TCH346, the failure of GDNF reported in the Lang and colleagues[204] trial followed robust evidence of efficacy in not only animal models,[208-211] but also the successful demonstration of efficacy in small, open label clinical trials.[212,213] This has led to questions about whether appropriate testing of the GDNF delivery system was performed in animal models to assure adequate exposure to the neurotrophic factor[214] prior to commencing the randomized trial reported by Lang and colleagues.[204]

The following section is aimed to provide a perspective on how new animal models need to be developed and/or characterized in order to discover and develop disease-modifying drugs for PD.

USE OF ANIMAL MODELS FOR TARGET IDENTIFICATION AND VALIDATION

As discussed above, the etiology of sporadic PD and specifically the mechanism underlying progressive cell death of dopaminergic neurons remain unclear. However, recent molecular genetic studies of PD provide conclusive evidence that Mendelian inheritance of mutations in genes encoding α-synuclein, *parkin*, DJ-1, PINK1, LRRK2 and ATP13A2, lead to rare, heritable PD (cf.,[215]). The identification of causative mutations provided the impetus to generate transgenic animal models for each genetic etiological factor in a number of species, including the fruit-fly (*Drosophila melanogaster*), nematode (*Caenorhabditis elegans*), and a number of mouse lines, as well as the rat and monkey models via viral-mediated gene transfer (as reviewed above). Together, these animal models provide a key resource to gain insights into the mechanisms of PD pathology, physiological and pharmacological functions of the genes responsible for familial PD as well as model systems to study interactions between environmental and genetic risk factors of the disease. Such insights, in turn, would drive identification and validation of new drug targets for PD. In particular, the animal models have the potential to uncover a convergent biochemical pathway(s) engaged by the various genetic and/or environmental risk factors that lead to PD pathology. Identification of such a pathway is a pre-requisite for the discovery of a potential disease-modifying therapy. Indeed, this is illustrated in the current, investigational therapeutic approaches for Alzheimer's disease. In Alzheimer's disease, dominant mutations in genes encoding three distinct proteins, the amyloid precursor protein, presenilin 1 and presenilin 2, appear to affect the production of the amyloid β peptide, $A\beta_{42}$, which is the primary component of the hallmark, extracellular plaque pathology in this disease. This convergence among genetic etiologic factors onto a key pathological player for the disease paved the way for identification of druggable targets in the amyloid precursor protein processing pathway. Thus β- and γ-secretase enzymes, which produce $A\beta_{42}$ through sequential processing of the amyloid precursor protein, represent major drug discovery targets for Alzheimer's disease; of course, their ultimate validity will have to await demonstration of efficacy in clinical studies.[x] For the PD-associated genetic etiology factors, such as convergent biochemical pathway has yet to emerge. However, it is noteworthy that studies of recessive, loss of function mutants in the model organism, *D. melanogaster*, have begun to provide promising clues suggesting that parkin, DJ-1 and PINK1 may function in a single or a discrete set of biochemical pathways. Thus loss of function mutations of PINK1 and parkin in *Drosophila* show similar phenotypes, and parkin can rescue the loss of *Drosophila* PINK1, suggesting that PINK1

---

[x] Please refer to Lindner *et al.*, Development, optimization and use of preclinical behavioral models to maximize the productivity of drug discovery for Alzheimer's disease in this volume for further discussion of the use of animal models for target identification and validation in Alzheimer's disease.

acts upstream of parkin in a common biochemical pathway[216,217] Similarly, PINK1 and DJ-1 knock-out flies show fertility defects and DJ-1 is known to suppress a regulator of PINK-1, Phosphatase and tensin homologue 1 (PTEN), further supporting the convergence on to a molecular pathway. The application of these findings to a vertebrate model has been hindered by the relatively mild phenotypes of the loss of function mutants in the mouse. Specifically, as discussed earlier the mouse knock-out models of parkin, DJ-1 or PINK1 do not show dopamine cell loss in the substantia nigra. However, these mice do show deficits in neuronal function and synaptic architecture. Together, these data raise the question whether different, though clinically relevant; phenotypes should be considered as evidence of pathological role of PD-linked recessive mutations in the mouse models. Indeed, for the dominant PD-linked gene, α-synuclein, studies of neuronal dysfunction and sensitive fine motor behavioral measures provide evidence of Parkinsonism in the presence[171,172] or absence of overt nigral dopaminergic cell loss[175,185] as detailed in the section above. Thus both vertebrate and invertebrate models of PD genetic etiological factors offer tools for identification and validation of novel drug targets.

To this end, the ease and efficiency of application of genetic modifier screens in model organisms such as *D. melanogaster*, *C. elegans* or yeast provide a powerful approach to identify biochemical pathways engaged by the genetic etiological factors of the disease. A successful example of such a strategy assessing pathological role of a single disease-linked gene, α-synuclein, can be seen in a recently published study by Cooper and colleagues who demonstrated that α-synuclein overexpression affects ER-to-Golgi trafficking, which can be rescued by the GTPase, Rab1.[218] A major strength of this paper was their use of multiple model organisms (yeast, fruit-fly and nematode) to confirm the findings, and thereby enhance the confidence in the relevance of the identified pathway in the disease pathophysiology. The ease of genetic manipulation in some model organisms such as the nematode offers the ability to perform studies on interactions between genes or genetic and environmental risk factors. This approach will be useful to determine whether the PD-linked dominant and recessive genes interact and converge onto a single biochemical pathway. Indeed, evidence of interactions between α-synuclein and parkin is implied in a recent *C. elegans* study where the pathology of a deletion mutant of the parkin orthologue, *pdr-1*, was exaggerated by expression of human mutant α-synuclein.[219] Similarly, PD-associated environmental toxins such as MPTP (or MPP$^+$) or rotenone induce greater toxicity in vertebrate and invertebrate animal models of PD.[220] These data have strengthened the hypothesis that sporadic PD results from an interaction between environmental toxicants, including pesticides, herbicides, neurochemicals and heavy metals and genetic susceptibility factors. An obvious next step is to perform genetic suppressor screens for the toxicity or neurodegeneration phenotype in a model organism to identify potential druggable targets in an unbiased way. Similarly, a compound screen may be performed to identify pharmacological modifiers of the toxicity followed by genetic modifier screens to identify the molecular target of the toxicity-modifying pharmacological agent. It is critical to understand that model organisms offer the first step in target identification. As alluded to above, it would be imperative to confirm the findings across multiple non-mammalian model systems but ultimately into a mammalian model such as a transgenic mouse or viral-mediated gene transduction in a rat or non-human primate species. This is required since, in some instances, a model organism may not express an orthologue of a disease-associated gene, raising concerns about the validity of assessing pathological role of a protein in an organism that does not express the specific protein normally. Thus studies of α-synuclein in yeast and *C. elegans* have come under criticism by some investigators since these organisms do not appear to have an α-synuclein orthologue.

A complementary approach to target identification using model organisms via genetic/pharmacological screening described above is to perform transcript and/or proteome profiling on genetically engineered models of PD.[221] This approach is particularly powerful if the transcriptome and proteome are profiled in multiple transgenic models at various time points during the progressive, age-related pathology in order to elucidate biochemical pathways triggering and/or responding to the pathology. Such unbiased approaches applied to animal models as well as post-mortem brain tissues from PD patients would complement the findings from the genetic screens to help elucidate physiological and pathological roles of a disease gene. Clearly, data from sporadic PD cases are critical to establish whether an overlap exists in etiopathological pathways identified from genetic etiology-based animal models and sporadic cases of PD.

ANIMAL MODELS TO DEVELOP A CLINICALLY TRANSLATABLE UNDERSTANDING OF PHARMACOKINETIC-PHARMACODYNAMIC RELATIONSHIPS

A major challenge in CNS drug development is related to selection of doses to assess efficacy in patients. Since brain is protected via the blood brain barrier, which regulates the entry of molecules via both active and passive processes, the estimation of an active dosage of a drug candidate in the brain tissue in human clinical trials is a non-trivial challenge. A standard approach has been to employ animal models of efficacy to derive plasma exposures associated with efficacy of a drug and then target to achieve a similar plasma exposure in human clinical trials. Indeed, the clinical trials of both TCH346 and CEP-1347 set human clinical doses on the basis of plasma exposures in animal models.[202,203] Of course, a thorough understanding of the pharmacokinetic profile of the drug candidate in animal models is conducted to generate a model prior to prediction of human clinical doses, which may be refined further following Phase I clinical studies. Despite this, the question of whether adequate doses of each drug were tested in the clinical trials that failed to show efficacy is never satisfactorily answered. This is because extrapolation of pharmacokinetic data provides no information on whether the drug was pharmacologically active. In other words, simply achieving a target exposure does not guarantee that the desired quality and quantity of a pharmacodynamic response was achieved in human subjects. This is because pharmacodynamic responses may be affected by physiological regulatory processes. Hence, the use of an appropriate pharmacodynamic response into an exposure–activity relationship model removes any ambiguity due to species differences, or other state-dependent (e.g., disease-related) factors and in turn, allows greater certainty in predicting active doses of a drug. A pharmacodynamic measure most proximal to the molecular target of the new drug molecule is likely to provide the most accurate prediction. Of course, the inaccessibility of brain tissue in clinical trials necessitates assessment of the pharmacodynamic measure in the CSF, plasma or urine from human studies. However, this will require that an understanding of the relationship between brain target occupancy by the drug candidate with the pharmacodynamic end-point in the accessible fluid be established in animal models prior to performing clinical studies. For certain targets, a proximal pharmacodynamic marker may not be intuitively identified. In this case, mass spectrometry or NMR-based unbiased proteomic and metabolomic approaches may be used early on in the drug discovery paradigm to identify the appropriate end-point for a drug. If such a measure was identified and found altered even in the peripheral fluid compartments (plasma or urine) in either the TCH346 or CEP-1347 trials, the trial results would have provided much more definitive lessons and conclusions that could be applied to future therapeutic strategies for PD progression.[xi]

ANIMAL MODELS FOR ASSESSMENT OF EFFICACY PREDICTIVE OF CLINICAL BENEFIT

The quest for animal models with high predictive validity is, of course, the holy grail of all drug discovery and development efforts and the most critical decision point that could reduce/mitigate the risk of clinical failures. The selection of an animal model in a drug discovery paradigm is based typically on the intended clinical use of the drug; that is, the aspect of the disease the drug is intended to treat. The main focus of therapeutic approaches for PD has been extrapyramidal motor deficits, even though there has been a recent surge in the recognition of other, non-motor symptomatology of PD such as dementia, depression, anxiety, constipation, etc. Thus PD therapeutic strategies, to date, have been aimed at: (a) palliative treatment of symptoms of dopamine dysfunction (i.e., Parkinsonism), (b) restoration of dopamine neuronal function via neurotrophic approaches and (c) neuroprotective therapies to halt the progressive loss of dopamine neurons. Interestingly, currently marketed drugs as well as major investigational approaches across the three categories listed above have relied primarily on demonstration of efficacy in animal models of neurotoxin (6-OHDA or MPTP)-induced loss of the dopaminergic pathways as shown in Table 5.1. A study of this table leads to the following major conclusions: (i) the successful clinical development of dopamine agonists (levodopa-based therapies, dopamine receptor agonists, and inhibitors of dopamine catabolism) for palliative treatment of PD on the basis of 6-OHDA and/or MPTP model indicates that the predictive validity of these models is high for the efficacy of newer, non-dopaminergic therapies aimed at treatment of the motor symptoms of PD; (ii) the 6-OHDA lesion models have been useful also for assessment of

---

[xi] Please refer to Cryan *et al.*, Developing more efficacious antidepressant medications: Improving and aligning preclinical detection and clinical assessment tools; Large *et al.*, Developing therapeutics for bipolar disorder: From animal models to the clinic, in Volume 1, Psychiatric Disorders; and Markou *et al.*, Contribution of animal models and preclinical human studies to medication development for nicotine dependence, in Volume 3, Reward Deficit Disorders, for further discussion on pharmacokinetic-pharmacodynamic relationships and drug response.

neurorestorative therapies (e.g., trophic factor administration); whether these agents intervene to halt the mechanism underlying disease progression remains to be determined; (iii) on the other hand, the recent clinical failure of CEP-1347 and TCH346 raises into question the value and predictive validity of the 6-OHDA and MPTP models for neuroprotective therapies, which by definition should interfere with the molecular mechanism associated progressive loss of dopamine. This is not surprising considering that both models suffer from several major limitations for application to neuroprotective therapeutic approaches as discussed above in the section discussing the etiopathology of PD. More importantly, although these models have reasonably good face validity, it is unclear whether the biochemical mechanisms underlying the dopaminergic toxicity induced by these toxins and treatment paradigms is the same as those leading to progressive dopamine cell death in idiopathic PD.[xii] Hence, further research is required to elucidate the pathways and biochemical processes associated with dopamine cell loss and/or Lewy body pathology in PD patients and animal models in order to determine the predictive validity of PD models for neuroprotective therapy.

As discussed above, the use of genetic etiology-based animal models coupled with studies of post-mortem brain tissue from PD patients will likely aid elucidation of these pathways. Animal models based on dysfunction of these pathways are likely to have greater predictive validity. In the mean time, the recent availability and detailed characterization of the α-synuclein transgenic mouse, rat and primate models (discussed above), provide an opportunity for assessment of CEP1347, TCH346 and other putative neuroprotective agents under development in these genetic etiology-based models. Evidence of efficacy of the clinically tested agents, CEP1347 and TCH346, in one of these models may strengthen the validation of the molecular targets of these drugs, while simultaneously raising issues regarding adequacy of clinically tested doses or species differences.[xiii] On the other hand, the lack of efficacy of these compounds in α-synuclein animal models would be consistent with the clinical findings and strengthen the rationale to use these models for other neuroprotective therapies. Since there are few clinical studies in PD whose results could be used opportunistically to test the validity of the animal models, it is imperative that CEP1347 and TCH346 be tested in the newer genetic etiology-based models to advance the field. Clearly, establishment of the validity of an animal model is an iterative process that

---

[xii] The authors allude to an important issue regarding the practice of validating a putative model of behavioral disorders by the response produced by a clinically active drug, or pharmacological isomorphism. The amelioration of abnormal behaviors present in the animal model by clinically effective drugs is an important, but not necessarily sufficient criterion for the establishment of the predictive validity of a particular model of a disorder as novel candidate drugs acting through different biochemical mechanisms of action than the clinically effective drug may be missed. Please refer to Steckler *et al.*, Developing novel anxiolytics: Improving preclinical detection and clinical assessment; Joel *et al.*, Animal models of obsessive–compulsive disorder: From bench to bedside via endophenotypes and biomarkers; Large *et al.*, Developing therapeutics for bipolar disorder: From animal models to the clinic, in Volume 1, Psychiatric Disorders; Lindner *et al.*, Development, optimization and use of preclinical behavioral models to maximize the productivity of drug discovery for Alzheimer's disease for further discussion of the strengths and limitations of pharmacological isomorphism in establishing model validity.

[xiii] See also Markou *et al.*, Contribution of animal models and preclinical human studies to medication: Development for nicotine dependence, in Volume 3, Reward Deficit Disorders.

integrates findings from basic science breakthroughs in genetics, biochemistry and pathophysiology of a disease to results of clinical trials of new therapeutic agents.

The genetic etiology-based models also provide an opportunity to assess non-motor, non-dopa responsive symptoms of PD since their amelioration remains a major unmet medical need. However, few researchers[170] focus their efforts at characterizing non-extrapyramidal behavioral and biochemical effects in the mouse models.

ANIMAL MODELS FOR DISCOVERY OF CLINICALLY TRANSLATABLE BIOMARKERS TO HELP SET THE DOSE RANGE AND ASSESS EFFICACY IN HUMAN CLINICAL TRIALS

From the discussion above, it should be apparent that for disease-modifying therapeutic approaches for PD, the available animal models have significant limitations. However, the critical need to address unmet medical need for PD mandates that a certain amount of known risk be taken to develop novel therapies for this debilitating disorder. One strategy to reduce the risk of failure in large, resource-intensive clinical trials of efficacy on disease progression is to discover and employ biomarkers that could provide objective data, based on which strategic go/no go decisions may be driven during the phase of early clinical trials. One of the key hurdles of translatability of results from animal models to the clinical setting is establishing and demonstrating the adequacy of the dose(s) of the drug candidate. To be specific, if the drug is thought to mediate its effects via a molecular target in the brain, it may not be sufficient to match the plasma drug concentration in human studies to that seen in animal models. An important consideration is whether the pharmacological agent is accessible to the intended target in the brain at sufficient concentrations and optimal duration to engage its proposed mechanism of action at clinically tolerated doses. Thus biomarkers of drug activity that can provide evidence of dose adequacy need to be discovered early on in appropriate animal models. A common example for such an application is determination of target occupancy by radioreceptor ligand imaging (PET or SPECT). This has been applied frequently to cell surface receptor targets, primarily G-protein coupled receptors. The first step in the translational approach is to establish drug target occupancy at doses that show efficacy in an animal model followed by the use of PET or SPECT imaging in human studies to set doses/dosing frequency on the basis of the dynamics of target occupancy. Indeed, in studies of selegiline, PET imaging demonstrated the irreversible nature of MAO inhibition by this drug, which led to a better understanding of the pharmacodynamic activity of this drug. Although powerful, target occupancy assessment is not always feasible since development of a selective and specific radiotracer poses many challenges, the severity of which is distinct for each target. An alternative approach is to identify a proximal biochemical marker in a clinically accessible tissue that reflects the engagement of the proposed mechanism of action of the therapeutic agent. It is noteworthy that this approach is much more powerful if the pharmacodynamic measure is also in the disease progression pathway. In this case, the pharmacodynamic measure offers the potential to be a surrogate biomarker of disease progression and modification. An example of such a marker may be CSF $A\beta_{42}$ levels for both β- and γ-secretase inhibitors. Similarly, for anti-inflammatory drugs such as COX inhibitors, levels of inflammatory prostaglandins (e.g., PGE2) in the CSF and/or plasma may provide the proximal pharmacological marker, whereas cytokine levels may provide a disease pathology-related marker with the potential to be a surrogate marker for clinical use. Needless to say, an understanding of the biochemical pathway of the molecular target engaged by an drug candidate in an animal model as well as the biochemical pathways associated with disease progression is required to identify pharmacodynamic measures of drug pharmacology as well as disease modification. For the latter, recent advances in proteomic and metabolomic technologies offer an opportunity to use unbiased biomarker discovery approaches on clinically accessible fluids, blood, urine and CSF. One barrier to this approach is the limited volume of CSF in rodents, especially the mouse, and the inability to sample the CSF serially from the same rodent.

In addition to discovery of biomarkers on the basis of pharmacodynamic or disease pathology-related response in animal models, appropriate models also offer the means to validate biomarkers used clinically. For example, the loss of dopaminergic neurons is monitored in the clinic by PET or SPECT imaging using ligands that reflect the functional integrity of the dopaminergic pathway. As discussed above, the most commonly used ligands target the dopamine transporter (e.g., $[^{123}I]\beta$CIT SPECT), an enzyme in the dopamine synthetic pathway, L aromatic acid decarboxylase (e.g., $[^{18}F]$fluorodopa PET) or the vesicular monoamine transporter, VMAT2 (e.g., $[^{11}C]$dihyrotetrabenazine PET). However, recent studies with dopaminergic therapies have raised questions regarding the validity of these imaging markers for dopamine neuronal integrity since some of the dopaminergic therapies may regulate the expression and/or function of the proteins targeted by the radiotracers (cf.,[44]). With the advent of microPET and SPECT technologies, it appears that the potential for the pharmacological regulation of the dopaminergic system by an investigative therapy may be studied in animal models using clinically applied radiotracers. These studies will help uncover potential confounds of the imaging markers to provide evidence of disease modification in clinical trials. Additionally, animal models provide the ability to characterize thoroughly alterations in a specific dopaminergic function monitored by a given imaging biomarker. Thus a recent study by Stephenson and colleagues demonstrates that presynaptic markers of the nigrostriatal dopaminergic neurons respond differentially to MPTP-induced toxicity as well as levodopa treatment following the intoxication, likely due to different compensatory changes in each marker.[223] Thus these data have direct implications for the selection of an imaging marker to monitor dopaminergic function in PD patients.

CONCLUDING REMARKS

PD therapeutic development is at a critical juncture to address key unmet medical needs by taking advantage of genetic breakthroughs, deeper understanding of the pathophysiology of the disease and clinical experience with new classes of putative disease-modifying agents. Specifically, recent research has presented unprecedented opportunities to develop and characterize animal models based on genetic etiology that could help identify and/or validate novel targets. Indeed a link exists between some familial PD mutations and disease pathology in humans. Commonality of mechanisms involved in mutation-induced disease and sporadic disease can be inferred from observations in post-mortem brains or peripheral cells from patients. For example, α-synuclein accumulates in the brain of patients with sporadic PD just as it accumulates in the brain of patients with α-synuclein mutations or gene multiplication.[10,131] Several mutations affect proteasomal function, which is also decreased in post-mortem brain of patients with PD.[141] Finally, several mutations occur in proteins related to the mitochondria and evidence of mitochondrial dysfunction has been obtained in PD.[198] Accordingly, one may hypothesize that identifying disease pathways in the genetic etiology-based animal models will lead to drug targets for the treatment of sporadic PD. The validity of this approach, however, can only be confirmed once a successful disease-modifying treatment has been developed for the disease. In the meantime, it is pragmatic to assume that the newly generated genetic models are also likely to possess greater predictive validity than the previous generation of toxin-based models for the clinical translatability of efficacy of new drug candidates.

REFERENCES

1. Dorsey, E.R., Constantinescu, R., Thompson, J.P., Biglan, K.M., Holloway, R.G., Kieburtz, K., Marshall, F.J., Ravina, B.M., Schifitto, G., Siderowf, A., and Tanner, C.M. (2007). Projected number of people with Parkinson disease in the most populous nations, 2005 through 2030. *Neurology*, 68:384–386.
2. Parkinson, J. (1817). *An Essay on the Shaking Palsy*. Neely and Jones, London, Sherwood.
3. Jankovic, J. (1992). Pathophysiology and clinical assessment of motor symptoms in Parkinson's disease. In Pahwa, R., Lyons, K., and Koller, W.C. (eds.), *Handbook of Parkinson's Disease*. Marcel Dekker, New York, pp. 129–158.
4. Zetusky, W.J., Jankovic, J., and Pirozzolo, F.J. (1985). The heterogeneity of Parkinson's disease: Clinical and prognostic implications. *Neurology*, 35:522–526.
5. Jankovic, J., McDermott, M., and Carter, J. (1990). Variable expression of Parkinson's disease: A base-line analysis of the DATATOP cohort. *Neurology*, 41:1529–1534.
6. Adler, C.H. (2005). Nonmotor complications in Parkinson's disease. *Mov Disord*, 20: S23–S29.
7. Hoehn, M. and Yahr, M. (1967). Parkinsonism: Onset, progression and mortality. *Neurology*, 17:427–442.
8. Gonera, E.G., van't, Hof M., Berger, H.J., van, Weel.C., and Horstink, M.W. (1997). Symptoms and duration of the prodromal phase in Parkinson's disease. *Mov Disord*, 12:871–876.
9. Montgomery, E.B., Lyons, K., and Koller, W.C. (2000). Early detection of probable idiopathic Parkinson's disease: II. A prospective application of a diagnostic test battery. *Mov Disord*, 15:474–478.
10. Braak, H., Del Tredici, K., Rüb, U., de Vos, R.A.I., Jansen Steur, E.N.H., and Braak, E. (2003). Staging of brain pathology related to sporadic Parkinson's disease. *Neurobiol Aging*, 24:197–211.
11. Hughes, A.J., Daniel, S.E., Kilford, L., and Lees, A.J. (1992). Accuracy of clinical diagnosis of idiopathic Parkinson's disease: A clinco-pathological study of 100 cases. *J Neuro Neurosurg Psychiatr*, 55:181–184.
12. Gelb, D.J., Oliver, E., and Gilman, S. (1999). Diagnostic criteria for Parkinson's disease. *Arch Neurol*, 56:33–39.

13. Jankovic, J., Rajput, A.H., McDermott, M., and Perl, D.P. (2000). The evolution of diagnosis in early Parkinson's disease. *Arch Neurol*, 57:369-372.

14. Hughes, A.J., Daniel, S.E., Ben-Shlomo, Y., and Lees, A.J. (2002). The accuracy of diagnosis of parkinsonian syndromes in a specialist movement disorder service. *Brain*, 125:861-870.

15. Morrish, P.K., Sawle, G.V., and Brooks, D.J. (1996). An [18F]dopa-PET and clinical study of the rate of progression in Parkinson's disease. *Brain*, 119:558-591.

16. Hilker, R., Schweitzer, K., Coburger, S., Ghaemi, M., Weisenbach, S., Jacobs, A.H., Rudolf, J., Herholz, K., and Heiss, W.D. (2005). Nonlinear progression of Parkinson's disease as determined by serial PET imaging of striatal [18F]fluorodopa activity. *Arch Neurol*, 62:378-382.

17. Marek, K., Innis, R., van Dyck, C., Fussell, B., Early, M., Eberly, S., Oakes, D., and Seibyl, J. (2001). [123I]β-CIT SPECT imaging assessment of the rate of Parkinson's disease progression. *Neurology*, 57:2089-2094.

18. Parkinson Study Group (2002). Dopamine transporter brain imaging to assess the effects of pramipexole vs levodopa on Parkinson's disease progression. *J Am Med Assoc*, 287:1653-1661.

19. Suchowersky, O., Gronseth, G., Perlmutter, J., Reich, S., Zesiewicz, T., and Weiner, W.J. (2006). Practice parameter: Neuroprotective strategies and alternative therapies for Parkinson's disease (an evidence-based review). *Neurology*, 66:976-982.

20. Fahn, S. (2006) Medical treatment of Parkinson's disease. In syllabus of the 16th annual course of a comprehensive review of movement disorders for the clinical practitioners, Edited by Fahn, S., Jankovic, J., Hallett, M., Jenner, P.G., 113-215.

21. Cotzias, G.C., Papavasiliou, P.S., and Gellene, R. (1969). Modification of parkinsonism chronic treatment with L dopa. *N Engl J Med*, 280:337-345.

22. Chase, T.N. (1998). Levodopa therapy: Consequences of the nonphysiologic replacement of dopamine. *Neurology*, 50:S17-S25.

23. Olanow, C.W., Agid, Y., Mizuno, Y., Albanese, A., Bonuccelli, U., Damier, P., De Yebenes, J., Gershanik, O., Guttman, M., Grandas, F., Hallett, M., Hornykiewicz, O., Jenner, P., Katzenschlager, R., Langston, W.J., LeWitt, P., Melamed, E., Mena, M.A., Michel, P.P., Mytilineou, C., Obeso, J.A., Poewe, W., Quinn, N., Raisman-Vozari, R., Rajput, A.H., Rascol, O., Sampaio, C., and Stocchi, F. (2004). Levodopa in the treatment of Parkinson's disease: Current controversies. *Mov Disord*, 19:997-1005.

24. Deep Brain Stimulation for Parkinson's Disease Study Group (2001). Deep brain Stimulation of the subthalamic nucleus or the pars interna of the globus pallidus in Parkinson's disease. *N Engl J Med*, 345:956-963.

25. Deuschl, G., Schade-Brittinger, C., Krack, P., Volkmann, J., Schäfer, H., Bötzel, K., Daniels, C., Deutschländer, A., Dillmann, U., Eisner, W., Gruber, D., Hamel, W., Herzog, J., Hilker, R., Klebe, S., Kloß, M., Koy, J., Krause, M., Kupsch, A., Lorenz, D., Lorenzl, S., Mehdorn, H.M., Moringlane, J.R., Oertel, W., Pinsker, M.O., Reichmann, H., Reuß, A., Schneider, G.H., Schnitzler, A., Steude, U., Sturm, V., Timmermann, L., Tronnier, V., Trottenberg, T., Wojtecki, L., Wolf, E., Poewe, W., Voges, J., for the German Parkinson Study Group (2006) Neurostimulation Section. A randomized trial of deep-brain stimulation for Parkinson's disease. N Engl J Med, 355: 896-908.

26. Nutt, J.G. (2007). Continuous dopaminergic stimulation: Is it the answer to the motor complications of levodopa. *Mov Disord*, 22:1-9.

27. Michel, P.P. and Hefti, F. (1990). Toxicity of 6-hydroxydopamine and dopamine for dopaminergic neurons in cultures. *J Neurosci Res*, 26:428-435.

28. Mytilineou, C., Han, S.K., and Cohen, G. (1993). Toxic and protective effects of L-dopa on mesencephalic cell cultures. *J Neurochem*, 61:1470-1478.

29. Mena, M.A., Davila, V., and Sulzer, D. (1997). Neurotrophic effects of L-DOPA in postnatal midbrain dopamine neuron/cortical astrocyte cocultures. *J Neurochem*, 69:1398-1408.

30. Murer, M.G., Dziewczapolski, G., Menalled, L.B., Garcia, M.C., Agid, Y., Gershanik, O., and Raisman-Vozari, R. (1998). Chronic levodopa is not toxic for remaining dopamine neurons, but instead promotes their recovery, in rats with moderate nigrostriatal lesions. *Ann Neurol*, 43:561–575.

31. Whone, A.L., Watts, R.L., Stoessl, A.J., Davis, M., Reske, S., Nahmias, C., Lang, A.E., Rascol, O., Ribeiro, M.J., Remy, P., Poewe, W.H., Hauser, R.A., and Brooks, D.J. (2003). REAL-PET Study Group. Slower progression of Parkinson's disease with ropinirole versus levodopa: The REAL-PET study. *Ann Neurol*, 54:93–101.

32. Fahn, S., Oakes, D., Shoulson, I., Kieburtz, K., Rudolph, A., Lang, A., Olanow, C.W., Tanner, C., and Marek, K. (2004). Parkinson Study Group. Levodopa and the progression of Parkinson's disease. *N Engl J Med*, 351:2498–2508.

33. Pahwa, R., Factor, S.A., Lyons, K.E., Ondo, W.G., Gronseth, G., Bronte-Stewart, H., Hallett, M., Miyasaki, J., Stevens, J., and Weiner, W.J. (2006). Practice parameter: Treatment of Parkinson's disease with motor fluctuations and dyskinesia (an evidence-based review). *Neurology*, 66:983–995.

34. Horstink, M., Tolosa, E., Bonuccelli, U., Deuschl, G., Friedman, A., Kanovsky, P., Larsen, J.P., Lees, A., Oertel, W., Poewe, W., Rascol, O., Sampaio, C. (2006). Review of the therapeutic management of Parkinson's disease. Report of a joint task force of the European Federation of Neurological Societies and the Movement Disorder Society-European Section. Part I: early (uncomplicated) Parkinson's disease. Part II: late (complicated) Parkinson's disease. *Eur J Neurol*, 13:1170–1185, 1186–1202.

35. National Collaborating Centre for Chronic Conditions. (2006). *Parkinson's Disease: National Clinical Guideline for Diagnosis and Management in Primary and Secondary Care*. Royal College of Physicians, London.

36. Ramaker, C., Marinus, J., Stiggelbout, A.M., and Van Hilten, B.J. (2002). Systematic evaluation of rating scales for impairment and disability in Parkinson's disease. *Mov Disord*, 17:867–876.

37. Biglan, K.M. and Holloway, R.G. (2003). Surrogate endpoints in Parkinson's disease research. *Curr Neurol Neurosci Rep*, 3:314–320.

38. Muenter, M.D. and Tyce, G.M. (1971). L-dopa therapy of Parkinson's disease: Plasma L-dopa concentration, therapeutic response, and side effects. *Mayo Clin Proc*, 46:231–239.

39. Nutt, J.G. and Holford, N.H. (1996). The response to levodopa in Parkinson's disease: Imposing pharmacological law, order. *Ann Neurol*, 39:561–573.

40. Stocchi, F. and Olanow, C.W. (2003). Neuroprotection in Parkinson's disease: Clinical trials. *Ann Neurol*, 53:S87–S97.

41. Leber, P. (1997). Slowing the progression of Alzheimer disease: Methodologic issues. *Alzheimer Dis Assoc Disord*, 11:S10–S21.

42. Mohr, E., Barclay, C.L., Anderson, R., Constant, J. (2004). Clinical trial design in the age of dementia treatment: challenges and opportunities. In Gauthier S., Scheltens P., Bonnett R. (eds), *Alzheimer's Disease and Related Disorders Annual 2004*, Taylor and Francis Group, London, pp. 109–113.

43. Michell, A.W., Lewis, S.J.G., Foltynie, T., and Barker, R.A. (2004). Biomarkers and Parkinson's disease. *Brain*, 127:1693–1705.

44. Ravina, B., Eidelberg, D., Ahlskog, J.E., Albin, R.L., Brooks, D.J., Carbon, M., Dhawan, V., Feigin, A., Fahn, S., Guttman, M., Gwinn-Hardy, K., McFarland, H., Innis, R., Katz, R.G., Kieburtz, K., Kish, S.J., Lange, N., Langston, J.W., Marek, K., Morin, L., Moy, C., Murphy, D., Oertel, W.H., Oliver, G., Palesch, Y., Powers, W., Seibyl, J., Sethi, K.D., Shults, C.W., Sheehy, P., Stoessl, A.J., and Holloway, R. (2005). The role of radiotracer imaging in Parkinson's disease. *Neurology*, 64:208–215.

45. Pate, B.D., Kawamata, T., Yamada, T., McGeer, E.G., Hewitt, K.A., Snow, B.J., Ruth, T.J., and Calne, D.B. (1993). Correlation of striatal fluorodopa uptake in the MPTP monkey with dopamine indices. *Ann Neurol*, 34:331–338.

46. Snow, B.J., Tooyama, I., McGeer, E.G., Yamada, T., Calne, D.B., Takahashi, H., and Kimura, H. (1993). Human positron emission tomography [18F]fluorodopa studies correlate with dopamine cell counts and levels. *Ann Neurol*, 34:324–330.
47. Marek, K., Jennings, D., and Seibyl, J. (2003). Parkinson Study Group. Long-term follow-up of patients with scans without evidence of dopaminergic deficit (SWEDD) in the ELLDOPA study. *Neurology*, 60:A298.
48. Eckert, T., Feigin, A., Lewis, D.E., Dhawan, V., Frucht, S., and Eidelberg, D. (2007). Regional metabolic changes in Parkinsonian patients with normal dopaminergic imaging. *Mov Disord*, 22:167–173.
49. Brooks, D.J., Frey, K.A., Marek, K.L., Oakes, D., Paty, D., Prentice, R., Shults, C.W., and Stoessl, A.J. (2003). Assessment of neuroimaging techniques as biomarkers of the progression of Parkinson's disease. *Exp Neurol*, 184:S68–S79.
50. Freeman, T.B., Vawter, D.E., Leaverton, P.E., Godbold, J.H., Hauser, R.A., Goetz, C.G., and Olanow, C.W. (1999). Use of placebo surgery in controlled trials of a cellular-based therapy for Parkinson's disease. *N Engl J Med*, 341:988–992.
51. Carlsson, A. (2002). Treatment of Parkinson's with L-DOPA. The early discovery phase, and a comment on current problems. *J Neural Transm*, 109:777–787.
52. Delfs, J.M., Ciaramitaro, V.M., Soghomonian, J.J., and Chesselet, M.F. (1996). Unilateral nigrostriatal lesions induce a bilateral increase in glutamate decarboxylase messenger RNA in the reticular thalamic nucleus. *Neuroscience*, 71:383–395.
53. Ungerstedt, U. (1968). 6-Hydroxy-dopamine induced degeneration of central monoamine neurons. *Eur J Pharmacol*, 5:107–110.
54. Ungerstedt, U. and Arbuthnott, G.W. (1970). Quantitative recording of rotational behavior in rats after 6-hydroxy-dopamine lesions of the nigrostriatal dopamine system. *Brain Res*, 24:485–493.
55. Przedborski, S., Levivier, M., Jiang, H., Ferreira, M., Jackson-Lewis, V., Donaldson, D., and Togasaki, D.M. (1995). Dose-dependent lesions of the dopaminergic nigrostriatal pathway induced by intrastriatal injection of 6-hydroxydopamine. *Neuroscience*, 67:631–647.
56. Rosenblad. D. Kirik, C., Devaux, B., Moffat, B., Phillips, H.S., and Bjorklund, A. (1999). Protection and regeneration of nigral dopaminergic neurons by neurturin or GDNF in a partial lesion model of Parkinson's disease after administration into the striatum or the lateral ventricle. *Eur J Neurosci*, 11:1554–1566.
57. Murray, T.K., Whalley, K., Robinson, C.S., Ward, M.A., Hicks, C.A., Lodge, D., Vandergriff, J.L., Baumbarger, P., Siuda, E., Gates, M., Ogden, A.M., Skolnick, P., Zimmerman, D.M., Nisenbaum, E.S., Bleakman, D., and O'Neill, M.J. (2003). LY503430, a novel alpha-amino-3-hydroxy-5-methylisoxazole-4-propionic acid receptor potentiator with functional neuroprotective and neurotrophic effects in rodent models of Parkinson's disease. *J Pharmacol Exp Ther*, 306:752–762.
58. Salin, P., Hajji, M.D., and Kerkerian-le Goff, L. (1996). Bilateral 6-hydroxydopamine-induced lesion of the nigrostriatal dopamine pathway reproduces the effects of unilateral lesion on substance P but not on enkephalin expression in rat basal ganglia. *Eur J Neurosci*, 8:1746–1757.
59. Costall, B., Naylor, R.J., and Pycock, C. (1975). The 6-hydroxydopamine rotational model for the detection of dopamine agonist activity: Reliability of effect from different locations of 6-hydroxydopamine. *J Pharm Pharmacol*, 27:943–946.
60. Kelly, P.H. (1975). Unilateral 6-hydroxydopamine lesions of nigrostriatal or mesolimbic dopamine-containing terminals and the drug-induced rotation of rats. *Brain Res*, 100:163–169.
61. Siever, L., Cohen, R., and Pert, A. (1981). Assessing pharmacologically induced dopamine receptor sensitivity changes with the Ungerstedt turning model. *Psychopharmacology (Berl)*, 75:212–213.

62. Kirik, D., Rosenblad, C., and Bjorklund, A. (1998). Characterization of behavioral and neuro-degenerative changes following partial lesions of the nigrostriatal dopamine system induced by intrastriatal 6-hydroxydopamine in the rat. *Exp Neurol*, 152:259–277.

63. Schallert, T., Upchurch, M., Lobaugh, N., Farrar, S.B., Spirduso, W.W., Gilliam, P., Vaughn, D., and Wilcox, R.E. (1982). Tactile extinction: distinguishing between sensorimotor and motor asymmetries in rats with unilateral nigrostriatal damage. *Pharmacol Biochem Behav*, 16:455–462.

64. Schallert, T., Upchurch, M., Wilcox, R.E., and Vaughn, D.M. (1983). Posture-independent sensorimotor analysis of inter-hemispheric receptor asymmetries in neostriatum. *Pharmacol Biochem Behav*, 18:753–759.

65. Schallert, T., Norton, D., Jones, T.A. (1992). A clinically relevant unilateral rat model of Parkinsonian akinesia. *J. Neural Transplant Plast*, 3: 332–333.

66. Schallert, T. and Tillerson, J.L. (2000). Intervention strategies for degeneration of DA neurons in Parkinsonism: Optimizing behavioral assessment of outcome. In Emerich, D.F., Dean III, R.L., and Sandberg, P.R. (eds.), *Central Nervous System Diseases*. Humana Press, Torowa, NJ.

67. Ariano, M.A., Grissell, A.E., Littlejohn, F.C., Buchanan, T.M., Elsworth, J.D., Collier, T.J., and Steece-Collier, K. (2005). Partial dopamine loss enhances activated caspase-3 activity: Differential outcomes in striatal projection systems. *J Neurosci Res*, 82:387–396.

68. Mehta, A. and Chesselet, M.F. (2005). Effect of GABA(A) receptor stimulation in the subthalamic nucleus on motor deficits induced by nigrostriatal lesions in the rat. *Exp Neurol*, 193:110–117.

69. Soghomonian, J.J. and Chesselet, M.F. (1992). Effects of nigrostriatal lesions on the levels of messenger RNAs encoding two isoforms of glutamate decarboxylase in the globus pallidus and entopeduncular nucleus of the rat. *Synapse*, 11:124–133.

70. Cenci, M.A. and Lundblad, M. (2005). Utility of 6-hydroxydopamine lesioned rats in the preclinical screening of novel treatments for Parkinson disease. In LeDoux, M. (ed.), *Animal Models of Movement Disorders*. Elsevier Academic Press, San Diego, CA, pp. 193–208.

71. Heikkila, R.E., Hess, A., and Duvoisin, R.C. (1984). Dopaminergic neurotoxicity of 1-methyl-4-phenyl-1,2,5,6-tetrahydropyridine in mice. *Science*, 224:1451–1453.

72. Jackson-Lewis, V., Jakowec, M., Burke, R.E., and Przedborski, S. (1995). Time course and morphology of dopaminergic neuronal death caused by the neurotoxin 1-methyl-4-phenyl-1,2,3,6-tetrahydropyridine. *Neurodegeneration*, 4:257–269.

73. Sedelis, M., Schwarting, R.K., and Huston, J.P. (2001). Behavioral phenotyping of the MPTP mouse model of Parkinson's disease. *Behav Brain Res*, 125:109–125.

74. Langston, J.W., Ballard, P., Tetrud, J.W., and Irwin, I. (1983). Chronic Parkinsonism in humans due to a product of meperidine-analog synthesis. *Science*, 219:979–980.

75. Przedborski, S. and Jackson-Lewis, V. (1998). Experimental developments in movement disorders: Update on proposed free radical mechanisms. *Curr Opin Neurol*, 11:335–339.

76. Giovanni, A., Sonsalla, P.K., and Heikkila, R.E. (1994). Studies on species sensitivity to the dopaminergic neurotoxin 1-methyl-4-phenyl-1,2,3,6-tetrahydropyridine. Part 2: Central administration of 1-methyl-4-phenylpyridinium. *J Pharmacol Exp Ther*, 270:1008–1014.

77. Staal, R.G., Hogan, K.A., Liang, C.L., German, D.C., and Sonsalla, P.K. (2000). *In vitro* studies of striatal esicles containing the vesicular monoamine transporter (VMAT2): Rat versus mouse differences in sequestration of 1-methyl-4-phenylpyridinium. *J Pharmacol Exp Ther*, 293:329–335.

78. Giovanni, A., Sieber, B.A., Heikkila, R.E., and Sonsalla, P.K. (1991). Correlation between the neostriatal content of the 1-methyl-4-phenylpyridinium species and dopaminergic neurotoxicity following 1-methyl-4-phenyl-1,2,3,6-tetrahydropyridine administration to several strains of mice. *J Pharmacol Exp Ther*, 257:691–697.

79. Muthane, U., Ramsay, K.A., Jiang, H., Jackson-Lewis, V., Donaldson, D., Fernando, S., Ferreira, M., and Przedborski, S. (1994). Differences in nigral neuron number and sensitivity to 1-methyl-4-phenyl-1,2,3,6-tetrahydropyridine in C57/bl and CD-1 mice. *Exp Neurol*, 126:195-204.
80. Jackson-Lewis, V. and Przedborski, S. (2007). Protocol for the MPTP mouse model of Parkinson's disease. *Nature Protocols*, 2:141-151.
81. Fornai, F., Schluter, O.M., Lenzi, P., Gesi, M., Ruffoli, R., Ferrucci, M., Lazzeri, G., Busceti, C.L., Pontarelli, F., Battaglia, G., Pellegrini,A., Nicoletti, F., Ruggieri, S., Paparelli,A., and Sudhof,T.C. (2005). Parkinson-like syndrome induced by continuous MPTP infusion: Convergent roles of the ubiquitin-proteasome system and alpha-synuclein. *Proc Natl Acad Sci USA*, 102:3413-3418.
82. Meredith, G.E. *et al.* (2002). Lysosomal malfunction accompanies alpha-synuclein aggregation in a progressive mouse model of Parkinson's disease. *Brain Res*, 956:156-165.
83. Sonsalla, P.K. and Heikkila, R.E. (1986). The influence of dose and dosing interval on MPTP-induced dopaminergic neurotoxicity in mice. *Eur J Pharmacol*, 129:339-345.
84. Tatton, N.A. and Kish, S.J. (1997). In situ detection of apoptotic nuclei in the substantia nigra compacta of 1-methyl-4-phenyl-1,2,3,6-tetrahydropyridine-treated mice using terminal deoxynucleotidyl transferase labelling and acridine orange staining. *Neuroscience*, 77:1037-1048.
85. Przedborski, S. and Vila, M. (2003). The 1-methyl-4-phenyl-1,2,3,6 tetrahydropyridine mouse model: A tool to explore the pathogenesis of Parkinson's disease. *Ann NY Acad Sci*, 991:189-198.
86. Furuya, T., Hayakawa, H., Yamada, M., Yoshimi, K., Hisahara, S., Miura, M., Mizuno, Y., and Mochizuki, H. (2004). Caspase-11 mediates inflammatory dopaminergic cell death in the 1-methyl-4-phenyl-1,2,3,6-tetrahydropyridine mouse model of Parkinson's disease. *J Neurosci*, 24:1865-1872.
87. Mizuno,Y., Sone, N., Suzuki, K., and Saitoh,T. (1988). Studies on the toxicity of 1-methyl-4-phenylpyridinium ion (MPP+) against mitochondria of mouse brain. *J Neurol Sci*, 86:97-110.
88. Nicklas, W.J., Youngster, S.K., Kindt, M.V., and Heikkila, R.E. (1987). MPTP, MPP+ and mitochondrial function. *Life Sci*, 40:721-729.
89. Przedborski, S., Jackson-Lewis,V., Djaldetti, R., Liberatore, G.,Vila, M.,Vukosavic, S., and Almer, G. (2000). The parkinsonian toxin MPTP: Action and mechanism. *Restor Neurol Neurosci*, 16:135-142.
90. Dauer, W. and Przedborski, S. (2003). Parkinson's Disease: Mechanisms and models. *Neuron*, 39:889-909.
91. Burns, R.S., Chiueh, C.C., Markey, S.P., Ebert, M.H., Jacobowitz, D.M., and Kopin, I.J. (1983). A primate model of parkinsonism: Selective destruction of dopaminergic neurons in the pars compacta of the substantia nigra by N-methyl-4-phenyl-1,2,3,6-tetrahydropyridine. *Proc Natl Acad Sci USA*, 80:4546-4550.
92. German, D.C., Dubach, M., Askari, S., Speciale, S.G., and Bowden, D.M. (1988). 1-Methyl-4-phenyl-1,2,3,6-tetrahydropyridine-induced parkinsonian syndrome in *Macaca fascicularis*: Which midbrain dopaminergic neurons are lost?. *Neuroscience*, 24:161-174.
93. Smith, R.D., Zhang, Z., Kurlan, R., McDermott, M., and Gash, D.M. (1993). Developing a stable bilateral model of parkinsonism in rhesus monkeys. *Neuroscience*, 52:7-16.
94. Bezard, E., Imbert, C., Deloire, X., Bioulac, B., and Gross, C.E. (1997). A chronic MPTP model reproducing the slow evolution of Parkinson's disease: Evolution of motor symptoms in the monkey. *Brain Res*, 766:107-112.
95. Elsworth, J.D.,Taylor, J.R., Sladek, J.R., Jr., Collier,T.J., Redmond, D.E., Jr., and Roth, R.H. (2000). Striatal dopaminergic correlates of stable parkinsonism and degree of recovery in old-world primates one year after MPTP treatment. *Neuroscience*, 95:399-408.

96. Doudet, D.J., Chan, G.L., Holden, J.E., Morrison, K.S., Wyatt, R.J., and Ruth, T.J. (1997). Effects of catechol-O-methyltransferase inhibition on the rates of uptake and reversibility of 6-fluoro-L-Dopa trapping in MPTP-induced parkinsonism in monkeys. *Neuropharmacology*, 36:363–371.

97. Jenner, P. (2003). The contribution of the MPTP-treated primate model to the development of new treatment strategies for Parkinson's Disease. *Parkinsonism Related Disord*, 9:131–137.

98. Benazzouz, A., Gross, C., Feger, J., Boraud, T., and Bioulac, B. (1993). Reversal of rigidity and improvement in motor performance by subthalamic high-frequency stimulation in MPTP-treated monkeys. *Eur J Neurosci*, 5:382–389.

99. Benabid, A.L., Chabardes, S., Seigneuret, E., Fraix, V., Krack, P., Pollak, P., Xia, R., Wallace, B., Sauter, F. (2006). Surgical therapy for Parkinson's disease. *J Neural Transm Suppl*. 383–392.

100. Petzinger, G.M., Fisher, B., Hogg, E., Abernathy, A., Arevalo, P., Nixon, K., and Jakowec, M.W. (2006). Behavioral motor recovery in the 1-methyl-4-phenyl-1,2,3,6-tetrahydropyridine-lesioned squirrel monkey (*Saimiri sciureus*): Changes in striatal dopamine and expression of tyrosine hydroxylase and dopamine transporter proteins. *J Neurosci Res*, 83:332–347.

101. Chade, A.R., Kasten, M. and Tanner, C.M. (2006). Nongenetic causes of Parkinson's Disease. *J Neural Transm Suppl*, 70:147–151.

102. Bove, J., Prou, D., Perier, C., and Przedborski, S. (2005). Toxin-induced models of Parkinson's disease. *NeuroRx*, 2:484–494.

103. Panov, A., Dikalov, S., Shalbuyeva, N., Taylor, G., Sherer, T., and Greenamyre, J.T. (2005). Rotenone model of Parkinson disease: Multiple brain mitochondria dysfunctions after short term systemic rotenone intoxication. *J Biol Chem*, 280:42026–42035.

104. Betarbet, R., Canet-Aviles, R.M., Sherer, T.B., Mastroberardino, P.G., McLendon, C., Kim, J.H., Lund, S., Na, H.M., Taylor, G., Bence, N.F., Kopito, R., Seo, B.B., Yagi, T., Yagi, A., Klinefelter, G., Cookson, M.R., and Greenamyre, J.T. (2006). Intersecting pathways to neurodegeneration in Parkinson's disease: Effects of the pesticide rotenone on DJ-1, alpha-synuclein, and the ubiquitin-proteasome system. *Neurobiol Dis*, 22:404–420.

105. Wang, X.F., Li, S., Chou, A.P., and Bronstein, J.M. (2006). Inhibitory effects of pesticides on proteasome activity: Implication in Parkinson's disease. *Neurobiol Dis*, 23:198–205.

106. Betarbet, R., Sherer, T.B., MacKenzie, G., Garcia-Osuna, M., Panov, A.V., and Greenamyre, J.T. (2000). Chronic systemic pesticide exposure reproduces features of Parkinson's Disease. *Nat Neurosci*, 3:1301–1306.

107. Zhu, C., Vourc'h, P., Fernagut, P.O., Fleming, S.M., Lacan, S., Dicarlo, C.D., Seaman, R.L., and Chesselet, M.F. (2004). Variable effects of chronic subcutaneous administration of rotenone on striatal histology. *J Comp Neurol*, 478:418–426.

108. Lapointe, N., St-Hilaire, M., Martinoli, M.G., Blanchet, J., Gould, P., Rouillard, C., and Cicchetti, F. (2004). Rotenone induces non-specific central nervous system and systemic toxicity. *Faseb J*, 18:717–719.

109. Hoglinger, G.U., Feger, J., Prigent, A., Michel, P.P., Parain, K., Champy, P., Ruberg, M., Oertel, W.H., and Hirsch, E.C. (2003). Chronic systemic complex I inhibition induces a hypokinetic multisystem degeneration in rats. *J Neurochem*, 84:491–502.

110. Alam, M. and Schmidt, W.J. (2002). Rotenone destroys dopaminergic neurons and induces parkinsonian symptoms in rats. *Behav Brain Res*, 136:317–324.

111. Sherer, T.B., Kim, J.H., Betarbet, R., and Greenamyre, J.T. (2003). Subcutaneous rotenone exposure causes highly selective dopaminergic degeneration and alpha-synuclein aggregation. *Exp Neurol*, 179:9–16.

112. Richter, F., Hamann, M., and Richter, A. (2007). Chronic rotenone treatment induces behavioral effects but no pathological signs of parkinsonism in mice. *J Neurosci Res*, 85:681–691.

113. Cicchetti, F., Lapointe, N., Roberge-Tremblay, A., Saint-Pierre, M., Jimenez, L., Ficke, B.W., and Gross, R.E. (2005). Systemic exposure to paraquat and maneb models early Parkinson's Disease in young adult rats. *Neurobiol Dis*, 20:360-371.

114. McCormack, A.L., Thiruchelvam, M., Manning-Bog, A.B., Thiffault, C., Langston, J.W., Cory-Slechta, D.A., and Monte, D.A. (2002). Environmental risk factors and Parkinson's Disease: Selective degeneration of nigral dopaminergic neurons caused by the herbicide paraquat. *Neurobiol Dis*, 10:119-127.

115. Fernagut, P.-O., Hutson, C.B., Fleming, S.M., Tetreaut, N., Salcedo, J., Masliah, E., Chesselet, M.F. (2007). Behavioral and histopathological consequences of paraquat intoxication in mice: Effects of alpha-synuclein overexpression, *Synapse*, 61(12):991-1001.

116. Cory-Slechta, D.A., Thiruchelvam, M., Barlow, B.K., and Richfield, E.K. (2005). Developmental pesticide models of the Parkinson disease phenotype. *Environ Health Perspect*, 113:1263-1270.

117. Li, A.A., Mink, P.J., McIntosh, L.J., Teta, M.J., and Finley, B. (2005). Evaluation of epidemiologic and animal data associating pesticides with. *J Occup Environ Med*, 47:1059-1087.

118. Hunter, R.L., Dragicevic, N., Seifert, K., Choi, D.Y., Liu, M., Kim, H.C., Cass, W.A., Sullivan, P.G., and Bing, G. (2007). Inflammation induces mitochondrial dysfunction and dopaminergic neurodegeneration in the nigrostriatal system. *J Neurochem*, 100:1375-1386.

119. Nass, R. and Blakely, R.D. (2003). The *Caenorhabditis elegans* dopaminergic system: Opportunities for insights into dopamine transport and neurodegeneration. *Annu Rev Pharmacol Toxicol*, 43:521-544.

120. Braungart, E., Gerlach, M., Riederer, P., Baumeister, R., and Hoener, M.C. (2004). *Caenorhabditis elegans* MPP+ model of for high-throughput drug screenings. *Neurodegener Dis*, 1:175-183.

121. Coulom, H. and Birman, S. (2004). Chronic exposure to rotenone models sporadic in *Drosophila melanogaster*. *J Neurosci*, 24:10993-10998.

122. Bonilla, E., Medina-Leendertz, S., Villalobos, V., Molero, L., and Bohorquez, A. (2006). Paraquat-induced oxidative stress in *Drosophila melanogaster*: Effects of melatonin, glutathione, serotonin, minocycline, lipoic acid and ascorbic acid. *Neurochem Res*, 31:1425-1432.

123. Greenamyre, J.T. and Hastings, T.G. (2004). Biomedicine. Parkinson's – divergent causes, convergent mechanisms. *Science*, 304:1120-1122.

124. Thiruchelvam, M., Brockel, B.J., Richfield, E.K., Baggs, R.B., and Cory-Slechta, D.A. (2000). Potentiated and preferential effects of combined paraquat and maneb on nigrostriatal dopamine systems: Environmental risk factors for Parkinson's Disease?. *Brain Res*, 873:225-234.

125. Mandel, S., Grunblatt, E., Riederer, P., Gerlach, M., Levites, Y., and Youdim, M.B. (2003). Neuroprotective strategies in Parkinson's Disease: An update on progress. *CNS Drugs*, 17:729-762.

126. Chan, C.S., Guzman, J.N., Ilijic, E., Mercer, J.N., Rick, C., Tkatch, T., Meredith, G.E., and Surmeier, D.J. (2007). Rejuvenation' protects neurons in mouse models of Parkinson's Disease. *Nature*, 447:1081-1086.

127. Polymeropoulos, M.H., Lavedan, C., Leroy, E., Ide, S.E., Dehejia, A., Dutra, A., Pike, B., Root, H., Rubenstein, J., Boyer, R., Stenroos, E.S., Chandrasekharappa, S., Athanassiadou, A., Papapetropoulos, T., Johnson, W.G., Lazzarini, A.M., Duvoisin, R.C., Di Iorio, G., Golbe, L.I., and Nussbaum, R.L. (1997). Mutation in the alpha-synuclein gene identified in families with Parkinson's Disease. *Science*, 276:2045-2047.

128. Kruger, R., Kuhn, W., Muller, T., Woitalla, D., Graeber, M., Kosel, S., Przuntek, H., Epplen, J.T., Schols, L., and Riess, O. (1998). Ala30Pro mutation in the gene encoding alpha-synuclein in Parkinson's Disease. *Nat Genet*, 18:106-108.

129. Singleton, A.B., Farrer, M., Johnson, J., Singleton, A., Hague, S., Kachergus, J., Hulihan, M., Peuralinna, T., Dutra, A., Nussbaum, R., Lincoln, S., Crawley, A., Hanson, M., Maraganore, D.,

Adler, C., Cookson, M.R., Muenter, M., Baptista, M., Miller, D., Blancato, J., Hardy, J., and Gwinn-Hardy, K. (2003). Alpha-Synuclein locus triplication causes Parkinson's Disease. *Science*, 302:841.

130. Chartier-Harlin, M.C., Kachergus, J., Roumier, C., Mouroux, V., Douay, X., Lincoln, S., Levecque, C., Larvor, L., Andrieux, J., Hulihan, M., Waucquier, N., Defebvre, L., Amouyel, P., Farrer, M., and Destee, A. (2004). Alpha-synuclein locus duplication as a cause of familial Parkinson's Disease. *Lancet*, 364:1167–1169.

131. Ibanez, P., Bonnet, A.M., Debarges, B., Lohmann, E., Tison, F., Pollak, P., Agid, Y., Durr, A., and Brice, A. (2004). Causal relation between alpha-synuclein gene duplication and familial. *Lancet*, 364:1169–1171.

132. Zarranz, J.J., Alegre, J., Gomez-Esteban, J.C., Lezcano, E., Ros, R., Ampuero, I., Vidal, L., Hoenicka, J., Rodriguez, O., Atares, B., Llorens, V., Tortosa Gomez, E., del Ser, T., Munoz, D.G., and de Yebenes, J.G. (2004). The new mutation, E46K, of alpha-synuclein causes Parkinson and Lewy body dementia. *Ann Neurol*, 55:164–173.

133. Spillantini, M.G., Schmidt, M.L., Lee, V.M., Trojanowski, J.Q., Jakes, R., and Goedert, M. (1997). Alpha-synuclein in Lewy bodies. *Nature*, 388:839–840.

134. Micieli, G., Tosi, P., Marcheselli, S., and Cavallini, A. (2003). Autonomic dysfunction in. *Neurol Sci*, 24 Suppl 1:S32–S34.

135. Clayton, D.F. and George, J.M. (1998). The synucleins: A family of proteins involved in synaptic function, plasticity, neurodegeneration and disease. *Trends Neurosci*, 21:249–254.

136. Ueda, K., Fukushima, H., Masliah, E., Xia, Y., Iwai, A., Yoshimoto, M., Otero, D.A., Kondo, J., Ihara, Y., and Saitoh, T. (1993). Molecular cloning of cDNA encoding an unrecognized component of amyloid in Alzheimer disease. *Proc Natl Acad Sci USA*, 90:11282–11286.

137. Feany, M.B. and Bender, W.W. (2000). A Drosophila model of Parkinson's Disease. *Nature*, 404:394–398.

138. Vekrellis, K., Rideout, H.J., and Stefanis, L. (2004). Neurobiology of alpha-synuclein. *Mol Neurobiol*, 30:1–21.

139. Galvin, J.E., Lee, V.M., and Trojanowski, J.Q. (2001). Synucleinopathies: Clinical and pathological implications. *Arch Neurol*, 58:186–190.

140. Kitada, T., Asakawa, S., Hattori, N., Matsumine, H., Yamamura, Y., Minoshima, S., Yokochi, M., Mizuno, Y., and Shimizu, N. (1998). Mutations in the parkin gene cause autosomal recessive juvenile parkinsonism. *Nature*, 392:605–608.

141. Lucking, C.B., Durr, A., Bonifati, V., Vaughan, J., De Michele, G., Gasser, T., Harhangi, B.S., Meco, G., Denefle, P., Wood, N.W., Agid, Y., and Brice, A. (2000). Association between early-onset and mutations in the parkin gene. *N Engl J Med*, 342:1560–1567.

142. Periquet, M., Latouche, M., Lohmann, E., Rawal, N., De Michele, G., Ricard, S., Teive, H., Fraix, V., Vidailhet, M., Nicholl, D., Barone, P., Wood, N.W., Raskin, S., Deleuze, J.F., Agid, Y., Durr, A., and Brice, A. (2003). Parkin mutations are frequent in patients with isolated early-onset parkinsonism. *Brain*, 126:1271–1278.

143. Olanow, C.W. and McNaught, K.S. (2006). Ubiquitin-proteasome system and Parkinson's Disease. *Mov Disord*, 21:1806–1823.

144. Leroy, E., Boyer, R., Auburger, G., Leube, B., Ulm, G., Mezey, E., Harta, G., Brownstein, M.J., Jonnalagada, S., Chernova, T., Dehejia, A., Lavedan, C., Gasser, T., Steinbach, P.J., Wilkinson, K.D., and Polymeropoulos, M.H. (1998). The ubiquitin pathway in Parkinson's Disease. *Nature*, 395:451–452.

145. Lincoln, S., Vaughan, J., Wood, N., Baker, M., Adamson, J., Gwinn-Hardy, K., Lynch, T., Hardy, J., and Farrer, M. (1999). Low frequency of pathogenic mutations in the ubiquitin carboxy-terminal hydrolase gene in familial Parkinson's Disease. *Neuroreport*, 10:427–429.

146. Abou-Sleiman, P.M., Healy, D.G., Quinn, N., Lees, A.J., and Wood, N.W. (2003). The role of pathogenic DJ-1 mutations in Parkinson's Disease. *Ann Neurol*, 54:283–286.

147. Bonifati, V., Rizzu, P., van Baren, M.J., Schaap, O., Breedveld, G.J., Krieger, E., Dekker, M.C., Squitieri, F., Ibanez, P., Joosse, M., van Dongen, J.W., Vanacore, N., van Swieten, J.C., Brice, A., Meco, G., van Duijn, C.M., Oostra, B.A., and Heutink, P. (2003). Mutations in the DJ-1 gene associated with autosomal recessive early-onset parkinsonism. *Science*, 299:256–259.

148. Hague, S., Rogaeva, E., Hernandez, D., Gulick, C., Singleton, A., Hanson, M., Johnson, J., Weiser, R., Gallardo, M., Ravina, B., Gwinn-Hardy, K., Crawley, A., St George-Hyslop, P.H., Lang, A.E., Heutink, P., Bonifati, V., and Hardy, J. (2003). Early-onset caused by a compound heterozygous DJ-1 mutation. *Ann Neurol*, 54:271–274.

149. Valente, E.M., Abou-Sleiman, P.M., Caputo, V., Muqit, M.M., Harvey, K., Gispert, S., Ali, Z., Del Turco, D., Bentivoglio, A.R., Healy, D.G., Albanese, A., Nussbaum, R., Gonzalez-Maldonado, R., Deller, T., Salvi, S., Cortelli, P., Gilks, W.P., Latchman, D.S., Harvey, R.J., Dallapiccola, B., Auburger, G., and Wood, N.W. (2004). Hereditary early-onset caused by mutations in PINK1. *Science*, 304:1158–1160.

150. Paisan-Ruiz, C., Jain, S., Evans, E.W., Gilks, W.P., Simon, J., van der Brug, M., Lopez de Munain, A., Aparicio, S., Gil, A.M., Khan, N., Johnson, J., Martinez, J.R., Nicholl, D., Carrera, I.M., Pena, A.S., de Silva, R., Lees, A., Marti-Masso, J.F., Perez-Tur, J., Wood, N.W., and Singleton, A.B. (2004). Cloning of the gene containing mutations that cause PARK8-linked Parkinson's Disease. *Neuron*, 44:595–600.

151. Zimprich, A., Biskup, S., Leitner, P., Lichtner, P., Farrer, M., Lincoln, S., Kachergus, J., Hulihan, M., Uitti, R.J., Calne, D.D., Stoessl, A.J., Pfeiffer, R.F., Patenge, N., Carbajal, I.C., Vieregge, P., Asmus, F., Muller-Myhsok, B., Dickson, D.W., Meitinger, T., Strom, T.M., Wszolek, Z.K., and Gasser, T. (2004). Mutations in LRRK2 cause autosomal-dominant parkinsonism with pleomorphic pathology. *Neuron*, 44:601–607.

152. Hernandez, D.G., Paisan-Ruiz, C., McInerney-Leo, A., Jain, S., Meyer-Lindenberg, A., Evans, E.W., Berman, K.F., Johnson, J., Auburger, G., Schaffer, A.A., Lopez, G.J., Nussbaum, R.L., and Singleton, A.B. (2005). Clinical and positron emission tomography of caused by LRRK2. *Ann Neurol*, 57:453–456.

153. Whaley, N.R., Uitti, R.J., Dickson, D.W., Farrer, M.J., Wszolek, Z.K. (2006). Clinical and pathologic features of families with LRRK2-associated. J Neural Transm Suppl., 221–229.

154. Clark, L.N., Wang, Y., Karlins, E., Saito, L., Mejia-Santana, H., Harris, J., Louis, E.D., Cote, L.J., Andrews, H., Fahn, S., Waters, C., Ford, B., Frucht, S., Ottman, R., and Marder, K. (2006). Frequency of LRRK2 mutations in early- and late-onset Parkinson disease. *Neurology*, 67:1786–1791.

155. Ozelius, L.J., Senthil, G., Saunders-Pullman, R., Ohmann, E., Deligtisch, A., Tagliati, M., Hunt, A.L., Klein, C., Henick, B., Hailpern, S.M., Lipton, R.B., Soto-Valencia, J., Risch, N., and Bressman, S.B. (2006). LRRK2 G2019S as a cause of in Ashkenazi Jews. *N Engl J Med*, 354:424–425.

156. Bras, J.M., Guerreiro, R.J., Ribeiro, M.H. *et al.* (2005). G2019S dardarin substitution is a common cause of Parkinson's disease in a Portuguese cohort. *Mov Disord*, 20:1653–1655.

157. Lesage, S., Durr, A., Tazir, M. *et al.* (2006). LRRK2 G2019S as a cause of Parkinson's disease in North African Arabs. *N Engl J Med*, 354:422–423.

158. Ramirez, A., Heimbach, A., Grundemann, J., Stiller, B., Hampshire, D., Cid, L.P., Goebel, I., Mubaidin, A.F., Wriekat, A.L., Roeper, J., Al-Din, A., Hillmer, A.M., Karsak, M., Liss, B., Woods, C.G., Behrens, M.I., and Kubisch, C. (2006). Hereditary parkinsonism with dementia is caused by mutations in ATP13A2, encoding a lysosomal type 5 P-type ATPase. *Nat Genet*, 38:1184–1191.

159. Fung, H.C., Scholz, S., Matarin, M., Simon-Sanchez, J., Hernandez, D., Britton, A., Gibbs, J.R., Langefeld, C., Stiegert, M.L., Schymick, J., Okun, M.S., Mandel, R.J., Fernandez, H.H., Foote, K.D., Rodriguez, R.L., Peckham, E., De Vrieze, F.W., Gwinn-Hardy, K., Hardy, J.A., and Singleton, A. (2006). Genome-wide genotyping in and neurologically normal controls: First stage analysis and public release of data. *Lancet Neurol*, 5:911–916.

160. Halperin, A., Elstein, D., and Zimran, A. (2006). Increased incidence of Parkinson disease among relatives of patients with Gaucher disease. *Blood Cells Mol Dis*, 36:426–428.

161. Machaczka, M., Rucinska, M., Skotnicki, A.B., and Jurczak, W. (1999). Parkinson's syndrome preceding clinical manifestation of Gaucher's disease. *Am J Hematol*, 61:216–217.
162. Tayebi, N., Callahan, M., Madike, V., Stubblefield, B.K., Orvisky, E., Krasnewich, D., Fillano, J. J., and Sidransky, E. (2001). Gaucher disease and parkinsonism: A phenotypic and genotypic characterization. *Mol Genet Metab*, 73:313–321.
163. Sidransky, E. (2006). Heterozygosity for a Mendelian disorder as a risk factor for complex disease. *Clin Genet*, 70:275–282.
164. Bandhyopadhyay, U. and Cuervo, A.M. (2007). Chaperone-mediated autophagy in aging and neurodegeneration: Lessons from alpha-synuclein. *Exp Gerontol*, 42:120–128.
165. Barbeau, A., Roy, M., Cloutier, T., Plasse, L., and Paris, S. (1987). Environmental and genetic factors in the etiology of Parkinson's Disease. *Adv Neurol*, 45:299–306.
166. Ritz, B. and Yu, F. (2000). Parkinson's Disease mortality and pesticide exposure in California 1984–1994. *Int J Epidemiol*, 29:323–329.
167. Dick, F.D. (2006). Parkinson's Disease and pesticide exposures. *Br Med Bull*, 79–80:219–231.
168. Zarow, C., Lyness, S.A., Mortimer, J.A., and Chui, H.C. (2003). Neuronal loss is greater in the locus coeruleus than nucleus basalis and substantia nigra in Alzheimer and Parkinson diseases. *Arch Neurol*, 60:337–341.
169. Fernagut, P.O. and Chesselet, M.F. (2004). Alpha-synuclein and transgenic mouse models. *Neurobiol Dis*, 17:123–130.
170. Fleming, S.M. and Chesselet, M.F. (2006a). Behavioral phenotypes and pharmacology in genetic mouse models of Parkinsonism. *Behav Pharmacol*, 17:383–391.
171. Richfield, E.K., Thiruchelvam, M.J., Cory-Slechta, D.A., Wuertzer, C., Gainetdinov, R.R., Caron, M.G., Di Monte, D.A., and Federoff, H.J. (2002). Behavioral and neurochemical effects of wild-type and mutated human alpha-synuclein in transgenic mice. *Exp Neurol*, 175:35–48.
172. Thiruchelvam, M.J., Powers, J.M., Cory-Slechta, D.A., and Richfield, E.K. (2004). Risk factors for dopaminergic neuron loss in human alpha-synuclein transgenic mice. *Eur J Neurosci*, 19:845–854.
173. Chen, L., Thiruchelvam, M.J., Madura, K., and Richfield, E.K. (2006). Proteasome dysfunction in aged human alpha-synuclein transgenic mice. *Neurobiol Dis*, 23:120–126.
174. Masliah, E., Rockenstein, E., Veinbergs, I., Mallory, M., Hashimoto, M., Takeda, A., Sagara, Y., Sisk, A., and Mucke, L. (2000). Dopaminergic loss and inclusion body formation in alpha-synuclein mice: Implications for neurodegenerative disorders. *Science*, 287:1265–1269.
175. Rockenstein, E., Mallory, M., Hashimoto, M., Song, D., Shults, C.W., Lang, I., and Masliah, E. (2002). Differential neuropathological alterations in transgenic mice expressing alpha-synuclein from the platelet-derived growth factor and Thy-1 promoters. *J Neurosci Res*, 68:568–578.
176. Hickey, M.A. and Chesselet, M.F. (2003). Apoptosis in Huntington's disease. *Prog Neuropsychopharmacol Biol Psych*, 27:255–265.
177. Tofaris, G.K., Garcia Reitbock, P., Humby, T., Lambourne, S.L., O'Connell, M., Ghetti, B., Gossage, H., Emson, P.C., Wilkinson, L.S., Goedert, M., and Spillantini, M.G. (2006). Pathological changes in dopaminergic nerve cells of the substantia nigra and olfactory bulb in mice transgenic for truncated human alpha-synuclein(1–120): Implications for Lewy body disorders. *J Neurosci*, 26:3942–3950.
178. Wakamatsu, M., Ishii, A., Iwata, S., Sakagami, J., Ukai, Y., Ono, M., Kanbe, D., Muramatsu, S.I., Kobayashi, K., Iwatsubo, T., Yoshimoto, M. (2006). Selective loss of nigral dopamine neurons induced by overexpression of truncated human alpha-synuclein in mice, *Neurobiol Aging*, 29(4):574–585.
179. Norris, E.H. and Giasson, B.I. (2005). Role of oxidative damage in protein aggregation associated with and related disorders. *Antioxid Redox Signal*, 7:672–684.
180. Lee, M.K., Stirling, W., Xu, Y., Xu, X., Qui, D., Mandir, A.S., Dawson, T.M., Copeland, N.G., Jenkins, N.A., and Price, D.L. (2002). Human alpha-synuclein-harboring familial-linked

Ala-53 → Thr mutation causes neurodegenerative disease with alpha-synuclein aggregation in transgenic mice. *Proc Natl Acad Sci USA*, 99:8968-8973.

181. Giasson, B.I., Duda, J.E., Quinn, S.M., Zhang, B., Trojanowski, J.Q., and Lee, V.M. (2002). Neuronal alpha-synucleinopathy with severe movement disorder in mice expressing A53T human alpha-synuclein. *Neuron*, 34:521-533.

182. van der Putten, H., Wiederhold, K.H., Probst, A., Barbieri, S., Mistl, C., Danner, S., Kauffmann, S., Hofele, K., Spooren, W.P., Ruegg, M.A., Lin, S., Caroni, P., Sommer, B., Tolnay, M., and Bilbe, G. (2000). Neuropathology in mice expressing human alpha-synuclein. *J Neurosci*, 20:6021-6029.

183. Kahle, P.J., Neumann, M., Ozmen, L., Muller, V., Jacobsen, H., Schindzielorz, A., Okochi, M., Leimer, U., van Der Putten, H., Probst, A., Kremmer, E., Kretzschmar, H.A., and Haass, C. (2000). Subcellular localization of wild-type and - associated mutant alpha - synuclein in human and transgenic mouse brain. *J Neurosci*, 20:6365-6373.

184. Cools, R., Lewis, S.J., Clark, L., Barker, R.A., and Robbins, T.W. (2007). L-DOPA disrupts activity in the nucleus accumbens during reversal learning in. *Neuropsychopharmacology*, 32:180-189.

185. Fleming, S.M., Salcedo, J., Hutson, C.B., Rockenstein, E., Masliah, E., Levine, M.S., and Chesselet, M.F. (2006b). Behavioral effects of dopaminergic agonists in transgenic mice overexpressing human wildtype alpha-synuclein. *Neuroscience*, 142:1245-1253.

186. Fleming, S.M., Tetreault, N.A., Masliah, E., and Chesselet, M.F. (2006c). Alterations in olfactory function in transgenic mice overexpressing human wild-type alpha synuclein. *Neurosci Abst*, 75:9.

187. Bohnen, N.I., Gedela, S., Kuwabara, H., Constantine, G.M., Mathis, C.A., Studenski, S.A., and Moore, R.Y. (2007). Selective hyposmia and nigrostriatal dopaminergic denervation in Parkinson's Disease. *J Neurol*, 254:84-90.

188. Kirik, D., Rosenblad, C., Burger, C., Lundberg, C., Johansen, T.E., Muzyczka, N., Mandel, R.J., and Bjorklund, A. (2002). Parkinson-like neurodegeneration induced by targeted overexpression of alpha-synuclein in the nigrostriatal system. *J Neurosci*, 22:2780-2791.

189. Von Coelln, R., Thomas, B., Savitt, J.M., Lim, K.L., Sasaki, M., Hess, E.J., Dawson, V.L., and Dawson, T.M. (2004). Loss of locus coeruleus neurons and reduced startle in parkin null mice. *Proc Natl Acad Sci USA*, 101:10744-10749.

190. Perez, F.A. and Palmiter, R.D. (2005). Parkin-deficient mice are not a robust model of parkinsonism. *Proc Natl Acad Sci USA*, 102:2174-2179.

191. Itier, J.M., Ibanez, P., Mena, M.A., Abbas, N., Cohen-Salmon, C., Bohme, G.A., Laville, M., Pratt, J., Corti, O., Pradier, L., Ret, G., Joubert, C., Periquet, M., Araujo, F., Negroni, J., Casarejos, M.J., Canals, S., Solano, R., Serrano, A., Gallego, E., Sanchez, M., Denefle, P., Benavides, J., Tremp, G., Rooney, T.A., Brice, A., and Garcia De, Y. (2003). JParkin gene inactivation alters behaviour and dopamine neurotransmission in the mouse. *Hum Mol Genet*, 12:2277-2291.

192. Palacino, J.J., Sagi, D., Goldberg, M.S., Krauss, S., Motz, C., Wacker, M., Klose, J., and Shen, J. (2004). Mitochondrial dysfunction and oxidative damage in parkin-deficient mice. *J Biol Chem*, 279:18614-18622.

193. Sato, S., Chiba, T., Nishiyama, S., Kakiuchi, T., Tsukada, H., Hatano, T., Fukuda, T., Yasoshima, Y., Kai, N., Kobayashi, K., Mizuno, Y., Tanaka, K., and Hattori, N. (2006). Decline of striatal dopamine release in parkin-deficient mice shown by *ex vivo* autoradiography. *J Neurosci Res*, 84:1350-1357.

194. Lu, X., Fleming, S.M., Chesselet, M.F., and Yang, W.X. (2006). A novel BAC transgenic mouse model of overexpressing human mutant parkin in dopaminergic neurons. *Neurosci Abst*, 612:3.

195. Chen, L., Cagniard, B., Mathews, T., Jones, S., Koh, H., Ding, Y.C., Carvey, P., Ling, Z.M., Kang, U., and Zhuang, X.J. (2005). Age-dependent motor deficits and dopaminergic dysfunction in DJ-1 null mice. *J Biol Chem*, 280:21418-21426.

196. Goldberg, M.S., Pisani, A., Haburcak, M., Vortherms, T.A., Kitada, T., Costa, C., Tong, Y., Martella, G., Tscherter, A., Martins, A., Bernardi, G., Roth, B., Pothos L, E.N., Calabresi, P., and Shen, J. (2005). Nigrostriatal dopaminergic deficits and hypokinesia caused by inactivation of the familial Parkinsonism-linked gene DJ-1. *Neuron*, 45:489–496.

197. Kim, R.H., Smith, P.D., Aleyasin, H., Hayley, S., Mount, M.P., Pownall, S., Wakeham, A., You-Ten, A.J., Kalia, S.K., Horne, P., Westaway, D., Lozano, A.M., Anisman, H., Park, D.S., and Mak, T.W. (2005). Hypersensitivity of DJ-1-deficient mice to 1-methyl-4-phenyl-1,2,3,6-tetra-hydropyrindine (MPTP) and oxidative stress. *Proc Natl Acad Sci USA*, 102:5215–5220.

198. Manning-Bog, A.B., Caudle, W.M., Perez, X.A., Reaney, S.H., Paletzki, R., Isla, M.Z., Chou, V.P., McCormack, A.L., Miller, G.W., Langston, J.W., Gerfen, C.r., Di Monte, D.A. Increased vulnerability of nigrostriatal terminals in dj-1-deficient mice is mediated by the dopamine transporter, *Neurobiol Dis*, 27(2):141–150.

199. Zhou, H., Falkenburger, B.H., Schulz, J.B., Tieu, K., Xu, Z., and Xia, X. (2007). Silencing of the *Pink1* gene expression by conditional RNAi does not induce dopaminergic neuron death in mice. *Int J Biol Sci*, 3:242–250.

200. Yang, Y., Gehrke, S., Imai, Y., Huang, Z., Ouyang, Y., Wang, J.W., Beal, L., Yang, M.F., Vogel, H., and Lu, B. (2006). Mitochondrial pathology and muscle and dopaminergic neuron degeneration caused by inactivation of Drosophila Pink1 is rescued by Parkin. *Proc Natl Acad Sci USA*, 103:10793–10798.

201. Cookson, M.R. (2005). The biochemistry of Parkinson's disease. *Ann Rev Biochem*, 74:29–52.

202. Olanow, C.W., Anthony, H., Schapira, V., LeWitt, P.A., Kieburtz, K., Sauer, D., Olivieri, G., Pohlmann, H., and Hubble, J. (2006). TCH346 as a neuroprotective drug in Parkinson's disease: A double-blind, randomised, controlled trial. *Lancet Neurol*, 5:1013–1020.

203. Waldmeier, P., Donna Bozyczko-Coyne, B., Michael Williams, B., and Jeffry Vaught, L. (2006). Recent clinical failures in Parkinson's disease with apoptosis inhibitors underline the need for a paradigm shift in drug discovery for neurodegenerative diseases. *Biochem Pharmacol*, 72:1197–1206.

204. Lang, A.E., Gill, S., Patel, N.K., Lozano, A., Nutt, J.G., Penn, R., Brooks, D.J., Hotton, G., Moro, E., Heywood, P., Brodsky, M.A., Burchiel, K., Kelly, P., Dalvi, A., Scott, B., Stacy, M., Turner, D., Wooten, V.G., Elias, W.J., Laws, E.R., Dhawan, V., Stoessl, A.J., Matcham, J., Coffey, R.J., and Traub, M. (2006). Randomized controlled trial of intraputamenal glial cell line-derived neurotrophic factor infusion in Parkinson disease. *Ann Neurol*, 59:459–466.

205. Saporito, M.S., Hudkins, R.L., and Maroney, A.C. (2002). Discovery of CEP-1347/KT-7515, an inhibitor of the JNK/SAPK pathway for the treatment of neurodegenerative diseases. *Prog. Med Chem*, 40:23–62.

206. Andringa, G., van Oosten, R.V., Unger, W. *et al.* (2000). Systemic administration of the propargylamine CGP 3466B prevents behavioural and morphological deficits in rats with 6-hydroxydopamine-induced lesions in the substantia nigra. *Eur J Neurosci*, 12:3033–3043.

207. Andringa, G., Eshuis, S., and Perentes, E. (2003). TCH346 prevents motor symptoms and loss of striatal FDOPA uptake in bilaterally MPTP treated primates. *Neurobiol Dis*, 14:205–217.

208. Kordower, J.H., Emborg, M.E., Bloch, J., Ma, S.Y., Chu, Y., Leventhal, L., McBride, J., Chen, E.Y., Palfi, S., Roitberg, B.Z., Brown, W.D., Holden, J.E., Pyzalski, R., Taylor, M.D., Carvey, P., Ling, Z., Trono, D., Hantraye, P., Deglon, N., and Aebischer, P. (2000). Neurodegeneration prevented by lentiviral vector delivery of GDNF in primate models of Parkinson's disease. *Science*, 290:767–773.

209. Ai, Y., Markesbery, W., Zhang, Z., Grondin, R., Elseberry, D., Gerhardt, G.A., and Gash, D.M. (2003). Intraputamenal infusion of GDNF in aged rhesus monkeys: Distribution and dopaminergic effects. *J Comp Neurol*, 461:250–261.

210. Gash, D.M., Zhang, Z., and Gerhardt, G. (1998). Neuroprotective and neurorestorative properties of GDNF. *Ann Neurol*, 44:S121–S125.

211. Kirik, D., Georgievska, B., and Bjorklund, A. (2004). Localized striatal delivery of GDNF as a treatment for Parkinson disease. *Nature Neurosci*, 7:105–110.

212. Gill, S.S., Patel, N.K., Hotton, G.R. *et al.* (2003). Direct brain infusion of glial cell line-derived neurotrophic factor in Parkinson disease. *Nat Med*, 9:589–595.

213. Slevin, J.T., Gerhardt, G.A., Smith, C.D., Gash, D.M., Kryscio, R., and Young, B. (2005). Improvement of bilateral motor functions in patients with Parkinson disease through the unilateral intraputaminal infusion of glial cell line-derived neurotrophic factor. *J Neurosurgery*, 102:216–222.

214. Salvatore, M.F., Ai, Y., Fischer, B., Zhang, A.M., Grondin, R.C., Zhang, Z., Gerhardt, G.A., and Gash, D.M. (2006). Point source concentration of GDNF may explain failure of phase II clinical trial. *Exper Neurol*, 202:497–505.

215. Hardy, J., Cai, H., Cookson, M., Gwinn-Hardy, K., and Singleton, A. (2006). Genetics of and Parkinsonism. *Ann Neurol*, 60:389–398.

216. Park, J., Lee, S.B., Lee, S., Kim, Y., Song, S., Kim, S., Bae, E., Kim, J., Shong, M., Kim, J.M., and Chung, J. (2006). Mitochondrial dysfunction in Drosophila PINK1 mutants is complemented by parkin. *Nature*, 441:1157–1161.

217. Clark, I.E., Dodson, M.W., Jiang, C., Cao, J.H., Huh, J.R., Seol, J.H., Yoo, S.J., Hay, B.A., and Guo, M. (2006). Drosophila pink1 is required for mitochondrial function and interacts genetically with parkin. *Nature*, 441:1162–1166.

218. Cooper, A.A., Gitler, A.D., Cashikar, A., Haynes, C.M., Hill, K.J., Bhullar, B., Liu, K., Xu, K., Strathearn, K.E., Liu, F., Cao, S., Caldwell, K.A., Caldwell, G.A., Marsischky, G., Kolodner, R.D., Labaer, J., Rochet, J.C., Bonini, N.M., and Lindquist, S. (2006). Alpha-synuclein blocks ER-Golgi traffic and Rab1 rescues neuron loss in Parkinson's models. *Science*, 313:324–328.

219. Springer, W., Hoppe, T., Schmidt, E., and Baumeister, R. (2005). A Caenorhabditis elegans Parkin mutant with altered solubility couples α-synuclein aggregation to proteotoxic stress. *Human Molecular Genetics*, 14:3407–3423.

220. Meulener, M., Whitworth, A.J., Armstrong-Gold, C.E. *et al.* (2005). Drosophila DJ-1 mutants are selectively sensitive to environmental toxins associated with Parkinson's disease. *Curr Biol*, 15:1572–1577.

221. Miller, R.M., Kiser, G.L., Kaysser-Kranich, T., Casaceli, C., Colla, E., Lee, M.K., Palaniappan, C., and Federoff, H.J. (2007). Wild-type and mutant α-synuclein induce a multi-component gene expression profile consistent with shared pathophysiology in different transgenic mouse models of PD. *Exper Neurol*, 204:421–432.

222. Lund, S., Na, H.M., Taylor, G., Bence, N.F., Kopito, R., Seo, B.B., Yagi, T., Yagi, A., Klinefelter, G., Cookson, M.R., and Greenamyre, J.T. (2006). Intersecting pathways to neurodegeneration in: Effects of the pesticide rotenone on DJ-1, alpha-synuclein, and the ubiquitin-proteasome system. *Neurobiol Dis*, 22:404–420.

223. Stephenson, D.T., Childs, M.A., Li, Q., Carvajal-Gonzalez, S., Opsahl, A., Tengowski, M., Meglasson, M.D., Merchant, K.M., and Emborg, M.E. (2007). Differential loss of presynaptic dopaminergic markers in Parkinsonian monkeys. *Cell Transplantation*, 16:229–244.

CHAPTER 6

Huntington Disease

Laura A. Wagner[1], Liliana Menalled[2], Alexander D. Goumeniouk[3], Daniela Brunner[2,4] and Blair R. Leavitt[1]

[1]Centre for Molecular Medicine and Therapeutics, Child and Family Research Institute, BC Children's Hospital, Department of Medical Genetics, University of British Columbia, Vancouver, BC, Canada
[2]PsychoGenics Inc., Tarrytown, NY, USA
[3]Department of Psychiatry, Department of Pharmacology and Therapeutics, University of British Columbia, Vancouver, BC, Canada
[4]Biopsychology Department, New York State Psychiatric Institute/Columbia University, New York, USA

Animal and Translational Models for CNS Drug Discovery,
Vol. 2 of 3: Neurological Disorders
Robert McArthur and Franco Borsini (eds), Academic Press, 2008

INTRODUCTION

Huntington Disease (HD) is a hereditary neurodegenerative disorder that is characterized by a triad of motor, cognitive, and psychiatric symptoms, which begin insidiously and progress over many years, eventually leading to death. HD is an autosomal dominant disorder, and each offspring of an affected individual has a 50% chance of inheriting the disease-causing allele. George Huntington was only 8 years old when he first observed patients with hereditary chorea; riding with his father (a physician) on his professional rounds around East Hampton, Long Island.[1] At the age of 21, George Huntington summarized the cardinal features of the disease that now bears his name in a report entitled "On Chorea," which appeared in the Medical and Surgical Reporter of Philadelphia on April 13, 1872.[2] This concise treatise outlined the distinctive choreiform movement disorder, the distinct hereditary nature of the chorea, and the frequent association of the chorea with psychiatric disease ("a tendency to insanity and suicide").

Initially there was considerable debate in the neurological literature about the validity of hereditary chorea as a distinct disorder, but the clinical entity was rapidly accepted and disseminated by the great Canadian physician Sir William Osler, and the name Huntington's chorea quickly gained acceptance as the eponymic designation of the disorder.[3] In 1983, the genetic defect in HD was mapped to chromosome 4p16.3,[4] and 10 years later linkage analysis identified an expansion in a CAG trinucleotide repeat region of the *HD gene* (initially called IT15) that was found to be the genetic mutation that causes HD.[5]

CLINICAL PRESENTATION OF HD

Signs and Symptoms

HD is found in populations around the world, with a prevalence as high as 1 in 10,000 in some populations of European ancestry, but up to a 10-fold reduced prevalence rate for HD in individuals of Asian or African descent.[6] The age of onset of HD is usually in the fourth or fifth decade, but is highly variable. The movement disorder in HD consists of both abnormal involuntary movements such as chorea and dystonia, as well as abnormalities of voluntary movement such as abnormal eye movements, bradykinesia (slowed voluntary movements), rigidity, dysphagia, dysarthria, and gait disturbance. Chorea, the hallmark clinical manifestation of HD, can be described as rapid irregular jerking, dancing or writhing movements of the face, limbs or trunk. Akathisia, an extremely uncomfortable internal sense of restlessness, often accompanies chorea. Many early-stage HD patients are not aware of their chorea, and appear to have little functional impairment at this stage. Early in the course of HD, chorea, hypotonia, and hyper-reflexia usually predominate, but as the disease progresses, rigidity and bradykinesia become progressively more severe and functional impairment increases.[7]

Juvenile-onset HD occurs in about 5–10% of patients and is characterized by onset under the age of 20 years. Classic juvenile HD often has an akinetic-rigid presentation with early and predominant spasticity, bradykinesia, and dystonia (the Westphal variant of HD) that is often complicated by myoclonus and seizures. Seizures are reported to occur in up to one-third of juvenile HD patients, but no increased frequency of seizures compared to the general population has ever been demonstrated in adult-onset HD.[8] Parkinsonian features may be the earliest abnormalities in juvenile-onset HD and often make clinical diagnosis difficult especially if no family history of HD is present. Chorea is a variable finding in Juvenile HD and often may not be present at all during the course of the illness. Rapid intellectual deterioration and school failures, apathy, personality changes, irritability, and violence are common features in Juvenile HD.

Cognitive defects in HD usually progress at a similar rate to the motor disturbances and memory recall is generally affected more than memory storage.[9] Cognitive changes usually begin with a subtle slowing of intellectual processes, personality changes, disinhibition, and reduced mental flexibility, but will eventually develop into a slowly progressive "subcortical dementia".[10] This form of dementia displays prominent and early loss of cognitive speed, flexibility, and concentration but aphasia and agnosia are uncommon.

George Huntington in his original description of the disorder identified "a tendency to insanity and suicide" in individuals with hereditary chorea.[2] Neuropsychiatric symptoms such as depression, apathy, suicidal ideation, and anxiety are common manifestations of HD, and can occur at any point in the course of the illness with little correlation to the stage of illness or motor progression.[11] Obsessive–compulsive symptoms and psychosis are relatively rare but can occur in HD as well. The presence of specific psychiatric features in HD often tends to run in families suggesting a role for environmental effects or genetic factors other than the HD mutation are involved.[12]

Common systemic features of HD include testicular degeneration,[13] sleep and circadian rhythm disorders,[14] and weight loss. Cachexia is an almost invariant feature of HD with a marked loss of body weight occurring as the disease progresses. The weight loss appears to be independent of dysphagia and occurs despite the maintenance of a normal caloric intake.[15] This has been taken as evidence that an underlying metabolic dysfunction may be involved in the basic pathogenesis of HD,[16] but direct evidence to confirm this hypothesis has been difficult to obtain.[17]

The formal diagnosis of HD remains clinical, and depends on the presence of a defined movement disorder (unexplained extrapyramidal movement disorder) in a patient with a family history of HD. The clinical diagnosis is generally confirmed by diagnostic testing for the gene mutation that causes HD.

Genetics of HD

HD is a monogenic disorder with autosomal dominant inheritance and the unusual non-mendelian feature of anticipation. The underlying genetic defect in HD is an expanded CAG trinucleotide repeat sequence in exon 1 of the HD gene that encodes for an expanded polyglutamine stretch near the N-terminus of the huntingtin (Htt) protein. Polyglutamine expanded mutant Htt protein appears to have altered physical and functional properties leading to a dominant toxic gain of function, although a role for loss of normal Htt function in HD pathogenesis remains a possibility. Expanded HD alleles containing greater than 35 CAG repeats are associated with selective neurodegeneration in specific brain regions and eventual development of the clinical phenotype of HD. A strong inverse correlation exists between the size of the CAG expansion and the age of onset (defined by motor signs) with earlier age of onset occurring with larger repeat sizes.[18] Overall, the CAG repeat size accounts for approximately 60–75% of the variance in age of onset. This relationship is complex, with greater variance in age of onset seen at lower CAG repeat sizes and less variance at higher CAG repeat sizes.[19]

Due to the inverse correlation of CAG repeat length with the age of onset of HD symptoms, CAG repeat sizes between 36 and 39 are associated with very late onset, leading to the appearance of reduced penetrance for this repeat range.[20] The CAG trinucleotide repeats expansion in the HD gene is a dynamic mutation with large CAG repeats sizes exhibiting greater instability. The CAG repeat in the HD gene is unstable during somatic development and during vertical transmission of the gene from parent to child. The unstable nature of the CAG expansion in HD provides the molecular basis for the clinical phenomenon of anticipation, defined as decreasing age of onset, or increasing severity of disease in successive generations. Intermediate alleles, defined as 27-35 CAG repeats, are not associated with a risk of developing HD, but can rarely expand into the pathogenic range during intergenerational transmission to cause HD in an offspring.[21] These intergenerational expansions from intermediate alleles often are identified as new HD probands (without a family history), and are more common than previously thought-being responsible for up to 10% of all HD cases.[22] Paternal transmission of the CAG repeat allele is more likely to result in expansion rather than contraction of the CAG repeat length and the majority of juvenile HD cases occur are due to paternal transmission of a large expanded allele.[23]

Neuropathology of HD

The hallmark neuropathological feature of HD is early and relatively selective neuronal loss in the caudate and putamen (collectively known as the striatum). Within the caudate, the medium-sized spiny neurons are selectively vulnerable to neurodegeneration in HD,[24] and cell loss tends to occur in a caudal to rostral pattern.[25] The enkephalinergic medium spiny neurons of the indirect striatal pathway are lost initially and then the substance P expressing medium spiny neurons of the direct pathway degenerate.[26] These neurons receive massive excitatory (glutamatergic) inputs from wide areas of neocortex and thalamus, and make efferent inhibitory projections (GABAergic) to the globus pallidus and substantia nigra.[27]

The other major cell type of the striatum, the aspiny cholinergic interneurons, are relatively resistant to degeneration in HD. Loss of pyramidal projection neurons in layers V and VI of the cerebral cortex[28] and the CA1 region of hippocampus[29] are also features of the selective neuronal cell death in HD. With disease progression degenerative changes generalize and include other brain regions such as the globus pallidus, and hypothalamus, subthalamic nucleus, substantia nigra, and thalamus.[24] Neurodegeneration in juvenile HD is less selective and cell loss is more generalized even in early stages of disease and can include cell loss in the cerebellum, a brain region usually relatively spared in HD.[30]

Nuclear and cytoplasmic intracellular inclusions are also a pathologic feature of HD and the other polyglutamine diseases; these inclusions are insoluble, ubiquitinated protein aggregates that sequester a variety of cellular proteins including full-length and truncated fragments of Htt. The presence of neuronal intranuclear Htt inclusions was first definitively recognized in transgenic mice.[31] Subsequent immunohistochemical analyses demonstrated the presence of neuronal Htt inclusions in post-mortem brain material from HD patients[32] and patients with other polyglutamine disorders.[33] Despite the presence of aggregates in these disorders their role in the pathogenesis of HD is unclear. In juvenile-onset HD, intranuclear inclusions are much more widespread and are present at earlier stages than in adult-onset HD.[32]

Pathogenic Mechanisms

Based on the well-defined clinical manifestations, genetics, and neuropathology of HD, any proposed mechanisms of HD pathogenesis must account for the regional selectivity of the neuropathology despite widespread expression of the mutant protein, include age-related factors that contribute to the late onset of the disease, and must explain the inverse correlation between age of onset and CAG repeat expansion size. Cellular changes observed in neurons expressing mutant Htt converge upon increased sensitivity to excitotoxicity and altered intracellular calcium homeostasis leading to the initiation of cell death pathways. Proteolysis of the Htt protein and the role of Htt aggregation and inclusion formation are also important features of HD that must be accounted for. Additional effects of mutant Htt observed in a variety of neuronal and other cell types include evidence for alterations in ubiquitin–proteasome system function, mitochondrial dysfunction, impaired axonal transport, and transcriptional dysregulation.[34]

Many years prior to the discovery of the causative mutation in the *HD gene,* it was found that injection of glutamate receptor agonists could reproduce many of the neurochemical, neuropathological, and behavioral features of HD in rodents and in non-human primates.[34,35] Recent studies in a mouse model expressing full-length human mutant Htt provided the first direct link between mutant Htt and increased intracellular calcium levels and sensitivity to glutamate excitotoxicity in HD.[36] In contrast to results, mouse models of HD that express only short fragments of mutant Htt have not shown enhanced vulnerability to glutamate-mediated excitotoxicity.[37] These data suggest that enhanced excitotoxicity is associated with expression of the full-length mutant HD gene, and are consistent with the hypothesis that glutamate-mediated excitotoxicity plays a role in selective striatal degeneration, since full-length transgenic mice show selective degeneration of striatal neurons similar to the neuropathology observed in human HD.[38,39]

In addition to the strong evidence for glutamate-mediated excitotoxicity in HD, there is data to indicate that other cellular pathways may also lead to altered neuronal calcium homeostasis. Mitochondria isolated from fibroblasts of humans with HD or the brains of full-length transgenic mice exhibit increased resting calcium, more depolarized resting membrane potentials, and lower thresholds for the calcium-induced permeability transition pore formation.[40] These mutant-Htt-mediated changes in mitochondrial function suggest that stimuli that increase neuronal intracellular calcium, including glutamate-mediated excitotoxicity, will have enhanced toxicity. An interaction between mutant Htt and inositol-3-phosphate receptors leading to an increased receptor sensitivity and increased calcium release has also been described.[41]

Intracellular inclusion bodies containing aggregated mutant Htt protein have been demonstrated in human HD brains, in transgenic rodent models of HD, and in cell cultures expressing mutant Htt.[31,32,42] These inclusions bodies can be found in the neuritis, cytoplasm and nucleus of neurons and contain ubiquitinated Htt and other proteins.[32] Htt aggregates have been suggested to impair many cellular functions including neurotransmitter release,[43,44] axonal transport[45,46] and may cause sequestration of transcription factors leading to a generalized dysregulation of gene transcription.[47]

The discovery of Htt inclusions initially suggested a direct role in HD pathogenesis[48] and prompted considerable work developing therapies to slow or prevent their formation, but the relevance of inclusions in HD is far from clear.[49] The distribution of inclusions in HD brain does not correlate well with regions of neuronal loss.[50,51] In several model systems, manipulations that decrease Htt inclusions actually promote cellular toxicity suggesting that the formation of inclusions of mutant Htt in cells may be part of a protective response to the misfolded mutant protein.[52,53] Despite these findings, no studies have yet been able to refute the hypothesis that aggregation at the submicroscopic level, in the form of soluble oligomers, may be the critical molecular species in HD pathogenesis.

A significant amount of evidence suggests that full-length mutant Htt undergoes proteolysis into smaller N-terminal fragments that are readily able to translocate to the nucleus and form oligomers.[54] Htt has been demonstrated to undergo proteolysis by a variety of enzymes including the caspases, calpains, and aspartyl proteases. Recent studies of full-length transgenic mice expressing mutant Htt modified to eliminate cleavage by a specific protease-caspase-6 – had complete amelioration of the HD behavioral and neuropathologic phenotype normally seen in this mouse model. In addition, striatal neurons from these caspase-6-resistant transgenic mice did not show increased sensitivity to glutamate-mediated excitotoxicity.[55] Together, these findings suggest a critical role for caspase-6 mediated cleavage of mutant Htt in HD pathogenesis, but it is clear that mutant Htt has a number of toxic effects in neurons and disrupts a wide variety of cellular functions in HD.

TREATMENT OPTIONS IN HD

While HD remains incurable, there are numerous pharmacotherapeutic options available, and judicious use of symptomatic agents can greatly improve the quality of life of patients and their care-givers.[56] These include treatments aimed at the symptom domains of HD and at altering its progression. In addition to the primary symptom domains of motor, psychiatric (behavioral), and cognitive symptoms, therapeutic strategies are available to address other specific symptoms affecting quality of life such as insomnia and weight loss. Unfortunately there is a dearth of quality evidence for treatments other than those focused on motor symptoms. Furthermore, even these controlled trials usually restrict the primary outcome measure to reduction of chorea. Nonetheless, the emergence of new agents, the novel or "atypical" antipsychotics most notably, has lead to the reporting of favorable effects in the form of small series of patients experiencing benefits in a variety of areas. No drug has been shown to improve cognitive dysfunction in HD, but clinical experience has shown that standard pharmacotherapy is generally very effective for the various neuropsychiatric manifestations in HD: depressed or obsessive–compulsive patients may respond to selective serotonin reuptake inhibitors (SSRIs) or the newer atypical antidepressant medications; benzodiazepines are useful adjuncts in anxious or agitated patients, and psychotic symptoms generally respond well to both classic and atypical neuroleptics (see below). Patients likely benefit from a multidisciplinary clinical approach including psychosocial, physical, speech, and occupational therapy. Supportive counseling for family members may also be helpful.

In terms of treatments altering disease progression, several compounds including riluzole, ethyl-eicosapentanoic acid, creatine, coenzyme Q10, and lamotrigine have been investigated in a randomized controlled fashion (see under section, "Disease modifying treatments"). Other compounds have been reported on as well. While it is beyond the scope of a discussion of pharmacotherapy, other therapeutic modalities such as transcranial magnetic stimulation (TMS), deep brain stimulation (DBS), and stem cells may prove to have a role modifying HD.

Symptomatic Treatments

Motor Symptoms

The motor symptoms of HD can be classified as being involuntary or manifesting themselves during voluntary acts. The former consist primarily of chorea while dystonia, rigidity, bradykinesia, abnormal gait, impaired balance, and fine motor control may cause difficulty with patients' voluntary movements such as walking, eating, and swallowing. The evidence for treatments of HD that is either randomized and/or controlled almost exclusively focuses on chorea as the primary endpoint.[57] This is particularly interesting insofar as chorea may be neither the first symptom to appear[58] nor subjectively distressing.[59]

The treatment of chorea in HD patients is achieved mainly by manipulating dopaminergic neurotransmission. This can be through using dopamine antagonists (such as the neuroleptics and atypical antipsychotics) or dopamine depleting compounds of which tetrabenazine is the prototypic agent.

Haloperidol (Haldol®) has been shown to improve chorea[60] in doses up to 10 mg/day. Olanzapine (Zyprexa®) demonstrated behavioral but not antichoreic effects at low doses (5 mg/day)[61] whereas high doses (30 mg/day) had significant effects reducing chorea by as much as 50%.[62]

Typical neuroleptics are associated with extrapyramidal symptoms and can therefore cause rigidity, dystonia, and bradykinesia.[63] Prolonged use is associated with abnormal involuntary movement disorders such as tardive dyskinesia.[63] Care must therefore be taken to distinguish HD motor symptoms from drug-induced side effects. The atypical antipsychotics are less prone to causing extrapyramidal side effects but are associated with an increased incidence of metabolic dysregulation such as weight gain, glucose abnormalities and dyslipidemia.[64]

The catecholamine-depleting effects of tetrabenazine are achieved by blocking VMAT-2, the vesicular monoamine transporter in the CNS. The efficacy of this compound has been demonstrated in HD patients.[65] As an attendant consequence of the mechanism of action of tetrabenazine, depression (a condition associated with monoamine depletion) is a potential side effect of its use. A previous history of depression may predict this side effect[66] which requires close clinical monitoring. Other side effects include somnolence and parkinsonism.[67]

Non-dopaminergic strategies with some benefit in reducing chorea include the benzodiazepines, including clonazepam (Klonopin®;[68,69]). These compounds have the risk of developing dependence and tolerance as well as causing cognitive and motor impairment.[67] Amantadine has also been shown in a randomized controlled trial to have an effect reducing chorea by 36–56% with reduction corresponding to plasma level but not CAG repeat length.[70] This effect is presumed by the authors to be due to amantadine's NMDA receptor antagonist effects.[70]

Cognitive Symptoms

As there are no randomized controlled trials with the assessment of cognitive function as a primary endpoint, this is an area which future research must address. Cognitive symptoms common in HD include specific deficits in such areas as attention, short-term memory and processing speed through more global problems such as executive dysfunction and impulsivity.[71]

The NMDA receptor antagonist/partial agonist memantine (Namenda®) was studied over 24 months in 27 patients in an open fashion. A trend toward delaying cognitive decline was seen.[72] Only small open studies and case reports exist for the cholinesterase inhibitors rivastigmine (Exelon®[73]), galantamine (Reminyl®[74]), and donepezil (Aricept®[75]).

Psychiatric Symptoms

HD patients exhibit the full spectrum of psychopathology seen in adult psychiatry.[71] Disorders amenable to pharmacotherapy include anxiety, depression, bipolar disorder, psychosis, and aggression. As there is no randomized controlled data to support the use of any specific agent in psychiatric syndromes in HD patients, conventional therapies will be listed with any particular aspects relevant to HD noted.

Aggression is also a common occurrence in HD patients. In one study, over 60% of 960 outpatients at a HD clinic reported a history of aggressive behavior at their baseline visit.[76] While there are reports of the use of neuroleptics such as haloperidol in the treatment of aggressive behavior,[77] Goedhard *et al.* reviewed this topic in general adult patients and concluded that atypical antipsychotics are superior to neuroleptics.[78] In HD patients, olanzapine showed a beneficial effect in reducing irritability.[79] Similarly, quetiapine (Seroquel®) improved agitation and irritability in a series of 5 HD patients without any motor effects.[80] Sodium valproate (Depakote®) was shown retrospectively to benefit dementia-related behavior problems in the elderly.[81] In view of the frequency of aggression in HD, anti-aggressive treatments warrant further controlled investigation.

Other Issues

The issue of weight loss in HD patients, particularly with significant chorea, can be a serious matter. Some of the aforementioned treatments are associated with weight gain. These include the atypical antipsychotics, most notably olanzapine and clozapine (Clozaril®[82]). The antidepressants paroxetine (Paxil®[83]) and mirtazapine (Remeron®[84]) also tend to cause weight gain in a significant percentage of patients. When caloric supplementation is inadequate and a psychiatric condition is comorbid, it may be a reasonable adjunctive measure to select a psychotropic associated with weight gain. A similar rationale would exist for psychiatric conditions and insomnia. Many agents used to treat psychiatric illness cause sedation (see Table 6.1). This may be advantageous particularly when the dosing is once daily at bedtime. The benzodiazepine clonazepam has been shown to have some antichoreic benefits[68,69] and may therefore be a reasonable choice in certain patients. Finally, to the extent that apathy and executive dysfunction may be caused by noradrenergic and dopaminergic dysregulation,[85] agents which modulate these neurotransmitters such as bupropion (Wellbutrin®), atomoxetine (Strattera®), modafinil (Provigil®), and pramipexole (Mirapex®) may warrant adequate clinical testing.

Disease Modifying Treatments

Insofar as HD is currently incurable, strategies and treatments aimed at altering the course and specifically slowing the progression of the illness have been investigated over the past decade. These include vitamin E (alpha-tocopherol),[86] lamotrigine

Table 6.1 Psychopharmacologic treatments[a]

Indication	Treatments	Special HD circumstances
Anxiety	SRI antidepressants	(+) treats comorbid depression
	Benzodiazepines	(−) dependence, tolerance (−) ataxia, cognitive impairment (+) antichoreic (clonazepam)
	Propranolol	(+) physical anxiety symptoms, tremor
Depression	SRI antidepressants	(+) anxiolytic (+) normalization of circadian rhythms
	Venlafaxine	(+) anxiolytic
	Mirtazapine	(+/−) sedating (+/−) weight gain
	Bupropion	(+/−) activating (+/−) no weight gain
	Amitriptyline	anticholinergic, (+/−) (−)sedating, (−) postural hypotension
Bipolar disorder	Lithium	need to be compliant and hydrated (+) ? neuroprotective
	Olanzapine	(+/−) weight gain (+) antipsychotic (+) antichoreic
	Quetiapine	(+/−) weight gain (+) antipsychotic (+/−) sedating, (−) postural hypotension
	Aripiprazole	(+) antipsychotic
	risperidone	(+) antipsychotic (+) antichoreic
Psychosis	Haloperidol	(+) antichoreic (+/−) sedating
	Chlorpromazine	(+/−) sedating
	Atypical antipsychotics	see bipolar disorder

SRI antidepressants include fluoxetine, paroxetine, citalopram, escitalopram, fluvoxamine, sertraline
(+) = benefit; (−) = detriment
[a]*Adapted from [63].*

(Lamictal®[87]), coenzyme Q10 and remacemide,[88] riluzole,[89] ethyl-eicosapentanoic acid (eEPA),[90] and creatine.[91]

The trial conducted by Peyser *et al.*[86] of D-alpha-tocopherol was placebo-controlled (*n* = 73) for a 1 year duration and failed to show any benefit to HD patients in terms of modifying chorea progression. Lamotrigine, a drug which inhibits the release of the potentially neuroexcitotoxic neurotransmitter glutamate, was investigated in a double-blinded placebo-controlled trial ($n = 64$) in HD patients with motor signs of less than 5 years duration for a study period of 30 months.[87] While there was no clear evidence that lamotrigine retarded HD progression objectively, 53.6% of treated patients reported symptomatic improvement (versus 14.8% of placebo treated, $P < 0.006$). There was a trend toward decreased chorea in the treated group ($P < 0.08$). A randomized, placebo-controlled, double-blind, 2×2 factorial trial of coenzyme Q10 (300 mg twice daily), remacemide (200 mg three times daily), both of these treatments or placebo was conducted with evaluations to 30 months ($n = 347$).[88] Patients were in stages I or II of illness with a total functional capacity (TFC) of 7 or higher. The primary outcome measure (slowing of decline in TFC) was not significantly affected by either (or both) treatments. There was a trend in slowing TFC decline (13%; 2.40 versus 2.74 point declines, $P < 0.15$) in the coenzyme Q10 group versus placebo.

Riluzole (Rilutek®), which decreases striatal glutamate and its neuroexcitotoxic consequences in animal models of HD showed some promise in an 8 week double-blind trial ($n = 63$) in reducing chorea.[89] Subjects received riluzole 100 mg/day or 200 mg/day or placebo. The 200 mg/day group showed a significant reduction in chorea and UHDRS total motor score (without improving TFC) at only 8 weeks. Nineteen subjects however had liver transaminase (ALT) elevations, seven of which were between 2 and 5 times the upper limit of normal. While the benefit to chorea over this comparatively short time frame is significant, the ALT elevations would require ongoing hepatic monitoring and might ultimately herald an unfavorable cost-benefit situation.

A series of case reports of an investigational product containing eicosapentanoic acid (EPA) lead to a randomized double-blind, placebo-controlled trial of ethyl-EPA.[90] Subjects received either placebo or 2 g of ethyl-EPA per day ($n = 135$) for 12 months. The UHDRS was used for assessment with the primary outcome measure being the Total Motor Score 4 subscale (TMS-4). One hundred twenty-two patients completed 12 months, 83 of these without any protocol violation ("per protocol group"). While the intent-to-treat (ITT) group which included all subjects randomized to treatment, showed no significant difference between eEPA and placebo on TMS-4, the per protocol group showed a significantly higher number of patients treated with eEPA to have stable or improved motor function. While the mechanism of action is uncertain, eEPA may stabilize mitochondrial function. Further investigation is ongoing.

Creatine is another compound, which may, among other things, stabilize mitochondrial function. Creatine was studied in a randomized, double-blind, placebo-controlled trial ($n = 64$) in which subjects received placebo or 8 g/day of creatine for 16 weeks.[91] It was found to be well tolerated and safe as well as bioavailable to the CNS. While UHDRS measures were unchanged compared to placebo, the trial was relatively short (16 weeks). Serum 8-hydroxy-2-deoxyguanosine (8OH2′dG), which are a marker of oxidative injury to DNA, were markedly elevated in HD patients at baseline (compared to normal subjects) and were significantly reduced in the HD patients who received creatine. Longer trials may prove this to be a biomarker for creatine's role in HD in regards to oxidative injury.

The authors of these trials and reviews of this area of disease modifying treatments[92] have correctly commented that most of these trials have been either underpowered or too short (or both) to detect clinically meaningful effects. Longer, larger studies may correct this.[i]

Other neuropsychiatric treatments, both traditional and novel, may hold promise. Lithium as a neuroprotective[93] agent has not been systematically evaluated in HD patients. The effect of antidepressants and atypical antipsychotics on brain-derived neurotrophic factor (BDNF)[94] may be currently contributing an unmeasured benefit to HD patients. Slow repetitive transcranial magnetic stimulation (1 Hz rTMS) has been shown to decrease chorea in HD patients.[95] The anticonvulsant levetiracetam (Keppra®) has been evaluated in an open trial and found to reduce chorea (but not improve TFC) in 22 patients.[96] Clearly more controlled trials of these treatments are warranted.

Clinical Conclusion

HD waits for a genetically mediated cure. In the meantime, treatments are available aimed at decreasing symptoms and improving quality of life. Unfortunately, other than chorea, few have good quality evidence to support their use. This is particularly true for psychiatric syndromes which, although extremely prevalent in HD, are virtually unexamined in any rigorous fashion.[92] Disease altering treatments have been limited by their power and duration but nonetheless have shown glimpses of promise. Larger, longer trials are needed (and, in some cases underway) to remedy this.

ANIMAL MODELS OF HD

Validity of Animal Models of HD

Mouse models of HD are important to the discovery and validation of drug targets for HD as well as central to proving drug efficacy preceding human therapeutic trials. The development and validation of an effective mouse model of disease is no trivial matter and requires extensive characterization and rigorous validation (see Table 6.2). The ideal mouse model for HD agrees in etiology, pathophysiology, symptomatology, and response to therapeutics when compared to the human condition. Originally, chemical models of HD were investigated based on their similar striatal neurodegenerative pattern as seen in human HD patients. These chemical models met the very basic symptomatology criterion alone. Since the discovery of the HD gene, however, more accurate gene models of HD have been developed as transgenic mice representing HD etiology, pathophysiology, and symptomatology. Although species differences complicate the exact phenotype comparisons that can be made, genetic HD mice overall recapitulate cognitive failure, motor dysfunction, and striatal neurodegeneration as seen in human HD patients.

Three basic design strategies have been applied in developing HD gene mouse models giving rise to three broad model categories including: (i) fragment models containing N-terminal fragments of the human mutant Htt protein in addition to both alleles of murine Hdh, (ii) full-length models containing the full-length human HD gene with

[i]Please refer to McEvoy and Freundenreich, Issues in the design and conductance of clinical trials, Volume 1, Psychiatric Disorders, for a comprehensive discussion regarding statistical power issues in clinical trials.

Table 6.2 Validation of animal models of disease[a]

Face validity- a superficial resemblance between the mouse model and human disease. A similarity seen in symptoms is a common justification in this case (e.g., chemical models of HD).

Predictive validity- the ability of a model to predict the performance of the condition being modeled. One example is a model's capacity to predict compound efficacy in therapeutic human trials.

Construct validity- a theoretical clarification of what a model is supposed to represent. This validation accounts for the inherent difference that may occur in a process when looking across species.

Etiological validity- in this case the model and the human condition must undergo identical etiologies. The simplest disease to model in this situation is that of a simple inheritance disease.

[a] Van Dam and De Deyn. (2006). *Drug discovery in dementia: The role of rodent models.* Nat Rev: Drug Discov 5:956–970.

an expanded polyglutamine tract in addition to both alleles of murine Hdh, and (iii) knock-in models of HD with pathogenic CAG expansions in murine Hdh. Individually these gene models are believed to represent certain aspects of HD based on their design and phenotype. These characteristics help define the strength of the model and its subsequent use in the field of HD research. Together these different gene models provide confirmatory proof of the dysfunction and disease caused by a Htt CAG expansion in mice. As a result, HD gene mouse models provide a powerful analysis for target validation and drug discovery preceding clinical trials. To date, the fourth criterion of an ideal HD mouse model, its predictive power in identifying effective drugs for HD awaits verification by emerging and ongoing human clinical trials.

Pre-Gene (Chemical) HD Models

Before the HD gene was mapped and more accurate gene models of HD were developed chemicals triggering neurodegeneration patterns similar to HD brain pathology were proposed as the originating models of HD. A mitochondrial toxin known as 3-nitroproprionic acid (3-NP) administered systemically induced striatal-specific lesions in many species including primates, rodents, and humans who accidentally consumed contaminated sugar cane.[97-100] An NMDA receptor antagonist, quinolinic acid (QA), when striatally injected into rats interestingly targeted GABAergic medium spiny neurons, the specific neuronal population as are affected in HD.[101] These observations surrounding both QA and 3-NP lead researchers to believe that these chemicals could represent possible models of HD. Although the discovery of the HD gene and subsequent development of HD gene transgenic models over-shadowed the significance of these chemicals as probable HD models, these chemicals prompted considerable research into specific pathophysiological mechanisms (i.e., mitochondrial dysfunction, NMDA receptor-mediated excitotoxicity) in HD gene models currently under investigation today.

HD Fragment Models

Fragment models were designed to express an N-terminal portion of the human HD gene containing an expanded CAG stretch within exon 1 in addition to endogenous murine htt. Identical sequence similarity exists between human and mouse Htt exon 1 outside the CAG expansion/polyproline stretch located 17 amino acids from the transcriptional start site. In humans 13-36 CAG repeats normally exist, whereas in mouse only 7 CAG repeats have been reported.[102] Fragment models were the first HD mouse models ever generated and were originally created as an alternative strategy to the technical challenges encountered when trying to develop transgenic mice expressing the notoriously large full-length HD gene. The strong phenotype of this initial fragment mouse model, however, provided evidence that a truncated N-terminal portion of expanded Htt could be used in replicating certain aspects of the HD disease process.[103] Subsequently a variety of HD fragment models have been generated independently.[103–106]

The best characterized of these models are the R6/2 and N171-82Q models which are routinely used in pre-clinical therapeutic drug trial. Additionally a conditional N-terminal mouse model, HD94-tet, was constructed which is useful in investigating the reversibility of the disease process (by shutting down the mutant Htt fragment) at different time-points in the disease. Although all fragment models share the unifying feature of containing a truncated N-terminal portion of expanded Htt, the variety of fragment models and mouse lines generated differ largely in construction with respect to strain background, regulatory promoter, CAG expansion size, fragment size, gene integration site, and gene dose (see Table 6.3). These construction differences have taught us that increasing CAG expansion size, Htt gene dose and/or decreasing fragment size are critical in accelerating the onset, severity, and progression of the disease phenotype.

R6 Model

The R6 mouse lines were the first HD gene mouse models ever generated. Multiple lines were created by microinjection of 1.9 kb of the human Htt genomic fragment containing promoter sequence (~1 kb of 5′ UTR) and Htt exon 1 carrying a (CAG)130 expansion. Originally four R6 mouse lines were created on the CBA × C57BL/6 J background strain, including R6/0, R6/1, R6/2, and R6/5 each with variable mutant Htt protein expression and CAG expansion size.[103] Of these lines, R6/2 is the best characterized and the most widely used because of its clear, strong phenotype and early disease-onset attributed to its large CAG expansion and high mutant protein expression.

N171-82Q

The N171-82Q mouse was created with a slightly longer N-terminal Htt fragment than the R6 line containing 82 polyglutamine repeats. N171-82Q is also on a C3H/HEJ × C57BL/6 J strain background and under the mouse prion protein promoter making it different from the R6 lines. Given its unique construction design and strain background the use of both the N171-82Q line and R6/2 lines is a practice of certain laboratories to confirm compound efficacy in HD pre-clinical therapeutic trials.[107–111]

Table 6.3 N-terminal mouse models of HD

Fragment model	Promoter	CAG repeats	Protein length	Expression of mutant Htt (%)	Earliest abnormal behavior	Lifespan	References
R6/1	IT15 (~1kb of 5′UTR)	115	63 aa	31	15–21 weeks (clasping)	32–40 weeks	103
R6/2	IT15 (~1kb of 5′UTR)	145	63 aa	75	5–6 weeks (motor deficit)	12–14 weeks	103,113,114
N171-18Q	Mouse prion protein	18	171 aa	10–20	None	Normal	105
N171-82Q	Mouse prion protein	82 (line 81)	171 aa	10–20	12 weeks (motor deficit)	24–30 weeks	105
HD94-tet	CAMKIIα-tTA; BiTetOCMV minimal	94	? (chimeric mouse/ human exon)1	?	4 weeks (clasping)	Normal	106,112

Tet/HD94

The Tet/HD94 conditional mice were generated containing a chimeric murine/human Htt exon 1 fragment including a 94 CAG repeats under a tetracycline regulated promoter.[106] Although not used in drug testing, these mice were critical in establishing the therapeutic potential of shutting-off the mutant Htt transgene both early in disease-onset (i.e., after neuropathological aggregate formation, but before motor deficit on the rotarod)[106] and late in disease progression (i.e., after motor deficit and showing slight neuronal loss).[112] Even in late-stage disease progression mice showed a 25% reduction in striatal neuronal loss and a complete recovery in motor function given a reduction in mutant Htt transgene expression.[112] These mice showed promise for therapeutic trials to be able to act both early and late in HD disease progression.

Phenotype of HD Fragment Models

N-terminal mouse models display the earliest disease onset and most rapid disease progression of any of the HD mouse models created. Both R6/2 and N171-82Q (line 81 and 100) exhibit HD-like features including motor deficits, severe weight loss, reduced brain weight, neuronal intranuclear inclusions, and premature death.[31,103,105,113-115] Of the N-terminal mouse models, the R6/2 line is the best characterized and most widely used in therapeutic trial because of the early onset of phenotypic abnormalities (motor deficits at 5–6 weeks) and premature death (starting at 10–13 weeks) enabling a rapid completion of therapeutic trials.[103] R6/2 transgenic mice show early learning impairments on cognitive tasks,[116] impairment in prepulse inhibition of startle[113] and progressive motor dysfunction including dystonic movement, declining motor performance and grip strength, gait abnormalities and clasping in the tail-suspension test.[113,114] Neuropathological features include a decrease in brain weight, volume, and neuronal counts,[31,103,114] as well as neuronal intranuclear inclusions.[31] Electrophysiological abnormalities are most pronounced in symptomatic R6/2 mice affecting corticostriatal pathways.[117] Furthermore, DNA damage has been noted in the brain late in the disease.[118] Originally R6/2 mice were described as having increased urination and handling-induced seizures,[103] however, these phenotypes have not manifested in other HD gene fragment mouse models.

Advantages/Disadvantages of HD Fragment Models

The most highly regarded advantage of the HD Fragment Models, particularly the R6/2 model, is their use in the rapid screening of therapeutics employing survival studies in under 3 months (see Table 6.3). The early and robust phenotype seen in these mice gives rise to low inter-animal variability permitting small testing cohorts.[119,120] Further early behavioral indicators of disease in the R6/2 model allows transgenic mice to be easily distinguished from normal littermate controls by behavioral tests at 5–6 weeks of age (see Table 6.3).[113] These pronounced survival and behavioral indications provide powerful outcome measures in designing effective pre-clinical therapeutic trials.

Despite its advantages in pre-clinical trial design, N-terminal mouse models do not display certain neuropathological features evident in HD. For example, the reduction in brain size and nuclear inclusion formation in these animals affects all CNS structures disagreeing with the predominant striatal cell loss seen in human patients.[103,120,121]

Some concern also exists that the phenotype of these mice could represent a defect caused by the polyglutamine expansion alone, and not a Htt context-specific polyglutamine expansion disorder. This was supported by the creation of a transgenic mouse containing a CAG expansion in the unrelated Hprt1 gene. These animals showed strong phenotypic overlap with the R6/2 model including seizures, tremors, and motor dysfunction.[122] Many subsequent studies however, have shown considerable overlap between R6/2 and other fragment and full-length HD models supporting its mutant Htt-specific effects. In addition, this model does not allow the study of early pathogenesis related to the cleavage of the Htt mutant protein.

HD Full-Length Models

Full-length models contain expanded human HD transgene in addition to endogenous murine Hdh. Transgenic full-length mouse models have been generated with either CAG expansions within the complete human HD gene using yeast artificial chromosome (YAC) vectors (YAC46, YAC72, and YAC128) or within human Htt cDNA (HD16, HD48, HD89, and PrP-tTA-6/iFL148Q). Similar to N-terminal mouse models, full-length mouse models differ with respect to strain background, regulatory promoter, CAG expansion size, gene integration site, and gene dose (see Table 6.4). The construction of full-length mouse models provided further confirmation that CAG expansion size and Htt gene dose are critical in accelerating the onset and progression of the disease phenotype even in the context of the full-length protein.[38,39,123,124]

Full-Length Gene Models

Using YAC a full-length model of HD was created containing the complete human HD gene including introns and endogenous promoter (~25 kb of upstream regulatory sequence). Three lines were created including YAC46,[38] YAC72,[38] and YAC128[39] containing 46, 72, and 128 CAG expanded repeats respectively within the human HD transgene. These mice exhibit an endogenous pattern of Htt expression (developmental and tissue-specific) given their IT15 promoter sequence.[38] Of these lines, the YAC128 model showed the earliest disease onset and largest disease severity leading to its use in pre-clinical trials.

cDNA Mouse Models

Two designs have been used in constructing full-length mutant HD cDNA mice. The first (HD48 and HD89) uses a constitutive CMV promoter showing widespread protein expression in brain,[123,125] while the second is an inducible model using a tetracycline regulated promoter in brain (PrP-tTA-6/iFL148Q).[126] The HD48 and HD89 mice showed interesting behavioral and neuropathological dysfunction, however, these transgenic lines were lost and no subsequent analysis can be performed. The PrP-tTA-6/iFL148Q mice show the weakest neuropathological similarities to human HD patients of any full-length mouse model. The use of its full-length myc-tagged Htt protein, however, does prove advantageous for *in vivo* Htt sub-cellular localization. This mouse line has similarly experienced difficulty in breeding and contracting of the CAG repeat.[126]

Table 6.4 Full-length mouse models of HD

Full-length models	Promoter	Brain expression pattern	CAG repeat length	Htt	Expression of mutant Htt (%)	Earliest abnormal behavior	Neuropathology	Nuclear Htt and/or aggregates	Comments	References
HD89	CMV	Widespread	89	cDNA	100–500	2 months – feet clasping	6 months – prominent striatal neuronal loss and astrocytosis	NII widespread	Line no longer available	123,123
YAC46	IT15 (~25kb)	Developmental	46	Gene	30–50	Normal up to 20 months	Normal up to 20 months	Normal		38
YAC72	IT15 (~25kb)	Developmental	72	Gene	30–50	7 months – hyperactivity	12 months – qualitative neuronal degeneration	Diffuse nuclear staining greatest in STR		38
YAC128	IT15 (~25kb)	Developmental	128	Gene	75	3 months – hyperactivity	9 months – striatal volume loss; 12 months – cortical volume loss	Diffuse nuclear staining greatest in STR	Used in pre-clinical trial	39,125
PrP-tTA-6/ iFL148Q	PrP-tTA; TRE-CMV	Widespread	148	cDNA	~100	6 months – trend toward motor dysfunction on rotarod	Astrocytosis and ventricular enlargement; no neuronal loss	NII widespread	c-myc tagged Htt protein very useful for protein localization studies	126

Phenotype of HD Full-Length Models

The best characterized and most widely used full-length mouse model is YAC128. Of the YAC mouse lines generated, this model displayed the earliest and most pronounced phenotype stimulating its application to pre-clinical therapeutic trials (see Table 6.4). YAC46 and YAC72 mice showed relatively weak, late-onset behavioral changes beginning at 7 months of age and subtle neuropathological changes by 12 months discouraging its use in pre-clinical trials.[38] Alternatively, YAC128 shows a spectrum of measurable behavioral, cognitive, motor, and neuropatholgical changes amenable to its use in therapeutic testing. Behavioral changes occur first at 3 months of age evident as hyperactivity and progress to hypoactivity by 12 months. Motor deficit is evident on the rotarod beginning at 6 months of age and progressively worsening with age. Neurodegeneration of specific brain regions also develops in the mice with striatal atrophy beginning at 9 months of age and cortical atrophy arising by 12 months.[39] These quantifiable motor and neurodegenerative changes make YAC128 a particularly suitable model for therapeutics testing.

HD full-length model neuropathology revealed the most interesting and unique findings for these mouse models. HD48 and HD89 mice were the first full-length models reported to show selective neuronal loss in the brain suggesting that the context of the CAG expansion in the full-length Htt protein is important to regional selectivity seen in HD brains.[123] This phenomenon was better characterized later in YAC128 where neuronal loss showed its greatest effects in the striatum, with less severe developments in the cortex, and virtually no effect in regions usually unaffected in HD such as the cerebellum.[39,125] Further an abnormal nuclear accumulation of Htt was shown to obey this same regional selectivity pattern with changes occurring as early as 2 months of age in YAC128 striatum.[125]

Advantages/Disadvantages of HD Full-Length Models

The generation of HD full-length models demonstrated the specificity of placing the CAG expansion within the context of the full-length human protein. By expressing human mutant Htt, HD full-length models produced a selective striatal neuronal loss and neuropathology not evident in other HD mouse models.[39,123,125] Further the YAC128 full-length model showed a consistent phenotype including motor dysfunction and neuronal loss providing effective outcome measures for conducting pre-clinical trials and drug testing.

Despite their interesting neuropathology, these mouse models display weaker phenotypes relative to N-terminal mouse models. This makes for longer pre-clinical trials (average 12 month trials), less dramatic outcome measurements, and wider mouse-to-mouse variability demanding larger testing cohorts (15 mice per treatment group) to reach statistical significance. Overall this increases the time and money required for each pre-clinical trial hindering many labs from using this model for therapeutic testing.

Knock-in Models

Murine and human Htt exhibit high conservation being 86% identical at the DNA level and 91% identical at the protein level.[102] As a result, multiple knock-in mouse lines were created by homologous recombination of either complete or partial human HD exon 1 containing expanded CAG repeats between 50 and 150 units with the mouse Htt gene (see Table 6.5).[127-132] This model is considered the most genetically accurate mouse model of HD existing in either the heterozygous or homozygous state.

CAG expansion less than 80

Within this category four mouse genotypes have been independently generated including HdhQ50,[127] Hdh6/Q72,[129] Hdh4/Q80,[128,129] CAG71,[128] and CHL1 (Hdh (CAG)80).[131] Of these mice none have been reported to exhibit any neuropathological abnormalities including brain weight, neuronal loss, or NIIs.[127,129,131] Furthermore behavior abnormalities were largely undetected in these mice.[129] Molecular abnormalities were detected *ex vivo*[128] suggesting that subtle irregularities may exist in these mice as a result of the expansion despite the absence of any gross phenotypic changes.

CAG expansion greater than 80

Within this category of knock-in mice at least 5 mouse genotypes have been generated to date including CAG94,[128] HdhQ92,[130] HdhQ111,[130] CAG140,[133] and CHL2 (Hdh (CAG)150).[131] Mouse lines with the largest CAG expanded tracts, >140 CAG repeats, including CAG140 and CHL2 mice are the most thoroughly characterized mice, with the most robust phenotype of all knock-in mice.

Phenotype of HD Knock-in Models

CAG140 or CHL2 mice both show progressive, more subtle behavior abnormalities. CAG140 mice have early hyperactivity preceding hypoactivity at 4 months of age and gait anomalies by 12 months of age. A proportion of homozygous CHL2 (Hdh (CAG)150/150) mice show inactivity, hind-limb clasping, and motor dysfunction on the rotarod before 10 months of age. A similar proportion of heterozygous CHL2 mice show these symptoms but at a later time-point before 20 months of age.[131] This developmental difference between homozygous and heterozygous CHL2 mice is interesting given that controversy still exists in human HD data as to whether phenotype differences may exist between homozygous and heterozygous HD patients.

Neuropathological observations of knock-in mice have revealed no visible loss of brain regions or decline in neuronal counts.[131] Most knock-in models with >80 CAG expansions have however, identified prominent diffuse nuclear Htt accumulation with age, and the subsequent formation of NII (ubiquitin and Htt positive) in the striatum, nucleus accumbens, and layers of the cortex.[130-132] This selective pattern of nuclear Htt accumulation parallels that seen in full-length HD mouse models confirming that the full-length expanded form of Htt is necessary for the selective pathology seen in HD. Behavioral abnormalities preceded neuropathological anomalies in the CAG140 model, adding to a growing body of evidence that suggests aggregates are not responsible for the early events triggered by the mutation.[132]

Advantages/Disadvantages of HD Knock-in Models

The weak phenotype observed in these mice was initially disappointing because this model exists as the most accurate genetic model of HD. Subsequently to its earliest characterizations, however, the development of knock-in mice with larger CAG

Table 6.5 Knock-in mouse models of HD

Knock-in model	CAG size	Zygosity	Earliest abnormal behavior	Neuropathology	Nuclear Htt and/or aggregates	References
HdhQ50	48	Homo.	None observed	None observed	Not reported	127
Hdh6/Q72	72	Hetero.	3 months – aggression	None observed	4 months – diffuse nuclear staining 11 months – nuclear microaggregates	129,179
Hdh4/Q80	80	Hetero.	3 months – aggression	None observed	Same as Hdh6/Q72	129,179
CAG71	71	Homo.	None observed	None observed	None observed	128
CHL1 (Hdh$^{(CAG)80}$)	80	Homo.	None observed	None observed	NII rare	131
HdhQ92	90	Homo.	None observed	None observed	5 months – diffuse nuclear staining 12 months – nuclear microaggregates and NII	130
CAG 94	94	Homo.	2 months – mild hyperkinesia	None observed	None observed	128
HdhQ111	109	Homo. And Hetero.	None observed	None observed	2.5 months – diffuse nuclear staining 5 months – microaggregates 16 months – NII	130
CAG140	140	Homo.	1 month – abnormal rearing and hyperactivity	None observed	2 months – diffuse nuclear staining 5 months – NII and microaggregates	132
CHL2 (Hdh$_{(CAG)150}$)	150	Homo. And Hetero.	~4–13 months shows motor deficits	Gliosis	7 months – diffuse nuclear staining 10 months – NII	131,139

tracts has proven very useful for the investigation of the early pathogenic events in HD. Additionally the knock-in model has provided valuable evidence of the behavioral and neuropathological differences surrounding homozygosity and heterozygosity of a mutant HD gene. In terms of pre-clinical trials, while these mouse models are used for compounds testing they are not as widely used as the full-length or N-terminal mouse models.

Other Models

While many of the models discussed above have been created with the purpose of studying the role of mutant Htt in HD, an alternative approach such as knocking-out the HD gene in mice is useful for studying the function of wild-type Htt. Complete loss of Hdh in mice results in embryonic lethality,[134] however, this lethality can be rescued by the presence of Htt in the extraembryonic tissue suggesting a critical role of Htt in development.[135] Adult Hdh +/− chimeras show neurological dysfunction,[136] while conditional Hdh knock-outs limited to the forebrain and testis show progressive neuronal degeneration and sterility.[137] YAC128 transgenic mice lacking endogenous Htt (YAC128 −/−) show motor abnormalities and effects on survival with no observable effects on striatal volume or neuronal counts.[138] Together this line of evidence suggests that wild-type Htt has a functional role in the adult brain, and that loss of wild-type Htt function may contribute to the neurological defects as seen in HD. Furthermore these mouse lines provide support toward a HD allele-specific therapy in selectively silencing the mutant HD gene, while maintaining wild-type Htt's expression and prosurvival function.

COMPARING HD MOUSE MODELS FOR PRE-CLINICAL TRIALS

Comparing HD gene mouse models reveals interesting features shared among these models in trying to recapitulate HD (see Table 6.6). Common to all mouse models are behavioral changes, motor dysfunction, and neurodegeneration attributed to a CAG expansion within either the full-length or fragment form of Htt. This provides good evidence to suggest that mutant Htt acts similarly in mice and humans to affect behavioral, motor, and neurological capacities. Still, differences in the severity and/or striatal specificity of human HD with current HD mouse models reminds us of the limitations of recapitulating a human disease in mice.

N-terminal mouse models undeniably exhibit the strongest, most rapid phenotype of all HD gene mouse models. With survival studies concluding in approximately 3–6 months, this feature makes it a common model for rapid therapeutic drug screening preceding human clinical trials. Full-length mouse models on the other hand exhibit a slower, progressive phenotype, which does not affect lifespan. Yet this model shows clear motor and neurodegenerative changes by 12 months of age providing reasonable outcome measures for pre-clinical therapeutic trials. Further the specificity of the model's neurodegeneration to striatal and cortical regions, as is seen in HD, makes it a very important mouse model for screening neuroprotective agents that could be effective against HD. Knock-in mice show the weakest phenotype and slowest

Table 6.6 Comparing HD mouse models for pre-clinical trials

	HD gene mouse models		
	N-terminal	**Full-length**	**Knock-in**
Course of Disease			
Onset	Rapid	Slow	Slow
Lifespan	Shortened	Normal	Normal
Genetics			
Mutant HD gene	Fragment	Full-length	Full-length
Expression	Over-expressed	Over-expressed	Endogenous
Source	Human	Human	Mouse
Phenotype			
Cognitive dysfunction	Yes	Yes	Yes
Behavioral changes	Yes	Yes	Yes
Motor defects	Yes	Yes	Yes
Progressive Changes			
Motor dysfunction	Yes	Yes	Yes
Weight loss	Yes	No	No
Neuropathology			
Atrophy	Yes	Yes (selective)	Yes (selective)
Neurodegeneration	Yes	Yes (selective)	No
Nuclear accumulation	No	Yes	Yes
Aggregates/NII	Yes	No	Yes
Uses			
Studies of pathogenesis	Yes	Yes	Yes
Therapeutic trials	Yes	Yes	Yes (few)

progression of all HD gene mouse models making it a time consuming model for pre-clinical therapeutic trials. The Hdh Q150/Q150 mice showed its strongest measures useful to pre-clinical trials at 24 months of age,[139] late in the lifespan of a mouse. Instead, knock-in mouse models like full-length mouse models are believed to be most useful in investigating the pathogenesis of the disease. Given that both models contain a full-length form of mutant Htt it is thought that these models may provide insight into mutant Htt cleavage and processing events responsible for the development and progression of the disease.

The different HD gene mouse models provide a needed tool for the investigation of HD pathogenesis and pre-clinical drug testing. Currently it is common practice to screen drug candidates in more than one HD gene mouse model to ensure testing accuracy and efficacy before moving forward into human clinical trials. This places a great deal of importance into the proper characterization of these mouse models and standardization of testing protocols across the HD field. Overall this will ensure a careful selection and prioritization of drug candidates for ongoing and future human clinical trials.

PRE-CLINICAL STUDIES IN HD MOUSE MODELS

Endpoints/Outcome Measures

Symptoms in both humans with HD and animal models of HD can be clustered into four categories including general health, motor control, mood/psychiatric health, and cognitive function. In terms of modeling symptoms of HD in animal models, these four categories are the main areas from which pre-clinical outcome measures are derived.

General Health

In mice, general health can be measured as changes in body weight and/or survival. In pre-clinical trials the definition of survival can differ from a lack of responsiveness to tactile stimulation, failure to right when turned sideways, to death. This definition difference can affect the outcome of a study, and therefore it is important to include a battery of tests in which survival is one additional measure. The R6/2 model provides a good example where body weight and survival are used as clear outcome measures. YAC128 does not show weight loss or changes in survival, however, so other functional measures are used in drug screens in this case.

The Irwin's test[140] can be used to assess aspects of neurological health by measuring basic reflexes such as escape to touch, righting, reaction to manipulation, the pinna reflex, and others. The test is very valuable for the detection of major or consistent abnormalities, however, lacks sufficient power for detecting mild phenotypes or drug effects.

Motor Control

The Rotarod test is one of the most widely used tests in mouse models of neurodegeneration as it is very sensitive to motor impairment.[141] Rotarod measures motor coordination and motor skill learning, which are important features in human HD.

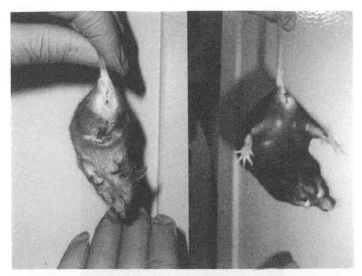

Figure 6.1   R6/2 (left) mice showing abnormal clasping of the hindlimbs and wild-type (right).

Both R6/2 and YAC128 use Rotarod testing to evaluate drug effects in pre-clinical trials. Untreated, R6/2 shows a clear motor deficit by 8 weeks of age,[119] while YAC128 shows motor decline beginning at 6 months of age.[39] Abnormal jerky movements, gait abnormalities, slowness of movement, and dystonia (clasping; see Figure 6.1) can additionally be monitored with Irwin's test.[140] The disadvantage of this test is that many of these measurements are analyzed with non-parametric statistics and therefore lack the statistical power needed for drug screening. The open field test provides a quick assessment of total activity and some indication of emotional reactivity to a novel and open environment. Despite its simplicity the dataset that can be obtained from this test is very rich. Typical measures of activity include total distance traveled, total number of movement bouts, and rearing.

The rearing-climbing test is a simple, high-throughput test that assesses spontaneous behavior in a novel environment. Mice are trapped under a mesh cup (see Figure 6.2) and the total number of rears and climbing activity is measured, in addition to the time and latency for each behavior.[142] This procedure can be easily automated providing fast measurement of activity. Measurements of rearing rate and total activity seem to be very sensitive to the motor dysfunction seen in animal models of HD.[142,143] Findings of early hyperactivity during disease progression in animal models of HD[132,144] have been interpreted as a recapitulation of the hyperkinesia seen in HD patients.

Cognitive Function

Cognitive and psychiatric symptoms of HD can be far more disruptive of normal life than HD-related motor deficits. CAG repeat size correlates with cognitive deficits[145,146] although some studies failed to show this correlation.[147,148] Cognitive deficits seem to be the result of dysfunction in fronto-striatal circuits and striatal areas rather than due

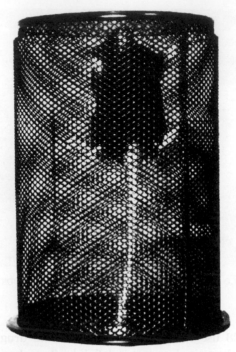

Figure 6.2 The rearing climbing test.

to a specific frontal deficit and therefore there is some correlation between motor and cognitive deficits as well.[149] Table 6.7 shows the most important cognitive dysfunctions in HD, some of which can be studied in animal models of HD. We will review below the tasks used currently in HD models.[ii]

T-maze reversal

Reversal of any task requires suppression of the previously learned task to allow learning of a new contingency. It is assumed that cortical input is required for this suppression, and thus strategy reversal has been monitored in the assessment of HD and in the study of animal models of HD.[150] One task, the two-choice swim tank has been used to study HD animal models. Both R6/2 and YAC128 have shown deficits in strategy reversal.[116,121]

Prepulse inhibition of startle

HD patients show reduced startle inhibition after being pre-warned with a weak stimulus (auditory or tactile) and then exposed to a larger, more intense stimulus. This startle response is known as prepulse inhibition.[151] Both R6/2[116,121] and YAC128[116,121]

[ii] For further description and discussion of tasks/procedures commonly used to assess cognitive function in rodents, please refer to Lindner *et al.*, Development, optimization and use of preclinical behavioral models to maximize the productivity of drug discovery for Alzheimer's disease, in this volume.

Table 6.7 Cognitive deficits in HD

Process	Subtypes	Psychological tasks with significant findings in HD
Executive function	Planning*, organize behavior, mental flexibility, attention set shifting*, parallel information processing	Tower of London Picture Ordering Task Wisconsin Card Sort Spatial Working Memory Task Verbal fluency tasks
Procedural memory		Rotary Pursuit Task
Psychomotor speed*		Stroop Digit Symbol substitution Trail Making Test Simple, Choice Reaction Time
Perceptual domain	Visuo-spatial attention	Peripheral Cueing Paradigm (Inhibition of Return Measure)
	Attention to Multiple Aspects of Stimuli Complex Visual Integration and Manipulation of Information	Perceptual Matching Discrimination Tasks Hooper Test of Perceptual Integration Facial Affect* Drawing
	Visual Task involving Planning and Organization Task involving complex imagery	Block Design Egocentric Spatial Location Mental Rotation
Sensory-motor	Gating	Prepulse-inhibition of Startle
Memory	Lack of active strategies for encoding Source Learning	Pair Associated Learning Task
Motor skill learning	Habit formation Sequence learning	Rotary Pursuit Tasks Serial Reaction Time Task

*indicates process found affected in presymptomatic HD carriers, also some impairments in category generation, spatial function, visual and verbal memory, picture sequencing, attention, learning. Based on [149].

show deficits in prepulse inhibition late in life. In R6/2 this startle deficit corresponds with hippocampal degeneration[113] consistent with the role of the septohippocampal system in prepulse inhibition in both humans[152] and rodents.[153]

Attention set shifting

This test entails learning a rule, such as classifying a sample based on color, and then learning a new rule based on a different stimulus, such as a number. It has been developed and validated for rats as dependent on the medial prefrontal cortex[154,155] and used in mice.[156] This test is based on the idea that an attention set is formed when attention is directed to a particular dimension of a stimulus, such as its color or shape. Switching between pairs of the same dimension (intra-dimensional shift, ID) is easier than switching to a new dimension (extra-dimensional shift, ED). Interestingly an ED deficit has been shown in Hdh$^{(CAG)150}$ knock-in mice[157] showing potential for cognitive assessment in HD animal models.

Morris Water Maze

Lesions of the striatum and hippocampus cause deficits in learning and knowledge acquisition in the Morris Water Maze.[158,159] Although there are different protocols for this task most include 4–5 days of training (4 trials/day) searching for an invisible escape platform in a pool of water. Preference for the platform location is indicative of learning. It has been suggested that different neural circuits direct learning this task. Procedural learning, "learning what to do," is probably governed by a circuit including the striatum;[160] whereas spatial memory, "learning where to go," is dependent on the hippocampus.[161] It would thus be expected that animal model of HD will show deficits in this task due to either procedural or spatial learning deficits. R6/2 mice show pathology in the hippocampus and a long-term potentiation deficit in the CA1 area, in addition to striatal pathology and therefore it is not surprising that they showed acquisition deficits in this task.[162] For animals with possible sensory and motor dysfunction a way to ensure that the deficit is cognitive is to run a standard visible platform phase. With a visible platform rodents do not need to use their memory and can simply approach the stimulus.

Mood Disturbances

Apart from the motor and cognitive symptoms described most HD patients suffer from other behavioral symptoms that can be described in three different axes seemingly reflecting clusters of apathy, depression, and irritability. Whereas in the study of animal models of HD symptoms homologous to apathy may well be apparent in standard test of motor function (i.e., as decreased rearing in the rearing-climbing prior to the onset of motor dysfunction,[142] the domains of depression and irritability have not been explored in animal models. This is certainly an area that deserves more attention and may provide additional experimental targets for drug screening.

PRE-CLINICAL TRIAL DESIGN

It is generally accepted in the HD field that drug candidates must be proven effective in more than one HD mouse model before moving forward into human clinical trials.

To successfully reproduce drug efficacy studies across mouse models and between different labs, however, demands rigorous standardization in standard operating procedures and pre-clinical trial design to be effective. To achieve this, trials must control for genetic or environmental factors that may influence phenotype and/or the progression of the disease. This includes standardized breeding, housing, and testing practices to reduce variability between subjects and across pre-clinical studies.

Breeding

It is known that litter size has a strong effect on behavior, eating patterns and body weight.[163] Culling litters to a given range can be used to reduce variability. Extensive literature also describes the effect of background strain and breeding strategies on transgenic mice phenotype.[164,165] Controlling CAG repeat size is a particular challenge when breeding transgenic and knock-in HD animal models. This is because intergeneration instability of the CAG tract has been reported in numerous HD mouse models, similar to the repeat instability seen in human HD. It is known for example, that colonies of R6/2 in different labs and commercial breeding facilities have considerable differences in the CAG repeat number.

Housing Conditions

It is well known that environmental enrichment is beneficial, for rodents and results in improved health and cognitive ability. Studies of the effects of environmental enrichment on R6/2 mice revealed changes in phenotype such as motor improvements on the rotarod provided limited cage enrichment (i.e., plastic tube) in the living environment.[166,167] Other changes in R6/2 have also been noted in weight loss and peristriatal cerebral volume provided environmental enrichment.[166,167] Figure 6.3 shows an example of a cage containing wild-type and R6/2 mice with enrichment elements (a plastic tube, shredded paper, rubber bone, and wet mush).

Accessibility to food and water can also become influential environmental factors on animal phenotype when working with animals of deteriorating health. In certain cases, for example, the animal's health may become so debilitating that accessibility to proper nourishment may confound the phenotype. As motor deficits become serious in R6/2 and R6/1 HD models a normal cage with food chow hanging from a basket may impose extra hardship, as affected mice may not be able to reach or effectively chew the food. In this case wet chow or food pellets on the floor of the cage may improve the animal's accessibility to adequate nourishment. A high or low water bottle spout may also impact the health and resultant phenotype of the mice. By properly controlling housing conditions, HD-specific phenotype instead of unrelated health symptoms (i.e., dehydration or malnourishment), will be better addressed in pre-clinical trials.

Further, the animal facilities within which the animals are kept must follow standardized animal unit guidelines to avoid inter-animal variability across HD mouse models. Careful controls must be placed on temperature and humidity of the living environment, the avoidance of viral and bacterial infections in the colony, the selection

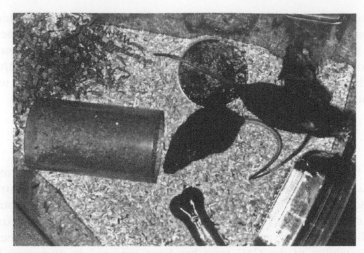

Figure 6.3   R6/2 mice and its wild-type control in an enriched housing environment. Two wild-type and an R6/2 mouse living in an enriched environment. Wet chow is added to the cage to ensure rearing deficits do not interfere with normal feeding. Other enrichment items can be added as shown in the picture (e.g., shredded paper, rubber bones, and tubes).

of standardized chow for the mice, and the levels of noise during testing and non-testing conditions.[168] R6/2 and wild-type YAC128 mice (FVB/N background strain) are particularly sensitive to noise and vibration. Excessive or unexpected noise may trigger seizures or abnormal phenotypes in these mice, and therefore extra care during animal husbandry and testing is needed.

Testing Protocol

As breeding and dosing are very costly components of a drug screening system, it is important to design a testing protocol that takes full advantage of testing cohorts. In order to make efficient use of mice then, testing batteries are employed to include a series of cognitive and motor tests over extended periods of time with each individual cohort. Motor tests that assess disease progression at different time-points are normal procedure for HD mouse models.[142] Tests of cognition can also be interspaced in between motor testing, with the proviso that tests involving learning and acquisition are not repeated. In this way testing protocols provide an assessment of early and late dysfunction. Initial assessment during a drug-free period is also important in assigning mice to treatment groups to minimize variability between groups.

This repeated testing although cost-effective, may confound phenotype or drug effect if testing batteries are staged too rigorously. In lines that deteriorate rapidly it could be a concern to employ too many tests in a short period of time. In this case factors such as fatigue and interference between tasks may shadow drug treatment effects in the mice. Furthermore, repeated motor testing will improve HD phenotype in mice just as environmental enrichment improves testing performance.[169] This would suggest that motor-testing regimes across facilities must be standardized for each HD mouse model to avoid inconsistencies among pre-clinical trials.

Optimal Allocation

The design of a drug screening strategy requires consideration of the number of drugs that need to be tested. If the number exceeds capacity an optimal allocation scheme can be used.[170] An optimal allocation design establishes multiple stages and a set of criteria for progression of a drug from one stage to the next. The final sample size is first calculated to ensure adequate power for detecting a drug effect $(1 - \beta)$. This final sample size is then divided into groups and assigned to the different stages. Although this could equate to numerous stages and unequal sample sizes per stage, a simple design would have two stages with half the subjects in each.

Having too many stages in the optimal allocation design can complicate breeding and drug dosing when conducting numerous trials. It is for this reason that a threshold must be set in deciding to progress from one stage to the next. Given that all drugs achieve this threshold for each stage, the trial will achieve the necessary power to show an overall drug effect when all stages are finally combined. Should a drug not achieve the threshold for any given stage then the trial will be concluded. This trial designs is currently used for clinical trials in cancer, where efficient trial design is mandatory for ethical reasons.[171] Similarly this trial design could be effective in preclinical research where limited resources and finances restrict the number and capacity of trials to be run. One disadvantage of the optimal allocation design is the time it takes to complete each trial. In this case a complete pre-clinical trial could be executed should the compound or drug target been previously validated by other HD mouse models.

PRE-CLINICAL TRIALS

Studies of HD pathogenesis have revealed many interesting drug targets for treatment of HD. Additionally, therapeutic strategies common to a number of different neurodegenerative diseases have been considered for treatment of HD. The treatment areas that have been considered include: energy metabolism, antioxidants, protease inhibitors, transglutaminase inhibitors, general enrichment of environment and nutrition, aggregate formation inhibitors, specific gene-targeted transcription (with viral vectors, drugs, transgenic over-expressors, or mouse knock-outs), excitotoxicity, and tissue transplants. Although many studies have shown positive results, few studies have been consistently replicated between research groups. Table 6.8 shows a comprehensive summary of all pre-clinical studies to date.

Energy Metabolism

HD has been suspected to be associated with bioenergetic deficits and thus both CoQ10 and creatine have been tested in pre-clinical trials with positive results in both

Table 6.8 Summary of therapeutic strategies evaluated in genetic mouse models of Huntington disease and their efficacy.

Target/Treatment	Mouse model	Dose/route/regime	Starting age of treatment (weeks)	Outcomes Survival	Body Weight Deficits	Behavior Motor coordination (rotarod)	Other	Neuropathology Brain and neuronal atrophy	Aggregates accumulation/size	Refs
Energy metabolism										
CoQ10	R6/2	1, 5, 10, 20, kg/kg/day DS (Chemco)	4	+ (2) (best: 5 kg/kg/day)	+	+ (best: 5 kg/day)	NS GS	+ brain & neuronal atrophy	+	180
		0.4, 1, 2 kg/kg/day DS (Tishcon)		+ (2) (best: 1 kg/kg/day)		+ (best: 1 kg/day)				
CoQ10	R6/2	0.2% DS	~4	+ (2) 14.6%				+ brain & neuronal atrophy	+	181
CoQ10	N171-82Q	500 mg/kg/day, SD	8	Decreased 17%						182
CoQ10	R6/2	0.2% DS	3	+ (3) 14.5%				v brain weight & atrophy		110
Creatine	R6/2	1% w/v SD	5	NS	NS	NS	NS (MWM, T-maze)		NS	183
Creatine	R6/2	2% SD	6	+ (5) 14.4%	+ (6 weeks of age)			+ brain weight, neuronal & brain atrophy + ATP & creatine levels	+	184
			8	+ (5) 9.7%	NS	NS		NS	NS	
			10	NS (5)	NS	NS		NS	NS	
Creatine	N171-82Q	2% SD	4 (3)	+ (3) 19%				+ brain weight & atrophy	+	108
Creatine	R6/2	1% SD	3	+ (4) 9.4%	+ 6.8%	+ 25%		+ brain & neuronal atrophy + NAA/choline ratio	+	109
		2% SD		+ (4) 17.4%	+ 10.3%	+ 33%				
		3% SD		+ (4) 4.4%	+ 6.5%	NS				

Antioxidant

Drug	Model	Dose/route	n	Survival	Weight	Motor	Neurochemistry	Neuropathology	Ref
Lipoic acid	N-171-82Q	0.05%, SD	4	+ (3) 8.2%	NS	+			107
	R6/2			+ (3) 7.1%	NS	NS			
S-PBN	R6/2	600 mg/l, DW		NS (3)	NS				185
BN82451	R6/2	300 mg/kg, daily PO or DS	4	+ 15%	+			+ brain & neuronal atrophy	
Ascorbate	R6/2	300 mg/kg, IP, 4 days per week	6			+ repetitive movements			186

Protease inhibitors

Drug	Model	Dose/route	n	Survival	Weight	Motor	Neurochemistry	Neuropathology	Ref
Minocycline	N171-82Q	10 g/kg, IP, daily	8	NS	NS		NS LA	NS brain atrophy	111
Minocycline	R6/2	5 mg/kg, IP, daily	~4	+ (2) 11.2%	NS	+		+ brain & neuronal atrophy Reduced reactive microglia	181
Minocycline	R6/2	1 & 5 mg/ml, DW	4	NS	NS	NS	NS GS	NS	187
Doxycycline		2 & 6 mg/ml, DW		NS	NS	NS	NS GS	NS	
Minocycline		5 mg/kg in 0.5 ml, IP, daily	6	+ 14%	NS	+		Decreased caspase 1 & 3 mRNA Decreased iNOS NS A2A, D1 or D2 receptors levels	NS
Tetracycline		5 mg/kg in 0.5 ml, IP, daily		NS	NS	NS			
zVAD-fmk	R6/2	100 ug/20g/28 d-ICV, osmotic minipump		+ (12.2%)	+	+			188
YVAD-cmk		50 ug/20g/28 d-ICV, osmotic minipump		NS					
DEVD-fmk		50 ug/20/28 d-ICV, osmotic minipump	7	NS					
zVAD-cmK & DEVD-fmk		50 ug/20g/28 d-ICV, osmotic minipump		+ (17.3%)	+				

(continued)

Table 6.8 (Continued)

Target/Treatment	Mouse model	Dose/route/regime	Starting age of treatment (weeks)	Survival	Body Weight Deficits	Motor coordination (rotarod)	Other	Brain and neuronal atrophy	Aggregates accumulation/size	Refs
Transglutaminase inhibitor										
Cystamine	R6/2	900 mg/l DW	prenatal	+	worsen	+	+ clasping			189
	R6/2x trans-glutaminase knock out		prenatal	+	worsen	+	+ clasping			
Cystamine	YAC128	900 mg/l DW	28		NS	NS	NS LA	+ striatal volume (11.4%) & atrophy Prevented cell loss & neuronal atrophy		190
			16		NS	+	NS LA	+ striatal neuropathology		191
Cystamine	R6/2	100 ul of 100M of cystamine, OP, daily	7	+	+	+ gait	+ clasping, tremors		NS	
Cystamine	R6/2	112 mg/kg, IP, daily	3	+ (2) 19.5%	+	+		+ brain & neuronal atrophy & brain weight Reduced transglutaminase activity	+ aggregates in striatum & cortex	192
		225 mg/kg, IP, daily		+ (2) 17%	+					
		900 mg/l DW	prenatal	+ (2) 16.8%	+					
Diet & enrichment										
Enrichment/exercise	R6/1	Running wheels	10			NS	Decreased LA & rearing + clasping + working memory	Frontal cortex BDNF levels+ BDNF mRNA+ in striatum		193
Enrichment environment	R6/1	Enriched environment	4					+ number of BrdU+ in dentate gyrus, irrespectively of genotpye		194

Intervention	Model	Duration			Findings	Ref
Enrichment environment	R6/1	4	+	+	NS brain weight + depleted BDNF levels in striatum & hippocampus & DARP levels in cortex	167
Enrichment environment	R6/1	4			Delayed loss of cannabinoid CB1 levels	195
Enrichment environment	N171-82Q, female	8	NS	NS		182
Enrichment environment	R6/2	4	NS	+	+ (marginal) GS	166
Highly enriched			NS	+	+ GS; NS striatal volume or brain weight+ (marginal) peristriatal volume; NS on aggregates on striatum or cingulated cortex	
Enrichment environment	R6/1	4	NS	+	+ clasping; + (marginal) striatum volume + peristriatal volume; NS	196
Environmental enrichment	R6/2	4	+	-	decreased rearing in open field	169
Enhanced diet			+			
Enhanced diet + Mixed housing genotypes			+	+		
Enhanced diet + Behavioral Testing		2.5	+	NS		
Enhanced diet + Breeding activity		4	+	NS		
Essential fatty acids	R6/1	254 mg, DS, QOD	prenatal	+	NS	+ clasping & LA; NS D_1 & D_2 receptor levels	197
Dietary restriction	N-171-82	8	+	+	Delay onset of disease; Reduced brain atrophyRestored BDNF & protein chaperone levels	198

(continued)

Table 6.8 (Continued)

Target/ Treatment	Mouse model	Dose/route/regime	Starting age of treatment (weeks)	Outcomes		Behavior		Neuropathology		Refs
				Survival	Body Weight Deficits	Motor coordination (rotarod)	Other	Brain and neuronal atrophy	Aggregates accumulation/ size	
Aggregate formation inhibitors										
Congo red	R6/2	33.33 mg/kg, IP, 3 times a week	6	NS (1)	+	NS	NS cognitive tests or clasping	NS	NS	199
Congo red	R6/2	1 mg/30g, IP, Q)D or ICV 4 ug/24 h	9	+	+	+	+ clasping & gait		+	200
Trehalose	R6/2	0.2% DW	3	+	+	+	+ clasping & gait	+ striatum & brain atrophy	+	201
		2% DW			+					
		5% DW			+					
Targeting gene transcription										
Sodium phenylbutyrate	N171-82Q	100 mg/kg, IP, 6 days weekly	10	+	NS	NS		+ brain & neuronal atrophy		202
Mithramycin A	R6/2	150 ug/kg, 100ul IP, daily	3	+ 29.1% (5)	+	+		+ brain & striatal atrophy	NS	203
Sodium Butyrate	R6/2	0.1–10 g/kg, IP, daily	3	+ (2) (effective doses 0.2–1.2 g/kg)	+ after 11 weeks of age	+ (effective doses 0.4– 1.2 mg/kg)		+ brain weight, brain & neuronal atrophy (at 1.2 mg/kg)	NS	204
SAHA	R6/2	0.67 mg/l, DW	4		Deleterious	+	NS GS	NS brain weight neuronal atrophy		205
Lithium	R6/2	2.3 mq/kg, sc, daily	5.3	NS	Decreased					206
			10.5	NS	+	+				
Targeting excitotoxicity										
Riluzole	R6/2	0.4 g/l DW	5	NS	NS	NS	NS LA GS	NS	NS	207
Riluzole	R6/2	10 mg/kg in 0.1 ml, PO, daily	3	+ (6) 10.2%	+	NS	Reduced hyperactivity observed at early ages	NS	NS on aggregates number. Less ubiquitinated	208

Treatment	Model	Dose	Age						Ref
Remacemide	N171-82Q	17.5 mg/kg/day SD	8	Decreased 22%		NS			182
Remacemide	R6/2	0.007% DS	3	+ (3) 15.5%	+	+		+ brain weight & atrophy	110
MPEP	R6/2	50 mg/kg, PO, BID	3.5	+ (6) 11%	Decreased	+	Reduced hyperactivity observed at early ages	NS	209
LY379268		1.2 mg/kg in 0.1 ml, PO daily		+ (6) 10.5%	NS	NS	Reduced hyperactivity observed at early ages	NS	
Repair strategies									
Striatal transplant	R6/2	E13-14 LGE striatal anlage	10	NS	NS	NS	+ (modest) LA		210
Anterior cingulate cortical transplant	R6/1	Birth			NS	NS	Delayed onset of clasping	NS striatal volume	211
Human umbilical cord–blood cells	R6/2	71–74 × 10(6) & 100–105 × 10(6)		+	+				212
Other drugs/therapies									
Metformin	R6/2	2 mg/ml DW	5	+ 20.1% (only in males)	NS	NS beam crossing	+ clasping males, NS gait		213
		5 mg/ml DW		NS	NS	NS			
Glibenclamide	R6/2	5 mg/kg, IP, daily	5.5	NS	NS	NS			214
Rosiglitazone		3 mg/kg, IP, daily		NS	NS	NS			
GDNF	N171-82Q	rAAV, striatum	5	+	+	+	+ clasping	NS striatal volume + neuronal number (NeuM +) & volume	215
GDNF	R6/2	Lentivirus, striatum	4–5	NS	NS	NS	NS clasping & LA	NS striatal neuronal volume, striatal atrophy or, cell proliferation in striatum, dentate gyrus, subventricular zone	216

(continued)

Table 6.8 (Continued)

Target Treatment	Mouse model	Dose/route/regime	Starting age of treatment (weeks)	Outcomes Survival	Body Weight Deficits	Behavior Motor coordination (rotarod)	Behavior Other	Neuropathology Brain and neuronal atrophy	Neuropathology Aggregates accumulation/size	Refs
CNTF	YAC72	Lentivirus	16				Normalized hyperactivity	Decreased the number of dark cells (+ GFAP immuno-reactivity)		217
Tacrine	R6/2	2.7 (all experiments) or 3.2 (T-maze) mg/kg, IP, daily	5	+	NS	NS	NS (MWM, T-maze)		NS	183
Fluoxetine	R6/1	20 mg/kg, IP, daily	10	NS	NS	NS	+ FST, cognitive function & spontaneous alternation	+ atrophy dentate gyrus Rescued deficits in neurogenesis in dentate gyrus		218
Moclobemide	R6/2	10 mg/kg, daily, IP	5	NS	NS	NS	NS MWM & T-maze		NS	183
Paroxetine	N171-82Q	5 mg/kg, sc, daily	8	+14%	+	+		+ brain atrophy		219
Alprazolam	R6/2	1 mg/kg	4	NS	NS	+	+ 2CSTNS zero mazeNS SHIRPA scores	+ circadian gene expression dysregulation		220
			9	+		+	+ 2CSTNS zero maze + SHIRPA scores			
Chloral hydrate		400 mg/kg	9	NS	worsen		+ 2CST			
Ethyl-EPA	YAC128	1% ethyl-EPA+ 4% coconut oil	28			+	+ LA	NS striatal volume, neuronal volume & cell loss		221
shRNA-Exon 1	R6/2	Striatum	5						+	222

Treatment	Model	Dose/Route							Ref
shRNA	HD190Q	rAA, striatum	12				+ DARPP-32 loss	+	223
siRNA-Exon 1	R6/2	HC-Ad, ICV	Birth (P2)	+	+	+ LA & clasping	+ brain atrophy	+ (close to injection site)	224
sHRNA-mutant htt	N171-82Q	AAV, Striatum/cerebellum	4	NS	+	+ stride length		+ (cerebellar injected animals)	225
DNA vaccine	R6/2	100ug plasmid, 2 doses 2 weeks apart	5						226
Clioquinol	R6/2	30mg/kg, PO, daily	3	+20%	+	+ clasping	+ brain atrophy	+	227
Celecoxib	N171-82Q	15000ppm	8	Decreased 41%	NS			NS	182
Acetylsalicylate	N171-82Q, R6/2	200mg/kg/day, DW	Weaning	Decreased (7) on R6/2. NS on N171-82Q	NS on R6/2. Decreased on N171-82Q	NS PPI deficit (N171-82Q)	NS striatal atrophy (N171-82Q)	NS (N171-82Q)	228
Rofecoxib	R6/2	15mg/kg/day		NS (7)	NS	NS LA		NS	
TUDCA	R6/2 male	500mg/kg, sc, every 3 days	6			+ LA	Decreased striatal atrophy. Decreased TUNEL positive cells	+	229
CCI-779	N171-82Q	20mg/kg, IP, 3 injection per week up to 16 weeks, then QOD up to 21 weeks	4	Decreased	+	+ GS, tremors	NS brain weight	+	230
Asialoerythropoetin	R6/2	80ug/kg, IP, daily	5	NS	NS	NS LA	NS striatal volume or neuronal size	NS	231
SCH 58261 (A2A antagonist)	R6/2	0.1mg/kg, IP, daily for 7 days	5	NS	NS	Decrease time spend in open arms EPM	Prevented abnormal NMDA response (corticostriatal slices)	NS	232
CGS21680 (A2A agonist)	R6/2 male	0.5ug/g, IP, daily	7	NS	NS	+ LA		+	233
		2.5ug/g, IP, daily		NS	+	NS	+ ventricle enlargement reduced	+	
		5ug/g, IP, daily		NS	NS	+ LA		+	

(continued)

Table 6.8 (Continued)

Target Treatment	Mouse model	Dose/route/regime	Starting age of treatment (weeks)	Outcomes Survival	Body Weight Deficits	Behavior Motor coordination (rotarod)	Behavior Other	Neuropathology Brain and neuronal atrophy	Neuropathology Aggregates accumulation/size	Refs
Combined therapies										
CoQ 10/minocycline	R6/2	0.2% DS/5 mg/kg, IP, daily	~4	+ (2) 18.2%	+	+		+ brain & neuronal atrophy. Reduced reactive microglia	+	181
CoQ 10/Remacemide	N171-82Q	0.2% & 0.007% DS	8	NS					NS	234
			5	NS	NS (males)	+ transiently				
CoQ 10/Remacemide	R6/2	0.2% & 0.007% DS	3	+ (3) 31.8%	+	+		+ brain weigh, brain & neuronal atrophy	+	110
CoQ 10/Remacemide	N171-82Q	0.2% & 0.007% DS		+ (3)	+	+				214
Glibenclamide/rosiglitazone	R6/2	5 mg/kg /3 mg/kg, IP, daily	5.5	NS	NS	NS				
Tacrine	R6/2	2.7 (all experiments) or 3.2 (T-maze) mg/kg, IP, daily	5	+	NS	NS	NS MWM & T-maze		NS	183
Tacrine & moclobemide	R6/2	2.7 (all experiments) mg/kg,/10 mg/kg, IP, daily	5	NS	NS	NS	+ MWM		NS	183
Tacrine and creatine		2.7 or 3.2 mg/kg, IP, daily /1% w/v SD		NS	NS	NS	NS MWM		NS	
Creatine & moclobemide		1% w/v SD/ 10 mg/ kg, daily, IP		NS	NS	NS	NS MWM		NS	
Tacrine, moclobemide & creatine		2.7 (all experiments) or 3.2 (T-maze mg/kg/10 mg/kg, IP, daily, 1% w/v, SD		+	NS	NS	+ MWM & T-maze	Partially recovery of gene expression	NS	

Double transgenic models

Treatment	Model								Ref
CHIP heterozygous knock out	N171-82Q		Worsen	Worsen	Worsen tremor & clasping		Increased		235
Overexpression of HSP27	R6/2	Conception	Worsen	NS	NS	NS GS & LA	NS markers of oxidative stress	NS	236
Transglutaminase knock out	R6/2	Conception	+	NS	+	NS clasping & LA			189
Sp1 heterozygous knock out	R6/2	Conception	+ (2)	NS	NS		NS striatum volume	NS	237
	N171-82Q		+ (2)		NS				
Overexpression of HSP104	N171-82Q	Conception	+ 20%	NS	NS	NS GS & wire maneuver		+	238
Overexpression of HSP70	R6/2	Conception	NS	+	NS	NS clasping	NS brain & neuronal atrophy	NS	239
Overexpression of Bcl-2	R6/2	Conception	+		+ (females)			+	240
Dominant negative of Caspase 1	R6/2	Conception	+ 20%	+ (females)	+	+ (females)	Restored A2A, D₁ or D₂ receptors levels	+ (onset)	241

+ = significant beneficial effect of the treatment; NS= not significant; CoQ10= coenzyme Q10; DW= drinking water; LS = diet supplemented; PO= oral gavage; IP= intraperitoneal; ICV= intracerebral ventricular; SC= subcutaneous; QOD: every other day

(1) Criteria of euthanasia: failure to rouse for the wash food in the morning for 2 hours.
(2) Criteria for euthanasia: failure to right within 30 seconds./failure to right
(3) Criteria for euthanasia: animal unable to initiate movement after being gentle prodded for 2 minutes
(4) Criteria for euthanasia: animal unable to initiate movement after being gentle prodded for 10 minutes.
(5) Criteria for euthanasia: animal unable to initiate movement after being gentle prodded for 20-30 seconds.
(6) Criteria for euthanasia: animal unable to raise from the side.
(7) Criteria for euthanasia; animal unable to right within 10 seconds. Most mice were found death before reaching this criteria.

MWM = Morris water maze; 2CST = two choice swim test; rAA = recombinant adenoassociated viral vector; GDNF = glial cell line-derived neurotrophic factor; CNTF = ciliary neurotrophic factor; shRNA = sorth hairpin siRNA; HC-Ad = high capacity adenoviral vector; AAV = adenoassociated virus; zVAD-fmk + Val-Ala-Asp-flucromethyl ketone; YVAD-cml = Tyr-Val-Ala-Asp-chloromethylketone; DEVD-fmk = Asp-Glu-Val-Asp-aldehyde-fmk; DARP = dopamine & cAMP regulated phosphoprotein (32kDa); S-PBN = sulpho-tert-phenylbutyinitrone; LGE = lateral ganglionic eminence; NAA = N-acetylaspartate; TUDCA = tauroursodeoxycholic acid; SAHA = suberoylanilide hydrozamic acid; EPM = elevated plus maze; R.R = Rotarod; GS = grip strength; LA = locomotor activity behavioral and neuropathological endpoints. CoQ10 however, did not produce a significant positive result in a clinical trial.[172] Both compounds, however, are taken as nutritional supplements as they are available over the counter.

Oxidative Damage and Excitotoxicity

Oxidative damage has been suggested as a possible culprit in the pathogenesis of HD. Compounds targeting excitotoxicity and free radical damage have been tested. Antioxidants have produced positive results, although not many studies have pursued this target and not much information has been collected regarding neuropathology. Compounds targeting excitotoxicity, such as remacemide, have not shown robust beneficial effect on neuropathology but some positive effects in behavioral and health domains, especially in combination with other compounds such as CoQ have been seen.

Protease Inhibitors

Several proteases can target Htt and lead to fragments that could contribute to aggregate formation. Under the hypothesis that the aggregates are toxic, protease inhibitors such as the antibiotics minocycline and tetracycline have been tested in the N171-82Q and R6/2 models. The results have been mostly negative with some positive effects on survival and motor function.

Transglutaminase Inhibitor

Htt is polymerized by the enzyme transglutaminase. Thus cystamine, which inhibits this enzyme, has been tested as an anti-aggregate therapy in both the R6/2 and YAC128 mouse models. The results were mixed with some positive effects on neuropathology but consistent behavioral and health effects were only observed in R6/2 mice.

Diet and Enrichment

As discussed above husbandry conditions such as diet and enrichment can have important effects on disease progression in HD models. Enrichment seems to have a consistent beneficial effect on motor function with variable positive effects on neuropathology.

Aggregate Formation Inhibitors

Although the casual relationship between disease and aggregate formation is controversial, under the hypothesis that aggregates are toxic, efforts have been spent screening agents that can decrease aggregate formation *in vitro*. Both trehalose and congo red have been tested in R6/2 mice and have shown positive effects in behavioral outcomes and pathology although replication of the congo red study failed.

Targeting Gene Transcription

The class of histone deacetylase inhibitors (HDAC inhibitors) is receiving increasing attention due to its potential to restore gene transcription. Although it is expected that newer, more specific HDACs will be the compounds to reach acceptable efficacy and safety, a number have already been tested in HD animal models. For example, the anti-cancer antibiotic mithramycin, which inhibits apoptosis, showed positive effects in the R6/2 mouse model, in both motor and health domains and in brain atrophy, although it did not affect aggregation. Other HDACs, such as butyrate, phenyl butyrate, and SAHA showed promised although the results were less consistent, and in the case of SAHA, even deleterious regarding body weight.

Tissue Transplantation

These strategies include transplant of tissue from the striatum and anterior cingulate cortex and injection of umbilical cord blood cells. Fetal striatal cells have been shown to integrate into a functional circuit and to alleviate motor and cognitive deficits.[173] These therapies have been tested with some encouraging results in humans although the studies have been carried out in a small scale due to the difficulties associated with these treatments.[174]

Other Drugs/Treatments

Antidiabetic drugs, such as metformin, have also been tested with some minor positive results in R6/2 mice. Another group of alternative treatments are the neurotrophic factors such as GDNF and CNTF and treatments that increase BDNF. Few pre-clinical trials have been completed with positive results that encourage more research in this area. Antidepressants such as serotonin reuptake inhibitors (SSRIs), fluoxetine (Prozac®) and paroxetine, have also been tested. SSRIs, which are widely used in the clinical treatment of HD, may have effects that go beyond regulation of neurotransmitter function and could alleviate brain atrophy, as shown pre-clinically, due to an indirect action on trophic factors and neurogenesis in particular.

Treatments aimed at reducing the load of abnormal Htt include short interfering RNA (siRNA) and small hairpin RNA (shRNA) have shown positive effects but must await developments in specificity and safety before humans can be treated. DNA vaccination has been used by introducing mutant Htt to stimulate the immune system and has been shown to ameliorate the diabetic phenotype of the R6/2 mice.

Metal chelators, such as clioquinol, may prove therapeutic as they form complexes with copper and zinc, therefore diminishing free ion concentrations. This may reduce brain excitability or help in the degradation of Htt.[175] Considering another aspect of the disorder, it has been long suspected that inflammatory processes have an important causative role in neurodegenerative disorders such as Alzheimer's and HD. Pre-clinical trials using the R6/2 mice however have failed to show positive effects using either aspirin or COX-2 inhibitors. A different type of protection, supported by a pre-clinical trial in R6/2 mice, may be given by tauroursodeoxycholic acid (TUDCA), a bile acid that has antioxidative action, mitigates mitochondrial insufficiency and prevents apoptosis.

The rapamycin analog CCI-779 has been used in flies and mice to test (and support) the hypothesis that inhibition of the kinase mTOR will decrease polyglutamine toxicity by decreasing Htt accumulation and increasing autophagy. Erythropoietin is one-of-a-kind cytokine that protects against excitotoxicity and promotes neurogenesis, making it a putative therapeutic drug for HD. An analog that lacks its pro-hematopoietic effects, asialoerythropoietin, however, did not show effects in the R6/2 mice.

In HD patients, caspase-1 is abnormally activated. Since caspase-1 cleaves Htt its inhibition could be beneficial through the reduction of toxic Htt fragments and may also elevate the levels of protective full-length normal Htt. Minocycline inhibits caspase-1 and -3 expression, and inducible nitric oxide synthetase activity, with the latter effect adding protection against free radical damage.

Adenosine A2A is a target for both HD and Parkinson's. Curiously both agonists and antagonists at this receptor are being investigated in HD, although the drug in trials for Parkinson's, KW6002 that aims at reducing the dosage of L-DOPA, is an antagonist. Other treatments include anticholinesterase inhibitors such as tacrine (Cognex®), used in Alzheimer's Disease, which show some but inconsistent effects in the R6/2 mouse.

Some studies have focused on the validation of targets for HD by crossing a model of HD with another transgenic mouse line to study its effect on the original phenotype by over- or under-expression of a second gene. The targets investigated using this strategy include CHIP, heat shock proteins, transglutaminase, Sp1, Bcl-2 and caspase11.

TRANSLATION FROM PRE-CLINICAL TO CLINICAL

Since the identification of the HD gene in 1993, the establishment of a wide variety of cellular and animal models have rapidly accelerated our understanding of the pathogenic mechanisms in HD. Studies in these models have provided many potential novel therapeutic targets. The challenge for the near future is to select the agents that will be brought forward to human clinical trials. It will be critical to choose effectively, because of the large number of subjects, time, and funding required to prove efficacy in slowing HD progression. Moreover, a wide variety of HD animal models are currently available, each with features that are similar as well as distinct from characteristics of human HD. The complexity of these models make decisions about prioritizing therapeutic agents based on individual animal models difficult, and therefore new therapeutic agents should have proven efficacy in several animal models prior to embarking on human clinical trials of any specific therapy.[119] A centralized system for prioritizing potential therapeutic agents for clinical testing in HD trials has been developed (SETHD; www.huntingtonproject.org) and it is hoped that in the future sufficient pre-clinical evaluation of agents will be performed to limit non-informative studies. Ultimately, the drugs that have been brought to clinical trial in HD to date, have been selected without the benefit of rigorous pre-clinical assessment, and were primarily selected based on a favorable safety profile, availability of the agent, and the presence of sufficient funding for clinical studies.

Despite incredible progress in identifying many potential therapeutic targets in HD, there has been no effective translation of these discoveries into effective therapies that have been clinically proven to slow or reverse the inexorable progression of disability and loss of function in HD.

Whereas research in the area of depression, anxiety, and schizophrenia has received intense attention from big Pharma and Academia, a number of less frequent disorders, such as HD, spinal muscular atrophy, and amyotrophic lateral sclerosis have almost been neglected by industry. The reason for the neglect is the high cost of drug discovery, marketing and distribution, which can reach 700 million dollars only to warrant a little over 10 years of market exclusivity. The market for the aforementioned disorders is huge, with more than 16 billion US dollars for depression in the United States of America alone, and therefore a blockbuster drug offsets this risk of development.

Many disorders, however, are not that prevalent and the cost-benefit equation is very different, discouraging any significant investment from big Pharma into the basic research that precedes drug development for rare genetic diseases. The World Health Organization defines a rare disorder as all pathological conditions affecting 0.65–1 out of every 1000 inhabitants. The European Union understands a rare disorder to be one with a prevalence of 5:10,000 Europeans; the United States of America defines it as an ailment affecting fewer than 200,000 Americans; Japan sets the limit at 50,000 Japanese patients; Australia at 2000 Australian patients.[176] However, when the unattended population is summed across the 6000 identified orphan disorders the number is a staggering 10–25 millions affected patients in the United States of America alone (NORD; http://www.rarediseases.org/).

The US Congress recognized this plea and enacted the orphan Drug Act (1983), which relaxed the regulatory constraints for the development of drugs that receive orphan drug designation, and also provided some financial and regulatory support for small companies pursuing treatments for an orphan disorder and provided 7 year of exclusivity after approval of the new drug for an orphan disorder. There is a similar mechanism in Europe through the European Medicines Agency that provides free drug approval protocol assistance, fee reductions for access to the centralized community procedures before and after marketing authorization, and 10 years of market exclusivity following drug approval.

Momentum for progress in the battle against HD is gaining popularity, primarily due to the effort of non-profit organizations to provide funding and support that encourages research leading to a cure or therapy for HD. Non-profit organizations are currently leading research for autism, amyotrophic lateral sclerosis, spinal muscular atrophy, Wilson's disease, and liposomal storage disorders. These institutions (e.g., CHDI, Cure Huntington's Disease Initiative; www.chdi-inc.org) sometimes act as small virtual biotech companies, outsourcing all components of a drug pipeline, such as chemistry, formulation, ADMET, *in vitro*, *in vivo* pre-clinical and clinical studies.

FUTURE DIRECTIONS

Considerable progress has been made in understanding the pathogenesis of HD and in identifying potential targets for therapeutic intervention. Pre-clinical efforts to evaluate potential agents directed against these targets continue to progress, and many compounds have been reported to result in beneficial effects when applied in various model systems of HD.[177] Despite progress in identifying pathogenic targets, developing compounds against these targets, and screening of compounds in pre-clinical models, the predictive value of a positive finding in any HD model system is still unknown. Improving the methods and outcome measures used in HD clinical trials is a critical step in translating advances in basic science into proven treatments for HD. A critical component of improved HD clinical trials will be the identification and validation of novel biological markers that track the course of HD (biomarkers).

Biomarkers that are sensitive measures of disease progression will be of paramount importance in future HD therapeutic trials, particularly in the pre-manifest HD population. To date there are a few putative biomarkers that have been evaluated in cross-sectional studies.[178] Some of these biomarkers have been examined in a limited number of subjects longitudinally, but at the current time there have not been good prospective studies of putative biomarkers in HD, in part due to the limited availability of prospectively collected, longitudinal samples, images and clinical data of sufficient quality and quantity. An example of one such prospective clinical study is TRACK-HD. This international multi-site study of early and pre-manifest HD (supported by the HighQ Foundation) was designed to evaluate a large number of phenotypic characteristics prospectively (using clinical rating scales, cognitive testing batteries, quantitative motor tasks, oculomotor testing, neuropsychiatric testing, neuroimaging, carefully collected biologic samples, and genetic information) over a 2-year period. The primary objective of this exciting study is to identify a combination of biomarkers (both "wet" and "dry") that will be sensitive for detecting change over the natural course of pre-manifest and early HD. The development and characterization of appropriate biomarkers in HD by studies, such as TRACK-HD, will improve the efficiency of future therapeutic trials by providing additional information on the effects of putative therapeutic agents in HD. Some clinical biomarkers (such as neuroimaging) may ultimately also become defined surrogate endpoints for HD clinical trials.

Developing effective treatments for human disease requires appropriate pre-clinical model systems in which to interrogate pathogenic mechanisms, and test novel therapeutic agents. For HD research a wide variety of disease models are already in place and despite the fact that the critical aspects of disease pathogenesis remain incompletely understood, the availability of these models for testing potential therapeutic compounds will be a critical element in finding the cure. To date, none of the drugs tested in human clinical trials had been previously demonstrated to be consistently effective across a variety of HD models, in systems as diverse as yeast, fly, worm, fish, mammalian cells, and transgenic mice. To encourage the appropriate selection of agents for human clinical trials it is imperative that the performance of any pre-clinical drug candidate be evaluated and compared in as wide a variety of systems as possible, since the capacity of any given model to predict the therapeutic potential of a compound has yet to be determined. The various pre-clinical models of HD that are currently being used to identify and test novel therapeutic compounds will only be validated once an agent has been shown to have proven efficacy in the clinic. Currently, efficacy in pre-clinical transgenic HD mouse trials is the single most decisive factor influencing the decision to take a given compound forward for development in the clinic.

The primary focus of this chapter has been to encourage the efficient screening of new therapeutic agents for the treatment of HD in pre-clinical transgenic mouse models, and to facilitate the translation of these studies into human clinical trials. Better animal disease models and more accurate pre-clinical evaluation of potential therapeutic agents will help prevent the massive expense and the disappointment of non-informative or unsuccessful clinical trials. The most promising new treatments that are effective in the various models of HD need to be rapidly evaluated for use in human clinical trials. Despite impressive recent advances in our understanding of the pathogenesis of HD, there are currently no known treatments that halt the progression or delay the clinical onset. Appropriate studies in pre-clinical models of HD will lead to the development of new treatments that prevent or slow down the progression of this devastating disease and will translate into improved quality of life, greater self-sufficiency, and longer more productive lives for individuals with HD.

REFERENCES

1. Hayden, M.R. (1981). *Huntington's Chorea*. Springer, Berlin.
2. Huntington, G. (1872). On Chorea. *The Medical and Surgical Reporter: A Weekly Journal*, 26(15):317-321.
3. Osler, W. (1894). *On Chorea and Choreiform Affections*. P. Blakston, Son & Co., Philadelphia.
4. Gusella, J.F., Wexler, N.S., Conneally, P.M., Naylor, S.L., Anderson, M.A., Tanzi, R.E., *et al.* (1983). A polymorphic DNA marker genetically linked to Huntingtons-disease, *Nature*, 306(5940) 234-238.
5. MacDonald, M.E., Ambrose, C.M., Duyao, M.P., Myers, R.H., Lin, C., Srinidhi, L. *et al.* (1993). A novel gene containing a trinucleotide repeat that is expanded and unstable on Huntingtons-disease chromosomes. *Cell Cell*, 72(6):971-983.
6. Harper, P.S. (1991). *Huntington's Disease*. WB Saunders Co., London.
7. Young, A.B., Shoulson, I., Penney, J.B., Starosta-Rubinstein, S., Gomez, F., Travers, H. *et al.* (1986). Huntington's disease in Venezuela: Neurologic features and functional decline. *Neurology*, 36(2):244-249.
8. van Dijk, J.G., van der Velde, E.A., Roos, R.A., and Bruyn, G.W. (1986). Juvenile Huntington disease. *Hum Genet*, 73(3):235-239.
9. Butters, N., Wolfe, J., Martone, M., Granholm, E., and Cermak, L.S. (1985). Memory disorders associated with Huntington's disease: Verbal recall, verbal recognition and procedural memory. *Neuropsychologia*, 23(6):729-743.
10. Zakzanis, K.K. (1998). The subcortical dementia of Huntington's disease. *J Clin Exp Neuropsychol*, 20(4):565-578.
11. Anderson, K.E. And Marder, K.S. (2001). An overview of psychiatric symptoms in Huntington's disease. *Curr Psychiatry Rep*, 3(5):379-388.
12. Lovestone, S., Hodgson, S., Sham, P., Differ, A.M., and Levy, R. (1996). Familial psychiatric presentation of Huntington's disease. *J Med Genet*, 33(2):128-131.
13. van Raamsdonk, J.M., Murphy, Z., Selva, D.M., Hamidizadeh, R., Pearson, J., Petersen, A. *et al.* (2007). Testicular degeneration in Huntington disease. *Neurobiol Dis*, 26(3):512-520.
14. Morton, A.J., Wood, N.I., Hastings, M.H., Hurelbrink, C., Barker, R.A., and Maywood, E.S. (2005). Disintegration of the sleep-wake cycle and circadian timing in Huntington's disease. *J Neurosci*, 25(1):157-163.
15. Sanberg, P.R., Fibiger, H.C., and Mark, R.F. (1981). Body-weight and dietary factors in Huntingtons-disease patients compared with matched controls. *Med J Aust*, 1(8):407-409.
16. Pratley, R.E., Salbe, A.D., Ravussin, E., and Caviness, J.N. (2000). Higher sedentary energy expenditure in patients with Huntington's disease. *Ann Neurol*, 47(1):64-70.

17. Gaba, A.M., Zhang, K., Marder, K., Moskowitz, C.B., Werner, P., and Boozer, C.N. (2005). Energy balance in early-stage Huntington disease. *Am J Clin Nutr*, 81(6):1335–1341.

18. Andrew, S.E., Goldberg, Y.P., Kremer, B., Telenius, H., Theilmann, J., Adam, S. *et al.* (1993). The relationship between trinucleotide (CAG) repeat length and clinical features of Huntington's disease. *Nat Genet*, 4(4):398–403.

19. Brinkman, R.R., Mezei, M.M., Theilmann, J., Almqvist, E., and Hayden, M.R. (1997). The likelihood of being affected with Huntington disease by a particular age, for a specific CAG size. *Am J Hum Genet*, 60(5):1202–1210.

20. Duyao, M., Ambrose, C., Myers, R., Novelletto, A., Persichetti, F., Frontali, M. *et al.* (1993). Trinucleotide repeat length instability and age of onset in Huntington's disease. *Nat Genet*, 4(4):387–392.

21. Semaka, A., Creighton, S., Warby, S., and Hayden, M.R. (2006). Predictive testing for Huntington disease: Interpretation and significance of intermediate alleles. *Clin Genet*, 70(4):283–294.

22. Falush, D., Almqvist, E.W., Brinkmann, R.R., Iwasa, Y., and Hayden, M.R. (2001). Measurement of mutational flow implies both a high new-mutation rate for Huntington disease and substantial under ascertainment of late-onset cases. *Am J Hum Genet*, 68(2):373–385.

23. Telenius, H., Kremer, H.P., Theilmann, J., Andrew, S.E., Almqvist, E., Anvret, M. *et al.* (1993). Molecular analysis of juvenile Huntington disease: The major influence on (CAG)n repeat length is the sex of the affected parent. *Hum Mol Genet*, 2(10):1535–1540.

24. Vonsattel, J.P., Myers, R.H., Stevens, T.J., Ferrante, R.J., Bird, E.D., and Richardson, E.P., Jr. (1985). Neuropathological classification of Huntington's disease. *J Neuropathol Exp Neurol*, 44(6):559–577.

25. Hedreen, J.C. And Folstein, S.E. (1995). Early loss of neostriatal striosome neurons in Huntington's disease. *J Neuropathol Exp Neurol*, 54(1):105–120.

26. Reiner, A., Albin, R.L., Anderson, K.D., D'Amato, C.J., Penney, J.B., and Young, A.B. (1988). Differential loss of striatal projection neurons in Huntington disease. *Proc Natl Acad Sci USA*, 85(15):5733–5737.

27. Albin, R.L., Young, A.B., and Penney, J.B. (1989). The functional anatomy of basal ganglia disorders. *Trends Neurosci*, 12(10):366–375.

28. Hedreen, J.C., Peyser, C.E., Folstein, S.E., and Ross, C.A. (1991). Neuronal loss in layers V and VI of cerebral cortex in Huntington's disease. *Neurosci Lett*, 133(2):257–261.

29. Spargo, E., Everall, I.P., and Lantos, P.L. (1993). Neuronal loss in the hippocampus in Huntington's disease: A comparison with HIV infection. *J Neurol Neurosurg Psychiatr*, 56(5):487–491.

30. Nance, M.A. And Myers, R.H. (2001). Juvenile onset Huntington's disease – clinical and research perspectives. *Ment Retard Dev Disabil Res Rev*, 7(3):153–157.

31. Davies, S.W., Turmaine, M., Cozens, B.A., Difiglia, M., Sharp, A.H., Ross, C.A. *et al.* (1997). Formation of neuronal intranuclear inclusions underlies the neurological dysfunction in mice transgenic for the HD mutation. *Cell Cell*, 90(3):537–548.

32. Difiglia, M., Sapp, E., Chase, K.O., Davies, S.W., Bates, G.P., Vonsattel, J.P. *et al.* (1997). Aggregation of huntingtin in neuronal intranuclear inclusions and dystrophic neurites in brain. *Science*, 277(5334):1990–1993.

33. Robitaille, Y., Lopes-Cendes, I., Becher, M., Rouleau, G., and Clark, A.W. (1997). The neuropathology of CAG repeat diseases: Review and update of genetic and molecular features. *Brain Pathol*, 7(3):901–926.

34. Ramaswamy, S., Shannon, K.M., and Kordower, J.H. (2007). Huntington's disease: Pathological mechanisms and therapeutic strategies. *Cell Transplant*, 16(3):301–312.

35. Fan, M.M. And Raymond, L.A. (2007). N-methyl-D-aspartate (NMDA) receptor function and excitotoxicity in Huntington's disease. *Prog Neurobiol*, 81(5–6):272–293.

36. Zeron, M.M., Hansson, O., Chen, N.S., Wellington, C.L., Leavitt, B.R., Brundin, P. *et al.* (2002). Increased sensitivity to N-methyl-D-aspartate receptor-mediated excitotoxicity in a mouse model of Huntington's disease. *Neuron*, 33(6):849–860.

37. Hansson, O., Petersen, A., Leist, M., Nicotera, P., Castilho, R.F., and Brundin, P. (1999). Transgenic mice expressing a Huntington's disease mutation are resistant to quinolinic acid-induced striatal excitotoxicity. *Proc Natl Acad Sci USA*, 96(15):8727–8732.

38. Hodgson, J.G., Agopyan, N., Gutekunst, C.A., Leavitt, B.R., LePiane, F., Singaraja, R. *et al.* (1999). A YAC mouse model for Huntington's disease with full-length mutant huntingtin, cytoplasmic toxicity, and selective striatal neurodegeneration. *Neuron*, 23(1):181–192.

39. Slow, E.J., van Raamsdonk, J., Rogers, D., Coleman, S.H., Graham, R.K., Deng, Y. *et al.* (2003). Selective striatal neuronal loss in a YAC128 mouse model of Huntington disease. *Hum Mol Genet*, 12(13):1555–1567.

40. Panov, A.V., Gutekunst, C.A., Leavitt, B.R., Hayden, M.R., Burke, J.R., Strittmatter, W.J. *et al.* (2002). Early mitochondrial calcium defects in Huntington's disease are a direct effect of polyglutamines. *Nat Neurosci*, 5(8):731–736.

41. Tang, T.S., Tu, H.P., Chan, E.Y.W., Maximov, A., Wang, Z.N., Wellington, C.L. *et al.* (2003). Huntingtin and Huntingtin-associated protein 1 influence neuronal calcium signaling mediated by inositol-(1,4,5) triphosphate receptor type 1. *Neuron*, 39(2):227–239.

42. Scherzinger, E., Lurz, R., Turmaine, M., Mangiarini, L., Hollenbach, B., Hasenbank, R. *et al.* (1997). Huntingtin-encoded polyglutamine expansions form amyloid-like protein aggregates *in vitro* and *in vivo*. *Cell Cell*, 90(3):549–558.

43. Edwardson, J.M., Wang, C.T., Gong, B., Wyttenbach, A., Bai, J.H., Jackson, M.B. *et al.* (2003). Expression of mutant huntingtin blocks exocytosis in PC12 cells by depletion of complexin II. *J Biol Chem*, 278(33):30849–30853.

44. Benn, C.L., Slow, E.J., Farrell, L.A., Graham, R., Deng, Y., Hayden, M.R. *et al.* (2007). Glutamate receptor abnormalities in the YAC128 transgenic mouse model of Huntington's disease. *Neuroscience*, 147(2):354–372.

45. Gunawardena, S., Her, L.S., Brusch, R.G., Laymon, R.A., Niesman, I.R., Gordesky-Gold, B. *et al.* (2003). Disruption of axonal transport by loss of huntingtin or expression of pathogenic PolyQ proteins in *Drosophila*. *Neuron*, 40(1):25–40.

46. Lee, W.C., Yoshihara, M., and Littleton, J.T. (2004). Cytoplasmic aggregates trap polyglutamine-containing proteins and block axonal transport in a *Drosophila* model of Huntington's disease. *Proc Natl Acad Sci USA*, 101(9):3224–3229.

47. Cha, J.H. (2000). Transcriptional dysregulation in Huntington's disease. *Trends Neurosci*, 23(9):387–392.

48. Ross, C.A. (1997). Intranuclear neuronal inclusions: A common pathogenic mechanism for glutamine-repeat neurodegenerative diseases?. *Neuron*, 19(6):1147–1150.

49. Slow, E.J., Graham, R.K., Osmand, A.P., Devon, R.S., Lu, G., Deng, Y. *et al.* (2005). Absence of behavioral abnormalities and neurodegeneration *in vivo* despite widespread neuronal huntingtin inclusions. *Proc Natl Acad Sci USA*, 102(32):11402–11407.

50. Gutekunst, C.A., Li, S.H., Yi, H., Mulroy, J.S., Kuemmerle, S., Jones, R. *et al.* (1999). Nuclear and neuropil aggregates in Huntington's disease: Relationship to neuropathology. *J Neurosci*, 19(7):2522–2534.

51. Kuemmerle, S., Gutekunst, C.A., Klein, A.M., Li, X.J., Li, S.H., Beal, M.F. *et al.* (1999). Huntingtin aggregates may not predict neuronal death in Huntington's disease. *Ann Neurol*, 46(6):842–849.

52. Saudou, F., Finkbeiner, S., Devys, D., and Greenberg, M.E. (1998). Huntingtin acts in the nucleus to induce apoptosis but death does not correlate with the formation of intranuclear inclusions. *Cell Cell*, 95(1):55–66.

53. Arrasate, M., Mitra, S., Schweitzer, E.S., Segal, M.R., and Finkbeiner, S. (2004). Inclusion body formation reduces levels of mutant huntingtin and the risk of neuronal death. *Nature*, 431(7010):805-810.

54. Leavitt, B.R., Wellington, C.L., and Hayden, M.R. (1999). Recent insights into the molecular pathogenesis of Huntington disease. *Semin Neurol*, 19(4):385-395.

55. Graham, R.K., Deng, Y., Slow, E.J., Haigh, B., Bissada, N., Lu, G. *et al.* (2006). Cleavage at the caspase-6 site is required for neuronal dysfunction and degeneration due to mutant huntingtin. *Cell Cell*, 125(6):1179-1191.

56. Grimbergen, Y.A. And Roos, R.A. (2003). Therapeutic options for Huntington's disease. *Curr Opin Investig Drugs*, 4(1):51-54.

57. Bonelli, R.M. And Hofmann, P. (2004). A review of the treatment options for Huntington's disease. *Expet Opin Pharmacother*, 5(4):767-776.

58. De Marchi, N. And Mennella, R. (2000). Huntington's disease and its association with psychopathology. *Harv Rev Psychiatr*, 7(5):278-289.

59. Vitale, C., Pellecchia, M.T., Grossi, D., Fragassi, N., Cuomo, T., Di Maio, L. *et al.* (2001). Unawareness of dyskinesias in Parkinson's and Huntington's diseases. *Neurolo Sci*, 22(1):105-106.

60. Barr, A.N., Fischer, J.H., Koller, W.C., Spunt, A.L., and Singhal, A. (1988). Serum haloperidol concentration and choreiform movements in Huntingtons-disease. *Neurology*, 38(1):84-88.

61. Squitieri, F., Cannella, M., Porcellini, A., Brusa, L., Simonelli, M., and Ruggieri, S. (2001). Short-term effects of olanzapine in Huntington disease. *Neuropsychiatr Neuropsychol Behav Neurol*, 14(1):69-72.

62. Bonelli, R.M. And Hofmann, P. (2002). Olanzapine for Huntington's disease: An open label study. *Eur Neuropsychopharmacol*, 12:S367.

63. Stahl, S. (2000). *Essential Psychopharmacology*, 2nd edition, Cambridge University Press, Cambridge.

64. Melkersson, K. And Dahl, M.L. (2004). Adverse metabolic effects associated with atypical antipsychotics – Literature review and clinical implications. *Drugs*, 64(7):701-723.

65. Marshall, F.J., Walker, F., Frank, S., Oakes, D., Plumb, S., Factor, S.A. *et al.* (2006). Tetrabenazine as antichorea therapy in Huntington disease – A randomized controlled trial. *Neurology*, 66(3):366-372.

66. Kenney, C., Hunter, C., Mejia, N., and Jankovic, J. (2006). Is history of depression a contraindication to treatment with tetrabenazine?. *Clin Neuropharmacol*, 29(5):259-264.

67. Compendium of Pharmaceuticals and Specialties (2002). 37th edition.

68. Peiris, J.B., Boralessa, H., and Lionel, N.D.W. (1976). Clonazepam in treatment of choreiform activity. *Med J Aust*, 1(8):225-227.

69. Stewart, J.T. (1988). Treatment of Huntingtons-disease with clonazepam. *South Med J*, 81(1):102.

70. Metman, L.V., Morris, M.J., Farmer, C., Gillespie, M., Mosby, K., Wuu, J. *et al.* (2002). Huntington's disease – A randomized, controlled trial using the NMDA-antagonist amantadine. *Neurology*, 59(5):694-699.

71. Folstein, S.E. (1989). The psychopathology of Huntingtons-disease. *J Nerv Ment Dis*, 177(10):645.

72. Beister, A., Kraus, P., Kuhn, W., Dose, M., Weindl, A., and Gerlach, M. (2004). The N-methyl-D-aspartate antagonist memantine retards progression of Huntington's disease. *J Neural Transm-Suppl*(68):117-122.

73. de Tommaso, M., Specchio, N., Sciruicchio, V., Difruscolo, O., and Specchio, L.M. (2004). Effects of rivastigmine on motor and cognitive impairment in Huntington's disease. *Mov Disord*, 19(12):1516-1518.

74. Petrikis, P., Andreou, C., Piachas, A., Bozikas, V.P., and Karavatos, A. (2004). Treatment of Huntington's disease with galantamine. *Int Clin Psychopharmacol*, 19(1):49-50.

75. Fernandez, H.H., Friedman, J.H., Grace, J., and Beason-Hazen, S. (2000). Donepezil for Huntington's disease. *Mov Disord*, 15(1):173-176.

76. Marder, K., Zhao, H., Myers, R.H., Cudkowicz, M., Kayson, E., Kieburtz, K. *et al.* (2000). Rate of functional decline in Huntington's disease. *Neurology*, 54(2):452–458.

77. Leonard, D.P., Kidson, M.A., Brown, J.G.E., Shannon, P.J., and Taryan, S. (1975). Double-blind trial of lithium-carbonate and haloperidol in Huntingtons-chorea. *Aust New Zeal J Psychiatr*, 9(2):115–118.

78. Goedhard, L.E., Stolker, J.J., Heerdink, E.R., Nijman, H.L.I., Olivier, B., and Egberts, T.C.G. (2006). Pharmacotherapy for the treatment of aggressive behavior in general adult psychiatry: A systematic review. J *Clin Psychiatr*, 67(7):1013.

79. Paleacu, D., Anca, M., and Giladi, N. (2002). Olanzapine in Huntington's disease. *Acta Neurol Scand*, 105(6):441–444.

80. Alpay, M. And Koroshetz, W.J. (2006). Quetiapine in the treatment of behavioral disturbances in patients with Huntington's disease. *Psychosomatics*, 47(1):70–72.

81. Meinhold, J.M., Blake, L.M., Mini, L.J., Welge, J.A., Schwiers, M., and Hughes, A. (2005). Effect of divalproex sodium on behavioural and cognitive problems in elderly dementia. *Drugs Aging*, 22(7):615–626.

82. Wirshing, D.A., Wirshing, W.C., Kysar, L., Berisford, M.A., Goldstein, D., Pashdag, J. *et al.* (1999). Novel antipsychotics: Comparison of weight gain liabilities. J *Clin Psychiatr*, 60(6):358–363.

83. Fava, M. (2000). Weight gain and antidepressants. J *Clin Psychiatr*, 61:37–41.

84. Montgomery, S.A., Reimitz, P.E., and Zivkov, M (1998). Mirtazapine versus amitriptyline in the long-term treatment of depression: A double-blind placebo-controlled study. *Int Clin Psychopharmacol*, 13(2):63–73.

85. Stahl, S.M., Zhang, L.S., Damatarca, C., and Grady, M. (2003). Brain-circuits determine destiny in depression: A novel approach to the psychopharmacology of wakefulness, fatigue, and executive dysfunction in major depressive disorder. J *Clin Psychiatr*, 64:6–17.

86. Peyser, C.E., Folstein, M., Chase, G.A., Starkstein, S., Brandt, J., Cockrell, J.R. *et al.* (1995). Trial of D-Alpha-Tocopherol in Huntingtons-Disease. *Am J Psychiatr*, 152(12):1771–1775.

87. Kremer, B., Clark, C.M., Almqvist, E.W., Raymond, L.A., Graf, P., Jacova, C. *et al.* (1999). Influence of lamotrigine on progression of early Huntington disease – A randomized clinical trial. *Neurology*, 53(5):1000–1011.

88. Kieburtz, K., Koroshetz, W., McDermott, M., Beal, M.F., Greenamyre, J.T., Ross, C.A. *et al.* (2001). A randomized, placebo-controlled trial of coenzyme Q(10) and remacemide in Huntington's disease. *Neurology*, 57(3):397–404.

89. Marshall, F.J., Cudkowicz, M., Hayden, M., Kieburtz, K., Zhao, H.W., Penney, J. *et al.* (2003). Dosage effects of riluzole in Huntington's disease – A multicenter placebo-controlled study. *Neurology*, 61(11):1551–1556.

90. Murck, H., Manku, M., Puri, B.K., Leavitt, B.R., Hayden, M.R., Ross, C.A. *et al.* (2005). Ethyl-EPA in Huntington's disease: A double blind, randomised, placebo controlled trial. J *Neurol Neurosurg Psychiatr*, 76.

91. Hersch, S.M., Gevorkian, S., Marder, K., Moskowitz, C., Feigin, A., Cox, M. *et al.* (2006). Creatine in Huntington disease is safe, tolerable, bioavailable in brain and reduces serum 8OH2' dG. *Neurology*, 66(2):250–252.

92. Bonelli, R.M., Hoedl, A., Kapfhammer, H.P., and Wenning, G.K. (2006). Psychiatric management of Huntington's disease: An evidence-based review. J *Neurol Sci*, 248(1-2):281.

93. Bauer, M., Alda, M., Priller, J., and Young, L.T. (2003). Implications of the neuroprotective effects of lithium for the treatment of bipolar and neurodegenerative disorders. *Pharmacopsychiatry*, 36:S250–sS254.

94. Aydemir, O., Deveci, A., and Taneli, F. (2005). The effect of chronic antidepressant treatment on serum brain-derived neurotrophic factor levels in depressed patients: A preliminary study. *Progr Neuro Psychopharmacol Biol Psychiatr*, 29(2):261–265.

95. Brusa, L., Versace, V., Koch, G., Bernardi, G., Iani, C., Stanzione, P. *et al.* (2005). Improvement of choreic movements by 1 Hz repetitive transcranial magnetic stimulation in Huntington's disease patients. *Ann Neurol*, 58(4):655–656.

96. de Tommaso, M., Sciruicchio, V., Specchio, N., Di Fruscolo, O., Cormio, C., Barulli, M. *et al.* (2005). Efficacy of levetiracetam in Huntington's disease. *J Neurol Sci*, 238:S503–S504.

97. Beal, M.F., Brouillet, E., Jenkins, B.G., Ferrante, R.J., Kowall, N.W., Miller, J.M. *et al.* (1993). Neurochemical and histologic characterization of striatal excitotoxic lesions produced by the mitochondrial toxin 3-nitropropionic acid. *J Neurosci*, 13(10):4181–4192.

98. Brouillet, E., Hantraye, P., Ferrante, R.J., Dolan, R., Leroywillig, A., Kowall, N.W. *et al.* (1995). Chronic mitochondrial energy impairment produces selective striatal degeneration and abnormal choreiform movements in primates. *Proc Natl Acad Sci USA*, 92(15):7105–7109.

99. Brouillet, E., Conde, F., Beal, M.F., and Hantraye, P. (1999). Replicating Huntington's disease phenotype in experimental animals. *Prog Neurobiol*, 59(5):427–468.

100. Ludolph, A.C., He, F., Spencer, P.S., Hammerstad, J., and Sabri, M. (1991). 3-Nitropropionic acid – exogenous animal neurotoxin and possible human striatal toxin. *Can J Neurol Sci*, 18(4):492–498.

101. Beal, M.F., Ferrante, R.J., Swartz, K.J., and Kowall, N.W. (1991). Chronic quinolinic acid lesions in rats closely resemble Huntingtons-disease. *J Neurosci*, 11(6):1649–1659.

102. Barnes, G.T., Duyao, M.P., Ambrose, C.M., Mcneil, S., Persichetti, F., Srinidhi, J. *et al.* (1994). Mouse Huntingtons-disease gene homolog (Hdh). *Somat Cell Mol Genet*, 20(2):87–97.

103. Mangiarini, L., Sathasivam, K., Seller, M., Cozens, B., Harper, A., Hetherington, C. *et al.* (1996). Exon 1 of the HD gene with an expanded CAG repeat is sufficient to cause a progressive neurological phenotype in transgenic mice. *Cell Cell*, 87(3):493–506.

104. Laforet, G.A., Sapp, E., Chase, K., McIntyre, C., Boyce, F.M., Campbell, M. *et al.* (2001). Changes in cortical and striatal neurons predict behavioral and electrophysiological abnormalities in a transgenic murine model of Huntington's disease. *J Neurosci*, 21(23):9112–9123.

105. Schilling, G., Becher, M.W., Sharp, A.H., Jinnah, H.A., Duan, K., Kotzuk, J.A. *et al.* (1999). Intranuclear inclusions and neuritic aggregates in transgenic mice expressing a mutant N-terminal fragment of huntingtin. *Hum Mol Genet*, 8(3):397–407.

106. Yamamoto, A., Lucas, J.J., and Hen, R. (2000). Reversal of neuropathology and motor dysfunction in a conditional model of Huntington's disease. *Cell Cell*, 101(1):57–66.

107. Andreassen, O.A., Ferrante, R.J., Dedeoglu, A., and Beal, M.F. (2001). Lipoic acid improves survival in transgenic mouse models of Huntington's disease. *Neuroreport*, 12(15):3371–3373.

108. Andreassen, O.A., Dedeoglu, A., Ferrante, R.J., Jenkins, B.G., Ferrante, K.L., Thomas, M. *et al.* (2001). Creatine increases survival and delays motor symptoms in a transgenic animal model of Huntington's disease. *Neurobiol Dis*, 8(3):479–491.

109. Ferrante, R.J., Andreassen, O.A., Jenkins, B.G., Dedeoglu, A., Kuemmerle, S., Kubilus, J.K. *et al.* (2000). Neuroprotective effects of creatine in a transgenic mouse model of Huntington's disease. *J Neurosci*, 20(12):4389–4397.

110. Ferrante, R.J., Andreassen, O.A., Dedeoglu, A., Ferrante, K.L., Jenkins, B.G., Hersch, S.M. *et al.* (2002). Therapeutic effects of coenzyme Q(10) and remacemide in transgenic mouse models of Huntington's disease. *J Neurosci*, 22(5):1592–1599.

111. Mievis, S., Ledent, C., and Blum, D. (2005). Lack of minocycline efficiency in genetic models of Huntington's disease. *J Neurol Neurosurg Psychiatr*, 76.

112. Diaz-Hernandez, M., Torres-Peraza, J., Salvatori-Abarca, A., Moran, M.A., Gomez-Ramos, P., Alberch, J. *et al.* (2005). Full motor recovery despite striatal neuron loss and formation of irreversible amyloid-like inclusions in a conditional mouse model of Huntington's disease. *J Neurosci*, 25(42):9773–9781.

113. Carter, R.J., Lione, L.A., Humby, T., Mangiarini, L., Mahal, A., Bates, G.P. *et al.* (1999). Characterization of progressive motor deficits in mice transgenic for the human Huntington's disease mutation. *J Neurosci*, 19(8):3248–3257.

114. Stack, E.C., Kubilus, J.K., Smith, K., Cormier, K., Del Signore, S.J., Guelin, E. *et al.* (2005). Chronology of behavioral symptoms and neuropathological sequela in R6/2 Huntington's disease transgenic mice. J *Comp Neurol*, 490(4):354-370.
115. Yu, Z.X., Li, S.H., Evans, J., Pillarisetti, A., Li, H., and Li, X.J. (2003). Mutant huntingtin causes context-dependent neurodegeneration in mice with Huntington's disease. J *Neurosci*, 23(6):2193-2202.
116. Lione, L.A., Carter, R.J., Hunt, M.J., Bates, G.P., Morton, A.J., and Dunnett, S.B. (1999). Selective discrimination learning impairments in mice expressing the human Huntington's disease mutation. J *Neurosci*, 19(23):10428-10437.
117. Cepeda, C., Hurst, R.S., Calvert, C.R., Hernandez-Echeagaray, E., Nguyen, O.K., Jocoy, E. *et al.* (2003). Transient and progressive electrophysiological alterations in the corticostriatal pathway in a mouse model of Huntington's disease. J *Neurosci*, 23(3):961-969.
118. Bogdanov, M.B., Andreassen, O.A., Dedeoglu, A., Ferrante, R.J., and Beal, M.F. (2001). Increased oxidative damage to DNA in a transgenic mouse model of Huntington's disease. J *Neurochem*, 79(6):1246-1249.
119. Hockly, E., Woodman, B., Mahal, A., Lewis, C.M., and Bates, G. (2003). Standardization and statistical approaches to therapeutic trials in the R6/2 mouse. *Brain Res Bull*, 61(5): 469-479.
120. Hersch, S.M. And Ferrante, R.J. (2004). Translating therapies for Huntington's disease from genetic animal models to clinical trials. *NeuroRx: The Journal of the American Society for Experimental NeuroTherapeutics*, 1:298-306.
121. van Raamsdonk, J.M., Pearson, J., Slow, E.J., Hossain, S.M., Leavitt, B.R., and Hayden, M.R. (2005). Cognitive dysfunction precedes neuropathology and motor abnormalities in the YAC128 mouse model of Huntington's disease. J *Neurosci*, 25(16):4169-4180.
122. Ordway, J.M., TallaksenGreene, S., Gutekunst, C.A., Bernstein, E.M., Cearley, J.A., Wiener, H.W. *et al.* (1997). Ectopically expressed CAG repeats cause intranuclear inclusions and a progressive late onset neurological phenotype in the mouse. *Cell Cell*, 91(6):753-763.
123. Reddy, P.H., Williams, M., Charles, V., Garrett, L., Pike-Buchanan, L., Whetsell, W.O. *et al.* (1998). Behavioural abnormalities and selective neuronal loss in HD transgenic mice expressing mutated full-length HD cDNA. *Nat Genet*, 20(2):198-202.
124. Graham, R.K., Slow, E.J., Deng, Y., Bissada, N., Lu, G., Pearson, J. *et al.* (2006). Levels of mutant huntingtin influence the phenotypic severity of Huntington disease in YAC128 mouse models. *Neurobiol Dis*, 21(2):444-455.
125. van Raamsdonk, J.M., Murphy, Z., Slow, E.J., Leavitt, B.R., and Hayden, M.R. (2005). Selective degeneration and nuclear localization of mutant huntingtin in the YAC128 mouse model of Huntington disease. *Hum Mol Genet*, 14(24):3823-3835.
126. Tanaka, Y., Igarashi, S., Nakamura, M., Gafni, J., Torcassi, C., Schilling, G. *et al.* (2006). Progressive phenotype and nuclear accumulation of an amino-terminal cleavage fragment in a transgenic mouse model with inducible expression of full-length mutant huntingtin. *Neurobiol Dis*, 21(2):381-391.
127. White, J.K., Auerbach, W., Duyao, M.P., Vonsattel, J.P., Gusella, J.F., Joyner, A.L. *et al.* (1997). Huntingtin is required for neurogenesis and is not impaired by the Huntington's disease CAG expansion. *Nat Genet*, 17(4):404-410.
128. Levine, M.S., Klapstein, G.J., Koppel, A., Gruen, E., Cepeda, C., Vargas, M.E. *et al.* (1999). Enhanced sensitivity to N-methyl-D-aspartate receptor activation in transgenic and knockin mouse models of Huntington's disease. J *Neurosci Res*, 58(4):515-532.
129. Shelbourne, P.F., Killeen, N., Hevner, R.F., Johnston, H.M., Tecott, L., Lewandoski, M. *et al.* (1999). A Huntington's disease CAG expansion at the murine Hdh locus is unstable and associated with behavioural abnormalities in mice. *Hum Mol Genet*, 8(5):763-774.
130. Wheeler, V.C., White, J.K., Gutekunst, C.A., Vrbanac, V., Weaver, M., Li, X.J. *et al.* (2000). Long glutamine tracts cause nuclear localization of a novel form of huntingtin in medium

spiny striatal neurons in Hdh(Q92) and Hdh(Q111) knock-in mice. *Hum Mol Genet*, 9(4):503–513.

131. Lin, C.H., Tallaksen-Greene, S., Chien, W.M., Cearley, J.A., Jackson, W.S., Crouse, A.B. *et al.* (2001). Neurological abnormalities in a knock-in mouse model of Huntington's disease. *Hum Mol Genet*, 10(2):137–144.

132. Menalled, L.B., Sison, J.D., Dragatsis, I., Zeitlin, S., and Chesselet, M.F. (2003). Time course of early motor and neuropathological anomalies in a knock-in mouse model of Huntington's disease with 140 CAG repeats. J *Comp Neurol*, 465(1):11–26.

133. Menalled, L.B. And Chesselet, M.F. (2002). Mouse models of Huntington's disease. *Trends Pharmacol Sci*, 23(1):32–39.

134. Zeitlin, S., Liu, J.P., Chapman, D.L., Papaioannou, V.E., and Efstratiadis, A. (1995). Increased apoptosis and early embryonic lethality in mice nullizygous for the Huntingtons-disease gene homolog. *Nat Genet*, 11(2):155–163.

135. Dragatsis, I., Efstratiadis, A., and Zeitlin, S. (1998). Mouse mutant embryos lacking huntingtin are rescued from lethality by wild-type extraembryonic tissues. *Development*, 125(8):1529–1539.

136. Reiner, A., Del Mar, N., Meade, C.A., Yang, H.T., Dragatsis, I., Zeitlin, S. *et al.* (2001). Neurons lacking huntingtin differentially colonize brain and survive in chimeric mice. J *Neurosci*, 21(19):7608–7619.

137. Dragatsis, I., Levine, M.S., and Zeitlin, S. (2000). Inactivation of Hdh in the brain and testis results in progressive neurodegeneration and sterility in mice. *Nat Genet*, 26(3):300–306.

138. van Raamsdonk, J.M., Pearson, J., Rogers, D.A., Bissada, N., Vogl, A.W., Hayden, M.R. *et al.* (2005). Loss of wild-type huntingtin influences motor dysfunction and survival in the YAC128 mouse model of Huntington disease. *Hum Mol Genet*, 14(10):1379–1392.

139. Woodman, B., Butler, R., Landles, C., Lupton, M.K., Tse, J., Hockly, E. *et al.* (2007). The Hdh(Q150/Q150) knock-in mouse model of HD and the R6/2 exon 1 model develop comparable and widespread molecular phenotypes. *Brain Res Bull*, 72(2–3):83–97.

140. Irwin, S. (1968). Comprehensive observational assessment: Ia. A systematic, quantitative procedure for assessing the behavioral and physiologic state of the mouse. *Psychopharmacologia*, 13(3):222–257.

141. Hamm, R.J., Pike, B.R., O'Dell, D.M., Lyeth, B.G., and Jenkins, L.W. (1994). The rotarod test: An evaluation of its effectiveness in assessing motor deficits following traumatic brain injury. J *Neurotrauma*, 11(2):187–196.

142. Hickey, M.A., Gallant, K., Gross, G.G., Levine, M.S., and Chesselet, M.F. (2005). Early behavioral deficits in R6/2 mice suitable for use in preclinical drug testing. *Neurobiol Dis*, 20(1):1–11.

143. van Raamsdonk, J.M., Metzler, M., Slow, E., Pearson, J., Schwab, C., Carroll, J. *et al.* (2007). Phenotypic abnormalities in the YAC128 mouse model of Huntington disease are penetrant on multiple genetic backgrounds and modulated by strain. *Neurobiol Dis*, 26(1):189–200.

144. Bolivar, V.J., Manley, K., and Messer, A. (2004). Early exploratory behavior abnormalities in R6/1 Huntington's disease transgenic mice. *Brain Res*, 1005(1–2):29–35.

145. Foroud, T., Siemers, E., Kleindorfer, D., Bill, D.J., Hodes, M.E., Norton, J.A. *et al.* (1995). Cognitive scores in carriers of Huntington's disease gene compared to noncarriers. *Ann Neurol*, 37(5):657–664.

146. Hahn-Barma, V., Deweer, B., Durr, A., Dode, C., Feingold, J., Pillon, B. *et al.* (1998). Are cognitive changes the first symptoms of Huntington's disease? A study of gene carriers. J *Neurol Neurosurg Psychiatr*, 64(2):172–177.

147. Gomez-Tortosa, E., del Barrio, A., Garcia Ruiz, P.J., Pernaute, R.S., Benitez, J., Barroso, A. *et al.* (1998). Severity of cognitive impairment in juvenile and late-onset Huntington disease. *Arch Neurol*, 55(6):835–843.

148. Berrios, G.E., Wagle, A.C., Markova, I.S., Wagle, S.A., Ho, L.W., Rubinsztein, D.C. *et al.* (2001). Psychiatric symptoms and CAG repeats in neurologically asymptomatic Huntington's disease gene carriers. *Psychiatr Res*, 102(3):217-225.

149. Craufurd, D. And Snowden, J. (2002). Neuropsychological and neuropsychiatric aspects of Huntington's disease. In Bates, G., Harper, P.S., and Jones, L. (eds.), *Huntington's Disease*, 3rd ed. Oxford University Press, Oxford, pp. 62-94.

150. Lange, K.W., Sahakian, B.J., Quinn, N.P., Marsden, C.D., and Robbins, T.W. (1995). Comparison of executive and visuospatial memory function in Huntington's disease and dementia of Alzheimer type matched for degree of dementia. *J Neurol Neurosurg Psychiatr*, 58(5):598-606.

151. Swerdlow, N.R., Paulsen, J., Braff, D.L., Butters, N., Geyer, M.A., and Swenson, M.R. (1995). Impaired prepulse inhibition of acoustic and tactile startle response in patients with Huntington's disease. *J Neurol Neurosurg Psychiatr*, 58(2):192-200.

152. Lange, K.W., Javoy-Agid, F, Agid, Y., Jenner, P., and Marsden, C.D. (1992). Brain muscarinic cholinergic receptors in Huntington's disease. *J Neurol*, 239(2):103-104.

153. Koch, M. (1996). The septohippocampal system is involved in prepulse inhibition of the acoustic startle response in rats. *Behav Neurosci*, 110(3):468-477.

154. Birrell, J.M. and Brown, V.J. (2000). Medial frontal cortex mediates perceptual attentional set shifting in the rat. *J Neurosci*, 20(11):4320-4324.

155. Tunbridge, E.M., Bannerman, D.M., Sharp, T., and Harrison, P.J. (2004). Catechol-o-methyltransferase inhibition improves set-shifting performance and elevates stimulated dopamine release in the rat prefrontal cortex. *J Neurosci*, 24(23):5331-5335.

156. Colacicco, G., Welzl, H., Lipp, H.P., and Wurbel, H. (2002). Attentional set-shifting in mice: Modification of a rat paradigm, and evidence for strain-dependent variation. *Behav Brain Res*, 132(1):95-102.

157. Brooks, S.P., Betteridgea, H., Truernan, R.C., Jones, L., and Dunnett, S.B. (2006). Selective extra-dimensional set shifting deficit in a knock-in mouse model of Huntington's disease. *Brain Res Bull*, 69(4):452-457.

158. Morris, R. (1984). Developments of a water-maze procedure for studying spatial learning in the rat. *J Neurosci Methods*, 11(1):47-60.

159. Block, F, Kunkel, M., and Schwarz, M. (1993). Quinolinic acid lesion of the striatum induces impairment in spatial learning and motor performance in rats. *Neurosci Lett*, 149(2):126-128.

160. Saint-Cyr, J.A., Taylor, A.E., and Lang, A.E. (1988). Procedural learning and neostriatal dysfunction in man. *Brain*, 111(Pt 4):941-959.

161. Micheau, J., Riedel, G., Roloff, E.L., Inglis, J., and Morris, R.G. (2004). Reversible hippocampal inactivation partially dissociates how and where to search in the water maze. *Behav Neurosci*, 118(5):1022-1032.

162. Murphy, K.P., Carter, R.J., Lione, L.A., Mangiarini, L., Mahal, A., Bates, G.P. *et al.* (2000). Abnormal synaptic plasticity and impaired spatial cognition in mice transgenic for exon 1 of the human Huntington's disease mutation. *J Neurosci*, 20(13):5115-5123.

163. Brunner, D., Buhot, M.C., Hen, R., and Hofer, M. (1999). Anxiety, motor activation, and maternal-infant interactions in 5HT1B knockout mice. *Behav Neurosci*, 113(3):587-601.

164. Gerlai, R. (1996). Gene-targeting studies of mammalian behavior: Is it the mutation or the background genotype? *Trends Neurosci*, 19(5):177-181.

165. Weller, A., Leguisamo, A.C., Towns, L., Ramboz, S., Bagiella, E., Hofer, M. *et al.* (2003). Maternal effects in infant and adult phenotypes of 5HT1A and 5HT1B receptor knockout mice. *Dev Psychobiol*, 42(2):194-205.

166. Hockly, E., Cordery, P.M., Woodman, B., Mahal, A., van Dellen, A., Blakemore, C. *et al.* (2002). Environmental enrichment slows disease progression in R61/2 Huntington's disease mice. *Ann Neurol*, 51(2):235-242.

167. Spires, T.L., Grote, H.E., Varshney, N.K., Cordery, P.M., van Dellen, A., Blakemore, C. *et al.* (2004). Environmental enrichment rescues protein deficits in a mouse model of Huntington's disease, indicating a possible disease mechanism. J *Neurosci*, 24(9):2270-2276.

168. Patterson-Kane, E.G., Farnworth, M.J. (2006). Noise exposure, music, and animals in the laboratory: A commentary based on laboratory Animal Refinement and Enrichment Forum (LAREF) discussions. J *Appl Animal Welfare Sci* 9(4):327-332.

169. Carter, R.J., Hunt, M.J., and Morton, A.J. (2000). Environmental stimulation increases survival in mice transgenic for exon I of the Huntington's disease gene. *Mov Disord*, 15(5):925-937.

170. Claxton, K. And Posnett, J. (1996). An economic approach to clinical trial design and research priority-setting. *Health Econ*, 5(6):513-524.

171. Chen, T.T. (1997). Optimal three-stage designs for phase II cancer clinical trials. *Stat Med*, 16(23):2701-2711.

172. Kieburtz, K., Koroshetz, W., McDermott, M., Beal, M.F., Greenamyre, J.T., Ross, C.A. *et al.* (2001). A randomized, placebo-controlled trial of coenzyme Q(10) and remacemide in Huntington's disease. *Neurology*, 57(3):397-404.

173. Farrington, M., Wreghitt, T.G., Lever, A.M.L., Dunnett, S.B., Rosser, A.E., and Barker, R.A. (2006). Neural transplantation in Huntington's disease: The NEST-UK donor tissue microbiological screening program and review of the literature. *Cell Transplant*, 15(4):279-294.

174. Gaura, V., Bachoud-Levi, A.C., Ribeiro, M.J., Nguyen, J.P., Frouin, V., Baudic, S. *et al.* (2004). Striatal neural grafting improves cortical metabolism in Huntington's disease patients. *Brain*, 127:65-72.

175. Ferrada, E., Arancibia, V., Loeb, B., Norambuena, E., Olea-Azar, C., and Huidobro-Toro, J.P. (2007). Stoichiometry and conditional stability constants of Cu(II) or Zn(II) clioquinol complexes; implications for Alzheimer's and Huntington's disease therapy. *Neurotoxicology*, 28(3):445-449.

176. Lavandeira, A. (2002). Orphan drugs: Legal aspects, current situation Haemophilia. *Haemophilia*, 8(3):194-198.

177. Bates, G.P. And Hockly, E. (2003). Experimental therapeutics in Huntington's disease: Are models useful for therapeutic trials?. *Curr Opin Neurol*, 16(4):465-470.

178. Henley, S.M.D., Bates, G.P., and Tabrizi, S.J. (2005). Biomarkers for neurodegenerative diseases. *Curr Opin Neurol*, 18(6):698-705.

179. Li, H., Li, S.H., Johnston, H., Shelbourne, P.F., and Li, X.J. (2000). Amino-terminal fragments of mutant huntingtin show selective accumulation in striatal neurons and synaptic toxicity. *Nat Genet*, 25(4):385-389.

180. Smith, K.M., Matson, S., Matson, W.R., Cormier, K., Del Signore, S.J., Hagerty, S.W. *et al.* (2006). Dose ranging and efficacy study of high-dose coenzyme Q10 formulations in Huntington's disease mice. *Biochim Biophys Acta*, 1762(6):616-626.

181. Stack, E.C., Smith, K.M., Ryu, H., Cormier, K., Chen, M., Hagerty, S.W. *et al.* (2006). Combination therapy using minocycline and coenzyme Q10 in R6/2 transgenic Huntington's disease mice. *Biochim Biophys Acta*, 1762(3):373-380.

182. Schilling, G., Savonenko, A.V., Coonfield, M.L., Morton, J.L., Vorovich, E., Gale, A. *et al.* (2004). Environmental, pharmacological, and genetic modulation of the HD phenotype in transgenic mice. *Exp Neurol*, 187(1):137-149.

183. Morton, A.J., Hunt, M.J., Hodges, A.K., Lewis, P.D., Redfern, A.J., Dunnett, S.B. *et al.* (2005). A combination drug therapy improves cognition and reverses gene expression changes in a mouse model of Huntington's disease. *Eur J Neurosci*, 21(4):855-870.

184. Dedeoglu, A., Kubilus, J.K., Yang, L., Ferrante, K.L., Hersch, S.M., Beal, M.F. *et al.* (2003). Creatine therapy provides neuroprotection after onset of clinical symptoms in Huntington's disease transgenic mice. J *Neurochem*, 85(6):1359-1367.

185. Klivenyi, P., Ferrante, R.J., Gardian, G., Browne, S., Chabrier, P.E., and Beal, M.F. (2003). Increased survival and neuroprotective effects of BN82451 in a transgenic mouse model of Huntington's disease. J *Neurochem*, 86(1):267-272.

186. Rebec, G.V., Barton, S.J., Marseilles, A.M., and Collins, K. (2003). Ascorbate treatment attenuates the Huntington behavioral phenotype in mice. *Neuroreport*, 14(9):1263-1265.

187. Smith, D.L., Woodman, B., Mahal, A., Sathasivam, K., Ghazi-Noori, S., Lowden, P.A. *et al.* (2003). Minocycline and doxycycline are not beneficial in a model of Huntington's disease. *Ann Neurol*, 54(2):186-196.

188. Chen, M., Ona, V.O., Li, M., Ferrante, R.J., Fink, K.B., Zhu, S. *et al.* (2000). Minocycline inhibits caspase-1 and caspase-3 expression and delays mortality in a transgenic mouse model of Huntington disease. *Nat Med*, 6(7):797-801.

189. Bailey, C.D. And Johnson, G.V. (2006). The protective effects of cystamine in the R6/2 Huntington's disease mouse involve mechanisms other than the inhibition of tissue transglutaminase. *Neurobiol Aging*, 27(6):871-879.

190. van Raamsdonk, J.M., Pearson, J., Bailey, C.D., Rogers, D.A., Johnson, G.V., Hayden, M.R., *et al.* (2005). Cystamine treatment is neuroprotective in the YAC128 mouse model of Huntington disease. *J Neurochem*, 95(1):210-220.

191. Karpuj, M.V., Becher, M.W., Springer, J.E., Chabas, D., Youssef, S., Pedotti, R. *et al.* (2002) Prolonged survival and decreased abnormal movements in transgenic model of Huntington disease, with administration of the transglutaminase inhibitor cystamine. *Nat Med*, 8(2):143-149.

192. Dedeoglu, A., Kubilus, J.K., Jeitner, T.M., Matson, S.A., Bogdanov, M., Kowall, N.W. *et al.* (2002). Therapeutic effects of cystamine in a murine model of Huntington's disease. J *Neurosci*, 22(20):8942-8950.

193. Pang, T.Y., Stam, N.C., Nithiananetharajah, J., Howard, M.L., and Hannan, A.J. (2006). Differential effects of voluntary physical exercise on behavioral and brain-derived neurotrophic factor expression deficits in Huntington's disease transgenic mice. *Neuroscience*, 141(2):569-584.

194. Lazic, S.E., Grote, H.E., Blakemore, C., Hannan, A.J., van Dellen, A., Phillips, W. *et al.* (2006). Neurogenesis in the R6/1 transgenic mouse model of Huntington's disease: effects of environmental enrichment. *Eur J Neurosci*, 23(7):1829-1838.

195. Glass, M., van Dellen, A., Blakemore, C., Hannan, A.J., and Faull, R.L. (2004). Delayed onset of Huntington's disease in mice in an enriched environment correlates with delayed loss of cannabinoid CB1 receptors. *Neuroscience*, 123(1):207-212.

196. van Dellen, A., Blakemore, C., Deacon, R., York, D., and Hannan, A.J. (2000). Delaying the onset of Huntington's in mice. *Nature*, 404(6779):721-722.

197. Clifford, J.J., Drago, J., Natoli, A.L., Wong, J.Y., Kinsella, A., Waddington, J.L. *et al.* (2002). Essential fatty acids given from conception prevent topographies of motor deficit in a transgenic model of Huntington's disease. *Neuroscience*, 109(1):81-88.

198. Duan, W., Guo, Z., Jiang, H., Ware, M., Li, X.J., and Mattson, M.P. (2003). Dietary restriction normalizes glucose metabolism and BDNF levels, slows disease progression, and increases survival in huntingtin mutant mice. *Proc Natl Acad Sci USA*, 100(5):2911-2916.

199. Wood, N.I., Pallier, P.N., Wanderer, J., and Morton, A.J. (2007). Systemic administration of Congo red does not improve motor or cognitive function in R6/2 mice. *Neurobiol Dis*, 25(2):342-353.

200. Sanchez, I., Mahlke, C., and Yuan, J. (2003). Pivotal role of oligomerization in expanded polyglutamine neurodegenerative disorders. *Nature*, 421(6921):373-379.

201. Tanaka, M., Machida, Y., Niu, S., Ikeda, T., Jana, N.R., Doi, H. *et al.* (2004). Trehalose alleviates polyglutamine-mediated pathology in a mouse model of Huntington disease. *Nat Med*, 10(2):148-154.

202. Gardian, G., Browne, S.E., Choi, D.K., Klivenyi, P., Gregorio, J., Kubilus, J.K. *et al.* (2005). Neuroprotective effects of phenylbutyrate in the N171-82Q transgenic mouse model of Huntington's disease. J *Biol Chem*, 280(1):556-563.

203. Ferrante, R.J., Ryu, H., Kubilus, J.K., D'Mello, S., Sugars, K.L., Lee, J. *et al.* (2004). Chemotherapy for the brain: the antitumor antibiotic mithramycin prolongs survival in a mouse model of Huntington's disease. J *Neurosci*, 24(46):10335–10342.

204. Ferrante, R.J., Kubilus, J.K., Lee, J., Ryu, H., Beesen, A., Zucker, B. *et al.* (2003). Histone deacetylase inhibition by sodium butyrate chemotherapy ameliorates the neurodegenerative phenotype in Huntington's disease mice. J *Neurosci*, 23(28):9418–9427.

205. Hockly, E., Richon, V.M., Woodman, B., Smith, D.L., Zhou, X., Rosa, E. *et al.* (2003). Suberoylanilide hydroxamic acid, a histone deacetylase inhibitor, ameliorates motor deficits in a mouse model of Huntington's disease. *Proc Natl Acad Sci USA*, 100(4): 2041–2046.

206. Wood, N.I. And Morton, A.J. (2003). Chronic lithium chloride treatment has variable effects on motor behaviour and survival of mice transgenic for the Huntington's disease mutation. *Brain Res Bull*, 61(4):375–383.

207. Hockly, E., Tse, J., Barker, A.L., Moolman, D.L., Beunard, J.L., Revington, A.P. *et al.* (2006). Evaluation of the benzothiazole aggregation inhibitors riluzole and PGL-135 as therapeutics for Huntington's disease. *Neurobiol Dis*, 21(1):228–236.

208. Schiefer, J., Landwehrmeyer, G.B., Luesse, H.G., Sprunken, A., Puls, C., Milkereit, A. *et al.* (2002). Riluzole prolongs survival time and alters nuclear inclusion formation in a transgenic mouse model of Huntington's disease. *Mov Disord*, 17(4):748–757.

209. Schiefer, J., Sprunken, A., Puls, C., Luesse, H.G., Milkereit, A., Milkereit, E. *et al.* (2004). The metabotropic glutamate receptor 5 antagonist MPEP and the mGluR2 agonist LY379268 modify disease progression in a transgenic mouse model of Huntington's disease. *Brain Res*, 1019(1–2):246–254.

210. Dunnett, S.B., Carter, R.J., Watts, C., Torres, E.M., Mahal, A., Mangiarini, L. *et al.* (1998). Striatal transplantation in a transgenic mouse model of Huntington's disease. *Exp Neurol*, 154(1):31–40.

211. van Dellen, A., Deacon, R., York, D., Blakemore, C., and Hannan, A.J. (2001). Anterior cingulate cortical transplantation in transgenic Huntington's disease mice. *Brain Res Bull*, 56(3–4):313–318.

212. Ende, N. And Chen, R. (2001). Human umbilical cord blood cells ameliorate Huntington's disease in transgenic mice. J *Med*, 32(3-4):231–240.

213. Ma, T.C., Buescher, J.L., Oatis, B., Funk, J.A., Nash, A.J., Carrier, R.L. *et al.* (2007). Metformin therapy in a transgenic mouse model of Huntington's disease. *Neurosci Lett*, 411(2):98–103.

214. Hunt, M.J. And Morton, A.J. (2005). Atypical diabetes associated with inclusion formation in the R6/2 mouse model of Huntington's disease is not improved by treatment with hypoglycaemic agents. *Exp Brain Res*, 166(2):220–229.

215. McBride, J.L., Ramaswamy, S., Gasmi, M., Bartus, R.T., Herzog, C.D., Brandon, E.P. *et al.* (2006). Viral delivery of glial cell line-derived neurotrophic factor improves behavior and protects striatal neurons in a mouse model of Huntington's disease. *Proc Natl Acad Sci USA*, 103(24):9345–9350.

216. Popovic, N., Maingay, M., Kirik, D., and Brundin, P. (2005). Lentiviral gene delivery of GDNF into the striatum of R6/2 Huntington mice fails to attenuate behavioral and neuropathological changes. *Exp Neurol*, 193(1):65–74.

217. Zala, D., Bensadoun, J.C., Pereira de Almeida, L., Leavitt, B.R., Gutekunst, C.A., Aebischer, P. *et al.* (2004). Long-term lentiviral-mediated expression of ciliary neurotrophic factor in the striatum of Huntington's disease transgenic mice. *Exp Neurol*, 185(1):26–35.

218. Grote, H.E., Bull, N.D., Howard, M.L., van Dellen, A., Blakemore, C., Bartlett, P.F. *et al.* (2005). Cognitive disorders and neurogenesis deficits in Huntington's disease mice are rescued by fluoxetine. *Eur J Neurosci*, 22(8):2081–2088.

219. Duan, W., Guo, Z., Jiang, H., Ladenheim, B., Xu, X., Cadet, J.L. *et al.* (2004). Paroxetine retards disease onset and progression in Huntingtin mutant mice. *Ann Neurol*, 55(4):590–594.

220. Pallier, P.N., Maywood, E.S., Zheng, Z.G., Chesham, J.E., Inyushkin, A.N., Dyball, R. *et al.* (2007). Pharmacological imposition of sleep slows cognitive decline and reverses dysregulation of circadian gene expression in a transgenic mouse model of huntington's disease. *J Neurosci*, 27(29):7869–7878.

221. van Raamsdonk, J.M., Pearson, J., Rogers, D.A., Lu, G., Barakauskas, V.E., Barr, A.M. *et al.* (2005). Ethyl-EPA treatment improves motor dysfunction, but not neurodegeneration in the YAC128 mouse model of Huntington disease. *Exp Neurol*, 196(2):266–272.

222. Huang, B., Schiefer, J., Sass, C., Landwehrmeyer, G.B., Kosinski, C.M., and Kochanek, S. (2007). High-capacity adenoviral vector-mediated reduction of huntingtin aggregate load *in vitro* and *in vivo*. *Hum Gene Ther*, 18(4):303–311.

223. Machida, Y., Okada, T., Kurosawa, M., Oyama, F., Ozawa, K., and Nukina, N. (2006). rAAV-mediated shRNA ameliorated neuropathology in Huntington disease model mouse. *Biochem Biophys Res Commun*, 343(1):190–197.

224. Wang, Y.L., Liu, W., Wada, E., Murata, M., Wada, K., and Kanazawa, I. (2005). Clinicopathological rescue of a model mouse of Huntington's disease by siRNA. *Neurosci Res*, 53(3):241–249.

225. Harper, S.Q., Staber, P.D., He, X., Eliason, S.L., Martins, I.H., Mao, Q. *et al.* (2005). RNA interference improves motor and neuropathological abnormalities in a Huntington's disease mouse model. *Proc Natl Acad Sci USA*, 102(16):5820–5825.

226. Miller, T.W., Shirley, T.L., Wolfgang, W.J., Kang, X.W., and Messer, A. (2003). DNA vaccination against mutant huntingtin ameliorates the HDR6/2 diabetic phenotype. *Mol Ther*, 7(5):572–579.

227. Nguyen, T., Hamby, A., and Massa, S.M. (2005). Clioquinol down-regulates mutant huntingtin expression *in vitro* and mitigates pathology in a Huntington's disease mouse model. *Proc Natl Acad Sci USA*, 102(33):11840–11845.

228. Norflus, F., Nanje, A., Gutekunst, C.A., Shi, G., Cohen, J., Bejarano, M. *et al.* (2004). Anti-inflammatory treatment with acetylsalicylate or rofecoxib is not neuroprotective in Huntington's disease transgenic mice. *Neurobiol Dis*, 17(2):319–325.

229. Keene, C.D., Rodrigues, C.M., Eich, T., Chhabra, M.S., Steer, C.J., and Low, W.C. (2002). Tauroursodeoxycholic acid, a bile acid, is neuroprotective in a transgenic animal model of Huntington's disease. *Proc Natl Acad Sci USA*, 99(16):10671–10676.

230. Ravikumar, B., Vacher, C., Berger, Z., Davies, J.E., Luo, S., Oroz, L.G. *et al.* (2004). Inhibition of mTOR induces autophagy and reduces toxicity of polyglutamine expansions in fly and mouse models of Huntington disease. *Nat Genet*, 36(6):585–595.

231. Gil, J.M., Leist, M., Popovic, N., Brundin, P., and Petersen, A. (2004). Asialoerythropoietin is not effective in the R6/2 line of Huntington's disease mice. *BMC Neurosci*, 5:17.

232. Dominici, M.R., Scattoni, M.L., Martire, A., Lastoria, G., Potenza, R.L., Borioni, A. *et al.* (2007). Behavioral and electrophysiological effects of the adenosine A(2A) receptor antagonist SCH 58261 in R6/2 Huntington's disease mice. *Neurobiol Dis*, 28(2):197–205.

233. Chou, S.Y., Lee, Y.C., Chen, H.M., Chiang, M.C., Lai, H.L., Chang, H.H. *et al.* (2005). CGS21680 attenuates symptoms of Huntington's disease in a transgenic mouse model. *J Neurochem*, 93(2):310–320.

234. Schilling, G., Coonfield, M.L., Ross, C.A., and Borchelt, D.R. (2001). Coenzyme Q10 and remacemide hydrochloride ameliorate motor deficits in a Huntington's disease transgenic mouse model. *Neurosci Lett*, 315(3):149–153.

235. Miller, V.M., Nelson, R.F., Gouvion, C.M., Williams, A., Rodriguez-Lebron, E., Harper, S.Q. *et al.* (2005). CHIP suppresses polyglutamine aggregation and toxicity *in vitro* and *in vivo*. *J Neurosci*, 25(40):9152–9161.

236. Zourlidou, A., Gidalevitz, T., Kristiansen, M., Landles, C., Woodman, B., Wells, D.J. *et al.* (2007). Hsp27 overexpression in the R6/2 mouse model of Huntington's disease: chronic neurodegeneration does not induce Hsp27 activation. *Hum Mol Genet*, 16(9):1078-1090.

237. Qiu, Z., Norflus, F., Singh, B., Swindell, M.K., Buzescu, R., Bejarano, M. *et al.* (2006). Sp1 is up-regulated in cellular and transgenic models of Huntington disease, and its reduction is neuroprotective. J *Biol Chem*, 281(24):16672-16680.

238. Vacher, C., Garcia-Oroz, L., and Rubinsztein, D.C. (2005). Overexpression of yeast hsp104 reduces polyglutamine aggregation and prolongs survival of a transgenic mouse model of Huntington's disease. *Hum Mol Genet*, 14(22):3425-3433.

239. Hansson, O., Nylandsted, J., Castilho, R.F., Leist, M., Jaattela, M., and Brundin, P. (2003). Overexpression of heat shock protein 70 in R6/2 Huntington's disease mice has only modest effects on disease progression. *Brain Res*, 970(1-2):47-57.

240. Zhang, Y., Ona, V.O., Li, M., Drozda, M., Dubois-Dauphin, M., Przedborski, S. et al. (2003). Sequential activation of individual caspases, and of alterations in Bcl-2 proapoptotic signals in a mouse model of Huntington's disease. J *Neurochem*, 87(5):1184-1192.

241. Ona, V.O., Li, M., Vonsattel, J.P., Andrews, L.J., Khan, S.Q., Chung, W.M. et al. (1999). Inhibition of caspase-1 slows disease progression in a mouse model of Huntington's disease. *Nature*, 399(6733):263-267.

Translational Research in ALS

Jacqueline Montes[1], Caterina Bendotti[2,3], Massimo Tortarolo[2], Cristina Cheroni[2], Hussein Hallak[4], Zipora Speiser[4], Sari Goren[4], Eran Blaugrund[4] and Paul H. Gordon[1]

[1]Department of Neurology, Columbia University, New York, NY, USA
[2]Laboratory of Molecular Neurobiology, Department Neuroscience, Instituto di Ricerche Farmacologiche Mario Negri, Milano, Italy
[3]Laboratory of Neurodegenerative Disorders, Fondazione Salvatore Maugeri, IRCCS, Pavia, Italy
[4]Global Research & Non-clinical Development Section, Global Innovative R&D, Teva Pharmaceutical Industries Ltd., Netanya, Israel

Animal and Translational Models for CNS Drug Discovery,
Vol. 2 of 3: Neurological Disorders
Robert McArthur and Franco Borsini (eds), Academic Press, 2008

INTRODUCTION

Amyotrophic lateral sclerosis (ALS) is an age-related neurodegenerative disease affecting motor neurons (MNs). There is no known cure and survival extends approximately 3 years on average from symptom onset.[1] Nearly two decades ago, the discovery that mutations in the Cu/Zn superoxide dismutase (SOD1) gene cause ALS in some families[2] led to the advent of a transgenic rodent model. Since then, several other chromosomal loci have been identified,[3] but the majority of ALS cases are thought to be sporadic.[4] Recent advances in the understanding of the pathogenesis have prompted numerous clinical trials of investigational agents, and advanced scientific methods are being used to examine the neuroprotective properties of large quantities of compounds. Yet, despite great strides in both the basic and clinical sciences, progress in ALS research so far has not translated into practical clinical applications.

History

Francois-Amilcar Aran is credited with the first clinical description of motor neuron disease (MND). In 1848, he reported a patient with progressive muscle weakness, and named the new syndrome progressive muscular atrophy (PMA).[5] Aran also gave one of the earliest accounts of ALS in describing a 33-year-old professional clown with weakness and hyperreflexia, and was probably also the first to report familial MND.[6]

Jean-Martin Charcot established clinical neurology as an autonomous discipline, but perhaps his greatest contribution was to that of ALS. He defined the clinical and pathological features,[7] demonstrating the association of weakness, fasciculation and spasticity, as well as the poor prognosis. By naming the disorder ALS, he implied that the disease begins in the upper motor neuron (UMN) and is transmitted to the lower motor neuron (LMN).

Sir William Richard Gowers, a neurologist in the 19th century England, suggested that PMA, progressive bulbar palsy and ALS are parts of one single motor system degeneration. He stated that all of his cases of PMA also had degeneration of the pyramidal tracts.[8] Following the lead of Gowers, W. Russell Brain, a renowned English neurologist, grouped PMA, progressive bulbar palsy and ALS into one disease, coining the term "motor neuron disease" which is still used in England instead of ALS.[9]

Epidemiology

ALS is considered a rare neurodegenerative disorder. In studies done through the mid-1990s, the incidence in Europe, the US, and Asia was reported between 0.4 and 2.6 per 100,000.[10-14] A recent observed increase in mortality may be in part due to more reliable reporting, increased awareness of the disease, and an aging general population.[15] ALS occurs most commonly in the fifth and sixth decades of life with the peak onset reported between 60 and 69 years of age.[16] There is evidence to suggest an increasing incidence in women; in several, mostly retrospective studies in the US, Europe, and Israel over the past 40 years, the male to female ratio has decreased from 2.6:1 to 1.3:1.[17]

Familial ALS

Approximately 10% of individuals with ALS have at least one other affected family member of familial ALS (FALS).[18] Of those with FALS, 5–10% have a Mendelian inheritance pattern with the Cu/Zn SOD1 gene as the cause in 10–15%.[19,20] Other mutations have been identified, the majority having autosomal dominant inheritance. Autosomal recessive inheritance is rare and mostly limited to juvenile-onset ALS.[21] FALS, particularly SOD1-linked ALS, usually presents with monmelic weakness, typically in the leg and is unlikely to have bulbar onset.[22] The mean age of onset is earlier with a higher probability of dying in the first months of the disease, but there are variations in disease onset and course in SOD1-related ALS that can be stratified by mutation type and location.[23]

Sporadic ALS

The majority of ALS cases have no family history and are considered to be sporadic ALS (SALS).[24] The cause of SALS is unknown, but the disease likely arises as a result of the interaction of multiple, as yet largely unidentified, different genes and environmental factors. Many environmental risk factors have been examined including physical activity; participation in sports; exposure to chemicals, heavy metals, cigarettes, or alcohol; diet; and trauma. In a review of five studies, three in the US and two in Europe, cigarette smoking was the only risk factor supported by class II epidemiological evidence, possibly accounting for the increasing incidence in women.[25] In more recent longitudinal and case-controlled studies, reported exposure to lead and pesticides was significantly associated with ALS but cigarette smoking, physical activity, and trauma were not associated.[26] There is an increased risk of ALS in Italian soccer players[27,28] and other athletes.[29] Speculative reasons include trauma to the neck, environmental exposures such as herbicides and pesticides, lifestyle risk factors such as the use of performance enhancing drugs, or possibly a genetic association between athleticism and disease predisposition. Although multiple environmental factors may contribute to SALS, underlying genetic susceptibility must also contribute. Recently, the first genome wide association studies in ALS were performed in people with SALS.[30] Numerous potential risk genes have been identified but require confirmation.

PATHOPHYSIOLOGY: MECHANISMS OF NEURODEGENERATION

ALS is characterized by progressive the UMN and LMN degeneration that affects the brainstem, cervical, thoracic, and lumbosacral regions. Although the mechanisms leading to MN degeneration are incompletely understood, free radical toxicity, glutamate excitotoxicity, mitochondrial dysfunction, and intermediate filament aggregation may lead to activation enzymes that regulate cell death pathways. Cell death seems to require an interaction between the MN and surrounding support cells,[31] and the process of cell death stimulates an inflammatory reaction. Inflammation may be linked to the etiology of ALS, or may be a secondary phenomenon that intensifies neuronal damage. Pro-inflammatory modulators, including microglia and astrocytes, interleukins, prostaglandins, and components of the complement cascade are activated in ALS.[32-39]

Oxidative toxicity is thought to arise from excess free radical production during the respiratory burst of inflammatory cells.[40] Free radicals are toxic to cellular organelles, and oxidative damage to organelles is found in MNs of ALS patients.[41-45] In some FALS models, SOD1, which converts superoxide anion to hydrogen peroxide, is overactive and produces greater than normal levels of free radicals, including superoxide, hydrogen peroxide, hydroxyl radicals, and peroxynitirite.[46]

Excitotoxicity may contribute to cell death in SALS. Levels of glutamate, the primary excitatory neurotransmitter in the central nervous system, are elevated in spinal fluid and brain of some ALS patients.[47,48] Increased concentrations of glutamate lead to surplus intracellular calcium, phosphorylation of intermediate filaments, and premature cell death.[49] Higher than normal levels may result from decreased transport by glial cells, responsible for glutamate reuptake.[50]

Abnormalities in complex I of the mitochondrial respiratory chain have also been identified in tissues of ALS subjects and transgenic ALS mice.[51,52] Mitochondrial dysfunction leads to energy store depletion rendering the cell less capable of detoxifying free radicals and of maintaining the cell membrane potential. Reduced cell membrane potential may activate glutamate receptors, enhancing excitotoxicity, and cytochrome dysfunction promotes activation of enzymes promoting cell death.[1,53]

Irrespective of the initial trigger, this cascade of events is associated with activation of cell death pathways.[54,55] Pro-inflammatory cytokines increase transcription of caspase enzymes, which in turn augment transcription of inflammatory modulators.[56] Hence, cell stressors leading to up-regulation of enzymes may promote cell death pathways via interrelated caspase enzyme-mediated and inflammatory mechanisms.[32,33,57]

CLINICAL PRESENTATION

El Escorial Criteria

There are no biomarkers for ALS, so the diagnosis and assessment of progression rely solely on clinical measures. The World Federation of Neurology developed diagnostic criteria[58] to establish the diagnosis of ALS and enhance clinical research. The diagnosis of ALS depend on a combination of LMN and UMN signs in one or more body regions defined as bulbar, cervical, thoracic and lumbosacral, in conjunction with the exclusion of other explanations for the neurological symptoms. These criteria, now revised,[59] have been used to enroll patients in treatment trials for over a decade.

ALS Phenotypes

The symptoms of ALS depend on the distribution of the MNs involved. UMN disease, which is the initial symptom in a minority of patients (1.3% to 6%), leads to spasticity and slowed movements.[60-62] Spasticity, caused by loss of the normal inhibition of LMN in the brainstem and spinal cord by degenerating UMNs, can be disabling; balance may be impaired, the gait may be labored, and slowed hand movements can reduce dexterity.[63] Some ALS patients develop jaw quivering or clenching, which can be precipitated by pain, anxiety, or cold.

Symptoms due to LMN degeneration, including weakness, atrophy, cramps and fasciculation, often overshadow those associated with UMN disease. Weakness is the initial symptom in 58% to 63% of patients,[64,65] beginning asymmetrically in the limbs in approximately 2/3 of patients, and in the bulbar region in about 1/3.[61,64-66] Arm weakness leads to difficulty performing tasks such as dressing, hygiene, and eating. Weakness in the hand causes loss of finger dexterity and trouble picking up small objects, writing, turning keys, and fastening buttons. Weakness of proximal arm muscles can lead to difficulty lifting, carrying, and reaching. As the symptoms progress, more function is lost leading to the eventual dependence on caregivers. Joint immobility can cause contractures, often in the fingers and the shoulders.

Weakness in the legs usually begins in the distal muscles, especially the dorsiflexors of the ankle; foot-drop is a frequent early symptom. While weakness in the legs can start unilaterally, it occurs in both legs simultaneously 13–20% of the time.[60,64] As the weakness ascends, difficulty going up stairs, stepping over curbs, and arising from chairs ensues. Falls and dependent edema are common. Eventually, walking, standing, and bearing weight for transfers become impossible. Weakness of the axial musculature leads to head drop and kyphosis, which can cause pain, imbalance due to change in the center of gravity, and interfere with activities such as eating and driving that require an upright posture.

In bulbar-onset ALS, dysarthria generally develops prior to dysphagia, with both UMN and LMN degeneration contributing to symptoms. UMN speech tends to be slow and effortful, with poor enunciation. Loss of LMNs in the brainstem can lead to breathiness to the voice and slurring of consonants.[67] In some, velopharyngeal incompetence causes air leakage through the nose and lends a hypernasal quality to the voice. With time, some patients become anarthric. Swallowing problems worsen with disease progression. Drooling, dehydration, malnutrition with weight loss, and aspiration are all associated with dysphagia. Sialorrhea occurs in 50% of ALS patients. Laryngospasm, due to adduction of the vocal cords, is usually caused by aspirated liquids or saliva, or acid reflux, and may cause stridor.

Dyspnea or other respiratory symptoms usually occur later in the disease course, but as many as 3% of patients have respiratory complaints as their initial symptom. Typical features of respiratory muscle weakness include dyspnea on exertion, dyspnea at rest, orthopnea, early morning headaches, poor vocal projection, and reduced cough strength. Survival in those with respiratory onset may not be different than that of those with bulbar-onset ALS.[68] Regardless of the site of onset, shortness of breath eventually occurs in most patients. Respiratory failure and pulmonary complications of bulbar paralysis, such as aspiration pneumonia, are the most common known causes of death in ALS.

Overt dementia is uncommon in ALS, but studies using formal neuropsychological tests have revealed deficits in frontal executive function in as many as 50% of ALS patients.[69,70] In a recent study of 279 patients with SALS, 51% of the patients had cognitive impairment compared to 5% of controls, and 41% met criteria for frontotemporal dementia.[71] The major protein component of ubiquitinated inclusions in the brains of patients with both FTD and ALS is now known to be TDP-43, linking the two disorders, and suggesting that they might exist on a continuous spectrum.[72] The frontotemporal cognitive abnormalities may lead to changes in personality, language, judgment, decision-making, and affect. The associated abulia and reduced judgment may render patients less able to participate in decisions about their medical treatments, and lead to shortened survival.[73]

Emotional liability, or pseudobulbar affect, due to interruption of neural pathways involved in emotion, respiration, vocalization and facial movements, may also be associated with UMN degeneration.[74] The characteristics of pseudobulbar affect, first described over 130 years ago, include uncontrolled laughter or crying. Episodes are usually inappropriate to the context of the situation, with uncontrolled crying being more common than laughter. The symptoms can limit social interactions and quality of life. Parvizi *et al.*,[75] reported that reciprocal pathways between motor cortex, brainstem, and cerebellum comprise a circuit that controls emotional responses appropriate for specific cognitive and social context. Disruption of the circuit disconnects centers that regulate perceived emotion from those that involve displayed emotion.

Fatigue and exercise intolerance are common symptoms in patients with ALS. Although fatigue is not a primary consequence of MN degeneration, it is often interpreted as advancing weakness. Fatigue can be caused by physical fatigue from over expenditure of energy; mental tiredness related to fear, stress or depression; anhedonia caused by depression; poor sleep from respiratory insufficiency, pain or depression; and side effects of medications.[76]

Constipation is also common in ALS, particularly when patients become less mobile. Constipation can be aggravated by anti-cholinergic medications used for sialorrhea or by narcotic medications used for pain or air hunger. Inadequate fluid intake due to dysphagia, arm weakness, or a desire to minimize trips to the bathroom can worsen the problem. In later stages of the disease, abdominal wall muscles may weaken to the point that patients are unable to push the stool out, even if it is soft.

Pain is often under recognized in ALS. Immobility, emotional distress, muscle spasms, edema, or the illness itself can all cause pain. Cramps and fasciculation, common symptoms in ALS, can also be bothersome to patients.

Heterogeneity in Rates of Progression

The rate of progression is widely variable in ALS, with survival time ranging from months to decades. An individuals' underlying rate of progression is probably the most important predictor of outcome in ALS.[77] This variability makes assessments of potential treatments difficult. Stratification of patients based on rate of disease progression at the first visit is now used in clinical trials to improve outcome measurement precision.[78] In clinical practice, patients presenting with rapidly progressing symptoms, even without a known family history of ALS, should be screened for SOD1 mutations, which can lead to the most fulminant disease course.

CURRENT TREATMENT OPTIONS

Riluzole (Rilutek®)

Currently, only one medication, riluzole, has been shown to slow the progression of ALS. Riluzole, first developed as an anti-epileptic agent, inhibits the presymptomatic release of glutamate, although its exact mechanism in ALS is not known. In two randomized placebo-controlled, clinical trials, riluzole was shown to modestly prolong survival by about 15%.[79,80] The first trial showed mild slowing in deterioration of muscle strength, but not the second. Neither study showed improvements in quality of life.[81,82] Post hoc analyses revealed slight prolongation in the time it took patients on riluzole to move from milder to more severe disability,[80] but the effect was not apparent to patients, family members, or physicians.[83]

The Cochrane Library conducted a meta-analysis of the results (Class I evidence)[84] of published trials of riluzole in ALS.[79,80,85] All examined tracheostomy-free survival and included a total of 876 riluzole-treated and 406 placebo-treated patients. The results of the meta-analysis indicated that riluzole 100 mg/day prolongs survival by approximately 2 months. The analysis was recently revised to include a fourth study[86] and showed similar results.[87]

The long-term safety of riluzole therapy has been established,[88] including in the elderly and those in advanced stages of the disease.[86] The most common side effects of riluzole are nausea, fatigue, vertigo, and somnolence. Serum transaminase elevation may occur, but rarely to levels that are clinically meaningful.

Symptomatic and Palliative Treatments

While ALS is still an incurable disease, many symptoms are amenable to supportive therapies, some of which may even improve the course of the illness. Neurologists are increasingly turning to published practice parameter guidelines, but there are few controlled trials of symptom management.[89] The lack of scientific data to guide the use of many therapies has led to a wide variety of management practice.[90]

There a several medications used for the treatment of spasticity Baclofen (Lioresal®), a gamma-amino-butyric acid (GABA) analog, facilitates MN inhibition.[91] Side effects include weakness, fatigue, and sedation. Reducing spasticity can also give patients a sense of looseness or weakness, which can be minimized by slow dose titration. Dantrolene sodium (Dantrium®) which reduces both rigidity and spasticity acts by blocking calcium release at the level of the sarcoplasmic reticulum. Dantrolene can be used in conjunction with baclofen; there may be a synergistic effect of the two drugs.[91] Tizanidine (Zanaflex®), an α2 receptor agonist, inhibits excitatory interneurons in the spinal cord, reduces rigidity as well as spasticity, and can be used in conjunction with other anti-spasticity medications. Side effects are similar to baclofen and optimal tolerance depend on slow dose titration. Benzodiazepines may be effective in treating painful spasms or cramps that accompany spasticity. The use of these drugs must be weighed against the potential for sedation and respiratory suppression. Stretching exercises can also reduce spasms associated with spasticity.[92]

If the maximum tolerated dose of oral medications is not effective, intrathecal baclofen is one alternative.[93] Direct administration of sterile baclofen into the CSF can minimize the side effects of oral administration. The concentration of the intrathecal dose is approximately 1/1000th the oral dose. Intrathecal administration allows a programmed variable dose delivery tailored to daily variation in symptoms. Botulinum toxin (BTX) injections have been reported to reduce spasticity due to other conditions but have not yet been formally studied in ALS. The risk of muscle paralysis may limit the use of BTX in large muscle groups in ALS.

Some patients, especially those with leg spasticity, can have urinary urgency or incontinence. The possibility of urinary tract infection or prostatism should be considered, but if no other cause can be identified, an empiric trial of a spasmolytic agent such as oxybutynin (Ditropan®) is indicated.

Jaw quivering or clenching can be treated with benzodiazepines such as clonazepam, diazepam, or lorazepam BTX injected at two sites within the masseter muscles may also be effective.

Cramps can often be reduced by stretching exercises, which patients can learn from a physical therapist. If physical measures are not adequate, quinine,[94] vitamins E and C,[95] and anti-spasticity agents such as baclofen[90] are often helpful. The treatment of fasciculation is less clear cut. Most patients are relieved by the reassurance that fasciculation do not mean that the disease is accelerating. For those who continue to be bothered, gabapentin[96] or anti-spasticity agents[90] can be tried.

The AAN practice parameter recommends both pharmacologic and non-pharmacologic interventions for sialorrhea.[89] Non-pharmacologic approaches include the use of suction machines and in-exsufflator or cough-assist devices. Treatment with anti-cholinergic medication is considered "first line" pharmacologic therapy, but the benefits can be self-limited, requiring additional medications after an initial improvement. Medication selection often depend upon the severity and frequency of the drooling. Sialorrhea associated with mealtimes or a particular time of day may be treated with as needed administration of hyoscyamine because of its transient benefit. Transdermal scopolamine, oral glycopyrolate, or tricyclic anti-depressant medications provide a more continuous effect.[91]

Several open-label trials indicate that injections of BTX into the salivary glands may help reduce sialorrhea.[97-100] BTX acts by blocking acetylcholine release from presynaptic cholinergic nerve terminals and reduces stimulation of the salivary glands. While there were no adverse events in these small studies, worsening of dysphagia, chewing difficulties, recurrent temporomandibular joint dislocation, and swelling of the base of tongue have been reported.[101-103] A multicenter controlled trial using BTX for sialorrhea is underway.

Radiotherapy may also reduce sialorrhea in ALS patients. In two separate open-label trials, effective control of drooling was achieved equally at different doses.[104,105] Controlled studies are needed to determine the actual benefit and optimal dosing regimens.

Thick mucous secretions may occur independently or co-exist with sialorrhea. Occasionally, treatment of sialorrhea can change the viscosity of saliva and produce thick phlegm. This problem can be exacerbated by inadequate water intake. Pharmacologic treatments that may be helpful include high-dose guaifenesin, nebulized acetylcysteine or saline, and beta blockers such as propranolol. An uncontrolled survey of alternative measures reported that dark grape juice, papaya tablets, sugar free citrus lozenges, and grapeseed oil can also be helpful.[106]

Laryngospasm is almost never life threatening, but if the episodes occur frequently, pharmacologic treatment is warranted since the attacks are usually anxiety provoking.[91] Concentrated liquid lorazepam applied sublingually generally provides relief. Antacids and proton pump inhibitors can be used for symptoms of gastroesophageal reflux disease. Since diaphragmatic weakness and overeating can worsen gastroesophageal reflux disease, patients with reduced vital capacity or who use a percutaneous endoscopic gastrostomy tube for nutrition may benefit from peristaltic agents, such as metochlorpropamide, and either antacids or proton pump inhibitors.

Selective serotonin reuptake inhibitors, tricyclic anti-depressants and some dopaminergic agents can be beneficial in treating pseudobulbar affect. Recently, a Phase III randomized controlled trial[107] showed that a combination of dextromethorphan hydrobromide (30 mg) and quinidine sulfate (30 mg) (DM/Q) was effective and fast acting for emotional liability. One hundred and forty patients received DM/Q or placebo twice daily for 4 weeks. DM/Q significantly reduced emotional lability, and improved quality of life and quality of relationship scores. Based on these and similar results from a trial in multiple sclerosis, DM/Q is currently under consideration for approval by the United States Food and Drug Administration.

Pharmacologic treatments can help relieve symptoms of fatigue, but the response to medications can be as idiosyncratic as the etiology of the fatigue. Medications that can have fatigue as a side effect should be stopped prior to adding new drugs. Off label use of pyridostigmine (Mestinon®) can reduce symptoms of weakness in some by enhancing neuromuscular junction transmission. Methylphenidate (Ritalin®) can also provide benefit in selected patients. Caution must be taken to monitor side effects of anorexia, restlessness, anxiety, or palpitations. Modafinil (Provigil®) can also be tried.

Initial management of constipation includes the use of stool softeners such as docusate or sennosides. Simply increasing fluid intake and substituting medications with fewer anti-cholinergic effects can also be effective. Increasing dietary fiber can help; a creative recipe for constipation consists of equal parts of prunes, prune juice, apple sauce, and bran.[108] Two tablespoons with each meal and at bedtime, along with adequate intake of fluids, fruits, and vegetables in the diet may be helpful. If not, milk of magnesia or bisacodyl tablets can be added to the regimen. In patients with a percutaneous endoscopic gastrostomy tube, lactulose can be administered as long as the patient is not impacted. Enemas or magnesium citrate can be used in urgent situations.

Early recognition of the common precipitants leading to discomfort is the first line of treatment for pain. Often pain can be treated without medication by directly treating the cause, including use of stretching and range of motion exercises, massage, physical therapy, and limb elevation as well as support hose to reduce edema. Medical managements may include non-steroidal anti-inflammatory drugs, benzodiazepines, and opioids. The latter are generally safe but may lead to constipation, respiratory depression in high doses, and tolerance. Liberal use of narcotics and anxiolytics is often necessary at the end stages of the illness to prevent suffering.

Published practice parameters also make recommendations for non-pharmacological treatment of dysphagia and respiratory insufficiency.[89] Percutaneous endoscopic gastrostomy tube placement for symptomatic dysphagia is recommended for patients before respiratory function measured by forced vital capacity (FVC) falls below 50% of predicted. Similarly, non-invasive ventilation (NIV) is recommended for those with symptoms of dyspnea or orthopnea and when FVC score falls below 50%.

CURRENT PRECLINICAL APPROACHES

ALS Models

The last decade has brought about tremendous progress in basic research on ALS thanks to the discovery of genes related to the familial forms of the disease, in particular that associated with SOD1 mutations. The major breakthrough came from development of robust animal models carrying SOD1 mutations. Although these models do not fully reflect the clinical and neuropathological processes leading to ALS, they are well suited to study basic mechanisms of selective vulnerability of MNs to degeneration and to test potential pharmacological approaches as candidates for therapy in human ALS. Genetically modified *in vitro* cell cultures have provided useful platforms for the discovery and development of potentially effective drugs. Nevertheless, disappointingly, this promising development in preclinical ALS research has not been followed by an effective therapy in clinical trials so far. The overall failure to validate the efficacy of developed treatment strategies raised a debate concerning the general predictive value of experimental modeling toward clinical efficacy. Hence, different groups started to conduct systematic reviews of preclinical research studies aimed at explaining such striking lack of success in translation from preclinical to clinical success. Very recently, a meta-analysis was performed on 167 studies in the transgenic mouse model of familial ALS carrying the mutant SOD1. This analysis demonstrates the limited methodological quality of most of the studies conducted, possibly leading to false-positive results, inflated size of effect and lack of reproducibility,[109] and is highly recommended for further reading. Keeping these limitations in mind, one of the aims of this section is to focus on the strengths and weaknesses of the most commonly used experimental cellular and animal models, and to consider factors in addition to poor methodological quality, that may have accounted for the low rate of success in clinical translation, such as ALS heterogeneity. The scope of this discussion is to put cellular and animal models in perspective and provide insights improving the translatability of results from these models to human pathology and consequently, improve the probability of drugs discovered and developed through these models to become effective therapeutics for this disorder.

In Vitro Models and High-Throughput Screens

Animal models are considered the best preclinical paradigms for testing drug therapies, but they present limitations in studying the fine pathogenic mechanisms at subcellular levels. Thus, the creation of simplified *in vitro* models consisting of cell or tissue cultures permits the study of specific cellular components under controlled conditions. Moreover, *in vitro* systems may be used to design cell-based high-throughput screening assays as a powerful strategy to identify compounds with potential neuroprotective effects.

So far several cellular models have been used for research studies in ALS, including purified primary MN, neuroblastoma–spinal cord-derived cell line cultures, cell co-cultures and tissue cultures, all showing important strengths and weaknesses when compared to each other.

The most simplified system is represented by isolated and purified MN cultures. This model allows the study of modifications occurring in precise biochemical pathways linked to specific insults such as transgene expression or toxic stimulation (oxidative stress, excitotoxicity, etc.). However, growing neurons and particularly MNs *in vitro* is often challenging as they require fundamental trophic support from neighbor non-neuronal cells and target tissues. Studies of primary MNs *in vitro* has highlighted some specific characteristics that can explain their selective vulnerability in ALS, that is, their preferential glutamate alpha-amino-3-hydroxy-5-methyl-4-isoxazoleproprionic acid (AMPA) receptor-mediated toxicity and mitochondrial depolarization in respect to other neuronal types.[110,111] Less clear is their vulnerability to the expression of familial ALS-linked SOD1 mutants that cause selective MN death in animal models and humans. In fact, despite one of the first reports demonstrating that only 50% of SOD^{G93A} expressing MNs survive after 6 days *in vitro* compared to wild-type cells,[112] more recent studies demonstrate that MNs carrying SOD1 mutant are not vulnerable under basal conditions, but they are more sensitive, than non-mutated cells, to toxic insults such as AMPA mediated excitotoxiciy, cyclosporin A stimulation or Fas-triggered death pathway activation.[113-116] Discrepancies concerning basal susceptibility of SOD1 mutant MNs *in vitro* can be attributed to different culturing conditions and environment. For instance, the presence or absence of co-cultured glial cells or the use of diverse nutrient components may influence MN survival, and the analysis of these factors may provide clues regarding the events that determine their selective vulnerability. In fact, *in vitro* and *in vivo* evidence indicates that a mechanism possibly involved in MN death is the activation of surrounding microglial cells. *In vitro* testing showed that microglia, activated by lipopolysaccharide (LPS) or by IgG complexes from ALS patients, can cause injury to cultured MN. Such effects were reduced by adding anti-oxidants and anti-glutamatergic agents to the culture.[117] Studies in primary cultures showed that microglia from adult SOD1 mutant mice secreted more TNF-alpha in response to LPS, as compared to microglial cultures from wild-type mice. These differences were not noted in microglial cells taken from embryonic wild type or mutant mice.[118] Moreover, studies in SOD1 mutant mice showed that a selective reduction in expression of the mutated gene in microglia and macrophages, significantly prolonged survival without changing the onset of the disease.[119] This suggests an involvement of the activated microglia and pro-inflammatory factors in the progression of the disease rather than its pathogenesis.

In support of this notion a remarkable activation of microglia and pro-inflammatory parameters was reported in the postmortem CNS of ALS patients.[35,120,121]

On the contrary, recent studies from co-cultures of astrocytes carrying human mutant SOD1 and embryonic mouse stem cell-derived MNs have suggested that astrocytes play a major role in the specific MN death.[122,123] These embryonic stem cell-based models were proposed as a powerful tool for studying the mechanism of neural degeneration. Nevertheless mechanisms involving Fas ligand or caspases cascade activation proposed to induce apoptosis of primary MNs in cultures or in SOD1 mutant mice[116,124] did not appear to play a role in this co-cultured model. This indicates that differences in cell death mechanisms may depend on the experimental paradigm used. Which *in vitro* model is the most reliable to the *in vivo* pathology needs to be defined.

To overcome the difficulties in preparing and using primary purified MNs, a number of laboratories use immortalized MN-like cells. Neuroblastoma–spinal cord (NSC) cell lines, obtained by the fusion of mouse neuroblastoma N18TG2 with mouse spinal MNs,[125] represent the *in vitro* model most used by research groups working on ALS. The NSC-34 clone is a good model for investigating sensitivity to different neurotoxic stimuli, with the exception of excitotoxicity, as these cells do not express functional glutamate receptors unless they grown in a serum free medium.[126,127] In particular, NSC-34 cells expressing different SOD1 mutants have been widely used to investigate mechanisms for gain of toxic function by this mutated enzyme. One of the major results obtained using this experimental paradigm regard the role of mitochondria in MN degeneration. It was demonstrated that mutated SOD1 induces swelling of these organelles, associated with decreased activity of complex II and IV of the electron transfer chain, cellular oxidative stress, alteration of voltage-dependent anion channel 2 (VDAC2), cytochrome C release and cell death.[128-131] Recently, Ferri *et al.*,[132] showed that 12 different familial ALS-mutant SOD1 proteins, with diverse biophysical properties, are more readily and selectively recruited by mitochondria in these cells than the wild-type enzyme. This effect is due to oxidation of Cys residues, occurring exclusively in NSC-34 mitochondria because of their peculiar pro-oxidant micro-environment. As a consequence of this process, mitochondria-associated SOD1 mutants cross-link oligomers, causing impairment of the respiratory complex and apoptotic death.[133] Other studies have demonstrated increased sensitivity to oxidative stress,[134] aggregate formation[135] and decreased expression of NFL and NFM mRNA and protein[136] in NSC-34 cell line expressing mutant SOD1. Importantly these cells do not die when expressing the mutant SOD1 under basal conditions, but like primary MNs, they become more sensitive to toxic stimuli. Therefore, both primary MNs and MN cell lines expressing mutant SOD1 can be a good cellular system to examine the potential environmental risk factors for ALS under a genetic predisposition.

Gene expression profiling and proteomic screening of the NSC-34 cell line has been carried out to identify which key components are altered through mutant SOD1 expression in these MN-like cells.[137,138] However, these results must be interpreted cautiously as the NSC-34 cell line consists of proliferating cells and therefore may not fully represent the pathophysiology of mature MNs.

A more complex *in vitro* system, in terms of cytoarchitecture and neuron-glia interactions is organotypic tissue cultures. These represent the *in vivo* situation more closely but also present aberrant modifications, such as circling neurite growth within the slice that can alter some parameters of study. This kind of model was initially used in preclinical ALS research to investigate the role of glutamate transporter impairment. Chronic blockade of glutamate uptake in cultured spinal cord slices led to slow MN death mediated by non-NMDA receptors.[139] Toxicity induced by sustained glutamate exposure is prevented by cyclooxygenase-2 (COX-2) inhibition.[140] Paradoxically, prostaglandin E2 (PGE2), an important prostaglandin downstream to COX-2 activation, was neuroprotective in the same system through the modulation of EP2 and EP3 receptors.[141] Various other studies have been carried out using this model. It was demonstrated that prolonged inhibition of ubiquitin-proteasome system in the whole slice determines the selective loss of MNs.[142] The same effect was obtained by long-lasting treatment with malonate, an inhibitor of mitochondrial complex II of the electron transport chain.[143]

Although the limitations of *in vitro* systems are well known, they provide an opportunity for mechanistic studies with the final goal of identifying potential targets for effective therapies. For example, setting up clear *in vitro* platforms of cells that are well characterized for their mechanism of death, can help screen large numbers of compounds or multidrug combinations. These platforms have the capacity to identify significantly more molecules with potential neuroprotective efficacy that would be worth testing *in vivo*. Similarly, testing the capacity of compounds to reduce SOD1 mutant aggregate formation[144] or identifying molecules that inactivate expression of the SOD1 gene or increase degradation of the SOD1 protein[145] could be an approach which, if successful, may be relevant to FALS patients carrying SOD1 mutations. As an example of such a high-throughput strategy using mechanistic-based *in vitro* models, one can refer to the studies of Rothstein *et al.*,[50] or Vincent *et al.*,[146] in which more that 1000 FDA approved drugs and nutritionals were screened in search of compounds capable of increasing expression of the astrocytic glutamate transporter (GLT1) or reducing glutamate-induced MN death. The first screen yielded several compounds that upregulated GLT1, of which the beta-lactam antibiotic family, specifically ceftriaxone, was selected for further testing. As such, various potential ALS drugs were shown to be effective in reducing MN death caused by various noxious stimuli in the *in vitro* models. However, these effects were partly translated in ALS animal models and not replicated in the clinical outcome. The reasons for such failure may be related to structural and biochemical differences between an adult and embryonic or postnatal MN and to the environment surrounding these cells, which is different from that of intact spinal cord or brain. Although culturing MNs from adult animals is a rather impossible task so far, improving the use of co-culture systems may provide a better chance to identify potential therapeutic approaches.

Transgenic SOD1 Models

Several transgenic mice were created by the introduction of the sequence coding for human mutant SOD1 under the control of a promoter that enables ubiquitous expression of the transgene; investigators have generated different lines overexpressing human SOD1 (hSOD1) with G93A, G37R or G85R mutations,[52,147,148] or mouse SOD1 (mSOD1) with G86R mutation.[149] These animals develop a phenotype that closely resembles ALS, with an adult onset progressive motor paralysis, muscle wasting, and reduced lifespan. Pathological changes mainly consist of depletion in MNs in the spinal cord, atrophy, gliosis, axonal swelling, and presence of ubiquitin-positive inclusions. By contrast, mice overexpressing wild-type hSOD1 remain clinically normal although they show some neurodegenerative changes at a late age.[150]

Transgenic mice carrying about 20 copies of hSOD1G93A was the first commercially available model.[52] These mice develop a motor system disorder prevalently affecting LMNs. Ultrastructural and microscopical analysis reveals that the earliest pathological feature in these mice is the swelling of mitochondria leading to vacuolization of large neurons of the anterior horns of the spinal cord.[151] As the disease progresses a widespread accumulation of ubiquitin is observed in the gray matter of the spinal cord,[152] and at the end stage, motor neuronal depletion is evident and hyaline, filamentous inclusions immunopositive for ubiquitin and neurofilaments are present in some of the surviving neurons.[52,153] Transgenic mice expressing low levels of mutant SOD1G37R show a motor disease restricted to LMNs, whereas higher copy number causes more severe abnormalities and affects a variety of other neuronal populations. The most obvious cellular abnormality is the presence of membrane-bounded vacuoles in axons and dendrites, which appear to be derived from degenerating mitochondria.[147]

Transgene expression of mutant hSOD1G85R or its murine counterpart SOD1G86R develop a very aggressive pathology with a rapid progression leading to paralysis and death within 2 weeks from the first symptoms. In SODG85R mice, MNs and astrocytes present immunopositive for ubiquitin and SOD1 inclusions as the most relevant pathological feature.[148] Differences in disease progression and survival in different SOD1 mice depend on the mutation and the copy number of the transgene.

Notwithstanding the availability of all these transgenic mouse lines, most preclinical trials aimed at identifying therapeutic interventions to be applied to humans, have been tested in SOD1G93A mice. Nevertheless, certain heterogeneity in terms of disease onset and life span duration has been reported for this mouse model depending on different factors such as the genetic background, number of transgenes, and gender. For example, backcrossing the SOD1G93A animals against a C57BL6 background increases their lifespan in respect to a SJL strain.[154] This can also influence the responses to drugs; for example, the immunomodulator copaxone shows a clear-cut therapeutic effect in one strain, but the effect is restricted to females when tested in a genetically more heterogeneous strain.[155] Thus, strain differences need to be considered in the reproducibility of the drug treatment responses.

More recently, transgenic technology has also permitted the creation of transgenic rats expressing the G93A mutant of SOD1. In this model, the onset of the disease occurs early and the rate of progression is very rapid. Pathological abnormalities are similar to those observed in the mouse model. Vacuolization and gliosis are evident before clinical onset and before MN death in the spinal cord and brainstem.[156] The advantage of this model is the size of the animals that allows the investigator to obtain more tissue for biochemical investigations, and applying treatment procedures that are not easily feasible in mice such as, that is, intracerebroventricular or intraspinal injections. Moreover, electrophysiologic and pathologic studies of the phrenic nerves in SOD1G93A rat model has demonstrated that this model recapitulate the process of respiratory failure due to diaphragmatic atrophy which is the usual mechanism for death in ALS patients.[157] This rat transgenic model is becoming more widely used to test new therapeutic strategies.[158,159]

Other Animal Models

Other models of MN degeneration have been discovered or developed in the last three decades, although only few of them have been used for therapy development. Some of them are associated with gene mutations found in human ALS or suggested risk factors for ALS or other MND, that is, dynein, alsin, VEGF-Hif1aRE,[160-162] they recapitulate only some features of the human disease. For example, most of them do not show lifespan reduction, which is considered one of the main outcome measures for assessing the efficacy of a treatment. Nevertheless, these models may provide useful insights in deciphering the mechanisms of selective MN degeneration as potential therapy targets.

Among the spontaneous mutant mice with MND phenotypes, wobbler mice have been largely used to assess potential therapeutic agents for human ALS. These mice are characterized by weakness and muscular atrophy restricted to the forelimbs that is associated with selective degeneration of MNs in the cervical tract of spinal cord.[163] These mice develop the disease in the early postnatal stage and consequently do not model the developmental progression of human ALS. Recently the genetic defect of these mice has been identified as a missense mutation in a vacuolar vesicular protein sorting (Vps54) involved in the transport of vesicles from late endosomes to the Golgi apparatus, indicating a new potential molecular mechanism for MND. Interestingly, most biochemical alterations found in the cervical spinal cord of these mice such as mitochondrial alterations, glutamate excitotoxicity, neuroinflammation, and oxidative injury are common to those found in SOD1 mutant mice. This indicates that these biochemical changes are independent from the initial cause of MND and possibly reflect the consequence of MN loss and glial reaction. Addressing these converging toxic mechanisms by combined treatment approaches may therefore result in a more effective therapeutic strategy, which may overcome the difficulties imposed by the heterogeneous nature of the disease.

REPRESENTATION OF MOTOR IMPAIRMENT

The extent of the disease in ALS mice is usually evaluated by tasks that measure locomotor activity, muscle strength and co-ordination such as recording limb tremors, latency to stay on a rotating bar, grip strength of hind and forelimbs, running wheel activity, and changes in gait. These measurements have been used to define the onset and the rate of progression of the disease and most of them are taken as the endpoints for testing therapies, in addition to the survival. However, the current methods of motor assessment are not directly comparable among the studies and this may produce different results depending on the methodologies used for testing the drug effect on disease onset and progression. For example, the criteria to define disease onset are rather variable and often based on subjective score systems, that is, extent of tremors or hindlimb adduction, rather than quantitatively defined parameters. The definition of symptom onset is relevant for establishing when to start a treatment. So far the vast majority of treatments in mice have been applied long before any signs of motor impairment are noted. Such an approach may provide useful information for proof-of-concept studies on pathogenic mechanisms of the disease, but has limited impact on the development of therapy for human ALS. In fact, patients at diagnosis already have clear signs of motor dysfunction and even worse, the lag-time between the first symptom and the true diagnosis which leads the patient to start a treatment is estimated to be between 12 and 17 months. Therefore, an effort has to be made, using preclinical studies, to define the progression of motor impairment in animal models better in relation to the human disease. This should be done in order to identify an interval for beginning of therapy which, in case of a positive response, could be worth proposing to human patients.

Survival is considered the main outcome measure for evaluation of treatment efficacy. Survival is also quite variable among groups, even within a similar mouse strain.

COGNITIVE ALTERATIONS IN MUTANT ALS MICE

The effect of ALS on MNs in the cortex, brainstem, and spinal cord has been extensively described,[164] but non-motor systems are affected as well.[165-169] Due to the severe and dramatic consequences of motor disability, effects on non-motor systems have not been the main focus of most clinical and non-clinical studies. Despite that, some reports describe cognitive impairment in a subgroup of ALS patients. A battery of neuropsychological tests has been used to diagnose cognitive impairment in 30–50% of ALS patients, ranging from mild impairment to frontotemporal dementia.[69-71] The main findings were executive dysfunction with deficits in verbal and non-verbal fluency and concept formation.[70,165,170-172] These studies indicated that in addition to motor cortex degeneration, the temporal and limbic areas also exhibited neuronal death.

The G93A SOD1 mouse mainly serves for motor function and survival testing,[52,173] but a few studies were performed in which these mice were also examined for behavioral and cognitive deficiencies. One major difference between cognitive testing in mutant mice versus ALS patients is that mice are examined during the presymptomatic stage while patients can be tested only after motor symptoms occur and the ALS diagnosis is made. The need to examine mutant mice at presymptomatic stages, before motor impairment occurs, stems from the fact that most cognitive tests like the water maze and passive or active avoidance require intact motor activity of experimental animals the mice must swim to find a hidden platform, jump in order to avoid electroshock, and explore objects, etc.

Two assumptions concerning cognitive and behavioral alterations in ALS were investigated using studies in presymptomatic G93A SOD1 mice:

1. Glutamate overactivity may cause hypofunction of the dopaminergic system leading to cognitive deficits.
2. Glutamate overactivity may enhance, rather than impair, some cognitive capabilities.

DOPAMINERGIC HYPOFUNCTION IN G93A MICE AND COGNITIVE PERFORMANCE

Several studies in ALS patients indicate dopaminergic hypofunction in the extrapyramidal area that is evident from a decrease in dopaminergic D_2 postsynaptic receptors in the striatum,[166,167] low striatal dopamine transporter levels,[168] and extrapyramidal symptoms in some ALS patients in which postmortem necropsy showed degeneration of the substantia nigra, globus pallidus, and thalamus.[169] Similarly, degeneration of substantia nigra and thalamus have also been reported in mutant G93A mice[174,175] associated with decreased levels of dopamine in the caudate-putaman and a decrease in tyrosine hydroxylase positive neuron staining in substantia nigra.[176]

The striatal dopaminergic system is involved in non-motor activities such as memory reward, sensory perception, and emotions[177-179] and is extensively innervated by glutamatergic fibers. It has been postulated that ALS-related glutamate excess may be involved in striatal damage, generating dopaminergic hypofunction, and cognitive deficits.[166,167]

Dopaminergic dysfunction in presymptomatic G93A mice was investigated by Geracitano *et al.*,[180] using electrophysiological and cognitive studies. Mice were tested in an active avoidance test, which is based on associative learning,[179] reflects functions of the subcortical nervous system and is dependent on the integrity of the dopaminergic system. Dopaminergic receptor antagonists cause poor performance in this test.[181-184] G93A mice had impaired avoidance in this task, compared to mice overexpressing wild-type SOD1 and wild-type controls.

In the same series of experiments, electrophysiological data revealed dopaminergic dysfunction by testing corticostriatal synaptic plasticity in brain slices of G93A mutant mice. Tetanic stimulation of the corticostriatal pathway generated an NMDA-dependent long-term potentiation (LTP) in these mice, in contrast to the long-term depression field potentials observed in brain slices obtained from control mice overexpressing the wild-type SOD and from normal controls. Perfusion of brain slices with dopamine, or the D_2 dopaminergic receptor agonist quinpirole, restored a normal long-term depression response to tetanic stimulation in G93A mice, indicating dopaminergic hypoactivity and dysfunction in the G93A brain.

GLUTAMATE OVERACTIVITY IN MUTANT ALS MICE AND COGNITIVE PERFORMANCE

Several lines of evidence implicate glutamate neurotoxicity in the pathogenesis of ALS patients and transgenic mice expressing the mutant SOD1 gene.[50,185,186] While glutamate excess may be the cause of MN death and of the dopaminergic hypofunction described above, it may also, under some circumstances, enhance cognitive capabilities in the presymptomatic stages. Testing such a hypothesis on ALS patients would be very difficult because they are identified only after disease diagnosis when significant neuronal damage has already taken place. One could think of retrospectively examining cognitive capabilities of such patients before they became ill, but to the best of our knowledge such a study was never performed. In contrast to patients, transgenic

ALS mice can be examined during presymptomatic stages of the disease. Spalloni et al.,[187] tested the hypothesis that increased CNS glutamate levels, present in G93A mutant mice, should be associated with an improvement in some cognitive aspects. In three interrelated studies, processes such as spatial learning and memory consolidation[179,188] were examined. Mutant G93A mice showed better spatial orientation and novel object recognition than wild-type control mice. Tetanic stimulation of Schaffer collaterals in brain hippocampal slices produced a stable increase of LTP in the CA-1 area of G93A mice relative to controls. Moreover, increased expression of glutamatergic AMPA receptor mRNA was found in the hippocampus of mutant mice, along with increased Glu R-1 protein. Indirectly, these results suggests that the improved learning and consolidation of memory in the mutant mice is related electrophysiologically to the strengthening of LTP and biochemically to the proteonomic changes in the hippocampus. This study therefore supports the notion that elevated glutamate activity in the brains of Cu/Zn SOD1 mutant G93A mice may enhance cognitive capabilities during the presymptomatic period, before the onset of significant neuronal damage.

To summarize, cognitive alterations have received much less attention than motor deficiencies in ALS, and both preclinical and clinical information is lacking. Dopaminergic hypofunction, found in both transgenic mice and some ALS patients may indeed be a factor contributing to cognitive decline. The possibility that glutamate excess may enhance cognition in presymptomatic stages of the disease is of interest but cannot be checked, at this stage, in ALS patients.

INTO THE FUTURE OF PRECLINICAL RESEARCH

Challenges in Representing a Heterogeneous Disease

ALS is the best characterized and most common of the MN disorders. Nevertheless, ALS patients cannot be considered as a homogeneous population, even when they are affected by familial forms of the disease.

Different risk and genetic factors might account for such heterogeneity and this may have an important impact on the result of a given therapeutic strategy. Molecular genetics has identified an increasing number of genes or loci associated with MN degeneration, although only few of them are related to the pure ALS phenotype in humans.[189] Developing animal models representative of the genetic heterogeneity may help to shed light on the mechanisms of MN death and eventually lead to the design of more specific therapeutic strategies for specific individuals or groups of patients with ALS.

As reported above, so far mutants, other than the transgenic SOD1 mice, have reproduced only some features of the human disease.[190] However, these mice representing etiologies for MN death, other than SOD1, can be useful to assess the efficacy of potential neuroprotective drugs in a spectrum of multifactorial mechanisms of neurodegeneration such is that hypothesized for ALS. Ideally, for each gene mutation or risk factor presumably involved in MN death, a new *in vitro* and *in vivo* model should be developed in order to create a battery of preclinical tests to search for the most promising therapeutic approaches.

DISCREPANCIES IN ANIMAL TESTING PROTOCOLS AND ALS CLINICAL TRIALS

There has been much discussion and description of the limitations of preclinical models of ALS. Although the mouse model is an excellent example for studying MND, questions still arise as to whether it is the best model of ALS for drug screening. The preclinical model has several limitations:[1] the model is based on the SOD1 mutation, which in humans represents only 2% of cases of ALS;[2] due to the nature of the animal model, it is difficult to determine if plasma concentrations required to show efficacy in the animal model are similar to those required in humans; and[3] the timing of the intervention, given that drugs are tried in presymptomatic animal models, whereas subjects in trials receive them at least months after symptom onset. Some studies, however, have demonstrated a good correlation between mouse model and human trial results. Riluzole use resulted in improvement in survival in both the mouse model and clinical trials [219]. Gabapentin showed a much smaller improvement in survival in the mouse model than did riluzole (6% versus 11%). In comparison, it was ineffective in a human trial.[191] Other compounds such as topiramate and TCH 346 were negative in the SOD1 model and also showed no efficacy in humans.[192-195 i] As such, one can conclude that in spite of the SOD1 model limitations, assessment of any potential candidate in this model is highly recommended. This is particularly true if the mechanism of action of the compound of interest revolves around the glutamate excitotoxicity hypothesis. Despite that, there are a considerable number of clinically failed compounds that showed some efficacy in animal models as will be discussed below.

GUIDELINES FOR FUTURE ANIMAL TRIAL DESIGN

The recent systematic review of more than 150 studies testing the efficacy of different drug treatments in the SOD1 mutant transgenic mice, mainly the SOD1G93A, has highlighted a clear deficit in the methodology used by different groups.[108] To overcome this problem, recently a group of basic researchers, clinicians, and drug company representatives participated in a workshop aimed to establish standard methods for drug testing in ALS models [204]. In principle, all the members of the workshop agreed to consider separately the studies performed to validate a hypothesis, where the drug is used as an investigational tool, and those specifically aimed to recommend a drug for use in humans. Such distinction refers to a series of recommendations that involve: the characteristic of the mouse model used (genetic background, gender, number of transgenes), treatment in the presymptomatic versus symptomatic phase, the primary and secondary endpoints to consider for the drug efficacy, the design of the study in terms of methods and dose response of drug application and the statistical analysis to be applied. These guidelines have been recently published.[196]

---

[i] Please refer to Merchant *et al.*, Animal models of Parkinson's disease to aid drug discovery and development, in this volume for further discussion on apparent lack of efficacy of experimental compounds in human clinical trials despite positive animal data.

BETWEEN PRECLINICAL AND CLINICAL TESTING

Most compounds clinically tested for ALS, showed some beneficial activities, either *in vitro* or, in most cases, *in vivo*. Despite that, in the past 6 years, large-scale trials of pentoxifylline, vitamin E, high-dose vitamin E, xaliproden, topiramate, gabapentin, two trials of creatine, celecoxib, TCH 346 and recently also minocycline have all failed, with some treatments even hastening disease progression or worsening symptoms. Thousands of patients have been enrolled and tens of millions of dollars invested.[197] Almost all papers announcing the results of a failed ALS clinical trial include some form of an analysis or editorial about the published results. For example, Cudkowicz *et al.*,[198] analyze the disappointing result of celecoxib and consider possible explanations why it may have failed, and what can be done in future trials. In this analysis the authors asked the following questions:

1. Was there sufficient underlying rationale, as well as experimental evidence from preclinical studies?
2. Was the dose level used in the clinical trial sufficient to reach the plasma concentrations required for efficacy based on the preclinical models?
3. Was the CNS penetration of the drug sufficient to exert the expected pharmacologic response?
4. How well do preclinical models of ALS predict the effect of treatment in humans with ALS?
5. What was the response of the marker of drug effect or a disease biomarker (that reflects a compound's mechanism of action) relative to efficacy?
6. Was the clinical study design and execution acceptable?

These questions asked in the celecoxib ALS clinical trial seem to be valid for all other failed ALS clinical trials. They may also be valid for future compounds in various stages of development for ALS in order to avoid some of the repeated failures observed since the year 2000.

In this section, we selected three out of many compounds developed for ALS and analyzed some aspects in their success or failure. These compounds are riluzole (Rilutek®), celecoxib (Celebrex®), and gabapentin (Neurontin®).

Riluzole

Preclinical

The riluzole package insert reports that the mode of action of riluzole is unknown. Its pharmacological properties include the following, some of which may be related to its effect:

1. An inhibitory effect on glutamate release.
2. Inactivation of voltage-dependent sodium channels.
3. Ability to interfere with intracellular events that follow transmitter binding at excitatory amino acid receptors.

In addition, it has been suggested that the glutamate transporter may be a target for the neuroprotective effect of riluzole. This agent, which possesses many potential modes of action including modulation of glutamate receptors and ion channel activity, has recently been shown to stimulate glutamate uptake in synaptosomes isolated from spinal cord.[199] Riluzole demonstrated a protective effect on cultured neurons and specifically on MN, attributed to its anti-glutamatergic effects on AMPA receptors[200-202] although other non-excitotoxic mechanisms were also proposed.[203]

The riluzole package insert also states that riluzole has also been shown, in a single study, to delay median time to death in the G93A SOD1 transgenic mouse model of ALS (http://www.sanofi-aventis.us/live/us/en/index.jsp). The percentage increase in survival is estimated to be approximately 11%.[204]

Clinical

Riluzole is currently the only FDA approved treatment for ALS, delaying death or tracheostomy by approximately 2 months. A Cochrane Library review states a 9% gain in the probability of surviving 1 year. In a secondary analysis of survival at separate time points, there was a significant survival advantage with riluzole 100 mg/day at 6, 9, 12, and 15 months, but not at 3 or 18 months.[84]

It is of interest to note that riluzole did not show a dose response profile in efficacy clinical trials. Fifty mg/day of riluzole could not be statistically distinguished from placebo and the results of 200 mg/day are essentially identical to 100 mg/day.

Open issues

It is still unclear which features of the riluzole mechanism of action are responsible for its modest efficacy in ALS, partly because other compounds having anti-glutamatergic mechanisms failed clinical trials (i.e., gabapentin and lamotrigine). There has been a surprising lack of effort to build on the modest success of riluzole and related benzothiazoles have not been tested in ALS animal models or patients. A call has been issued for a collaborative effort between academic scientists and industry to rejuvenate development of this drug class.[205]

Riluzole has a linear pharmacokinetic profile and good brain penetration but still there is no dose response in efficacy between the 100 and 200 mg/day doses. Two concepts have been put forward to explain the development of pharmaco-resistance. The transporter hypothesis contends that the expression or function of multidrug transporters in the brain is augmented, leading to impaired access of drug to CNS targets. In other words, is it possible that riluzole is a substrate to a transporter at the blood–brain barrier that gets saturated between the 100 and 200 mg/day dose levels? The target hypothesis holds that changes in the properties of the drug targets themselves may result in reduced drug sensitivity.[206] This implies that the riluzole mechanism of action involves some saturable process that may stop responding with increasing dose. No information is currently available to explain either scenario. Investigation of such concepts may help shed some light on possible new drug discovery efforts in the field of ALS.

Celecoxib

Preclinical

Celecoxib is a COX-2 inhibitory agent, for various inflammatory conditions, that blocks prostaglandin synthesis. Selective COX-2 inhibitors were shown to protect MN in organotypic spinal cord cultures against excitotoxicity[140] and attenuate MN-like cell death when exposed LPS-treated macrophages.[207] Inhibition of COX-2 interferes with two processes thought to play important roles in ALS pathogenesis; glutamate-induced excitotoxicity and inflammation. Inhibitors of COX-2 have been preclinically shown to reduce astrocytic glutamate release markedly and should therefore reduce the deleterious effects of this major source of the excitotoxic neurotransmitter. In addition, COX-2 activity also results in inflammation and the production of free radicals that may play an important role in the pathogenesis of ALS. Importantly, reported studies of postmortem spinal cords of 29 patients who died of ALS, and of mice with the mutant SOD1 G93A transgenic form of ALS, showed markedly increased levels of mRNA for COX-2, COX-2 protein, and/or increased levels of PGE2.

When transgenic mice with human mutant SOD1 were treated with celecoxib, a delay in the onset of weakness and weight loss, and prolonged survival (more than 25%) were observed. Celecoxib treatment also inhibited the production of PGE2 in the spinal cords of these mice. The observation that COX-2 inhibitors have beneficial effects in SOD mutant transgenic mouse models of ALS has been confirmed in several laboratories using celecoxib, rofecoxib, or nimesulide.

Clinical

A double-blind, placebo-controlled, clinical trial was conducted and 300 subjects with ALS were randomized (2:1) to receive celecoxib (800 mg/day) or placebo for 12 months.[198] Results indicate that celecoxib did not slow the decline in muscle strength, vital capacity, motor unit number estimates, ALS Functional Rating Scale-Revised (ALSFRS-R), or affect survival. Celecoxib was well tolerated and was not associated with an increased frequency of adverse events. The authors conclude that further studies of celecoxib at a dosage of 800 mg/day in ALS are not warranted.

It was examined whether plasma concentration of celecoxib measured in subjects was comparable to plasma concentration in the mouse model. Plasma levels of celecoxib in mice fed the chow ad libitum were 0.68 to 1.35 μg/ml, which is similar to the serum levels in celecoxib-treated subjects at 4 (1.28 μg/ml) and 8 months (1.21 μg/ml). Thus, the dosage used in this study produced circulating levels of celecoxib comparable with those in the mouse studies.

To determine whether celecoxib treatment was effective in inhibiting COX-2 in the CNS of subjects with ALS in this study, the authors sought to use CSF levels of PGE2, a main product of COX-2 activity, as a surrogate marker for the pharmacological effect of celecoxib treatment. Based on two previous studies, it was expected that PGE2 levels would be elevated in the CSF of ALS subjects and it was anticipated that effective inhibition of COX-2 in the CNS should result in reduction of CSF PGE2. However, there was no reduction in PGE2 levels in patients treated with celecoxib. When baseline PGE2 CSF levels were compared to PGE2 levels in previous reports, it was determined that PGE2 was not elevated in the CSF of ALS patients in this study.

Open issues

Celecoxib is lipophilic, and has been shown to penetrate into the CNS in rodents and humans. Its penetration into the CNS of transgenic SOD mutant mice was sufficient to inhibit PGE2 production in the spinal cord. The discrepancy in results between the recent celecoxib subject group and those previously reported remains unexplained. Because PGE2 levels were not elevated at baseline in this large sample of patients, COX-2 inhibition would not be expected to result in further lowering of the levels. This leaves open the question of whether celecoxib treatment actually exerted its pharmacological effect of inhibiting COX-2 in the CNS, which remains the most problematic aspect of this study. The fact that elevated levels of PGE2 were not found in CSF samples from this group of ALS patients may either suggest a low degree of inflammation at this disease stage, or indicate that CSF levels of PGE2 do not necessarily reflect COX-2 activity in the CNS.

The rationale for a pathogenic role of PGE2 in ALS was the basic premise for the celecoxib clinical trial.[207] However, prostaglandins (PGE2 and prostaglandin D2) may also have a paradoxical neuroprotective function, which has been demonstrated in the *in vitro* "excitotoxic" model of ALS and in stroke models. It is therefore theoretically possible that PGE2 production could actually be protective in ALS, whereas inhibition might be harmful. However, the celecoxib-treated patients in the study did not have a faster progressing course as compared to control patients, largely discounting this possibility.

This clinical study with celecoxib[207] used rigorous and accurate measures of disease progression, previously shown to be reliable in ALS studies. It was powered to detect a 35% decrease in the rate of arm strength decline, with a probability of 81%.[ii] In the mouse model, celecoxib treatment resulted in approximately a 25% prolongation of survival, and a smaller delay in onset of reduced rotarod function. However, that neither the primary outcome measure nor any of the secondary measures showed even a trend toward benefit makes it highly improbable that an important therapeutic effect was missed.

Genetic discoveries have clearly shown that ALS is more than one disease,[206] so maybe there is a need to better match the models with the clinical populations that they were designed to simulate. If COX-2 inhibitors were effective in ALS mice carrying mutations in Cu/Zn SOD1, should the clinical trial have been performed first in a familial SOD1 ALS population?

[ii] Please refer to McEvoy and Freundenreich, Issues in the design and conductance of clinical trials, Volume 1, Psychiatric Disorders, for a comprehensive discussion regarding statistical power issues in clinical trials.

Gabapentin

Preclinical

Interest in gabapentin as a possible treatment option for ALS was first presented in the form of a hypothesis.[208] While riluzole inhibits glutamate release, gabapentin is hypothesized to decrease the rate of formation of glutamate derived from the branched-chain amino acids (BCAAs) leucine, isoleucine, and valine. The proposed decrease in formation of glutamate from BCAAs may decrease the pool of glutamate and therefore compensate for diminished glutamate uptake capacity and/or abnormal glutamate metabolism in patients with ALS.[208] It is now realized that gabapentin binding to the calcium channel alpha-2–delta (α_2–δ) subunit represents a site of action for gabapentin. There is evidence that presynaptic inhibition of neurotransmitter release (presumably of glutamate) is the critical effect that emerges from gabapentin binding to α_2–δ-1.[209]

Gabapentin was tested *in vivo* in SOD1 transgenic mouse model. The effect was extremely small, an approximate 6% prolongation of survival.[210] In addition, gabapentin was tested in tissue cultures and the effect appeared to be more pronounced than *in vivo*.[191]

Clinical

Prior to initiation of the efficacy trial, two smaller studies were performed, both showing some trends toward a beneficial effect of gabapentin on ALS patients. A randomized clinical trial was initiated using a gabapentin dose of 3600 mg/day for 9 months. Of the 204 patients enrolled, 128 completed the study.[191] The study found no significant difference in the rate of decline of the arm scores between the treated and untreated groups. In fact, a combined analysis of all studies revealed a more rapid rate of decline of the FVC in the patients treated with gabapentin compared with the combined placebo groups ($P = 0.04$). The authors concluded that there was no beneficial effect of gabapentin on disease progression in ALS.[191]

Open issues

The three clinical trials described above evaluated a wide range of gabapentin dose levels staring from 500 mg/day to 1, 1.5, 2.4, and 3.6 g/day. One can assume that in the last efficacy study, the maximum possible dose was administered in order to provide the drug with the maximum likelihood of success. Yet from a pharmacokinetic stand point gabapentin appears to have non-linear kinetics with increasing dose (http://www.pfizer.com/pfizer/download/uspi_neurontin.pdf). For example, gabapentin bioavailability is not dose proportional; that is, as dose is increased, bioavailability decreases. Bioavailability of gabapentin is approximately 60%, 47%, 34%, 33%, and 27% following 900, 1200, 2400, 3600, and 4800 mg/day given in three divided doses, respectively. As such the assumption that with increasing dose one might get a proportional increase in exposure, does not apply for gabapentin. It is possible that gabapentin pharmacokinetic characteristics may have limited the ability of the investigators to get high enough exposure of gabapentin to reach the desired outcome of decreasing glutamate excitotoxicity either by decreasing glutamate synthesis or release.

The reason for the lack of dose proportionality with gabapentin exposure is believed to be the fact that gabapentin is a substrate for the large neutral amino acid system L (leucine) transporter. In fact, the system L transporter is required for oral absorption and for active transport into the brain.[209] Gabapentin has been shown to be a substrate for the system L transporter with high affinity and low capacity.[211] As such, saturation of system L transporter might provide an explanation for the lack of dose proportionality with increasing dose.

In recent years Pfizer has introduced pregabalin (Lyrica®), which is a three-substituted analog of GABA and a compound related to gabapentin. Like gabapentin, pregabalin is an α_2–δ ligand. So from a pharmacology stand point, one might expect pregabalin to inhibit presynaptic glutamate release.[209] In addition, pregabalin is also a substrate for system L transporter with one key difference: pregabalin appears to be a low affinity high-capacity substrate. This difference presumably explains why pregabalin exposure is linear with increasing dose.[211] Pregabalin oral bioavailability is ≥90%, is independent of dose and has a linear pharmacokinetic profile (http://www.pfizer.com/pfizer/download/uspi_lyrica.pdf).

Considering the pregabalin pharmacokinetics and pharmacodynamic profile, one might wonders if it might be a reasonable candidate worth testing in preclinical models of ALS and in ALS patients.

TRIAL DESIGN

An important aspect of studying new interventions is the design of the clinical trial. Successful trials provide valid and easily interpretable data. A trial should be appealing to patients, so that enrollment is complete and dropout is minimal, but it cannot sacrifice validity for the sake of patient interests. Several different designs are used in trials for ALS.

In an open-label study, all participants receive the active medication. Open-label studies are appealing to patients who wish to try any potentially beneficial medication, but unless the drug produces an overwhelming effect, studies without a control group are often uninterpretable; the data cannot provide evidence of efficacy.[212] A control group must be used to negate placebo effects and detect side effects of an experimental drug that mimic symptoms of ALS (weakness, fatigue, weight loss, or respiratory failure).[212] Consequently, open-label trials are currently considered only for early phase studies.

One potential use is the single-arm futility study, which screens drugs before proceeding to efficacy trials. In this design, the null hypothesis states that a drug's effect is superior to a minimally acceptable outcome.[213] If the null hypothesis is rejected, futility of the therapy is established. Conversely, if futility is not shown, then the study can proceed to a Phase III trial. The rationale for this design is to study a drug with a minimum number of subjects in a one-sample design, thereby avoiding exposure of large numbers of patients to a potentially futile treatment. The futility design allows investigators to protect against falsely concluding that a drug is ineffective due to underpowering, while at the same time providing reassurance of a reasonable likelihood of success in a well-powered efficacy trial.

The futility design is being used in a Phase II trial of coenzyme Q10 (CoQ10), in which the null hypothesis of superiority is tested using the ALSFRS-R.[214] This trial uses a placebo group and has two stages. The first stage is a dose selection phase where two doses are tested against placebo. The second stage compares the preferred dose against placebo. The data from the preferred dose in the first stage are used in the analysis of the second stage. If the decline in the ALSFRS-R is less than a predetermined percentage, then the null hypothesis of superiority is not rejected and inadequate evidence of futility is concluded, thereby justifying the selected dose of the drug eligible for a Phase III trial.

A selection trial design can also be conducted between two or more active treatment arms, with the aim of choosing the empirically superior treatment at the end of the study.[215] This design also used in the first stage of the CoQ10 trial, differs from a conventional Phase II trial which requires proof of a statistically significant difference between arms. The selection design screens multiple agents in small sample size trials before proceeding to large efficacy trials with the agents most likely to provide benefit.

The randomized, double-blind, placebo-controlled trial is the accepted standard for Phase III efficacy studies. It gives data that are unbiased as well as simple to interpret, and is required for licensing of a new medication.[216] Typically, patients are randomly assigned to one of two groups. One group receives the drug to be tested, and the other group receives a placebo (or the standard treatment). The effects of different dose levels can be investigated with multiple parallel groups included in a randomized, controlled trial. Randomization balances known and unknown confounders between groups and negates selection bias with regards to treatment assignment.

Challenges of Recruitment and Retention

ALS is rare, so enrolling adequate numbers of patients in a short period of time requires recruitment enhancing strategies such as the use of multicenter consortia. The larger the sample size, the greater the number of clinical centers necessary. In the recent past, patients have become activists.[217] They share information on the internet, advocate using multiple medications, and they seek new, ostensibly more effective clinical trials. Patients with ALS are motivated, but the situation can change when their disease progresses; they may become depressed or lose interest in a trial. They may drop out of a trial to participate in a more recently publicized study, or they may secretly use other available investigational agents. Establishing and maintaining a study population is difficult under these circumstances.

Once a trial starts, it is necessary to monitor adherence and to implement strategies to prevent dropout,[217] including treatment of depression and other palliative measures. Study nurses and physicians spend time with patients, discussing various issues and difficulties patients face while participating in the study. Prior to enrollment, a discussion of the importance of scientific research and the need for complete data in testing medications, helps patients understand their role in the process. Other ways to minimize dropout, include easy administering outcomes, infrequent patient visits, and home visits if necessary.

Measuring Progression and Outcome Measures

Currently, there are no biomarkers of disease progression in ALS, so investigators use potential surrogate markers, which measure disease progression, if not the drug's direct impact on MNs. A variety of outcome measures have been used in clinical trials.[218,219] Measurement techniques should be relevant, valid, reliable, simple and sensitive to change.[220] Each technique carries its own set of problems that impact trial design, including expense, variability, and difficulty in administration.

Outcomes in ALS trials are chosen to detect symptomatic improvement, reduced rate of deterioration, prolonged survival time, and reduced mortality.[221] The primary outcome should be clinically relevant to patients, and ideally, the effects of the treatment on the primary outcome should impact medical practice. In ALS, loss of muscle function, respiratory failure, or death are usually chosen as primary outcomes. Which primary outcome measure is selected will affect the sample size and study design. Secondary outcome measures are chosen to complement the primary outcome in assessing safety and disease progression but are of less clinical or medical importance.[222]

The results of all relevant analyses of outcomes should be reported, whether or not they are statistically or clinically significant, clearly specifying which were planned a *priori* and which were done post hoc. Selective reporting can bias the conclusions. Post hoc analysis should be identified so that the reader can determine whether the relationships make clinical sense. To ensure accurate data reporting, investigators need to have full access to data from industry sponsored trials,[223] and all results should be reported accurately, completely, and in context.

Survival time has been used as the primary outcome measure in past clinical trials.[80] Mortality is a robust measure of effect in this rapidly progressive terminal disease, but there are disadvantages to using it as a primary outcome measure. Survival is influenced by varying clinical practices at different centers, and the trials must be large and long for adequate power. The use of NIV, gastrostomy as well as opioid treatments change survival, and longevity in ALS depend on the level of general medical care, the presence or absence of other systemic diseases, the qualities of the caregiver and of the home, the availability of mobility aids, the provision of services, and a variety of personality factors that determine coping ability.[224] The use of antibiotics for bronchitis or aspiration pneumonia, and aggressive general care can prolong life. Patients who are involved in clinical trials are generally cared for by highly motivated caregivers and health care professionals who are interested and concerned about patients' well-being. Tracheostomy for permanent ventilator care postpones death, and this procedure is often considered equivalent to death for the purpose of defining survival time.[225] The strongest argument against using death as the primary outcome may be the size of the study required. The median survival time after the onset of symptoms ranges from 23 to 52 months, with 50% survival somewhere between 3 and 4 years after disease onset. Adequate power may require at least 1000 subjects followed over 3 years, which greatly increases the cost of the trial. A recent trial of creatine used continuous data monitoring and stopped the trial once the statistical ability to detect efficacy was impossible; the design helped reduce the length and cost of this survival trial.[226]

Clinical surrogates for survival are often used as outcome measures to improve trial efficacy. The ALS Functional Rating Scale (ALSFRS) measures four components of physical functioning: bulbar function, arm function and ability to perform activities of daily living, leg function, and respiratory function. It was first designed to augment the standard outcome measures of mortality, muscle strength and pulmonary function in clinical trials of ALS.[227] It was modeled after the ALS Severity Scale, already validated, which itself was designed using the Unified Parkinson Disease Rating Scale.[228]

The ALSFRS was initially validated in two studies,[229] and was then assessed in a large clinical trial of ciliary neurotrophic factor.[227,230] The test-retest reliability and internal consistency were confirmed in the 245 patients in the placebo group. The baseline ALSFRS score was correlated with other outcome measures, and with survival. Change in ALSFRS over time paralleled change in muscle testing, FVC, Schwab and England scale and global clinical impression reports.

One weakness of the original scale was that it weighted limb and bulbar function over respiratory function. During the course of a clinical trial of brain-derived neurotrophic factor (BDNF),[231] three additional questions that evaluate the progression of respiratory dysfunction were developed and tested. The addition of the respiratory symptom ratings resulted in a scale that better predicted survival and was more sensitive to change than the original ALSFRS.[232] The revised ALSFRS-R has strong internal consistency and construct validity.[232] The ALSFRS-R has also been shown to predict survival in an ALS clinic population.[233]

One advantage of using a functional rating scale over other primary outcome measures is ease of administration, which could reduce subject dropout from trials. The ALSFRS-R can be administered to patients or caregivers, in-person or over the telephone.[234,235] The scale has now been used as a primary outcome measure in Phase II[214,236] and Phase III trials.[237] Extensive evaluator training has been used to ensure reliable data acquisition in trials, but a self-administered version of the ALSFRS-R has also been shown to be reliable.[238]

Assessments of strength testing, including manual muscle testing (MMT) and maximum voluntary isometric contraction (MVIC), are sensitive and reproducible endpoints in ALS trials[239] and are a familiar procedure in neurological clinics. MVIC was developed as part of the Tufts Quantitative Neuromuscular Evaluation (TQNE).[240] MVIC requires a strain gauge (a force displacement transducer), a strap to hold the limb being tested, a special examining table to position the patient's joints and to fix the strain gauge at a proper angle, and a computer to process the data. MVIC quantifies isometric muscle strength and has been used as a primary outcome in many trials during the past 10 years.[192,231,241] Its range and sensitivity have been validated by several natural history studies.[58,218,242,243] However, the reliability of the test can be low unless the examiner is well trained, and there has been excessive dropout of data from trials using MVIC because of the difficulty patients with advanced ALS have in performing the test.[191,192] MVIC is no longer considered the ideal primary outcome measure it once was because of the needed equipment and space, and the high degree of loss to follow-up.

MMT, a global assessment of strength has also been used in most treatment trials, often in conjunction with MVIC. MMT of 34 muscle groups is as sensitive as MVIC in measuring change in strength, and is less expensive to perform.[239] MMT has several disadvantages,[244] including the need for physical therapists to obtain the high degree of precision necessary to minimize variability in the test. MMT has now being used as a primary outcome measure in an ongoing trial of insulin-like growth factor-1.

Respiratory function tests such as negative inspiratory pressure, or maximum inspiratory pressure, and FVC assess diaphragm strength. The FVC (percent predicted) is easily administered, is often used as part of enrollment criteria[245] and is a standard secondary outcome measure in trials of ALS. FVC produces linear, consistent and reliable data in longitudinal studies of ALS patients.[191]

Potential Biomarkers

There is a clear need for identification of biomarkers, laboratory measures of the disease process that can be used to show a treatment effect at the biological level. Potential markers of UMN function include transcranial magnetic stimulation, magnetic resonance imaging, and spectroscopy. In patients with ALS and UMN syndromes, *N*-acetyl-aspartate concentrations in the primary cortex differ from controls on MR spectroscopic imaging, and central motor conduction time is prolonged on transcranial magnetic stimulation.[246] Unfortunately, neither test has been shown to correlate well with disease progression.[247] Biochemical markers are also being studied as secondary outcomes in trials of ALS. Potential biomarkers include indices of oxidative injury,[44,248,249] levels of matrix metalloproteinase-9,[250] and transforming growth factor-1.[251] Other potential biomarkers include a proteomic approach used to reveal protein biomarkers in blood or CSF[252,253] and inflammatory markers, such as COX-2 or prostaglandin levels in the CNS.[254]

Electrodiagnostic studies can provide information on disease progression not readily available from measurement of muscle strength or clinical functional scales. Motor unit number estimation (MUNE) gives a quantitative assessment of an LMN survival and loss, by estimating the number of functioning motor units.[255] MUNE has its greatest utility in tracking motor unit loss over time via longitudinal studies in the same muscle group. MUNE declined reliably in 80 patients during a clinical trial of ciliary neurotrophic factor.[227] In trials of creatine[256] and topiramate[192] the number of motor units declined predictably in both treated patients and controls. However, the statistical method used may not have been sensitive enough to reliably measure progression of ALS due to motor unit instability.[257] Of the several methods available, the most sensitive and reliable has yet to be determined, but in a longitudinal natural history study of 64 patients with ALS, multiple-point stimulation MUNE correlated with clinical measures, was sensitive to changes over time and detected LMN loss before clinical manifestations appeared.[246]

Slowing Disease Progression

The benefit of riluzole has been replicated in several trials, but patients cannot perceive the 11% effect. About 40% of patients in the US do not take riluzole, in part because many do not believe the response is meaningful. Greater numbers of more powerful agents are needed to build on the benefit of riluzole. Given the current state of knowledge, however, it is not yet possible to affect a cure in ALS; preclinical screening and treatment trials still assess medications that slow, not reverse, the progression of the disease. Which outcome measures best assess slowing of progression and how much of an effect is clinically meaningful is debated. Data from one trial suggest that patients cannot perceive a difference in the ALSFRS-R until it reaches nine points or more.[258] The World Federation of Neurology, Airlie House Guidelines recommend consideration of quality of life measures in addition to survival when determining the efficacy and benefit of a new treatment.[259]

CONCLUSION AND FUTURE DIRECTIONS

ALS researchers are working toward innovative models testing new mechanisms of cell degeneration, genome wide screens, and novel therapies for the future. *In vitro* and murine models allow for studies of new agents prior to trials in patients. However, to date, there has not been translation of a truly clinically effective therapy. Improved communication between preclinical and clinical scientists and a standardized, preclinical approach will enhance translation from models to patients and ensure that the best drugs progress to clinical trials. Animal studies that give treatment after symptom onset, in doses and regimen that can be emulated in humans and that study spinal fluid pharmacokinetics can enhance the effective translation to human studies. Different genes may influence susceptibility and disease phenotype, even in those with apparently SALS, and pharmacogenomic studies could aid in tailoring new therapies to individual patients based on their genetic profile.[260] Other new technologies such as retrograde viral delivery of a medication, RNA interference of abnormal gene products, and cell replacement therapy show promise for the future but are still in the early stages of development. Improved techniques in human trials, including easy-to-administer outcome measures that minimize dropout, adequate power, and sufficient statistical planning will maximize the likelihood of success once promising agents reach the clinical trial phase.

ALS offers the chance of proof-of-concept studies faster than other disorders. The rapidly progressive disease course makes ALS a good testing ground for new therapies. Milestones for outcomes are reached earlier, providing results sooner than is possible in other neurodegenerative disorders. Once an agent is shown to slow neurodegeneration in ALS, it might also be indicated for and could be tested in other neurodegenerative disorders. One day soon, advances in both the basic and clinical sciences will lead to effective new treatments for ALS, and the implications will be felt across all neurodegenerative diseases.

ACKNOWLEDGEMENTS

Caterina Bendotti, Cristina Cheroni and Massimo Tortarolo are supported by grants from the Italian Ministry for Health (Ricerca Finalizzata, Malattie Neurodegenerative), Telethon, Fondazione Cariplo and Fondazione Vialli e Mauro per la Ricerca e lo Sport.

REFERENCES

1. Rowland, L.P. and Shneider, N.A. (2001). Amyotrophic lateral sclerosis. *N Engl J Med*, 344(22):1688–1700.

2. Siddique, T., Figlewicz, D.A., Pericak-Vance, M.A., Haines, J.L., Rouleau, G., Jeffers., A.J. *et al.* (1991). Linkage of a gene causing familial amyotrophic lateral sclerosis to chromosome 21 and evidence of genetic-locus heterogeneity. *N Engl J Med*, 324(20):1381–1384.

3. Boillee, S., Vande Velde, C., and Cleveland, D.W. (2006). ALS: A disease of motor neurons and their nonneuronal neighbors. *Neuron*, 52(1):39–59.

4. Bruijn, L.I., Miller, T.M., and Cleveland, D.W. (2004). Unraveling the mechanisms involved in motor neuron degeneration in ALS. *Annu Rev Neurosci*, 27:723–749.

5. Aran, F. (1850). Recherches sur une maladie non encore decrite du systeme musculaire (atrophie musculaire progressive). *Arch Gen Med*, 24:15–35.

6. Aran, F. (1848). Revue clinique des hopitaux et hospices, *Un Med 2*, 553–554, 7–8.

7. Rowland, L.P. (2001). How amyotrophic lateral sclerosis got its name: the clinical-pathologic genius of Jean-Martin Charcot. *Arch Neurol*, 58(3):512–515.

8. Gowers, W. (1899). *A Manual of Diseases of the Nervous System*, 3rd ed. Blakiston, Philadelphia.

9. Brain, W. and Walton, J. (1969). *Brain's Disease of the Nervous System*. Oxford University Press, London.

10. Roman, G.C. (1996). Neuroepidemiology of amyotrophic lateral sclerosis: Clues to aetiology and pathogenesis. *J Neurol Neurosurg Psychiatr*, 61(2):131–137.

11. Alcaz, S., Jarebinski, M., Pekmezovic, T., Stevic-Marinkovic, Z., Pavlovic, S., and Apostolski, S. (1996). Epidemiological and clinical characteristics of ALS in Belgrade, Yugoslavia. *Acta Neurol Scand*, 94(4):264–268.

12. Chancellor, A.M. and Warlow, C.P. (1992). Adult onset motor neuron disease: worldwide mortality, incidence and distribution since 1950. *J Neurol Neurosurg*, 55(12):1106–1115.

13. Cuadrado-Gamarra, J.I., Sevillano-García, M.D., and de Pedro- Cuesta, J. (1999). Motoneuron disease in Spain: differential epidemiological features. *Rev. Neurol.*, 29(9):887–889.

14. Govoni, V., Granieri, E., Capone, J., Manconi, M., and Casetta, I. (2003). Incidence of amyotrophic lateral sclerosis in the local health district of Ferrara. *Neuroepidemiology*, 22(4):229–234.

15. Beghi, E., Logroscino, G., Chio, A., Hardiman, O., Mitchell, D., Swingler, R. *et al.* (2006). The epidemiology of ALS and the role of population-based registries. *Biochim Biophys Acta*, 1762(11–12):1150–1157.

16. Sorenson, E.J., Stalker, A.P., Kurland, L.T., and Windebank, A.J. (2002). Amyotrophic lateral sclerosis in Olmsted County, Minnesota, 1925 to 1998. *Neurology*, 59(2):280–282.

17. Incidence of ALS in Italy: Evidence for a uniform frequency in Western countries. (2001). *Neurology*, 56(2):239–244.

18. Mitsumoto, H., Przedborski, S., and Gordon, P. (eds.), (2006). *Familial ALS and Genetic Approaches to ALS.* Taylor & Francis, New York, London.

19. Deng, H.X., Hentati, A., Tainer, J.A., Iqbal, Z., Cayabyab, A., Hung, W.Y. *et al.* (1993). Amyotrophic lateral sclerosis and structural defects in Cu,Zn superoxide dismutase. *Science*, 261(5124):1047–1051.

20. Rosen, D.R., Siddique, T., Patterson, D., Figlewicz, D.A., Sapp, P., Hentati, A. *et al.* (1993). Mutations in Cu/Zn superoxide dismutase gene are associated with familial amyotrophic lateral sclerosis. *Nature*, 362(6415):59–62.

21. Mitsumoto, H., Przedborski, S., and Gordon, P. (eds.) (2006). *Classification, Diagnosis, and Presentation of Diagnosis of ALS.* Taylor & Francis, New York, London.

22. Juneja, T., Pericak-Vance, M.A., Laing, N.G., Dave, S., and Siddique, T. (1997). Prognosis in familial amyotrophic lateral sclerosis: Progression and survival in patients with glu100gly and ala-4val mutations in Cu,Zn superoxide dismutase. *Neurology*, 48(1):55–57.

23. Cudkowicz, M.E., McKenna-Yasek, D., Sapp, P.E., Chin, W., Geller, B., Hayden, D.L. *et al.* (1997). Epidemiology of mutations in superoxide dismutase in amyotrophic lateral sclerosis. *Ann Neurol*, 41(2):210–221.

24. Siddique, T., Pericak-Vance, M.A., Brooks, B.R., Roos, R.P., Hung, W.Y., Antel, J.P. *et al.* (1989). Linkage analysis in familial amyotrophic lateral sclerosis. *Neurology*, 39(7):919–925.

25. Armon, C. (2003). An evidence-based medicine approach to the evaluation of the role of exogenous risk factors in sporadic amyotrophic lateral sclerosis. *Neuroepidemiology*, 22(4):217–228.

26. Qureshi, M.M., Hayden, D., Urbinelli, L., Ferrante, K., Newhall, K., Myers, D. *et al.* (2006). Analysis of factors that modify susceptibility and rate of progression in amyotrophic lateral sclerosis (ALS). *Amyotroph Lateral Scler*, 7(3):173–182.

27. Beretta, S., Carri, M.T., Beghi, E., Chio, A., and Ferrarese, C. (2003). The sinister side of Italian soccer. *Lancet Neurol*, 2(11):656–657.

28. Chio, A., Benzi, G., Dossena, M., Mutani, R., and Mora, G. (2005). Severely increased risk of amyotrophic lateral sclerosis among Italian professional football players. *Brain*, 128(Pt 3):472–476.

29. Scarmeas, N., Shih, T., Stern, Y., Ottman, R., and Rowland, L.P. (2002). Premorbid weight, body mass, and varsity athletics in ALS. *Neurology*, 59(5):773–775.

30. Schymick, J.C., Scholz, S.W., Fung, H.C., Britton, A., Arepalli, S., Gibbs, J.R. *et al.* (2007). Genome-wide genotyping in amyotrophic lateral sclerosis and neurologically normal controls: First stage analysis and public release of data. *Lancet Neurol*, 6(4):322–328.

31. Clement, A.M., Nguyen, M.D., Roberts, E.A., Garcia, M.L., Boillee, S., Rule, M. *et al.* (2003). Wild-type nonneuronal cells extend survival of SOD1 mutant motor neurons in ALS mice. *Science*, 302(5642):113–117.

32. Hirano, A. (1991). Cytopathology of amyotrophic lateral sclerosis. *Adv Neurol*, 56:91–101.

33. Schiffer, D., Cordera, S., Cavalla, P., and Migheli, A. (1996). Reactive astrogliosis of the spinal cord in amyotrophic lateral sclerosis. *J Neurol Sci*, 139:27–33.

34. Almer, G., Guegan, C., Teismann, P., Naini, A., Rosoklija, G., Hays, A.P. *et al.* (2001). Increased expression of the pro-inflammatory enzyme cyclooxygenase-2 in amyotrophic lateral sclerosis. *Ann Neurol*, 49(2):176–185.

35. Yasojima, K., Tourtellotte, W.W., McGeer, E.G., and McGeer, P.L. (2001). Marked increase in cyclooxygenase-2 in ALS spinal cord: Implications for therapy. *Neurology*, 57(6):952–956.

36. Wong, N.K. and Strong, M.J. (1998). Nitric oxide synthase expression in cervical spinal cord in sporadic amyotrophic lateral sclerosis. *Eur J Cell Biol*, 77(4):338–343.

37. Martin, L.J., Price, A.C., Kaiser, A., Shaikh, A.Y., and Liu, Z. (2000). Mechanisms for neuronal degeneration in amyotrophic lateral sclerosis and in models of motor neuron death (review). *Int J Mol Med*, 5(1):3–13.

38. Engelhardt, J.I., Tajti, J., and Appel, S.H. (1993). Lymphocytic infiltrates in the spinal cord in amyotrophic lateral sclerosis. *Arch Neurol*, 50(1):30–36.

39. Almer, G., Teismann, P., Stevic, Z., Halaschek-Wiener, J., Deecke, L., Kostic, V. *et al.* (2002). Increased levels of the pro-inflammatory prostaglandin PGE2 in CSF from ALS patients. *Neurology*, 58(8):1277–1279.

40. Klegeris, A. and McGeer, P.L. (1994). Rat brain microglia and peritoneal macrophages show similar responses to respiratory burst stimulants. *J Neuroimmunol*, 53(1):83–90.

41. Ferrante, R.J., Shinobu, L.A., Schulz, J.B., Matthews, R.T., Thomas, C.E., Kowall, N.W. *et al.* (1997). Increased 3-nitrotyrosine and oxidative damage in mice with a human copper/zinc superoxide dismutase mutation. *Ann Neurol*, 42(3):326–334.

42. Floyd, R.A. and Carney, J.M. (1992). Free radical damage to protein and DNA: Mechanisms involved and relevant observations on brain undergoing oxidative stress. *Ann Neurol*, 32:S22–S27.

43. Shaw, P.J., Ince, P.G., Falkous, G., and Mantle, D. (1995). Oxidative damage to protein in sporadic motor neuron disease spinal cord. *Ann Neurol*, 38(4):691–695.

44. Beal, M.F., Ferrante, R.J., Browne, S.E., Matthews, R.T., Kowall, N.W., and Brown, R.H., Jr. (1997). Increased 3-nitrotyrosine in both sporadic and familial amyotrophic lateral sclerosis. *Ann Neurol*, 42(4):644–654.

45. Shibata, N., Nagai, R., Uchida, K., Horiuchi, S., Yamada, S., Hirano, A. *et al.* (2001). Morphological evidence for lipid peroxidation and protein glycoxidation in spinal cords from sporadic amyotrophic lateral sclerosis patients. *Brain Res*, 917(1):97–104.

46. Wiedau-Pazos, M., Goto, J.J., Rabizadeh, S., Gralla, E.B., Roe, J.A., Lee, M.K. *et al.* (1996). Altered reactivity of superoxide dismutase in familial amyotrophic lateral sclerosis. *Science*, 271(5248):515–518.

47. Plaitakis, A. and Caroscio, J.T. (1987). Abnormal glutamate metabolism in amyotrophic lateral sclerosis. *Ann Neurol*, 22(5):575–579.

48. Spreux-Varoquaux, O., Bensimon, G., Lacomblez, L., Salachas, F., Pradat, P.F., Le Forestier, N. *et al.* (2002). Glutamate levels in cerebrospinal fluid in amyotrophic lateral sclerosis: A reappraisal using a new HPLC method with coulometric detection in a large cohort of patients. *J Neurol Sci*, 193(2):73–78.

49. Choi, D.W. (1988). Glutamate neurotoxicity and diseases of the nervous system. *Neuron*, 1(8):623–634.

50. Rothstein, J.D., Martin, L.J., and Kuncl, R.W. (1992). Decreased glutamate transport by the brain and spinal cord in amyotrophic lateral sclerosis. *N Engl J Med*, 326(22):1464–1468.

51. Wiedemann, F.R., Winkler, K., Kuznetsov, A.V., Bartels, C., Vielhaber, S., Feistner, H. *et al.* (1998). Impairment of mitochondrial function in skeletal muscle of patients with amyotrophic lateral sclerosis. *J Neurol Sci*, 156:65–72.

52. Gurney, M.E., Pu, H., Chiu, A.Y., Dal Canto, M.C., Polchow, C.Y., Alexander, D.D. *et al.* (1994). Motor neuron degeneration in mice that express a human Cu,Zn superoxide dismutase mutation. *Science*, 264(5166):1772–1775.

53. Guegan, C., Vila, M., Rosoklija, G., Hays, A.P., and Przedborski, S. (2001). Recruitment of the mitochondrial-dependent apoptotic pathway in amyotrophic lateral sclerosis. *J Neurosci*, 21(17):6569–6576.

54. Friedlander, R.M. (2003). Apoptosis and caspases in neurodegenerative diseases. *N Engl J Med*, 348(14):1365–1375.

55. Yoshihara, T., Ishigaki, S., Yamamoto, M., Liang, Y., Niwa, J., Takeuchi, H. *et al.* (2002). Differential expression of inflammation- and apoptosis-related genes in spinal cords of a mutant SOD1 transgenic mouse model of familial amyotrophic lateral sclerosis. *J Neurochem*, 80(1):158–167.

56. Gurney, M.E., Tomasselli, A.G., and Heinrikson, R.L. (2000). Neurobiology. Stay the executioner's hand. *Science*, 288(5464):283–284.

57. Cheng, A., Chan, S.L., Milhavet, O., Wang, S., and Mattson, M.P. (2001). p38 MAP kinase mediates nitric oxide-induced apoptosis of neural progenitor cells. *J Biol Chem*, 276(46):43320–43327.

58. Brooks, B.R. (1994). El Escorial World Federation of Neurology criteria for the diagnosis of amyotrophic lateral sclerosis. Subcommittee on Motor Neuron Diseases/Amyotrophic Lateral Sclerosis of the World Federation of Neurology Research Group on Neuromuscular Diseases and the El Escorial "Clinical limits of amyotrophic lateral sclerosis" workshop contributors. *J Neurol Sci*, 124Suppl:96–107.

59. Ross, M.A., Miller, R.G., Berchert, L., Parry, G., Barohn, R.J., Armon, C. *et al.* (1998). Toward earlier diagnosis of amyotrophic lateral sclerosis: Revised criteria, rhCNTF ALS Study Group. *Neurology*, 50(3):768–772.

60. Caroscio, J.T., Mulvihill, M.N., Sterling, R., and Abrams, B. (1987). Amyotrophic lateral sclerosis. Its natural history. *Neurol Clin*, 5(1):1–8.

61. Li, T.M., Alberman, E., and Swash, M. (1990). Clinical features and associations of 560 cases of motor neuron disease. *J Neurol Neurosurg Psychiatr*, 53(12):1043–1045.

62. Rowland, L.P. (1998). Diagnosis of amyotrophic lateral sclerosis. *J Neurol Sci*, 160(Suppl 1):S6–S24.

63. Nardone, A., Galante, M., Lucas, B., and Schieppati, M. (2001). Stance control is not affected by paresis and reflex hyperexcitability: The case of spastic patients. *J Neurol Neurosurg Psychiatr*, 70(5):635–643.

64. Gubbay, S.S., Kahana, E., Zilber, N., Cooper, G., Pintov, S., and Leibowitz, Y. (1985). Amyotrophic lateral sclerosis. A study of its presentation and prognosis. *J Neurol*, 232:295–300.

65. Jokelainen, M. (1977). Amyotrophic lateral sclerosis in Finland. II: Clinical characteristics. *Acta Neurol Scand*, 56(3):194–204.

66. Traynor, B.J., Codd, M.B., Corr, B., Forde, C., Frost, E., and Hardiman, O.M. (2000). Clinical features of amyotrophic lateral sclerosis according to the El Escorial and Airlie House diagnostic criteria: A population-based study. *Arch Neurol*, 57(8):1171–1176.

67. Hillel, A.D. and Miller, R. (1989). Bulbar amyotrophic lateral sclerosis: Patterns of progression and clinical management. *Head Neck*, 11(1):51–59.

68. Shoesmith, C.L., Findlater, K., Rowe, A., and Strong, M.J. (2007). Prognosis of amyotrophic lateral sclerosis with respiratory onset. *J Neurol Neurosurg Psychiatr.*, 78(6):629–631.

69. Massman, P.J., Sims, J., Cooke, N., Haverkamp, L.J., Appel, V., and Appel, S.H. (1996). Prevalence and correlates of neuropsychological deficits in amyotrophic lateral sclerosis. *J Neurol Neurosurg Psychiatr*, 61(5):450–455.

70. Lomen-Hoerth, C., Murphy, J., Langmore, S., Kramer, J.H., Olney, R.K., and Miller, B. (2003). Are amyotrophic lateral sclerosis patients cognitively normal? *Neurology*, 60(7):1094–1097.

71. Ringholz, G.M., Appel, S.H., Bradshaw, M., Cooke, N.A., Mosnik, D.M., and Schulz, P.E. (2005). Prevalence and patterns of cognitive impairment in sporadic ALS. *Neurology*, 65(4):586–590.

72. Neumann, M., Sampathu, D.M., Kwong, L.K., Truax, A.C., Micsenyi, M.C., Chou, T.T. *et al.* (2006). Ubiquitinated TDP-43 in frontotemporal lobar degeneration and amyotrophic lateral sclerosis. *Science*, 314(5796):130–133.

73. Olney, R.K., Murphy, J., Forshew, D., Garwood, E., Miller, B.L., Langmore, S. *et al.* (2005). The effects of executive and behavioral dysfunction on the course of ALS. *Neurology*, 65(11):1774–1777.

74. Haymaker, W., and Hartwif, K. (1988). Disorders of the brainstem and its cranial nerves, In Baker, A. and Joynt, R. (eds.), *Clinical Neurology*. J.B. Lippincott Company, Philadelphia.

75. Parvizi, J., Anderson, S.W., Martin, C.O., Damasio, H., and Damasio, A.R. (2001). Pathological laughter and crying: A link to the cerebellum. *Brain*, 124(Pt 9):1708–1719.

76. Krupp, L. (2004). *Fatigue in Multiple Sclerosis: A guide to diagnosis and management.* Demos, New York.

77. Armon, C., Graves, M.C., Moses, D., Forte, D.K., Sepulveda, L., Darby, S.M. *et al.* (2000). Linear estimates of disease progression predict survival in patients with amyotrophic lateral sclerosis. *Muscle Nerve*, 23(6):874–882.

78. Gordon, P.H. and Cheung, Y.K. (2006). Progression rate of ALSFRS-R at time of diagnosis predicts survival time in ALS. *Neurology*, 67(7):1314–1315. author reply 5.

79. Bensimon, G., Lacomblez, L., and Meininger, V. (1994). A controlled trial of riluzole in amyotrophic lateral sclerosis. ALS/Riluzole Study Group. *N Engl J Med*, 330(9):585–591.

80. Lacomblez, L., Bensimon, G., Leigh, P.N., Guillet, P., and Meininger, V. (1996). Dose-ranging study of riluzole in amyotrophic lateral sclerosis. Amyotrophic Lateral Sclerosis/Riluzole Study Group II. *Lancet*, 347(9013):1425–1431.

81. Rowland, L.P. (1994). *Riluzole for the treatment of amyotrophic lateral sclerosis - too soon to tell? N Engl J Med*, 330(9):636-637.

82. Sojka, P., Andersen, P.M., and Forsgren, L. (1997). Effects of riluzole on symptom progression in amyotrophic lateral sclerosis. *Lancet*, 349(9046):176-177.

83. Practice advisory on the treatment of amyotrophic lateral sclerosis with riluzole: Report of the Quality Standards Subcommittee of the American Academy of Neurology. (1997). *Neurology*, 49(3):657-659.

84. Miller, R.G., Mitchell, J.D., and Lyon, M. (2002). D.H. Moore. Riluzole for amyotrophic lateral sclerosis (ALS)/motor neuron disease (MND). *Cochrane Database Syst Rev*, 2. CD001447

85. Meininger, V., Dib, M., Aubin, F., Jourdain, G., and Zeisser, P. (1997). The Riluzole Early Access Programme: Descriptive analysis of 844 patients in France. ALS/Riluzole Study Group III. *J Neurol*, 244(Suppl 2):S22-S25.

86. Bensimon, G., Lacomblez, L., Delumeau, J.C., Bejuit, R., Truffinet, P., and Meininger, V. (2002). A study of riluzole in the treatment of advanced stage or elderly patients with amyotrophic lateral sclerosis. *J Neurol*, 249(5):609-615.

87. Miller, R., Mitchell, J., Lyon, M., and Moore, D. (2007). Riluzole for amyotrophic lateral sclerosis (ALS)/motor neuron disease (MND). *Cochrane Database Syst Rev*, 1. CD001447

88. Lacomblez, L., Bensimon, G., Leigh, P.N., Debove, C., Bejuit, R., Truffinet, P. *et al.* (2002). Long-term safety of riluzole in amyotrophic lateral sclerosis. *Amyotroph Lateral Scler Other Motor Neuron Disord*, 3(1):23-29.

89. Miller, R.G., Rosenberg, J.A., Gelinas, D.F., Mitsumoto, H., Newman, D., Sufit, R. *et al.* (1999). Practice parameter: the care of the patient with amyotrophic lateral sclerosis (an evidence-based review): Report of the Quality Standards Subcommittee of the American Academy of Neurology: ALS Practice Parameters Task Force. *Neurology*, 52(7):1311-1323.

90. Forshew, D.A. and Bromberg, M.B. (2003). A survey of clinicians' practice in the symptomatic treatment of ALS. *Amyotroph Lateral Scler Other Motor Neuron Disord*, 4(4):258-263.

91. Mitsumoto, H., Przedborski, S., and Gordon, P. (eds.) (2006). *Symptomatic Pharmacotherapy: Bulbar and Constitutional Symptoms.* Taylor & Francis, New York, London.

92. Ashworth, N.L., Satkunam, L.E., and Deforge, D. (2004). Treatment for spasticity in amyotrophic lateral sclerosis/motor neuron disease. *Cochrane Database Syst Rev*, 1. CD004156

93. Marquardt, G. and Seifert, V. (2002). Use of intrathecal baclofen for treatment of spasticity in amyotrophic lateral sclerosis. *J Neurol Neurosurg Psychiatr*, 72(2):275-276.

94. Connolly, P.S., Shirley, E.A., Wasson, J.H., and Nierenberg, D.W. (1992). Treatment of nocturnal leg cramps. A crossover trial of quinine vs vitamin E. *Arch Intern Med*, 152(9):1877-1880.

95. Khajehdehi, P., Mojerlou, M., Behzadi, S., and Rais-Jalali, G.A. (2001). A randomized, double-blind, placebo-controlled trial of supplementary vitamins E, C and their combination for treatment of haemodialysis cramps. *Nephrol Dial Transplant*, 16(7):1448-1451.

96. Romano, J.G. (1996). Reduction of fasciculations in patients with amyotrophic lateral sclerosis with the use of gabapentin. *Arch Neurol*, 53(8):716.

97. Giess, R., Naumann, M., Werner, E., Riemann, R., Beck, M., Puls, I. *et al.* (2000). Injections of botulinum toxin A into the salivary glands improve sialorrhoea in amyotrophic lateral sclerosis. *J Neurol Neurosurg Psychiatr*, 69(1):121-123.

98. Porta, M., Gamba, M., Bertacchi, G., and Vaj, P. (2001). Treatment of sialorrhoea with ultrasound guided botulinum toxin type A injection in patients with neurological disorders. *J Neurol Neurosurg Psychiatr*, 70(4):538-540.

99. Manrique, D. (2005). Application of botulinum toxin to reduce the saliva in patients with amyotrophic lateral sclerosis. *Rev Bras Otorrinolaringol (Engl Ed)*, 71(5):566-569.

100. Contarino, M.F., Pompili, M., Tittoto, P., Vanacore, N., Sabatelli, M., Cedrone A. *et al.* (2007). Botulinum toxin B ultrasound-guided injections for sialorrhea in amyotrophic lateral sclerosis and Parkinson's disease, *Parkinsonism Relat Disord.*, 13(5):299-303.

101. Winterholler, M.G., Erbguth, F.J., Wolf, S., and Kat, S. (2001). Botulinum toxin for the treatment of sialorrhoea in ALS: Serious side effects of a transductal approach. *J Neurol Neurosurg Psychiatr*, 70(3):417–418.

102. Bhatia, K.P., Munchau, A., and Brown, P. (1999). Botulinum toxin is a useful treatment in excessive drooling in saliva. *J Neurol Neurosurg Psychiatr*, 67(5):697.

103. Tan, E.K., Lo, Y.L., Seah, A., and Auchus, A.P. (2001). Recurrent jaw dislocation after botulinum toxin treatment for sialorrhoea in amyotrophic lateral sclerosis. *J Neurol Sci*, 190(1–2):95–97.

104. Stalpers, L.J. and Moser, E.C. (2002). Results of radiotherapy for drooling in amyotrophic lateral sclerosis. *Neurology*, 58(8):1308.

105. Harriman, M., Morrison, M., Hay, J., Revonta, M., Eisen, A., and Lentle, B. (2001). Use of radiotherapy for control of sialorrhea in patients with amyotrophic lateral sclerosis. *J Otolaryngol*, 30(4):242–245.

106. I. Foulsum, (ed.), (1999). Secretion management in motor neuron disease, *10th International Symposium on ALS/MND ALS and Other Motor Neuron Disorders*.

107. Brooks, B.R., Thisted, R.A., Appel, S.H., Bradley, W.G., Olney, R.K., Berg, J.E. *et al.* (2004). Treatment of pseudobulbar affect in ALS with dextromethorphan/quinidine: A randomized trial. *Neurology*, 63(8):1364–1370.

108. Mitsumoto, H. and Munsat, T. (eds.) (2001). *Treating the Symptoms of ALS*, Second ed. Demos, New York.

109. Benatar, M. (2007). Lost in translation: Treatment trials in the SOD1 mouse and in human ALS. *Neurobiol Dis*, 26(1):1–13.

110. Carriedo, S.G., Yin, H.Z., and Weiss, J.H. (1996). Motor neurons are selectively vulnerable to AMPA/kainate receptor-mediated injury in vitro. *J Neurosci*, 16(13):4069–4079.

111. Carriedo, S.G., Sensi, S.L., Yin, H.Z., and Weiss, J.H. (2000). AMPA exposures induce mitochondrial Ca(2+) overload and ROS generation in spinal motor neurons in vitro. *J Neurosci*, 20(1):240–250.

112. Azzouz, M., Poindron, P., Guettier, S., Leclerc, N., Andres, C., Warter, J.M. *et al.* (2000). Prevention of mutant SOD1 motoneuron degeneration by copper chelators in vitro. *J Neurobiol*, 42(1):49–55.

113. Van Den Bosch, L., Storkebaum, E., Vleminckx, V., Moons, L., Vanopdenbosch, L., Scheveneels, W. *et al.* (2004). Effects of vascular endothelial growth factor (VEGF) on motor neuron degeneration. *Neurobiol Dis*, 17(1):21–28.

114. Spalloni, A., Pascucci, T., Albo, F., Ferrari, F., Puglisi-Allegra, S., Zona, C. *et al.* (2004). Altered vulnerability to kainate excitotoxicity of transgenic-Cu/Zn SOD1 neurones. *Neuroreport*, 15(16):2477–2480.

115. Dewil, M., Dela Cruz, V.F., Van Den Bosch, L., and Robberecht, W. (2007). Inhibition of p38 mitogen activated protein kinase activation and mutant SOD1(G93A)-induced motor neuron death, *Neurobiol Dis.*, 26(2):332–341.

116. Raoul, C., Estevez, A.G., Nishimune, H., Cleveland, D.W., deLapeyriere, O., Henderson, C.E. *et al.* (2002). Motoneuron death triggered by a specific pathway downstream of Fas potentiation by ALS-linked SOD1 mutations. *Neuron*, 35(6):1067–1083.

117. Zhao, W., Xie, W., Le, W., Beers, D.R., He, Y., Henkel, J.S. *et al.* (2004). Activated microglia initiate motor neuron injury by a nitric oxide and glutamate-mediated mechanism. *J Neuropathol Exp Neurol*, 63(9):964–977.

118. Weydt, P., Yuen, E.C., Ransom, B.R., and Moller, T. (2004). Increased cytotoxic potential of microglia from ALS-transgenic mice. *Glia*, 48(2):179–182.

119. Boillee, S., Yamanaka, K., Lobsiger, C.S., Copeland, N.G., Jenkins, N.A., Kassiotis, G. *et al.* (2006). Onset and progression in inherited ALS determined by motor neurons and microglia. *Science*, 312(5778):1389–1392.

120. Henkel, J.S., Engelhardt, J.I., Siklos, L., Simpson, E.P., Kim, S.H., Pan, T. *et al.* (2004). Presence of dendritic cells, MCP-1, and activated microglia/macrophages in amyotrophic lateral sclerosis spinal cord tissue. *Ann Neurol*, 55(2):221–235.

121. Kawamata, T., Akiyama, H., Yamada, T., and McGeer, P.L. (1992). Immunologic reactions in amyotrophic lateral sclerosis brain and spinal cord tissue. *Am J Pathol*, 140(3):691–707.

122. Nagai, M., Re, D.B., Nagata, T., Chalazonitis, A., Jessell, T.M., Wichterle, H. *et al.* (2007). Astrocytes expressing ALS-linked mutated SOD1 release factors selectively toxic to motor neurons. *Nat Neurosci*, 10(5):615–622.

123. Di Giorgio, F.P., Carrasco, M.A., Siao, M.C., Maniatis, T., and Eggan, K. (2007). Non-cell autonomous effect of glia on motor neurons in an embryonic stem cell-based ALS model. *Nat Neurosci*, 10(5):608–614.

124. Li, M., Ona, V.O., Guegan, C., Chen, M., Jackson-Lewis, V., Andrews, L.J. *et al.* (2000). Functional role of caspase-1 and caspase-3 in an ALS transgenic mouse model. *Science*, 288(5464):335–339.

125. Cashman, N.R., Durham, H.D., Blusztajn, J.K., Oda, K., Tabira, T., Shaw, I.T. *et al.* (1992). Neuroblastoma x spinal cord (NSC) hybrid cell lines resemble developing motor neurons. *Dev Dyn*, 194(3):209–221.

126. Durham, H.D., Dahrouge, S., and Cashman, N.R. (1993). Evaluation of the spinal cord neuron X neuroblastoma hybrid cell line NSC-34 as a model for neurotoxicity testing. *Neurotoxicology*, 14(4):387–395.

127. Eggett, C.J., Crosier, S., Manning, P., Cookson, M.R., Menzies, F.M., McNeil, C.J. *et al.* (2000). Development and characterisation of a glutamate-sensitive motor neurone cell line. *J Neurochem*, 74(5):1895–1902.

128. Menzies, F.M., Cookson, M.R., Taylor, R.W., Turnbull, D.M., Chrzanowska-Lightowlers, Z.M., Dong, L. *et al.* (2002). Mitochondrial dysfunction in a cell culture model of familial amyotrophic lateral sclerosis. *Brain*, 125(Pt 7):1522–1533.

129. Liu, R., Li, B., Flanagan, S.W., Oberley, L.W., Gozal, D., and Qiu, M. (2002). Increased mitochondrial antioxidative activity or decreased oxygen free radical propagation prevent mutant SOD1-mediated motor neuron cell death and increase amyotrophic lateral sclerosis-like transgenic mouse survival. *J Neurochem*, 80(3):488–500.

130. Rizzardini, M., Mangolini, A., Lupi, M., Ubezio, P., Bendotti, C., and Cantoni, L. (2005). Low levels of ALS-linked Cu/Zn superoxide dismutase increase the production of reactive oxygen species and cause mitochondrial damage and death in motor neuron-like cells. *J Neurol Sci*, 232(1–2):95–103.

131. Fukada, K., Zhang, F., Vien, A., Cashman, N.R., and Zhu, H. (2004). Mitochondrial proteomic analysis of a cell line model of familial amyotrophic lateral sclerosis. *Mol Cell Proteomics*, 3(12):1211–1223.

132. Ferri, A., Cozzolino, M., Crosio, C., Nencini, M., Casciati, A., Gralla, E.B. *et al.* (2006). Familial ALS-superoxide dismutases associate with mitochondria and shift their redox potentials. *Proc Natl Acad Sci USA*, 103(37):13860–13865.

133. Sathasivam, S., Grierson, A.J., and Shaw, P.J. (2005). Characterization of the caspase cascade in a cell culture model of SOD1-related familial amyotrophic lateral sclerosis: expression, activation and therapeutic effects of inhibition. *Neuropathol Appl Neurobiol*, 31(5):467–485.

134. Cookson, M.R., Menzies, F.M., Manning, P., Eggett, C.J., Figlewicz, D.A., McNeil, C.J. *et al.* (2002). Cu/Zn superoxide dismutase (SOD1) mutations associated with familial amyotrophic lateral sclerosis (ALS) affect cellular free radical release in the presence of oxidative stress. *Amyotroph Lateral Scler Other Motor Neuron Disord*, 3(2):75–85.

135. Obata, Y., Niikura, T., Kanekura, K., Hashimoto, Y., Kawasumi, M., Kita, Y. *et al.* (2005). Expression of N19S-SOD1, an SOD1 mutant found in sporadic amyotrophic lateral sclerosis patients, induces low-grade motoneuronal toxicity. *J Neurosci Res*, 81(5):720–729.

136. Menzies, F.M., Grierson, A.J., Cookson, M.R., Heath, P.R., Tomkins, J., Figlewicz, D.A. *et al.* (2002). Selective loss of neurofilament expression in Cu/Zn superoxide dismutase (SOD1) linked amyotrophic lateral sclerosis. *J Neurochem*, 82(5):1118-1128.

137. Allen, S., Heath, P.R., Kirby, J., Wharton, S.B., Cookson, M.R., Menzies, F.M. *et al.* (2003). Analysis of the cytosolic proteome in a cell culture model of familial amyotrophic lateral sclerosis reveals alterations to the proteasome, antioxidant defenses, and nitric oxide synthetic pathways. *J Biol Chem*, 278(8):6371-6383.

138. Kirby, J., Menzies, F.M., Cookson, M.R., Bushby, K., and Shaw, P.J. (2002). Differential gene expression in a cell culture model of SOD1-related familial motor neurone disease. *Hum Mol Genet*, 11(17):2061-2075.

139. Rothstein, J.D., Jin, L., Dykes-Hoberg, M., and Kuncl, R.W. (1993). Chronic inhibition of glutamate uptake produces a model of slow neurotoxicity. *Proc Natl Acad Sci USA*, 90(14):6591-6595.

140. Drachman, D.B. and Rothstein, J.D. (2000). Inhibition of cyclooxygenase-2 protects motor neurons in an organotypic model of amyotrophic lateral sclerosis. *Ann Neurol*, 48(5):792-795.

141. Bilak, M., Wu, L., Wang, Q., Haughey, N., Conant, K., St Hillaire, C. *et al.* (2004). PGE2 receptors rescue motor neurons in a model of amyotrophic lateral sclerosis. *Ann Neurol*, 56(2):240-248.

142. Tsuji, S., Kikuchi, S., Shinpo, K., Tashiro, J., Kishimoto, R., Yabe, I. *et al.* (2005). Proteasome inhibition induces selective motor neuron death in organotypic slice cultures. *J Neurosci Res*, 82(4):443-451.

143. Kaal, E.C., Vlug, A.S., Versleijen, M.W., Kuilman, M., Joosten, E.A., and Bar, P.R. (2000). Chronic mitochondrial inhibition induces selective motoneuron death *in vitro*: A new model for amyotrophic lateral sclerosis. *J Neurochem*, 74(3):1158-1165.

144. Corcoran, L.J., Mitchison, T.J., and Liu, Q. (2004). A novel action of histone deacetylase inhibitors in a protein aggresome disease model. *Curr Biol*, 14(6):488-492.

145. Broom, W.J., Auwarter, K.E., Ni, J., Russel, D.E., Yeh, L.A., Maxwell, M.M. *et al.* (2006). Two approaches to drug discovery in SOD1-mediated ALS. *J Biomol Screen*, 11(7):729-735.

146. Vincent, A.M., Backus, C., Taubman, A.A., and Feldman, E.L. (2005). Identification of candidate drugs for the treatment of ALS. *Amyotroph Lateral Scler Other Motor Neuron Disord*, 6(1):29-36.

147. Wong, P.C., Pardo, C.A., Borchelt, D.R., Lee, M.K., Copeland, N.G., Jenkins, N.A. *et al.* (1995). An adverse property of a familial ALS-linked SOD1 mutation causes motor neuron disease characterized by vacuolar degeneration of mitochondria. *Neuron*, 14(6):1105-1116.

148. Bruijn, L.I., Becher, M.W., Lee, M.K., Anderson, K.L., Jenkins, N.A., Copeland, N.G. *et al.* (1997). ALS-linked SOD1 mutant G85R mediates damage to astrocytes and promotes rapidly progressive disease with SOD1-containing inclusions. *Neuron*, 18(2):327-338.

149. Ripps, M.E., Huntley, G.W., Hof, P.R., Morrison, J.H., and Gordon, J.W. (1995). Transgenic mice expressing an altered murine superoxide dismutase gene provide an animal model of amyotrophic lateral sclerosis. *Proc Natl Acad Sci USA*, 92(3):689-693.

150. Jaarsma, D., Haasdijk, E.D., Grashorn, J.A., Hawkins, R., van Duijn, W., Verspaget, H.W. *et al.* (2000). Human Cu/Zn superoxide dismutase (SOD1) overexpression in mice causes mitochondrial vacuolization, axonal degeneration, and premature motoneuron death and accelerates motoneuron disease in mice expressing a familial amyotrophic lateral sclerosis mutant SOD1. *Neurobiol Dis*, 7(6 Pt B):623-643.

151. Bendotti, C., Calvaresi, N., Chiveri, L., Prelle, A., Moggio, M., Braga, M. *et al.* (2001). Early vacuolization and mitochondrial damage in motor neurons of FALS mice are not associated with apoptosis or with changes in cytochrome oxidase histochemical reactivity. *J Neurol Sci*, 191(1-2):25-33.

152. Cheroni, C., Peviani, M., Cascio, P., Debiasi, S., Monti, C., and Bendotti, C. (2005). Accumulation of human SOD1 and ubiquitinated deposits in the spinal cord of SOD1G93A mice during motor neuron disease progression correlates with a decrease of proteasome. *Neurobiol Dis*, 18(3):509–522.

153. Migheli, A., Atzori, C., Piva, R., Tortarolo, M., Girelli, M., Schiffer, D. *et al.* (1999). Lack of apoptosis in mice with ALS. *Nat Med*, 5(9):966–967.

154. Heiman-Patterson, T.D., Deitch, J.S., Blankenhorn, E.P., Erwin, K.L., Perreault, M.J., Alexander, B.K. *et al.* (2005 Sep 15). Background and gender effects on survival in the TgN(SOD1-G93A)1Gur mouse model of ALS. *J Neurol Sci*, 236(1–2):1–7.

155. Angelov, D.N., Waibel, S., Guntinas-Lichius, O., Lenzen, M., Neiss, W.F., Tomov, T.L. *et al.* (2003). Therapeutic vaccine for acute and chronic motor neuron diseases: implications for amyotrophic lateral sclerosis. *Proc Natl Acad Sci USA*, 100(8):4790–4795.

156. Howland, D.S., Liu, J., She, Y., Goad, B., Maragakis, N.J., Kim, B. *et al.* (2002). Focal loss of the glutamate transporter EAAT2 in a transgenic rat model of SOD1 mutant-mediated amyotrophic lateral sclerosis (ALS). *Proc Natl Acad Sci USA*, 99(3):1604–1609.

157. Llado, J., Haenggeli, C., Pardo, A., Wong, V., Benson, L., Coccia, C. *et al.* (2006). Degeneration of respiratory motor neurons in the SOD1 G93A transgenic rat model of ALS. *Neurobiol Dis*, 21(1):110–118.

158. Klein, S.M., Behrstock, S., McHugh, J., Hoffmann, K., Wallace, K., Suzuki, M. *et al.* (2005). GDNF delivery using human neural progenitor cells in a rat model of ALS. *Hum Gene Ther*, 16(4):509–521.

159. Storkebaum, E., Lambrechts, D., Dewerchin, M., Moreno-Murciano, M.P., Appelmans, S., Oh, H. *et al.* (2005). Treatment of motoneuron degeneration by intracerebroventricular delivery of VEGF in a rat model of ALS. *Nat Neurosci*, 8(1):85–92.

160. Oosthuyse, B., Moons, L., Storkebaum, E., Beck, H., Nuyens, D., Brusselmans, K. *et al.* (2001). Deletion of the hypoxia-response element in the vascular endothelial growth factor promoter causes motor neuron degeneration. *Nat Genet*, 28(2):131–138.

161. Hafezparast, M., Klocke, R., Ruhrberg, C., Marquardt, A., Ahmad-Annuar, A., Bowen, S. *et al.* (2003). Mutations in dynein link motor neuron degeneration to defects in retrograde transport. *Science*, 300(5620):808–812.

162. Hadano, S., Hand, C.K., Osuga, H., Yanagisawa, Y., Otomo, A., Devon, R.S. *et al.* (2001). A. gene encoding a putative GTPase regulator is mutated in familial amyotrophic lateral sclerosis 2. *Nat Genet*, 29(2):166–173.

163. Mitsumoto, H. and Bradley, W.G. (1982). Murine motor neuron disease (the wobbler mouse): Degeneration and regeneration of the lower motor neuron. *Brain*, 105(Pt 4):811–834.

164. Dib, M. (2003). Amyotrophic lateral sclerosis: progress and prospects for treatment. *Drugs*, 63:289–310.

165. Abrahams, S., Goldstein, L.H., Suckling, J., Ng, V., Simmons, A., Chitnis, X. *et al.* (2005). Frontotemporal white matter changes in amyotrophic lateral sclerosis. *J Neurol*, 252(3):321–331.

166. Vogels, O.J., Oyen, W.J., van Engelen, B.G., Padberg, G.W., and Horstink, M.W. (1999). Decreased striatal dopamine-receptor binding in sporadic ALS: Glutamate hyperactivity?. *Neurology*, 52(6):1275–1277.

167. Vogels, O.J., Veltman, J., Oyen, W.J., and Horstink, M.W. (2000). Decreased striatal dopamine D2 receptor binding in amyotrophic lateral sclerosis (ALS) and multiple system atrophy (MSA): D2 receptor down-regulation versus striatal cell degeneration. *J Neurol Sci*, 180(1–2):62–65.

168. Borasio, G.D., Linke, R., Schwarz, J., Schlamp, V., Abel, A., Mozley, P.D. *et al.* (1998). Dopaminergic deficit in amyotrophic lateral sclerosis assessed with [I-123] IPT single photon emission computed tomography. *J Neurol Neurosurg Psychiatr*, 65(2):263–265.

169. Desai, J. and Swash, M. (1999). Extrapyramidal involvement in amyotrophic lateral sclerosis: Backward falls and retropulsion. *J Neurol Neurosurg Psychiatr*, 67(2):214–216.

170. Schreiber, H., Gaigalat, T., Wiedemuth-Catrinescu, U., Graf, M., Uttner, I., Muche, R. *et al.* (2005). Cognitive function in bulbar- and spinal-onset amyotrophic lateral sclerosis. A longitudinal study in 52 patients. *J Neurol*, 252(7):772–781.

171. Rippon, G.A., Scarmeas, N., Gordon, P.H., Murphy, P.L., Albert, S.M., Mitsumoto, H. *et al.* (2006). An observational study of cognitive impairment in amyotrophic lateral sclerosis. *Arch Neurol*, 63(3):345–352.

172. Kilani, M., Micallef, J., Soubrouillard, C., Rey-Lardiller, D., Demattei, C., Dib, M. *et al.* (2004). A longitudinal study of the evolution of cognitive function and affective state in patients with amyotrophic lateral sclerosis. *Amyotroph Lateral Scler Other Motor Neuron Disord*, 5(1):46–54.

173. Battistini, S., Giannini, F., Greco, G., Bibbo, G., Ferrera, L., Marini, V. *et al.* (2005). SOD1 mutations in amyotrophic lateral sclerosis. Results from a multicenter Italian study. *J Neurol*, 252(7):782–788.

174. Leichsenring, A., Linnartz, B., Zhu, X.R., and Lubbert, H. (2006). C.C. Stichel. Ascending neuropathology in the CNS of a mutant SOD1 mouse model of amyotrophic lateral sclerosis. *Brain Res*, 1096(1):180–195.

175. Andreassen, O.A., Ferrante, R.J., Klivenyi, P., Klein, A.M., Shinobu, L.A., Epstein, C.J. *et al.* (2000). Partial deficiency of manganese superoxide dismutase exacerbates a transgenic mouse model of amyotrophic lateral sclerosis. *Ann Neurol*, 47(4):447–455.

176. Kostic, V., Gurney, M.E., Deng, H.X., Siddique, T., Epstein, C.J., and Przedborski, S. (1997). Midbrain dopaminergic neuronal degeneration in a transgenic mouse model of familial amyotrophic lateral sclerosis. *Ann Neurol*, 41(4):497–504.

177. Calabresi, P., Pisani, A., Mercuri, N.B., and Bernardi, G. (1996). The corticostriatal projection: From synaptic plasticity to dysfunctions of the basal ganglia. *Trends Neurosci*, 19(1):19–24.

178. Calabresi, P., De Murtas, M., and Bernardi, G. (1997). The neostriatum beyond the motor function: Experimental and clinical evidence. *Neuroscience*, 78(1):39–60.

179. Carlson, N.G., Bacchi, A., Rogers, S.W., and Gahring, L.C. (1998). Nicotine blocks TNF-alpha-mediated neuroprotection to NMDA by an alpha-bungarotoxin-sensitive pathway. *J Neurobiol*, 35(1):29–36.

180. Geracitano, R., Paolucci, E., Prisco, S., Guatteo, E., Zona, C., Longone, P. *et al.* (2003). Altered long-term corticostriatal synaptic plasticity in transgenic mice overexpressing human CU/ZN superoxide dismutase (GLY(93)→ALA) mutation. *Neuroscience*, 118:399–408.

181. Arnt, J. (1982). Pharmacological specificity of conditioned avoidance response inhibition in rats: Inhibition by neuroleptics and correlation to dopamine receptor blockade. *Acta Pharmacol Toxicol (Copenh)*, 51(4):321–329.

182. Beninger, R.J., Phillips, A.G., and Fibiger, H.C. (1983). Prior training and intermittent retraining attenuate pimozide-induced avoidance deficits. *Pharmacol Biochem Behav*, 18(4):619–624.

183. Brown, R., David, J.N., and Carlsson, A. (1973). Dopa reversal of hypoxia-induced disruption of the conditioned avoidance response. *J Pharm Pharmacol*, 25(5):412–414.

184. Brown, R.M., Kehr, W., and Carlsson, A. (1975 Mar 7). Functional and biochemical aspects of catecholamine metabolism in brain under hypoxia. *Brain Res*, 85(3):491–509.

185. Rothstein, J.D. (1995). Excitotoxic mechanisms in the pathogenesis of amyotrophic lateral sclerosis. *Adv Neurol*, 68:7–20. discussion 1–7

186. Rothstein, J.D., Van Kammen, M., Levey, A.I., Martin, L.J., and Kuncl, R.W. (1995). Selective loss of glial glutamate transporter GLT-1 in amyotrophic lateral sclerosis. *Ann Neurol*, 38(1):73–84.

187. Spalloni, A., Geracitano, R., Berretta, N., Sgobio, C., Bernardi, G., Mercuri, N.B. *et al.* (2006). Molecular and synaptic changes in the hippocampus underlying superior spatial abilities in pre-symptomatic G93A +/+ mice overexpressing the human Cu/Zn superoxide dismutase (Gly93 → ALA) mutation. *Exp Neurol*, 197(2):505–514.

188. Kandel, E.R. and Squire, L.R. (2000). Neuroscience: Breaking down scientific barriers to the study of brain and mind. *Science*, 290(5494):1113–1120.

189. James, P.A. and Talbot, K. (2006). The molecular genetics of non-ALS motor neuron diseases. *Biochim Biophys Acta*, 1762(11–12):986–1000.

190. Carri, M.T., Grignaschi, G., and Bendotti, C. (2006). Targets in ALS: Designing multidrug therapies. *Trends Pharmacol Sci*, 27(5):267–273.

191. Miller, R.G., Moore, D.H., II., Gelinas, D.F., Dronsky, V., Mendoza, M., Barohn, R.J. *et al.* (2001). Phase III randomized trial of gabapentin in patients with amyotrophic lateral sclerosis. *Neurology*, 56(7):843–848.

192. Cudkowicz, M.E., Shefner, J.M., Schoenfeld, D.A., Brown, R.H., Jr., Johnson, H., Qureshi, M. *et al.* (2003). A randomized, placebo-controlled trial of topiramate in amyotrophic lateral sclerosis. *Neurology*, 61(4):456–464.

193. Kaufmann, P. and Lomen-Hoerth, C. (2003). ALS treatment strikes out while trying for a homer: The topiramate trial. *Neurology*, 61(4):434–435.

194. Groeneveld, G.J., van der Tweel, I., Wokke, J.H., and van den Berg, L.H. (2004). Sequential designs for clinical trials in amyotrophic lateral sclerosis. *Amyotroph Lateral Scler Other Motor Neuron Disord*, 5(4):202–207.

195. Miller, T.M. and Cleveland, D.W. (2005). Medicine. Treating neurodegenerative diseases with antibiotics. *Science*, 307(5708):361–362.

196. Ludolph, A., Bendotti, C., Blaugrund, E., Hengerer, B., Löffler, J., Martin, J. *et al.* (2007). Guidelines for the preclinical in vivo evaluation of pharmacological active drugs for ALS/MND: Report on the 142nd ENMC International Workshop, *Amyotroph Lateral Scler* (in press).

197. Johnston, S.C. and Hauser, S.L. (2006). Basic and clinical research: What is the most appropriate weighting in a public investment portfolio? *Ann Neurol*, 60(1):9A–11A.

198. Cudkowicz, M.E., Shefner, J.M., Schoenfeld, D.A., Zhang, H., Andreasson, K.I., Rothstein, J.D. *et al.* (2006). Trial of celecoxib in amyotrophic lateral sclerosis. *Ann Neurol*, 60(1):22–31.

199. Azbill, R.D., Mu, X., and Springer, J.E. (2000). Riluzole increases high-affinity glutamate uptake in rat spinal cord synaptosomes. *Brain Res*, 871(2):175–180.

200. Hubert, J.P., Burgevin, M.C., Terro, F., Hugon, J., and Doble, A. (1998). Effects of depolarizing stimuli on calcium homeostasis in cultured rat motoneurones. *Br J Pharmacol*, 125(7):1421–1428.

201. Van Westerlaak, M.G., Joosten, E.A., Gribnau, A.A., Cools, A.R., and Bar, P.R. (2001). Differential cortico-motoneuron vulnerability after chronic mitochondrial inhibition in vitro and the role of glutamate receptors. *Brain Res*, 922(2):243–249.

202. Albo, F., Pieri, M., and Zona, C. (2004). Modulation of AMPA receptors in spinal motor neurons by the neuroprotective agent riluzole. *Neurosci Res*, 78:200–207.

203. Koh, J.Y., Kim, D.K., Hwang, J.Y., Kim, Y.H., and Seo, J.H. (1999). Antioxidative and proapoptotic effects of riluzole on cultured cortical neurons. *J Neurochem*, 72(2):716–723.

204. Rothstein, J.D. (2003). Of mice and men: reconciling preclinical ALS mouse studies and human clinical trials. *Ann Neurol*, 53(4):423–426.

205. Traynor, B.J., Bruijn, L., Conwit, R., Beal, F., O'Neill, G., Fagan, S.C. *et al.* (2006). Neuroprotective agents for clinical trials in ALS: A systematic assessment. *Neurology*, 67(1):20–27.

206. Remy, S. and Beck, H. (2006). Molecular and cellular mechanisms of pharmacoresistance in epilepsy. *Brain*, 129(Pt 1):18–35.
207. Huang, Y., Liu, J., Wang, L.Z., Zhang, W.Y., and Zhu, X.Z. (2005). Neuroprotective effects of cyclooxygenase-2 inhibitor celecoxib against toxicity of LPS-stimulated macrophages toward motor neurons. *Acta Pharmacol Sin*, 26(8):952–958.
208. Welty, D.F., Schielke, G.P., and Rothstein, J.D. (1995). Potential treatment of amyotrophic lateral sclerosis with gabapentin: A hypothesis. *Ann Pharmacother*, 29(11):1164–1167.
209. Löscher, W. and Schmidt, D. (2006). New horizons in the development of antiepileptic drugs: Innovative strategies. *Epilepsy Res*, 69:183–272.
210. Gurney, M.E., Cutting, F.B., Zhai, P., Doble, A., Taylor, C.P., Andrus, P.K. *et al.* (1996). Benefit of vitamin E, riluzole, and gabapentin in a transgenic model of familial amyotrophic lateral sclerosis. *Ann Neurol*, 39(2):147–157.
211. Su, T.Z., Feng, M.R., and Weber, M.L. (2005). Mediation of highly concentrative uptake of pregabalin by L-type amino acid transport in Chinese hamster ovary and Caco-2 cells. *J Pharmacol Exp Ther*, 313(3):1406–1415.
212. Mitsumoto, H., Chad, D., and Pioro, E. (1998). *Treatment trials. Amyotrophic Lateral Sclerosis*. FA Davis Co, Philadelphia.
213. Palesch, Y.Y. and Tilley, B.C. (2004). An efficient multi-stage, single-arm Phase II futility design for ALS. *Amyotroph Lateral Scler Other Motor Neuron Disord*, 5(Suppl 1):55–56.
214. Levy, G., Kaufmann, P., Buchsbaum, R., Montes, J., Barsdorf, A., Arbing, R. *et al.* (2006). A two-stage design for a phase II clinical trial of coenzyme Q10 in ALS. *Neurology*, 66(5):660–663.
215. Cheung, Y.K., Gordon, P.H., and Levin, B. (2006). Selecting promising ALS therapies in clinical trials. *Neurology*, 67(10):1748–1751.
216. Rose, F. (ed.) (1994). *The need for double-blind controlled trials in amyotrophic lateral sclerosis*. Smith-Gordon, London.
217. Haynes, R.B. and Dantes, R. (1987). Patient compliance and the conduct and interpretation of therapeutic trials. *Control Clin Trials*, 8(1):12–19.
218. Brooks, B.R., Sufit, R.L., DePaul, R., Tan, Y.D., Sanjak, M., and Robbins, J. (1991). Design of clinical therapeutic trials in amyotrophic lateral sclerosis. *Adv Neurol*, 56:521–546.
219. Bromberg, M.B. (2002). Diagnostic criteria and outcome measurement of amyotrophic lateral sclerosis. *Adv Neurol*, 88:53–62.
220. Rose, F. (ed.) (1990). *Critique of assessment methodology in amyotrophic lateral sclerosis*. Demos, New York.
221. Rose, F. (ed.) (1994). *Longitudinal clinical assessments in motor neurone disease. Relevance to clinical trials*. Smith-Gordon, London.
222. Meinert, C. (1986). *Clinical trials*. Oxford University Press, New York.
223. Rosenberg, R.N., Aminoff, M., Boller, F., Soerensen, P.S., Griggs, R.C., Hachinski, V. *et al.* (2002). Reporting clinical trials: Full access to all the data. *Brain*, 125(Pt 3):i–iii.
224. Munsat, T.L., Andres, P.L., Finison, L., Conlon, T., and Thibodeau, L. (1988). The natural history of motoneuron loss in amyotrophic lateral sclerosis. *Neurology*, 38(3):409–413.
225. Drachman, D.B., Chaudhry, V., Cornblath, D., Kuncl, R.W., Pestronk, A., Clawson, L. *et al.* (1994). Trial of immunosuppression in amyotrophic lateral sclerosis using total lymphoid irradiation. *Ann Neurol*, 35(2):142–150.
226. Groeneveld, G.J., Veldink, J.H., van der Tweel, I., Kalmijn, S., Beijer, C., de Visser, M. *et al.* (2003). A randomized sequential trial of creatine in amyotrophic lateral sclerosis. *Ann Neurol*, 53(4):437–445.
227. The Amyotrophic Lateral Sclerosis Functional Rating Scale. Assessment of activities of daily living in patients with amyotrophic lateral sclerosis. The ALS CNTF treatment study (ACTS) phase I-II Study Group (1996). *Arch Neurol*, 53(2):141–147.

228. Fahn, S., Elton, R. and Committee MotUD. (1987). *Unified Parkinson's Disease Rating Scale*, In Fahn, S. Marsden, C. Calne, D. Goldstein, M. (eds.), Macmillan Healthcare Information, Florham Park.

229. Cedarbaum, J.M. and Stambler, N. (1997). Performance of the Amyotrophic Lateral Sclerosis Functional Rating Scale (ALSFRS) in multicenter clinical trials. *J Neurol Sci*, 152(Suppl 1):S1–S9.

230. A phase I study of recombinant human ciliary neurotrophic factor (rHCNTF) in patients with amyotrophic lateral sclerosis. The ALS CNTF Treatment Study (ACTS) Phase I-II Study Group. (1995 Dec). *Clin Neuropharmacol*, 18(6): 515–532.

231. A controlled trial of recombinant methionyl human BDNF in ALS: The BDNF Study Group (Phase III). (1999). *Neurology*, 52(7): 1427–1433.

232. Cedarbaum, J.M., Stambler, N., Malta, E., Fuller, C., Hilt, D., Thurmond, B. *et al.* (1999). The ALSFRS-R: A revised ALS functional rating scale that incorporates assessments of respiratory function. BDNF ALS Study Group (Phase III). *J Neurol Sci*, 169(1-2):13–21.

233. Kaufmann, P., Levy, G., Thompson, J.L., Delbene, M.L., Battista, V., Gordon, P.H. *et al.* (2005). The ALSFRSr predicts survival time in an ALS clinic population. *Neurology*, 64(1):38–43.

234. Kasarskis, E.J., Dempsey-Hall, L., Thompson, M.M., Luu, L.C., Mendiondo, M., and Kryscio, R. (2005). Rating the severity of ALS by caregivers over the telephone using the ALSFRS-R. *Amyotroph Lateral Scler Other Motor Neuron Disord*, 6(1):50–54.

235. Kaufmann, P., Levy, G., Montes, J., Buchsbaum, R., Barsdorf, A.I., Battista, V. *et al.* (2007). Excellent inter-rater, intra-rater, and telephone-administered reliability of the ALSFRS-R in a multicenter clinical trial. *Amyotroph Lateral Scler*, 8(1):42–46.

236. Scelsa, S.N., MacGowan, D.J., Mitsumoto, H., Imperato, T., LeValley, A.J., Liu, M.H. *et al.* (2005). A pilot, double-blind, placebo-controlled trial of indinavir in patients with ALS. *Neurology*, 64(7):1298–1300.

237. Gordon, P.H., Moore, D.H., Miller, R.G., Florence, J.M., Verheijde, J.L., Doorish, C. *et al.* (2007). Efficacy of minocycline in patients with amyotrophic lateral sclerosis: A phase III randomised trial. *Lancet Neurol*, 6(12):1045–1053.

238. Montes, J., Levy, G., Albert, S., Kaufmann, P., Buchsbaum, R., Gordon, P.H. *et al.* (2006). Development and evaluation of a self-administered version of the ALSFRS-R. *Neurology*, 67(7):1294–1296.

239. Great Lakes ALS Study Group (2003). A comparison of muscle strength testing techniques in amyotrophic lateral sclerosis. *Neurology*, 61(11): 1503–1507.

240. Andres, P.L., Finison, L.J., Conlon, T., Thibodeau, L.M., and Munsat, T.L. (1988). Use of composite scores (megascores) to measure deficit in amyotrophic lateral sclerosis. *Neurology*, 38(3):405–408.

241. A double-blind placebo-controlled clinical trial of subcutaneous recombinant human ciliary neurotrophic factor (rHCNTF) in amyotrophic lateral sclerosis. ALS CNTF Treatment Study Group. (1996). *Neurology*, 46(5): 1244–1249.

242. Brooks, B., Lewis, D. and Rawling, J. (1994). *The Natural History of Amyotrophic Lateral Sclerosis*, In Williams, A. (ed.), Chapman and Hall Medical, London.

243. Ringel, S.P., Murphy, J.R., Alderson, M.K., Bryan, W., England, J.D., Miller, R.G. *et al.* (1993). The natural history of amyotrophic lateral sclerosis. *Neurology*, 43(7):1316–1322.

244. Andres, P.L., Skerry, L.M., Thornell, B., Portney, L.G., Finison, L.J., and Munsat, T.L. (1996). A comparison of three measures of disease progression in ALS. *J Neurol Sci*, 139:64–70.

245. Schmidt, E.P., Drachman, D.B., Wiener, C.M., Clawson, L., Kimball, R., and Lechtzin, N. (2006). Pulmonary predictors of survival in amyotrophic lateral sclerosis: use in clinical trial design. *Muscle Nerve*, 33(1):127–132.

246. Mitsumoto, H., Ulug, A.M., Pullman, S.L., Gooch, C.L., Chan, S., Tang, M.X. *et al.* (2007). Quantitative objective markers for upper and lower motor neuron dysfunction in ALS. *Neurology*, 68(17):1402–1410.

247. Kaufmann, P., Pullman, S.L., Shungu, D.C., Chan, S., Hays, A.P., Del Bene, M.L. *et al.* (2004). Objective tests for upper motor neuron involvement in amyotrophic lateral sclerosis (ALS). *Neurology*, 62(10):1753–1757.

248. Bogdanov, M., Brown, R.H., Matson, W., Smart, R., Hayden, D., O'Donnell, H. *et al.* (2000). Increased oxidative damage to DNA in ALS patients. *Free Radic Biol Med*, 29(7):652–658.

249. Simpson, E.P., Henry, Y.K., Henkel, J.S., Smith, R.G., and Appel, S.H. (2004). Increased lipid peroxidation in sera of ALS patients: A potential biomarker of disease burden. *Neurology*, 62(10):1758–1765.

250. Beuche, W., Yushchenko, M., Mader, M., Maliszewska, M., Felgenhauer, K., and Weber, F. (2000). Matrix metalloproteinase-9 is elevated in serum of patients with amyotrophic lateral sclerosis. *Neuroreport*, 11(16):3419–3422.

251. Houi, K., Kobayashi, T., Kato, S., Mochio, S., and Inoue, K. (2002). Increased plasma TGF-beta1 in patients with amyotrophic lateral sclerosis. *Acta Neurol Scand*, 106(5):299–301.

252. Ramstrom, M., Ivonin, I., Johansson, A., Askmark, H., Markides, K.E., Zubarev, R. *et al.* (2004). Cerebrospinal fluid protein patterns in neurodegenerative disease revealed by liquid chromatography-Fourier transform ion cyclotron resonance mass spectrometry. *Proteomics*, 4(12):4010–4018.

253. Ranganathan, S., Williams, E., Ganchev, P., Gopalakrishnan, V., Lacomis, D., Urbinelli, L. *et al.* (2005). Proteomic profiling of cerebrospinal fluid identifies biomarkers for amyotrophic lateral sclerosis. *J Neurochem*, 95(5):1461–1471.

254. McGeer, P.L. and McGeer, E.G. (2002). Inflammatory processes in amyotrophic lateral sclerosis. *Muscle Nerve*, 26(4):459–470.

255. McComas, A.J., Fawcett, P.R., Campbell, M.J., and Sica, R.E. (1971). Electrophysiological estimation of the number of motor units within a human muscle. *J Neurol Neurosurg Psychiatr*, 34(2):121–131.

256. Shefner, J.M., Cudkowicz, M.E., Schoenfeld, D., Conrad, T., Taft, J., Chilton, M. *et al.* (2004). A clinical trial of creatine in ALS. *Neurology*, 63(9):1656–1661.

257. Shefner, J.M., Cudkowicz, M.E., Zhang, H., Schoenfeld, D., and Jillapalli, D. (2007). Revised statistical motor unit number estimation in the Celecoxib/ALS trial. *Muscle Nerve*, 35(2):228–234.

258. Gordon, P.H., Cheng, B., Montes, J., Doorish, C., Albert, S.M., and Mitsumoto, H. (2007). Outcome measures for early phase clinical trials. *Amyotroph Lateral Scler*, 8(5):270–273.

259. World Federation of Neurology Research Group on Neuromuscular Diseases Subcommittee on Motor Neuron Disease. Airlie House guidelines. Therapeutic trials in amyotrophic lateral sclerosis. Airlie House "Therapeutic Trials in ALS" Workshop Contributors. (1995). *J Neurol Sci*, 129: 1–10.

260. Maimone, D., Dominici, R., and Grimaldi, L.M. (2001). Pharmacogenomics of neurodegenerative diseases. *Eur J Pharmacol*, 413(1):11–29.

CHAPTER 8

Animal and Translational Models of the Epilepsies

Henrik Klitgaard[1], Alain Matagne[1], Steven C. Schachter[2] and H. Steve White[3]

[1]Preclinical CNS Research, UCB Pharma SA, Chemin du Foriest, Braine-l'Alleud, Belgium
[2]Department of Neurology, Harvard Medical School and Beth Israel Deaconess Medical Center, Boston, USA
[3]Anticonvulsant Drug Development Program, Department of Pharmacology and Toxicology, Salt Lake City, USA

Animal and Translational Models for CNS Drug Discovery,
Vol. 2 of 3: Neurological Disorders
Robert McArthur and Franco Borsini (eds), Academic Press, 2008

INTRODUCTION

Epilepsy is one of the most common brain disorders, affecting an estimated 2 to 4 million people in the US, including 1 of every 50 children, 1 of 100 adults, and 1 million women of childbearing age.[1,2] The annual incidence of epilepsy is approximately 50 to 70 per 100,000, or 200,000 newly diagnosed patients every year.[3] Approximately, 50 million persons have epilepsy worldwide, and the majority cannot afford medications or do not have access to medical facilities. The annual incidence is higher in developing countries than in developed countries, largely because of traumatic brain injuries during birth and acquired central nervous system (CNS) infections.

Although epilepsy can develop at any age, a disproportionate number of cases begin in childhood and after the age of 65. The causes of epilepsy vary according to the age of onset. Common etiologies in children and young adults are congenital brain malformations, inborn errors of metabolism, brain trauma, brain tumors, intracranial infection, and vascular malformations. Etiologies in the elderly are Alzheimer's disease and other degenerative brain disorders, stroke, brain tumors, head injuries, and alcohol or drug abuse.[4] However, up to half of patients with epilepsy do not have an identifiable underlying cause.

Epilepsy is associated with an increased risk of mortality and injuries, such as fractures and burns, particularly in patients whose seizures are not fully controlled. Causes of death among persons with epilepsy include accidental deaths (e.g., asphyxiation and drowning), sudden and unexplained death in epilepsy (SUDEP; which is diagnosed when no other cause is found), status epilepticus (a condition of repeated seizures without recovery of consciousness), underlying brain disease (such as brain tumors), and suicide.

DIAGNOSIS OF EPILEPSY

An epileptic seizure is a sudden change in behavior due to transient, pathological hypersynchronization of neuronal networks in the brain, and is the primary symptom of epilepsy. Not all sudden changes in behavior are seizures, however, and not all seizures are epileptic seizures. Non-epileptic seizures resemble epileptic seizures and may result from an otherwise normal brain responding to a systemic physiological change, such as hypoxia, or may be associated with an underlying psychiatric disorder (termed psychogenic non-epileptic seizures).

Although epilepsy is generally diagnosed once a patient has had two or more epileptic seizures, the medical evaluation typically begins after the first seizure to search for conditions that cause non-epileptic seizures and determine if there is an underlying brain lesion on neuroimaging studies (computed tomography or magnetic resonance imaging). Electroencephalograms (EEGs) are useful to support a diagnosis of epilepsy and to help classify a patient's seizure type as generalized or partial, as discussed below. However, EEGs are insensitive and may be normal in over half of patients with epilepsy.

Seizures are classified by physicians as partial or generalized based on their behavioral semiology as related by the patient and witnesses to the seizure, and the associated EEG findings. Besides identifying the type(s) of seizure a patient has, the physician determines whether the patient has an identifiable epilepsy syndrome, which is defined by specific seizure types, age of epilepsy onset, family history, response to particular antiepileptic drugs (AEDs), and prognosis.

Generalized seizures affect both sides of the brain simultaneously when the seizure begins and are usually not associated with identifiable brain pathology. Generalized seizures are further subdivided into absence seizures, myoclonic seizures, and generalized tonic–clonic seizures (also called convulsions).

- Absence seizures are characterized by the sudden onset of staring with impaired consciousness. They typically begin in childhood, last between 5 and 10 s, and may occur dozens if not hundreds of times a day, particularly when patients are not mentally stimulated or are hyperventilating. Up to 90% of patients with childhood absence epilepsy have a spontaneous remission of their seizures before reaching adulthood.
- Myoclonic seizures consist of sudden, brief, shock-like contractions affecting the arms, legs, face or trunk, often occurring in the early morning and generally with retained consciousness.
- Generalized tonic–clonic seizures (previously called grand mal seizures or convulsions) usually begin with a loud noise as air is forcibly expelled from the lungs. The arms and legs stiffen (tonic phase), the patient falls to the ground, and the lips and skin appear dusky in color (cyanotic). After 60 to 90 s, the arms and legs start to jerk, eventually in unison, for an additional 1 to 2 min (clonic phase). Bloody, frothy sputum may be seen coming from the mouth. After the clonic phase ends, the patient appears to be in a deep sleep, and then gradually returns to consciousness over minutes to hours, appearing sleepy and confused, and often complaining of a severe, throbbing headache.

In contrast to generalized seizures, partial seizures affect a restricted area of cerebral cortex at their onset, usually due to an underlying brain lesion, whether or not apparent on neuroimaging studies. Symptoms that patients with partial seizures experience and remember are called simple partial seizures – "simple" means that consciousness is not impaired. Patients often refer to these as auras. Typical symptoms of simple partial seizures are fear, nausea, jerking of the arm and leg on one side of the body, or a metallic taste, though many other symptoms may occur, and usually in a stereotyped fashion for each patient.

Other patients may not be consciously aware of their partial seizures because they abruptly lose consciousness, which is called a complex partial seizure ("complex" means that consciousness is impaired). Complex partial seizures (known in the past as temporal lobe seizures and psychomotor seizures) are the most common type of seizures in adults with epilepsy. During complex partial seizures, patients typically appear awake, but do not meaningfully interact with people or objects around them and do not respond as expected to instructions or questions. They appear to stare off into space and either remain still or exhibit repetitive non-purposeful behaviors called automatisms such as chewing motions, lip smacking, repeating words or phrases, aimless walking or running, or undressing. If patients are forcibly restrained or re-directed during complex partial seizures or during the postictal period, they may resist and become aggressive.

Complex partial seizures typically last less than 3 min and may be immediately preceded by a simple partial seizure or followed by a generalized tonic–clonic seizure. After complex partial seizures, patients may be confused or somnolent, and may complain of a headache. Because their consciousness is impaired during complex partial seizures, patients have no or incomplete memory of what takes place during their occurrence.

PRINCIPLES OF TREATMENT

The goals of treating epilepsy are to address the underlying cause, when known, and to enable the patient to lead a lifestyle consistent with his or her capabilities by minimizing seizures and avoiding significant treatment-related side effects. Achieving this goal requires the patient to report the occurrence of their seizures accurately, which may be difficult for patients with complex partial seizures, as well as the frequency and severity of side effects they experience.

Primary care physicians or emergency room physicians often make the initial diagnosis of epilepsy and begin therapy. If the patient's seizures are not controlled, then he or she is often referred to a neurologist or epileptologist for further diagnostic evaluation and additional therapeutic trials.

AEDs are generally not started until after the second seizure and epilepsy is diagnosed, though some experts recommend beginning AEDs after the first seizure if the initial medical evaluation suggests that the patient has a high risk for additional epileptic seizures. Risk factors for recurrent seizures include previous brain injury (e.g., head injury, stroke, encephalitis), a brain lesion seen on neuroimaging studies, abnormalities on the neurological examination suggesting a brain lesion, a partial seizure or an absence or myoclonic seizure as the first seizure, and an EEG that demonstrates epileptiform abnormalities.

AEDs are selected based on a number of factors, including the patient's seizure type, the pharmacokinetic profile of the drug, the patient's age and co-morbid medical and psychiatric conditions, whether the patient is a woman of childbearing potential, the potential for adverse effects and drug–drug interactions, and drug costs. The selection of AEDs for women who of childbearing potential is particularly important because all AEDs can potentially cause birth defects, especially when taken in combination.

Therapy is generally initiated with a single AED (monotherapy), which enhances compliance, provides a greater therapeutic window, and is more cost effective than combination therapy. With the exception of medical emergencies, when a loading dose is given, therapy is usually initiated with a low dose and increased slowly until seizures are completely controlled, unless bothersome side effects occur that persist, at which time the dose is lowered to minimize side effects, and consideration is given to a second drug as monotherapy or to combination therapy. Because AEDs suppress seizures but are not disease-modifying, the patient's adherence to the AED dosing schedule on a daily basis is crucial for maintaining seizure control. Nonetheless, noncompliance is common, often leading to an increase in seizures and/or medication side effects, especially in patients with frequent seizures, memory dysfunction, and complicated AED regimens, or in patients who willfully disregard their physicians' treatment plans or are unable to pay for medications.

The number of US Food and Drugs Administration (FDA)-approved AEDs has dramatically increased over the past 15 years, as shown in Table 8.1, presenting clinicians with numerous options. Several other agents under development for epilepsy during this period were either associated with animal toxicity in pre-clinical studies or were ineffective in clinical trials. Guidelines from the American Academy of Neurology and the American Epilepsy Society for the use of the newer AEDs in the treatment of new-onset and medically refractory seizures are based on published studies of efficacy, tolerability and safety in adults and children.[5,6] However, these publications may not be helpful to clinicians who must individualize treatment decisions based on clinical variables that are often exclusion criteria for published drug trials. Published expert opinion provides some guidance in these situations.[7]

If a prescribed AED does not control seizures at a tolerable dose, then the usual strategy is to start a second AED that is also appropriate for the patient's seizure type(s). The second AED is usually titrated to a tolerable and potentially effective dosage before the first AED is tapered and stopped, unless the first AED caused a side effect requiring immediate discontinuation, or the first AED provided some degree of therapeutic benefit. Some patients have better seizure control on combinations of AEDs than on individual drugs.

AEDs frequently cause dose-related side effects such as sedation, diplopia, nystagmus, dysarthria, ataxia, incoordination, tremor, mood alteration, dizziness, headache, and cognitive impairment. Combination AED therapy may be associated with increased AED side effects compared to monotherapy. Consequently, side effects are a major cause of medication intolerance and noncompliance, particularly during titration. Clinicians should attempt to modify a patient's dosage and dosing schedule to alleviate peak-level side effects when possible, and use AED serum concentrations as a guide but not absolute determinant of daily doses.

When AEDs are withdrawn, whether for lack of efficacy, intolerable side effects or because the patient has presumably undergone a remission, special caution is warranted, because abrupt AED discontinuation may increase the risk of seizures, including potentially life-threatening status epilepticus. This is particularly the case for sedative drugs such as Phenobarbital (PB) and the benzodiazepines (BZDs), which should be tapered over weeks to months.

The psychosocial consequences of epilepsy, including mood disorders such as depression and anxiety, unemployment, inability to drive, and stigma may require evaluation and interventions from other specialists, including psychiatrists, psychologists, neuropsychologists, social workers, and vocational counselors.

PHARMACOLOGICAL AND NON-PHARMACOLOGICAL THERAPIES

AEDs are the mainstay of therapy, and vary from one another based on their mechanisms of action on brain neurons, the seizure type(s) they effectively control, pharmacokinetic properties, side effect profile, teratogenicity, and propensity for drug–drug interactions. These drugs work primarily by inhibiting the initiation, propagation and maintenance of abnormally synchronized neuronal electrical activity, the underlying pathophysiological basis of epileptic seizures. The molecular targets for most of the marketed AEDs appear to be either voltage-gated or ligand-gated ion channels. Drugs such as phenytoin (Dilantin®, PHT) that are active in the maximal electroshock (MES) animal model of epilepsy prolong inactivation of voltage-dependent sodium channels, thereby preventing neurons from firing at rates above those needed for normal function but insufficient for sustaining a seizure. Similarly, other AEDs act on T-type calcium channels to reduce firing, while still others;

- bind to or enhance the function of γ-aminobutyric acid (GABA-A) receptors, which raises the threshold for initiation of an action potential, or
- reduce excitatory transmission between neurons in sequence by interfering with the binding of glutamate to *N*-methyl-D-aspartate (NMDA) or α-amino-3-hydroxy-5-methylisonozole-4-proprionitic acid (AMPA) receptors.

Antiepileptic Drugs

Since the introduction of PB in 1912, a number of AEDs have been introduced into the market and are listed and described in Table 8.1.

Outcome

Overall, nearly two in three patients become seizure-free with AED treatment, typically with their first or second AED. Risk factors for continuing seizures in the remaining patients are a known etiology for the epilepsy, frequent seizures before AEDs were started, partial-onset seizures, epileptiform activity on the EEG, family history of epilepsy, and co-morbid psychiatric history. Patients with medically refractory seizures usually require numerous trials of AEDs, typically in combinations, and often live with significant dose-related side effects. Some children with benign epilepsy syndromes are eventually able to discontinue AEDs and remain seizure-free.

Non-Pharmacological Therapies

Non-pharmacological therapies, generally considered as adjuncts to AEDs for patients who do not become seizure-free with AEDs alone, include brain surgery, vagus nerve stimulation, diets such as the ketogenic diet and the modified Atkins diet, and a variety of stress-reduction techniques. Among these options, brain surgery for carefully selected patients offers the greatest potential for complete seizure control. The ketogenic diet is a high-fat, low-protein, and very low-carbohydrate diet that came into clinical use for epilepsy in the 1920s. Its mechanism of action is unknown, but it is presumed to be related in some way to the induction of ketosis. The modified Atkins diet produces similar metabolic changes but is easier to follow.

Table 8.1 Description and use of common AEDs

AED and year of approval	Mechanism of action	Anti-seizure activity	Treatment regimen in adults	Side-effects and contra-indications
Phenytoin (PHT) 1937	Blocks sodium-dependent action potentials; reduces neuronal calcium uptake	Partial seizures and generalized tonic–clonic seizures	Initiated at 15 mg/kg (not more than 50 mg/min) if given intravenously; 15 mg/kg in three divided doses over 9–12 h if given orally; 5 mg/kg/day maintenance.	Systemic side-effects: gingival hypertrophy, body hair increase, rash, and lymphadenopathy Neurotoxic side-effects: confusion, slurred speech, double vision, ataxia, and neuropathy (with long-term use) Possible idiosyncratic side-effects: agranulocytosis, Stevens-Johnson syndrome, aplastic anemia, hepatic failure, dermatitis/rash, and serum sickness
Primidone (PRM) 1954; Phenobarbital (PB) 1912	Prolongs GABA-mediated chloride-channel openings	Partial seizures and generalized tonic–clonic seizures–	1–5 mg/kg/day	Systemic side-effects: nausea and rash Neurotoxic side-effects: alteration of sleep cycles, sedation, lethargy, behavioral changes, hyperactivity, ataxia, and dependence Possible idiosyncratic side-effects: agranulocytosis, Stevens-Johnson syndrome, hepatic failure, dermatitis/rash, and serum sickness
Ethosuximide (ESM) 1960	Reduces T-type calcium currents	Absence seizures	Starting dose is initiated at 250 to 500 mg daily, with 250 mg dose increments over 2 to 3 weeks as needed	Systemic side-effects: nausea and vomiting Neurotoxic side-effects: sleep disturbance, drowsiness, and hyperactivity Possible idiosyncratic side-effects: agranulocytosis, Stevens-Johnson syndrome, aplastic anemia, dermatitis/rash, and serum sickness
Carbamazepine (CBZ) 1974	Blocks voltage-dependent sodium channels	Partial seizures and generalized tonic–clonic seizures	Initiated at 100 to 200 mg daily and increased by 100 to 200 mg every 3 to 14 days over a period of 1 to 2 months	Drug-drug interactions are common Systemic side-effects: nausea, vomiting, diarrhea, hyponatremia, rash, pruritus, and fluid retention Neurotoxic side-effects: drowsiness, and dizziness, blurred or double vision, lethargy, and headache Possible idiosyncratic side-effects: agranulocytosis, Stevens-Johnson syndrome, aplastic anemia, hepatic failure, dermatitis/rash, serum sickness, and pancreatitis

(continued)

Table 8.1 (Continued)

AED and year of approval	Mechanism of action	Anti-seizure activity	Treatment regimen in adults	Side-effects and contra-indications
Valproate (VPA) 1978	Reduces high-frequency neuronal firing; possibly blocks sodium-dependent action potentials; enhances GABA effects on CNS.	All forms of generalized seizures and partial seizures	Initiated at 15 mg/kg/day in three divided doses; increased by 5–10 mg/kg/day every week as needed and tolerated	Systemic side-effects: weight gain, nausea, vomiting, hair loss, and easy bruising Neurotoxic side-effects: tremor Possible idiosyncratic side-effects: agranulocytosis, Stevens–Johnson syndrome, aplastic anemia, hepatic failure, dermatitis/rash, serum sickness, and pancreatitis
Felbamate (FBM) 1993	Several mechanisms of action including: – blockade of voltage-gated Na^+ currents; – inhibition of voltage-gated Ca^{2+} channels; – limits glutamate mediated excitation by blocking NMDA receptors; – enhances GABA-mediated inhibition	Partial seizures as well as generalized seizures that occur in association with Lennox–Gastaut syndrome[a]	Initiated at 1200 mg/day, with gradual titration to 1800–4800 mg daily as needed and tolerated	Drug–drug interactions are common Side-effects include: insomnia, headache, nausea and vomiting, decreased appetite, weight loss, and dizziness Association with an elevated risk of potentially fatal bone marrow suppression and hepatitis, which cannot be predicted based on routine monitoring of blood counts and liver function tests
Gabapentin (GBP) 1993	Binds to alpha2/delta auxillary subunits of voltage-gated calcium channels	Partial seizures	Initiated at 300 mg daily, with 300 mg increments every several days as needed[b]	Side-effects: Drowsiness, dizziness, weight gain, fluid retention, and ataxia
Lamotrigine (LTG) 1994	Inhibition of voltage-dependent sodium channels, resulting in decreased release	Partial seizures and generalized tonic–clonic seizures; myoclonic seizures	For patients taking an enzyme-inducing AED: 25 mg bid titrated upward by 50 mg increments every 1–2 weeks as	Systemic side-effects: rash and nausea Neurotoxic side-effects: dizziness and somnolence

Drug	Mechanism of action	Indications	Dosage	Side-effects
	of the excitatory neurotransmitters glutamate and aspartate		needed. For patients taking VPA: 25 mg every other day with increases of 25 to 50 mg every 2 weeks as needed to a maximum of 300 to 500 mg/day	Possible idiosyncratic side-effects: Stevens-Johnson syndrome and hypersensitivity syndrome
Topiramate (TPM) 1996	Blocks sodium-dependent action potentials; attenuates kainate-induced responses; enhances GABAergic transmission	Partial seizures and generalized tonic–clonic seizures; myoclonic seizures	Initiated at 25–50 mg/day; with increases of 25–50 mg/day every 1–2 weeks until 100–1000 mg/day maintenance in two divided doses	Systemic side-effects: anorexia and weight loss. Neurotoxic side-effects: confusion, cognitive slowing dysphasia, dizziness, fatigue and paresthesias. Possible idiosyncratic side-effects: nephrolithiasis
Tiagabine (TGB) 1997	Inhibits neuronal and glial reuptake of GABA	Partial seizures	Initiated at 4–10 mg/day; with increases of 8–12 mg/day each 4 weeks until 20–60 mg/day maintenance in 2–4 divided doses	Neurotoxic side-effects: dizziness, weakness, ataxia nervousness, tremor and somnolence
Levetiracetam (LEV) 1999	Binds to the synaptic vesicle protein 2 A; oppose zinc-induced inhibition of GABA- and glycine currents; inhibits N-type calcium channels and intracellular calcium release	Partial seizures and generalized tonic–clonic seizures; myoclonic seizures	Initiated at 1000 mg/day; with increases of 1000 mg/day every 2 weeks until 1000–4000 mg/day in two divided doses[b]	Systemic side-effects: anorexia. Neurotoxic side-effects: somnolence, dizziness, headache and nervousness
Oxcarbazepine (OXC) 2000	Blocks sodium-dependent action potentials; reduces neuronal calcium uptake	Partial seizures and generalized tonic-clonic seizures	Initiated at 150–300 mg/day; with increases of 300 mg/day every 3–5 days until 900–2700 mg/day maintenance in 2–3 divided doses	Systemic side-effects: nausea, vomiting, hyponatremia, and rash. Neurotoxic side-effects: drowsiness, dizziness, headache, double vision, and ataxia

(continued)

Table 8.1 (Continued)

AED and year of approval	Mechanism of action	Anti-seizure activity	Treatment regimen in adults	Side-effects and contra-indications
Zonisamide (ZNS)2000	Blocks voltage-dependent sodium and T-type calcium channels; inhibits release of excitatory neurotransmitters	Partial seizures; infantile spasms; progressive myoclonic epilepsy	Initiated at 100 mg/day; with increases by 100 mg/day every 2 weeks until 400–600 mg/day in 1–2 divided doses	Systemic side-effects: anorexia Neurotoxic side-effects: dizziness, ataxia, fatigue, somnolence, and confusion Possible idiosyncratic side-effects: nephrolithiasis
Pregabalin (PGB) 2005	Binds to alpha2/delta auxiliary subunits of voltage-gated calcium channels	Partial seizures	Initiated at 75 mg twice daily or 50 mg 3 times a day, with gradual increases as tolerated to 600 mg/day[b]	Side-effects: drowsiness, dizziness, and weight gain, fluid retention, and ataxia

[a] The use of FBM is now primarily limited to patients, for example, those with Lennox–Gastaut syndrome, for whom the benefits of treatment are judged by their physicians to outweigh the risks of FBM.

[b] Target doses are lower in patients with renal dysfunction.

UNMET MEDICAL NEEDS

Despite unprecedented growth in the number of FDA-approved pharmacotherapies, seizures in approximately 30% of patients with epilepsy remain refractory, and many others have unacceptable medication-related side effects. Because only a small fraction of these patients are candidates for brain surgery, there continues to be an unmet medical need for effective and tolerable treatments for epilepsy.

Currently available AEDs suppress seizures, but do not resolve the pathophysiological process underlying a patient's epilepsy, nor do they prevent the development of seizures in patients without epilepsy but at high risk, such as those who suffer a serious brain injury. There is therefore a need for drugs that are antiepileptogenic.[8]

ANIMAL MODELS FOR AED DISCOVERY

With the exception of levetiracetam (Keppra®; LEV), the majority of the AEDs approved since 1993 were identified and developed as a result of their ability to block acute evoked seizures in rodent models of epilepsy. However, as noted above, there continues to be a significant unmet need for the patient with therapy-resistant epilepsy and thus the discovery and development of more efficacious and less toxic AEDs. Regardless of the process by which a new AED is conceived, it must always demonstrate some degree of efficacy in one or more animal seizure or epilepsy models before it is likely to proceed down the drug development pathway and ultimately validated in well-controlled randomized clinical trials.

In Vivo Testing

Since the era of Merritt and Putnam,[9] a new investigational AED is likely to be evaluated in a battery of well-established animal seizure and epilepsy models that have varying degrees of face validity when it comes to predicting clinical efficacy. Having said this, it is important to note that no single laboratory test will establish the presence or absence of anticonvulsant activity or fully predict the clinical utility of an investigational AED. Historically, the successful identification of PHT using the cat MES test by Merritt and Putnam[9] and the subsequent acceptance of PHT as an effective drug in the management of human generalized tonic–clonic seizures provided the validation required to consider the MES test as a useful model of human generalized tonic–clonic seizures. In addition to the MES test, the subcutaneous pentylenetetrazol (sc PTZ) test, and the electrical kindling model represent two other important *in vivo* model systems that have played an important role over the last 40 years in the early identification and characterization of AEDs.[10,11]

Advances in our understanding at the molecular and genetic level have led to the development of newer mouse models that incorporate known genetic defects that resemble the human condition more closely. By taking advantage of a growing number of these mutant mouse strains, we will likely gain greater insight into the role of various molecular targets in ictogenesis and epileptogenesis. In addition, mutant mouse models represent important tools for evaluating those drugs that evolve from a mechanistic-based discovery program and they will likely play an important role in our efforts to develop personalized medicines for those patients with a known genetic mutation.

CORRELATION OF ANIMAL ANTICONVULSANT PROFILE AND CLINICAL UTILITY

The MES and Kindled Rat Models

The MES test and the kindling model represent two highly predictive models that are useful in the characterization of a drug's potential utility against generalized tonic–clonic and partial seizures, respectively (Table 8.2). The kindling model of partial epilepsy has, over the last 20 plus years, been used with increasing frequency in the AED development process. Kindling refers to the process whereby there is a progressive increase in electrographic and behavioral seizure activity in response to repeated stimulation of a limbic brain region such as the amygdala or hippocampus with an initially subconvulsive current.[12] Kindling is associated with a progressive increase in seizure severity and duration, a decrease in focal seizure threshold, and neuronal degeneration in limbic brain regions that resemble human temporal lobe epilepsy. Unlike the MES and sc PTZ tests, the kindling model is a model of focal epilepsy and one that displays a pharmacological profile consistent with human partial epilepsy. Moreover, the kindled rat is the one model that accurately predicted the clinical utility of LEV (Table 8.2). This one example demonstrates the importance of employing a battery of models in an initial screening protocol to avoid inadvertently "missing" a potentially important new therapy. In addition to LEV, the kindling model accurately predicts the clinical utility of all of the AEDs currently employed in the treatment of partial epilepsy (Table 8.2).

The sc PTZ Seizure Model

In addition to the MES and kindling models, the sc PTZ test has played an important role in differentiating the anticonvulsant profile of investigational drugs.[10] Early on, efficacy in the sc PTZ test was considered suggestive of a drug's potential utility against generalized absence seizures. This interpretation, which was based primarily on the finding that drugs active in the clinic against spike-wave seizures (i.e., ethosuximide (Zarontin®, ESM), trimethadione, valproic acid (Depakene®, VPA), and BZDs) were able to block clonic seizures induced by sc PTZ; whereas drugs such as PHT and carbamazepine (Tegretol®, CBZ), which are both inactive against human spike-wave seizures are also ineffective against sc PTZ seizures in animals. Moreover, PHT and CBZ are also capable of exacerbating human spike-wave seizures. As summarized in Table 8.2, the sc PTZ test would also suggest that barbiturates and tiagabine (Gabitril®, TGB) should also possess efficacy against generalized absence. For the barbiturates (and possibly TGB), this is in direct opposition to what has been reported clinically. For example PB, like PHT and CBZ, worsens human spike-wave discharges.[13] In contrast, PB is useful for the management of myoclonic seizures. Thus, the sc PTZ test may have greater utility in the identification of drugs with activity against myoclonic seizures.[14]

Table 8.2 Correlation between anticonvulsant efficacy and clinical utility of the established and second generation AEDs in experimental animal models[a]

Experimental model	Clinical seizure type			
	Tonic and/or clonic generalized seizures	Myoclonic/generalized absence seizures	Generalized absence seizures	Partial seizures
MES (Tonic extension)[b]	CBZ, PHT, VPA, PB(FBM, GBP, LTG, TPM, ZNS)			
sc PTZ (Clonic seizures)[b]		ESM, VPA, PB[c], BZD(FBM, GBP, TGB, VGB[c])		
Spike-wave discharges(Absence seizures)[d]			ESM, VPA, BZD(LTG, TPM, LEV)	
Electrical kindling(Focal seizures)				CBZ, PHT, VPA, PB, BZD(FBM, GBP, LTG, TPM, TGB, ZNS, LEV, VGB)

[a] BZD, benzodiazepines; CBZ, carbamazepine; ESM, ethosuximide; FBM, felbamate; GBP, gabapentin; LTG, lamotrigine; LEV, levetiracetam; PB, phenobarbital; PHT, phenytoin; TGB, tiagabine; TPM, topiramate; VPA, valproic acid; ZNS, zonisamide; VGB, vigabatrin.

[b] Data summarized from White et al., 2002AUQ1.

[c] PB, TGB, and VGB block clonic seizures induced by sc PTZ but are inactive against generalized absence seizures and may exacerbate spike wave seizures.

[d] Data summarized from (Hosford and Wang 1997[17]; Hosford et al. 1997[18]; Marescaux and Vergnes 1995[16]; Snead 1992[15]).

Models of Spike-Wave Seizures

In recent years, there have been three other animal models emerge that are more predictive than the sc PTZ test for the identification of drugs effective against generalized absence seizures. These include spike-wave seizures induced by the chemoconvulsant γ-butyrolactone,[15] the genetic absence epileptic rat of Strasbourg (GAERS[16]), and, the lethargic (*lh/lh*) mutant mouse.[17,18] The *lh/lh* mouse displays spontaneous spike-and-wave discharges that are blocked by AEDs clinically effective in reducing spike-wave activity (e.g., the BZDs, ESM, VPA, and lamotrigine (Lamictal®, LTG)). In addition, drugs that elevate GABA levels (e.g., vigabatrin (VGB) and TGB), drugs that directly activate the GABA-B receptor, and the barbiturates potentiate spike-wave seizures in all three models. As such, these three models should be employed when evaluating any drug that is under development for the treatment of spike-wave seizures.

Models for Adverse Effect Testing

A crucial parameter deciding the clinical utility of AEDs is the therapeutic index (TI) expressing the margin between anticonvulsant and adverse effects. With respect to assessing CNS-related adverse effects, pre-clinical testing include behavioral observations, activity measurements and models evaluating the potential impact of an AED on motor function in rodents. Among the latter models, the rotarod test is commonly used to quantify TI.[19] The rotarod test consists of a rotating rod upon which drug-treated animals are placed. The extent treatment by which an AED deteriorates the ability of the animals to remain on the rotating rod within a certain time period is recorded. A therapeutic index (TI) can be established by comparing the minimum dose of an AED that induces impaired performance of the animals in the rotarod against the minimum anticonvulsant dose in the same species.

The validity of using normal animals for pre-clinical adverse effect testing and adverse effect predictions in epilepsy patients is questionable and it is advised to include fully limbic kindled rodents.[20] When testing a series of NMDA antagonists in fully amygdala kindled rats, Löscher and Hönack observed more marked ataxia, hyperactivity, and stereotypic behaviors than in normal rats.[21] From this finding it was predicted that NMDA antagonists would induce more severe adverse effects in epilepsy patients than in healthy volunteers.[22] This was subsequently confirmed in man when the potential antiepileptic properties of the competitive NMDA antagonist D-CPPene was tested.[23] D-CPPene was shown to be well-tolerated in healthy volunteers in doses up to 2000 mg/day. In contrast, when used as add-on therapy in eight patients with refractory complex partial epilepsy, doses of 500–1000 mg/day induced severe adverse effects consisting of confusion, hallucination, ataxia, impaired concentration, and sedation. This led to premature termination of the trial. The plasma concentrations following administration of similar doses of D-CPPene in healthy volunteers and epilepsy patients revealed higher exposure levels in the healthy volunteers. These results indicate that pharmacodynamic factors were mainly responsible for the severe adverse effects observed in the epilepsy patients.

The enhanced susceptibility of fully amygdala kindled rats to the behavioral adverse effects of NMDA antagonists was later observed with several AEDs[24] and appear to also include the ability of AEDs to impair cognitive function.[20] This pattern has been reproduced in other models of limbic kindling[25] but is absent after chemical kindling.[20] Thus, this phenomenon appears to represent a permanent reactivity specific for limbic kindling and correlate several complications with AED use in man being linked to an interaction with the dysfunction of the brain imposed by the epileptic condition. The importance of using fully limbic kindled animals in pre-clinical testing of adverse effects in order to predict the clinical utility of a new AED appropriately is strongly recommended; especially as several AED candidates often involve novel or unknown molecular mechanisms.

STRATEGIES FOR AED DISCOVERY

The identification of candidate AEDs for development has largely been based on three different approaches. These consist of (1) random screening of new chemical entities for anticonvulsant activity; (2) structural variation leading to derivatives of existing AEDs; and (3) rational, target-based drug discovery.

The first drug for epilepsy was potassium bromide, introduced by Sir Charles Locock in 1857. Nearly six decades later, Hauptmann identified the antiepileptic properties of PB. The discovery of these two AEDs did not involve any pre-clinical testing, their antiepileptic potential were disclosed by introducing them to epilepsy patients. Following potassium bromide and PB, all established AEDs have been discovered principally by random screening in pre-clinical models or by variation of the structure of known AEDs. However, the past three decades have witnessed an increased understanding of the molecular mechanisms involved in the pathophysiology of epilepsy and has revealed mechanisms crucial for the antiepileptic properties of most AEDs. This has nourished an emphasis on rational, target-based drug discovery.

Random Screening of New Chemical Entities

During their search for a non-sedating analog of PB, Merrit and Putman discovered PHT in 1937 by its ability to suppress seizure activity in the MES model in cats.[9] Thereby PHT became the first AED discovered by its activity in a pre-clinical model. Using this MES model, CBZ was discovered two decades later in the laboratories of Geigy during structure activity studies aimed at optimizing the anticonvulsant activity of a new chemical scaffold. This was followed by the discovery of Eymard of the antiepileptic potential of VPA due to its activity in the sc PTZ model in rodents. Because of the early success with the MES and sc PTZ models, they have been used extensively for random screening of new AEDs during the last 40 years. This has resulted in the discovery of a significant number of additional, 2nd generation AEDs as well as AED candidates currently in clinical development. However, the limitations in focusing exclusively on these two models, involving acute seizures evoked in normal rodents, were emphasized by the experience with LEV.

LEV is the (S)-enantiomer of the ethyl analog of the nootropic drug piracetam. LEV was synthesized in 1974 in an attempt to identify a second generation agent of piracetam. LEV did not show any consistent nootropic activity but revealed potent and general anti-seizure activity in sound-susceptible mice.[26] Regardless, LEV was devoid of seizure protection in both the MES and sc PTZ model in rodents.[19,27] Likewise, LEV did not possess a mechanism of action typically associated with an AED, that is, inhibition of Na^+ - and low-voltage operated (T-type) Ca^{2+} channels or direct enhancement of GABA-mediated inhibition.[28] Based on this unconventional profile, LEV should not have been pursued as a potential AED candidate.

Despite these confounding results, LEV was assessed further in amygdala kindled rats. In this model, LEV showed anti-seizure activity in fully amygdala kindled rats and a marked and persistent ability to inhibit kindling acquisition.[27,29] Testing in a variety of genetic animal models of epilepsy also revealed protection against postural stimulation-induced seizures in epilepsy-like mice,[30] against seizures induced by acoustic stimulation in sound-sensitive rats and against spontaneous spike-and-wave discharges in GAERS rats.[31]

The experience with LEV illustrates the limitations of relying solely upon the use of acute seizures evoked by MES and sc PTZ in normal animals as a valid screening procedure for drugs targeting a disease characterized by a chronic epileptic condition resulting in the appearance of spontaneous repetitive seizures. This experience highlights rather the need to use a battery of models during random screening of new chemical entities that include animal models with (a) an acquired, kindled, alteration in seizure threshold and (b) animals with induced or natural mutations associated with an altered seizure threshold or spontaneous seizure expression.[32]

Derivatives of Existing AEDs

The most productive strategy for AED discovery has been structural variation of existing AEDs. The successful discovery of PHT in the MES model stimulated early on an interest in molecular structures related to this AED. As an outcome, trimethadone and ESM were identified as AEDs although their mechanism of action and antiepileptic properties are different from that of PHT. However, a structurally more close derivative of PHT, fosphenytoin, has also been introduced as an AED as well as oxcarbazepine, a derivative of CBZ.

Structural variation of second generation AEDs has also been devoted significant attention. With the purpose to improve the limited bioavailability of GBP, both PGB and XP-13512 was produced. In an attempt to improve pharmacokinetics and safety of LTG, JZP-4 was identified. Two derivatives of LEV, brivaracetam and seletracetam has also been discovered and introduced into clinical development. They derive from efforts focusing primarily on improving the antiepileptic efficacy of LEV and, secondarily, on enhancing potency and tolerability.

Rational, Target-Based Drug Discovery

During the last three decades, the pharmaceutical industry has concentrated on target-based drug discovery as a natural extension of increased understanding of the molecular mechanisms involved in the pathophysiology of epilepsy. These drug discovery efforts have focused primarily on approaches enhancing inhibitory GABAergic or reducing excitatory glutamatergic, neurotransmission. A major assumption behind these efforts has been that epileptic seizures reflect exaggerated aspects of normal cell physiology.

The most successful rational strategy for target-based AED discovery concentrated on enhancing GABAergic inhibition. Indeed, it has long been recognized that alterations in GABAergic inhibition alter neuroexcitability and thereby the probability for seizure activity. Originally, this was observed by Killam and Bain who showed that GABA is the only cerebral amino acid that is significantly affected by convulsive hydrazides.[33] Subsequently, it was discovered that locally or intravenously applied GABA could stop hydrazide-induced seizures, and that GABA administered at high doses was an effective anticonvulsant therapy in some epilepsy patients.[34] Consistent with these observations, several established AEDs, including VPA, barbiturates and BZDs, are known to mediate their antiepileptic properties, at least partly, by an ability to enhance GABAergic inhibition. Irreversible inhibition of GABA aminotransferase or GABA re-uptake led to the discovery of VGB and TGB, for example.

A major limitation of the rational, target-based AED discovery conducted so far has been its reliance on mechanisms potentially involved in exaggerated aspects of normal cell physiology. This reliance does not take into account evidence that epileptic disorders involve heterogenous pathophysiological mechanisms and the presumed multifactorial nature of AED resistance.[35] Resistance to AEDs is a major unmet need. More complete understanding of the biology of this phenomenon and development of systems modeling pharmacoresistance, including new animal models, is crucial for the success of rational, target-based AED discovery.

MODELS OF PHARMACORESISTANCE

The models summarized in Table 8.2 have been successfully used to identify effective therapies for the treatment of human epilepsy. Moreover, those drugs found effective in one or more of these models can be expected to be clinically effective against partial, generalized, and secondarily generalized seizures. Unfortunately, in spite of their utility in screening for effective therapies for the symptomatic treatment of seizures, there still remains a substantial need for the identification of therapies for the patient with refractory seizures. In this respect, one might argue that the models summarized in Table 8.2 are not predictive of efficacy in those patients with refractory epilepsy. Thus, the identification and characterization of one or more model systems that would predict efficacy in the pharmacoresistant patient population would be a valuable asset to the epilepsy community. In addition to being useful for therapy development, the ability to segregate animals on the basis of their responsiveness or lack of sensitivity to a given AED would be: (a) useful for attempting to understand the molecular mechanisms underlying pharmacoresistance; (b) an asset for those studies designed to assess whether it is possible to reverse drug resistance; and (3) useful for identification of surrogate markers that might be able to predict which patient will remit and become pharmacoresistant. Unfortunately, a model will only become clinically validated at the time that a drug is found markedly to reduce the incidence of therapy-resistant epilepsy in patients with epilepsy. In the mean time, drugs in development for the treatment of epilepsy should be evaluated in as many proposed models of pharmacoresistance as feasible. At the time that a new drug is introduced into the market that substantially reduces the percentage of patients with refractory epilepsy, we will hopefully be able to identify the one or more model system(s) retrospectively that would predict efficacy against refractory seizures.

At the present time, there are a number of potentially interesting model systems of therapy resistance available. Before briefly discussing the salient features of those models that have emerged in recent years, it is first important to define AED "pharmacoresistance" from a model development perspective. The participants of two NIH/NINDS/AES-sponsored Workshops on Animal Models held in 2001 and 2002 agreed that any proposed model of "pharmacoresistant" epilepsy should meet certain criteria. For example, human experience dictates that "pharmacoresistance" can be defined as persistent seizure activity that does not respond to monotherapy at tolerable doses with at least two current AEDs.[36,37] Thus, the "demonstrated resistance" to two or more of the first line AEDs employed in the treatment of partial epilepsy was considered pivotal. Ideally, it can be hoped that any proposed model will lead to the identification of a new therapy that will ultimately be highly effective in humans resistant to existing AEDs.

In recent years there have been several *in vivo* model systems described that display a phenotype consistent with pharmacoresistant epilepsy (see[38] for review). These include: the PHT-resistant kindled rat,[39,40] the LTG-resistant kindled rat,[41-44] the 6 Hz psychomotor seizure model of partial epilepsy,[45] post-status epileptic models of temporal lobe epilepsy,[46-51] and the methylazoxymethanol acetate (MAM) *in utero* model of nodular heterotopias.[52] All of these models have some utility when attempting to differentiate an investigational drugs anticonvulsant profile from existing AEDs. This is not to imply that other approaches using *in vitro* systems are of any less value and the reader is referred to references[53] and[54] for review and references. The remainder of this section will briefly discuss some of the unique features of the PHT- and LTG-resistant kindled rat models, the 6 Hz psychomotor seizure model, and the post-seizure models as they relate to their utility for early differentiation of new therapies.

PHT-Resistant Kindled Rat Model

Löscher *et al.*, have conducted extensive pharmacological evaluations in the kindled rat model over the years and were among the first to demonstrate that kindled seizures were less sensitive to anticonvulsant treatment than MES-induced generalized tonic extension seizures.[55,56] Subsequently, Rundfeldt *et al.*, found that the pharmacological response to a challenge dose of PHT within a population of kindled rats could be differentiated on the basis of whether a particular rat was a responder or a non-responder.[57] For example, they observed two population of rats; that is, those that consistently responded to a challenge dose of PHT and those that never responded. This observation became the cornerstone of numerous studies designed to evaluate the effectiveness of "established" and "investigational" AEDs in PHT responders and non-responders.

One particular advantage of the PTS-resistant kindled rat is that it permits an investigator to conduct comparative studies in two separate populations of rats; that is, sensitive and resistant. Although more labor-intensive than the acute evoked seizure models (MES, sc PTZ, and others), the kindled rat, unlike the spontaneous seizure models (discussed below), does not require continuous video-EEG monitoring.

LTG-Resistant Kindled Rat Model

The LTG-resistant kindled rat model of partial epilepsy was first described by Postma *et al.*[41] Unlike the PHT-resistant kindled rat, resistance to LTG is induced when a rat is exposed to low-dose LTG during the kindling acquisition phase. Thus, exposure to a low dose (5 mg/kg) of LTG during kindling development leads to reduced efficacy of LTG when administered to the fully kindled rat.[41] A similar phenomenon has been observed for CBZ.[58] Perhaps more importantly, is the observation that LTG-resistant rats are also refractory to CBZ, PHT, and topiramate (Topamax®, TPM) but not VPA or the investigational KCNQ2 activator retigabine.[42-44]

The LTG-resistant kindled rat may offer a practical advantage over the PHT-resistant rat in that it is not necessary to pre-screen a population of rats in order to identify those animals that are pharmacoresistant. In this regard, it might serve as an early model of drug-resistant epilepsy to differentiate novel AEDs from PHT, LTG, CBZ, and TPM for further evaluation in more extensive model systems including the PHT-resistant kindled rat.

The Low-Frequency (6 Hz) Electroshock Seizure Model

In many respects, the 6 Hz seizure model offers many of the same advantages of the MES test. For example, the 6 Hz seizure test, like the MES test, is an acute electrically evoked seizure using standard corneal electroshock. Moreover, it is high-throughput, and requires minimal technical expertise. The main difference between the 6 Hz and MES tests is the frequency (6 Hz versus 50 Hz) and duration (3 s versus 0.2 s) of the stimulation employed. The low-frequency, long-duration stimulus results in a seizure that is characterized by immobility, forelimb clonus, Straub tail, and facial automatisms and is thought to more closely model human limbic seizures.[45,59,60] Interestingly, the pharmacological profile of the 6 Hz model is somewhat dependent on the intensity of the stimulation (Table 8.3). For example, at a convulsive current (CC) sufficient to induce a prototypical seizure in 97% of the population tested (i.e., the CC_{97}), the 6 Hz seizure test is relatively non-discriminating; that is, the large majority of AEDs evaluated (PHT, LTG, ESM, LEV, and VPA) are effective in blocking the acute seizure. As the current intensity is increased to a level that is 1.5 times the CC_{97}, several of the AEDs lose their ability to protect against a 6 Hz seizure. At a current equivalent to 2 times the CC_{97}, only VPA and LEV retained their ability to block 6 Hz seizures; albeit, the potency of both drugs at 2 times the CC_{97} was markedly reduced.[45] The finding that LEV was found to be active at a specific stimulus intensity where other anticonvulsants display little to no efficacy illustrates the use of the 6 Hz model as a screen for novel anticonvulsant compounds; particularly when one considers that LEV was inactive in the acute seizure models such as the MES and sc PTZ seizure tests.[19] Thus, the incorporation of a simple acute screen that would minimize the chances of "missing" a unique drug like LEV should be an important consideration when setting up an anticonvulsant testing protocol to evaluate investigational AEDs.

Table 8.3 Effect of stimulus intensity on the anticonvulsant efficacy of phenytoin, lamotrigine, ethosuximide, levetiracetam, and valproic acid in the 6 Hz seizure test[a]

Antiepileptic drug	ED_{50} (mg/kg, i.p.) and 95% C.I.[b]		
	22 mA	32 mA	44 mA
Phenytoin	9.4 (4.7–14.9)	>60	>60
Lamotrigine	4.4 (2.2–6.6)	>60	>60
Ethosuximide	86.9 (37.8–156)	167 (114–223)	>600
Levetiracetam	4.6 (1.1–8.7)	19.4 (9.9–36.0)	1089 (787–2650)
Valproate	41.5 (16.1–68.8)	126 (94.5–152)	310 (258–335)

[a] *From Barton et al., 2001* [45], *with permission.*
[b] *Confidence interval shown in parentheses.*

Post-Status Epilepticus Models of Temporal Lobe Epilepsy

Post-status epilepticus models of refractory epilepsy are beginning to emerge as an important tool in the differentiation of investigational AEDs. These models of pharmacoresistant epilepsy differ significantly from the AED-resistant kindled rat and the 6 Hz seizure model in that seizures are spontaneously evolving and not evoked. This adds yet another level of complexity to the pharmacological evaluation of an investigational drug but yields potentially important information about its relative efficacy compared to existing AEDs.

The development and characterization of this model system for pharmacological testing has resulted from a focused effort of the epilepsy community to identify clinically relevant models of chronic epilepsy.[36,37] In many respects, the post-status models described thus far fulfill one very important characteristic of the ideal model system; that is, spontaneous recurrent seizures (SRS) following a species-appropriate latent period.[36,37] The post-status epileptic rat is particularly useful in that this model permits the investigator the opportunity to evaluate the efficacy of a given treatment on seizure frequency, seizure type (i.e., focal or generalized), and the liability for tolerance development following chronic treatment. Unfortunately, by their very nature, drug trials in rats with spontaneous seizures take on another level of complexity. They are extremely laborious and time consuming, and require a greater level of technical expertise. As such there have only been a few pharmacological studies conducted to date.[46,48-51] Having said this, the advantages that this model provides for differentiating a given compound from the established AEDs is well-worth the investment. All of these models are being used with increasing frequency in the search for novel AEDs. They can play an important role in efforts to differentiate investigational drugs from existing

AEDs. Unfortunately, none of these models have been validated clinically and thus, it is too early to say whether any of these models, will lead to the identification of the next generation AED. Furthermore, it is also important to note that the use of these models has led to the development of novel drug-testing protocols in animals that resemble human clinical protocols more closely. Moreover, each of these models provide a biological system that will likely lead to a greater understanding of the mechanisms underlying pharmacoresistant epilepsy. As such, they can be used to test novel approaches designed to overcome or reverse therapy resistance, and to perhaps identify appropriate surrogate markers of pharmacoresistance. One can envision the day when we will be able to identify the patient at risk for developing therapy-resistant epilepsy and institute a prophylactic therapy that prevents the emergence of pharmacoresistance.

BIOMARKERS OF THERAPEUTIC RESPONSE

While the selection and use of currently available AEDs based on an accurate diagnosis and assessment of seizure type will lead to seizure freedom in the majority of patients with epilepsy, there is no method, at present, for individualizing the choice of AEDs, whether at treatment initiation or during a course of therapy. This limitation has been recognized and ongoing efforts in pharmacogenomics offers the eventual possibility of avoiding AEDs in patients at high risk of idiosyncratic reactions or in selecting AEDs for particular genetically defined epilepsy syndromes. Further, the only way to gauge whether an AED will be effective and well-tolerated is to monitor the patient over time on treatment. Therefore, there is a need for biomarkers that reliably predict efficacy, safety and tolerability of an AED early in its course, thereby potentially avoiding ineffective treatments and dose-related or idiosyncratic side effects. While emerging proof-of-concept clinical models such as the photosensitivity model may be useful to screen AEDs before launching lengthy and expensive clinical development programs, they do not yet appear able to predict which patients will benefit from specific AEDs.

SUMMARY AND CONCLUDING REMARKS

This chapter described the epidemiology, clinical manifestations and diagnosis of epilepsy, as well as its response to pharmacological and non-pharmacological treatments. The treatment of epilepsy is symptomatic; preventive treatments are not known. New drugs are being discovered and developed with the help of a variety of animal models of seizures and epilepsy. Novel compounds that appear to have a favorable therapeutic window in these models, show no significant pre-clinical toxicity and have potential therapeutic benefit in other conditions such as neuropathic pain or mood disorders are generally moved forward into clinical epilepsy trials, typically assessed as add-on therapy in patients with refractory partial-onset seizures. However, because as many as one in three patients with partial-onset seizures remains refractory to available AEDs, there is a need to move beyond conventional animal models and to explore other animal models and mechanisms of action by which neuronal hyperexcitability may be reduced. The introduction of LEV is an example of an effective AED that was unimpressive in conventional animal models. The objective of this chapter, therefore, was to examine the characteristics of newly emerging animal models of pharmacoresistance as well as the framework within which candidate drugs for epilepsy are discovered and developed.

REFERENCES

1. Hauser, W.A. and Hesdorffer, D.C. (1990). *Epilepsy: Frequency, Causes and Consequences*. Demos, New York.

2. Devinsky, O. and Yerby, M.S. (1994). Women with epilepsy. Reproduction and effects of pregnancy on epilepsy. *Neurol Clin N Am*, 12:479–495.

3. Schachter, S.C. (2004). Seizure disorders. *Prim Care Clin Office Pract*, 31:85–94.

4. Hommet, C., Hureaux, R., Barre, J., Constans, T., and Berrut, G. (2007). Epileptic seizures in clinically diagnosed Alzheimer's disease: Report from a geriatric medicine population. *Aging Clin Exp Res*, 19:430–431.

5. French, J.A., Kanner, A.M., Bautista, J. *et al.* (2004). Efficacy and tolerability of the new antiepileptic drugs I: Treatment of new onset epilepsy: Report of the Therapeutics and Technology Assessment Subcommittee and Quality Standards Subcommittee of the American Academy of Neurology and the American Epilepsy Society. *Neurology*, 62:1252–1260.

6. French, J.A., Kanner, A.M., Bautista, J. *et al.* (2004). Efficacy and tolerability of the new antiepileptic drugs II: Treatment of refractory epilepsy: Report of the Therapeutics and Technology Assessment Subcommittee and Quality Standards Subcommittee of the American Academy of Neurology and the American Epilepsy Society. *Neurology*, 62:1261–1273.

7. Karceski, S., Morrell, M.J., and Carpenter, D. (2005). Treatment of epilepsy in adults: Expert opinion. *Epilepsy Behav*, 7(Suppl 1):S1–S64.

8. Schachter, S.C. (2002). Drug-mediated antiepileptogenesis in humans. *Neurology*, 59(suppl 5):S34–S35.

9. Putnam, T.J. and Merritt, H.H. (1937). Experimental determination of the anticonvulsant properties of some phenyl derivatives. *Science*, 85:525–526.

10. White, H.S., Johnson, M., Wolf, H.H., and Kupferberg, H.J. (1995). The early identification of anticonvulsant activity: Role of the maximal electroshock and subcutaneous pentylenetetrazol seizure models. *Ital J Neurol Sci*, 16:73–77.

11. White, H.S., Wolf, H.H., Woodhead, J.H., and Kupferberg, H.J. (1998). The National Institutes of Health Anticonvulsant Drug Development Program: Screening for efficacy. In French, J., Leppik, I., and Dichter, M.A. (eds.), *Antiepileptic Drug Development. Advances in Neurology*, Vol. 76. Lippincott-Raven Publishers, Philadelphia, pp. 29–39.

12. Goddard, G.V., McIntyre, D.C., and Leech, C.K. (1969). A permanent change in brain function resulting from daily electrical stimulation. *Exp Neurol*, 25(3):295–330.

13. Mattson, R.H. (1995). General principles: Selection of antiepileptic drug therapy. In Levy, R.H., Mattson, R.H., and Meldrum, B.S. (eds.), *Antiepileptic Drugs*, 4th edition. Raven Press, New York, pp. 123–135.

14. Löscher, W., Hönack, D., Fassbender, C.P., and Nolting, B. (1991). The role of technical, biological and pharmacological factors in the laboratory evaluation of anticonvulsant drugs. 3. Pentylenetetrazole seizure models. *Epilepsy Res*, 8:171–189.

15. Snead, O.C. (1992). Pharmacological models of generalized absence seizures in rodents. *J Neural Transm*, 35:7–19.

16. Marescaux, C. and Vergnes, M. (1995). Genetic absence epilepsy in rats from Strasbourg (GAERS). *Ital J Neurol Sci*, 16:113–118.
17. Hosford, D.A. and Wang, Y. (1997). Utility of the lethargic (lh/lh) mouse model of absence seizures in predicting the effects of lamotrigine, vigabatrin, tiagabine, gabapentin, and topiramate against human absence seizures. *Epilepsia*, 38:408–414.
18. Hosford, D.A., Clark, S., Cao, Z., Wilson, W.A.J., Lin, F., Morrisett, R.A., and Huin, A. (1992). The role of GABAB receptor activation in absence seizures of lethargic (lh/lh) mice. *Science*, 257:398–401.
19. Klitgaard, H., Matagne, A., Gobert, J., and Wulfert, E. (1998). Evidence for a unique profile of levetiracetam in rodent models of seizures and epilepsy. *Eur J Pharmacol*, 353(2–3):191–206.
20. Klitgaard, H., Matagne, A., and Lamberty, Y. (2002). Use of epileptic animals for adverse effect testing. *Epilepsy Res*, 50:55–65.
21. Löscher, W. and Hönack, D. (1991). Anticonvulsant and behavioral effects of two novel competitive *N*-methyl-ᴅ-aspartic acid receptor antagonists, CGP 37849 and CGP 39551, in the kindling model of epilepsy. Comparison with MK-801 and carbamazepine. *J Phamacol Exp Ther*, 256:432–440.
22. Löscher, W. and Hönack, D. (1991). The novel competitive *N*-methyl-ᴅ-aspartate (NMDA) antagonist CGP 37849 preferentially induces phencyclidine-like behavioral effects in kindled rats: Attenuation by manipulation of dopamine, alpha-1 and serotonin 1A receptors. *J Pharmacol Exp Ther*, 257:1146–1153.
23. Sveinbjornsdottir, S., Sander, J.W.A.S., Upton, D. *et al.* (1993). The excitatory amino acid antagonist D-CPPene (SDZ EAA-494) in patients with epilepsy. *Epilepsy Res*, 16:165–174.
24. Hönack, D. and Löscher, W. (1995). Kindling increases the sensitivity of rats to adverse effects of certain antiepileptic drugs. *Epilepsia*, 36(8):763–771.
25. Matagne, A. and Klitgaard, H. (1998). Validation of corneally kindled mice: A sensitive screening model for partial epilepsy in man. *Epilepsy Res*, 31:59–71.
26. Gower, A.J., Noyer, M., Verloes, R., Gobert, J., and Wulfert, E. (1992). ucb L059, a novel anticonvulsant drug: Pharmacological profile in animals. *Eur J Pharmacol*, 222(2–3):193–203.
27. Löscher, W. and Hönack, D. (1993). Profile of ucb L059, a novel anticonvulsant drug in models of partial and generalized epilepsy in mice and rats. *Eur J Pharmacol*, 232:147–158.
28. Margineanu, D.G. and Klitgaard H. (2002). Levetiracetam mechanisms of action, *Antiepileptic Drugs*, 5th edition, Chapter 40, 419–427.
29. Löscher, W., Hönack, D., and Rndfeldt, C. (1998). Antiepileptogenic effects of the novel anticonvulsant levetiracetam (ucb L059) in the kindling model of temporal lobe epilepsy. *J Pharmacol Exp Ther*, 284:474–479.
30. De Deyn, P.P., Kabatu, H., D'Hooge, R., and Mori, A. (1992). Protective effect of ucb L059 against postural stimulation-induced seizures in EL Mice. *Neurosciences*, 18(suppl 2):187–192.
31. Gower, A.J., Hirsch, E., Boehrer, A., Noyer, M., and Marescaux, C. (1995). Effects of levetiracetam, a novel antiepileptic drug, on convulsant activity in two genetic rat models of epilepsy. *Epilepsy Res*, 22:207–213.
32. Klitgaard, H. (2001). Levetiracetam: The preclinical profile of a new class of antiepileptic drugs? *Epilepsia*, 42(suppl. 4):13–18.
33. Killam, K.F. and Bain, J.A. (1957). Convulsant hydrazides. I. *In vitro* and *in vivo* inhibition of vitamin B6 enzyms by convulsant hydrazides. *J Pharmacol Exp Ther*, 119:255–262.
34. Killam, K.F., Dasgupta, S.R., and Killam, E.K. (1960). Studies on the action of convulsant hydrazides as vitamin B6 antagonists in the central nervous system. In Roberts, E. (ed.), *Inhibition in the Nervous System and Gamma-Aminobutyric Acid*. Pergamon Press, New York, NY, pp. 302–316.
35. Perucca, E., French, J., and Bialer, M. (2007). Development of new antiepileptic drugs: Challenges, incentives, and recent advances. *Lancet Neurol*, 6:793–804.

36. Stables, J.P., Bertram, E., Dudek, F.E., Holmes, G., Mathern, G., Pitkanen, A. *et al.* (2003). Therapy discovery for pharmacoresistant epilepsy and for disease-modifying therapeutics: Summary of the NIH/NINDS/AES models II workshop. *Epilepsia*, 44(12):1472–1478.
37. Stables, J.P., Bertram, E.H., White, H.S., Coulter, D.A., Dichter, M.A., Jacobs, M.P. *et al.* (2002). Models for epilepsy and epileptogenesis: Report from the NIH workshop, Bethesda, Maryland. *Epilepsia*, 43(11):1410–1420.
38. Löscher, W., Jackel, R., and Czuczwar, S.J. (1986). Is amygdala kindling in rats a model for drug-resistant partial epilepsy? *Exp Neurol*, 93(1):211–226.
39. Löscher, W., Rundfeldt, C., and Honack, D. (1993). Pharmacological characterization of phenytoin-resistant amygdala-kindled rats, a new model of drug-resistant partial epilepsy. *Epilepsy Res*, 15(3):207–219.
40. Rundfeldt, C. and Löscher, W. (1993). Anticonvulsant efficacy and adverse effects of phenytoin during chronic treatment in amygdala-kindled rats. *J Pharmacol Exp Ther*, 266(1):216–223.
41. Postma, T., Krupp, E., Li, X.L., Post, R.M., and Weiss, S.R. (2000). Lamotrigine treatment during amygdala-kindled seizure development fails to inhibit seizures and diminishes subsequent anticonvulsant efficacy. *Epilepsia*, 41(12):1514–1521.
42. Srivastava, A., Woodhead, J.H., and White, H.S. (2003). Effect of lamotrigine, carbamazepine and sodium valproate on lamotrigine-resistant kindled rats. *Epilepsia*, 44(Suppl. 9):42.
43. Srivastava, A., Franklin, M.R., Palmer, B.S., and White, H.S. (2004). Carbamazepine, but not valproate, displays pharmaco-resistance in lamotrigine-resistant amygdala kindled rats. *Epilepsia*, 45(Suppl 7):12.
44. Srivastava, A. and White, H.S. (2005). Retigabine decreases behavioral and electrographic seizures in the lamotrigine-resistant amygdala kindled rat model of pharmacoresistant epilepsy. *Epilepsia*, 46(Suppl 8):217–218.
45. Barton, M.E., Klein, B.D., Wolf, H.H., and White, H.S. (2001). Pharmacological characterization of the 6 Hz psychomotor seizure model of partial epilepsy. *Epilepsy Res*, 47:217–227.
46. Brandt, C., Volk, H.A., and Loscher, W. (2004). Striking differences in individual anticonvulsant response to phenobarbital in rats with spontaneous seizures after status epilepticus. *Epilepsia*, 45(12):1488–1497.
47. Glien, M., Brandt, C., Potschka, H., and Loscher, W. (2002). Effects of the novel antiepileptic drug levetiracetam on spontaneous recurrent seizures in the rat pilocarpine model of temporal lobe epilepsy. *Epilepsia*, 43(4):350–357.
48. Leite, J.P. and Cavalheiro, E.A. (1995). Effects of conventional antiepileptic drugs in a model of spontaneous recurrent seizures in rats. *Epilepsy Res*, 20(2):93–104.
49. Grabenstatter, H.L. and Dudek, F.E. (2005). The effect of carbamazepine on spontaneous seizures in freely-behaving rats with kainate-induced epilepsy. *Epilepsia*, 46(Suppl. 8):287.
50. Grabenstatter, H.L., Ferraro, D.J., Williams, P.A., Chapman, P.L., and Dudek, F.E. (2005). Use of chronic epilepsy models in antiepileptic drug discovery: The effect of topiramate on spontaneous motor seizures in rats with kainate-induced epilepsy. *Epilepsia*, 46(1):8–14.
51. van Vliet, E.A., van Schaik, R., Edelbroek, P.M., Redeker, S., Arionica, E., Wadman, W.J., Marchi, N., Vezzani, A., and Gorter, J.A. (2006). Inhibition of the multidrug transporter *P*-glycoprotein improves seizure control in phenytoin-treated chronic epileptic rats. *Epilepsia*, 47(4):672–680.
52. Smyth, M.D., Barbaro, N.M., and Baraban, S.C. (2002). Effects of antiepileptic drugs on induced epileptiform activity in a rat model of dysplasia. *Epilepsy Res*, 50(3):251–264.
53. Dichter, M.A. and Pollard, J. (2006). Cell culture models for studying epilepsy. In Pitkanen, A., Schwartzkroin, P.A., and Moshe, S.L. (eds.), *Models of Seizures and Epilepsy*. Elsevier Academic Press, New York, pp. 23–34.
54. Heinemann, U., Kann, O., and Schuchmann, S. (2006). An overview of in vitro seizure models in acute and organotypic slices. In Pitkanen, A., Schwartzkroin, P.A., and Moshe, S.L. (eds.), *Models of Seizures and Epilepsy*. Elsevier Academic Press, New York, pp. 35–44.

55. Löscher, W. (2006). Animal models of drug-refractory epilepsy. In Pitkanen, A., Schwartzkroin, P.A., and Moshe, S.L. (eds.), *Models of Seizures and Epilepsy*. Elsevier Academic Press, New York, pp. 551–567.

56. Löscher, W. (1986). Experimental models for intractable epilepsy in non-primate animal species. In Schmidt, D. and Morselli, P.L. (eds.), *Intractable Epilepsy: Experimental and Clinial Aspects*. Raven Press, New York, pp. 25–37.

57. Rundfeldt, C., Honack, D., and Loscher, W. (1990). Phenytoin potently increases the threshold for focal seizures in amygdala-kindled rats. *Neuropharmacology*, 29(9):845–851.

58. Weiss, S.R. and Post, R.M. (1991). Development and reversal of contingent inefficacy and tolerance to the anticonvulsant effects of carbamazepine. *Epilepsia*, 32(1):140–145.

59. Barton, M.E., Peters, S.C., and Shannon, H.E. (2003). Comparison of the effect of glutamate receptor modulators in the 6 Hz and maximal electroshock seizure models. *Epilepsy Res*, 56(1):17–26.

60. Brown, W.C., Schiffman, D.O., Swinyard, E.A., and Goodman, L.S. (1953). Comparative assay of an antiepileptic drugs by psychomotor seizure test and minimal electroshock threshold test. *J Pharmacol Exp Ther*, 107(3):273–283.

Translational Models for the 21st Century: Reminiscence, Reflections, and Some Recommendations

Paul Willner[1], Franco Borsini[2] and Robert A. McArthur[3]

[1]Department of Psychology, Swansea University, Swansea, Wales, UK
[2]sigma-tau S.p.A., Pomezia, Roma, Italy
[3]McArthur and Associates GmbH, Ramsteinerstrasse, Basel, Switzerland

INTRODUCTION

This series has provided a systematic overview of translational research in psychopharmacology that integrates the perspectives of academics, industrial pharmacologists, and clinicians, in therapeutic areas representing three broad therapeutic domains, neurological disorders, psychiatric disorders, and reward/impulse control disorders. An earlier attempt to systematize translational research in psychopharmacology summarized the scope of the endeavor as follows:

> *The problem of using animal behavior to model human mental disorders is, explicitly or implicitly, the central preoccupation of psychopharmacology. The idea that psychiatric disorders might be modeled in animals provides the basis for a substantial proportion of current research; and research that does not employ behavioral models directly is usually justified by reference to its eventual benefits, in terms of an understanding of the human brain and the development of more effective and safer therapies.[1]*

In effect, the principle that translation from animals to humans is both possible and necessary underpins and justifies the whole field of preclinical psychopharmacology.

The forerunner to the present series, *Behavioural Models in Psychopharmacology: Academic, Theoretical and Industrial Perspectives*[2] was intended to generalize an approach first outlined in a more focused earlier review of animal models of depression.[3] These publications introduced four significant ideas: that drug screening tests should not be thought of as models and differ in their practical and evidential requirements; that academics, industrial pharmacologists, and clinicians view preclinical behavioral models from different perspectives, based on their different professional aspirations; that it is important to establish, or at least, estimate, the validity of animal models of psychiatric disorders; and that this is best achieved by considering validity from different aspects that reflect different bodies of evidence.

In the 20 or so years since these ideas were first introduced, they have achieved a wide degree of acceptance, and the first two are very apparent in the structure and

Animal and Translational Models for CNS Drug Discovery,
Vol. 2 of 3: Neurological Disorders
Robert McArthur and Franco Borsini (eds), Academic Press, 2008

337

content of the present series. The three approaches to the validation of animal models that were outlined in these publications, using terms borrowed from the realm of psychometric testing, were predictive validity ("performance in the test predicts performance in the condition being modeled"), face validity ("there are phenomenological similarities between the two"), and construct validity ("the model has a sound theoretical rationale").[2] This analysis has since become standard, as seen, for example, in recent reviews of animal models of anxiety[4] and schizophrenia.[5] Indeed, these principles are now so well established that many contributors to the present series begin their discussions by considering the face, predictive, and construct validity of the models used and being developed in their therapeutic areas.[i] The extent to which these concepts have become absorbed into the language of psychopharmacology is demonstrated by the fact that they are now almost always used without attribution to the original publications.

Much has changed in terms of model development in the last 20 years; particularly in neurology. As has been discussed in the neurological therapeutic areas surveyed in this series, much of the work has been developed more recently, and it is noticeable that these chapters tend to have a different flavor to those chapters surveying psychiatric and reward deficit disorders, being heavily dominated by genetic and genomic models. In psychiatry, on the other hand, while these areas have also been heavily influenced by the genomic revolution, in behavioral terms, models of depression, anxiety, schizophrenia, or substance abuse have seen relatively little development. That is not to say that there have not been developments in the procedures by which models of depressed-like, anxious-like, schizophrenic-like or substance-abuse-like behaviors can be assessed. Indeed, there is now a significantly greater choice of procedures. However, the newer developments are largely more sophisticated variants on procedures that were well established prior to 1990.

Schizophrenia represents perhaps the one major therapeutic area where a significant shift in emphasis has been evident over the past 20 years. From the discovery of neuroleptics in the early 1950s[6,7] and the establishment of the dopamine hypothesis of schizophrenia,[8] drug discovery and development of pharmaceuticals used to treat the positive, that is, psychotic, symptoms of schizophrenia have centered around impairment of excessive dopaminergic function. Effects of mesolimbic dopaminergic imbalance have been relatively straightforward to model, mainly using changes in locomotion.[ii] Notwithstanding the importance of dopamine in schizophrenia,

---

[i] For further and detailed discussions regarding criteria of validity, the reader is invited to refer to discussions, for example, by Steckler *et al.*, Developing novel anxiolytics: Improving preclinical detection and clinical assessment; Large *et al.*, Developing therapeutics for bipolar disorder: From animal models to the clinic; Joel *et al.*, Animal models of obsessive–compulsive disorder: From bench to bedside via endophenotypes and biomarkers, in Volume 1, *Psychiatric Disorders*; Lindner *et al.*, Development, optimization and use of preclinical behavioral models to maximize the productivity of drug discovery for Alzheimer's Disease; Merchant *et al.*, Animal models of Parkinson's Disease to aid drug discovery and development, in Volume 2, *Neurologic Disorders*; Koob, The role of animal models in reward deficit disorders: Views from academia; Markou *et al.*, Contribution of animal models and preclinical human studies to medication development for nicotine dependence, in Volume 3, *Reward Deficit Disorders*.

[ii] Please refer to Jones et al., Developing new drugs for schizophrenia: From animals to the clinic, in Volume 1, Psychiatric Disorders. For further discussion regarding models and procedures in schizophrenia research.

awareness of the influence of other neurotransmitters such as serotonin, glutamate and GABA has led to considerable research into the role of these and their interactions with dopamine.[9,10] Pharmaceutical interest in glutamate in schizophrenia has been particularly fruitful with the development of the metabotropic glutamate$_{2/3}$ (mGlu$_{2/3}$) receptor agonist LY2140023, which appears to be as effective as olanzapine (Zyprexa®) as an antipsychotic in a Phase II trial.[11,12] mGlu$_{2/3}$ receptor agonists have been discovered and characterized using classical locomotor activity procedures or pharmacological interaction studies,[13-15] but it is interesting to note that they also show positive effects on newer procedures that have been developed to assess drug effects on models of negative (i.e., social withdrawal, lack of affect and drive, poverty of speech) and cognitive symptoms of schizophrenia.[15,16] Such procedures include sensory gating and pre-pulse inhibition,[17] sustained or focused attention,[18,19] and impaired social interaction.[20] Furthermore, greater awareness of neurodevelopmental and environmental factors of schizophrenia has led to the establishment of models such as neo-natal hippocampal lesions,[21] and to attempts to model effects of peri-partum complications as risk factors of schizophrenia.[22]

Stress as a predisposing factor, the role of the hypothalamo-pituitary-adrenal (HPA) axis and reactions to stress influenced by the environment and development, are themes discussed not only in the chapters of the Psychiatry volume, such as depression,[23] anxiety,[24] bipolar disorders,[25] and attention deficit hyperactivity disorder (ADHD),[26] but also the chapters representing the reward and impulse deficit disorders; disorders that share a high psychiatric component.[27-29] Consequently, major efforts have been made to model the effects of chronic stress and influences of development on psychiatric, reward deficit, and impulse control disorders. Behavioral developments in these areas are concerned almost exclusively with the ways in which stressors are applied and their effects evaluated. The procedures used to evaluate these changes have not changed markedly in the past 20 years. However, the way in which these procedures are used has been greatly influenced by the "endophenotypic" approach to considering psychiatric disorders and how to model aspects of these disorders.[23,24,iii] Similarly, models of reward and impulse disorders continue to be dominated by self-administration and place conditioning procedures. There is certainly a greater use of more sophisticated procedures, such as second order or progressive ratio reinforcement schedules[30,iv] but the procedures themselves have been well established for decades.[31]

Nevertheless, despite the relatively minor changes in the behavioral methodologies, research in these "traditional" areas of translational modeling is markedly different from 20 years, ago, since they too have been transformed by the genomic revolution, which now dominates and largely determines directions of change, dwarfing developments in behavioral technologies. Almost every chapter in this series bears witness to the

---

iii Please refer to McArthur and Borsini, preface to this volume, "What do *you* mean by translational research? An enquiry through animal and translational models for CNS drug discovery," and references within for further discussion on endophenotypes and deconstructing behavioral syndromes.

iv See also Koob, The role of animal models in reward deficit disorders: Views from academia; and Rochas *et al.*, Development of medications for heroin and cocaine addiction and regulatory aspects of abuse liability testing in Volume 3, *Reward Deficit Disorders*.

fact that current research is highly productive in proposing new models of aspects of psychiatric and impulse control disorders that, like the new neurological models, are based almost exclusively on the use of genetically modified animals.[32,33] Molecular biology has also had a huge impact on the understanding of intracellular processes, particularly in relation to those intracellular sequelae of transmitter–receptor interactions that result in changes in gene expression. These developments were driven in part by the recognition that successful pharmacotherapy for psychiatric disorders – depression in particular – often requires chronic drug treatment. Consequently, there is an increasing use in preclinical studies of chronic dosing strategies modeled on the time course of clinical action, leading to a search for the biochemical mechanisms that underlie slowly developing neuroadaptive changes and the identification of a plethora of novel intracellular targets.[34-38]

A similar dynamic is apparent in relation to the understanding of brain structure and function, which serves as the context for translational research Twenty years ago, psychopharmacology was preoccupied almost exclusively with neurotransmitters; specifically the monoamines dopamine, norepinephrine and serotonin, acetylcholine and GABA, and their receptors. There had been a shift away from the original paradigm that saw the brain as a "biochemical soup," with a recognition that the anatomical site of action was also a crucial consideration, but little attention was paid to the underlying neural circuitry. Over the past 20 years, progress in understanding neurotransmitters and their receptors has been slowly incremental, particularly in relation to glutamatergic and peptidergic systems, as well as the cannabinoid systems, which represent the only major truly novel development. On the other hand, the understanding of brain circuitry has increased exponentially. The importance of dopamine and the mesolimbic and nigrostriatal systems in terms of movement (Parkinson's) and mood (schizophrenia), helped focus research on a more "neural systems" approach. Subsequently, examination of the relationships and interactions between neurotransmitter and neuromodulators within discrete neural circuits has helped to clarify neural substrates of behavioral processes, with the result that the basic operating principles of the brain are being increasingly well understood.[39-41] The parallel development of cognitive neuroscience has been accompanied by technological innovations, most notably, brain scanning methodologies, which have promoted a substantial growth of studies in human participants that complement the traditional work in animal models.

Over the past two decades, then, it is the dramatic developments in molecular biology and in behavioral and cognitive neuroscience, rather than developments in psychopharmacology itself, that have had the major impact on both the theory and practice of translational research, as exemplified by the contributions that comprise the present series. And the fundamental dilemma of psychopharmacology was already apparent 20 years ago, and remains so today: that following an early "golden age" all of the investment in academic and industrial research has produced tiny returns by way of novel pharmacotherapies. For 30, perhaps 40, years now, psychopharmacological research has not substantially changed the pharmacological armamentarium with which to treat devastating and life-threatening behavioral disorders. It has often been pointed out, but bears repeating, that it was 1958, now half a century ago, when the first publication appeared on the clinical efficacy of tricyclic[42] and monoamine oxidase inhibiting[43] antidepressants which, together with neuroleptics a few years earlier[6,7] and benzodiazepines a few years later,[44,45] completed the triad of innovations that have dominated clinical psychopharmacology ever since. Shortly afterwards, basic pharmacotherapy for neurologic disorders was revolutionized by the elucidation of the role of dopamine in Parkinson's disease[46,47] followed by the use of L-dopa in its treatment.[48] The concept of neurologic disorders related to neurotransmitter deficiency and its treatment by replacement of the neurotransmitter was one of the driving forces behind the research into acetylcholine potentiation by cholinesterase inhibitors in Alzheimer's disease,[49] which culminated with the registration of tacrine (Cognex®), a pro-cholinergic drug for dementia, in 1993.

Subsequent clinical developments following all of these innovations have been disappointingly unimpressive. For example, second or third generation antidepressants cannot be claimed as pharmacological innovations, since they target known properties of tricyclics, that is, serotonin and/or noradrenergic inhibition; furthermore, the efficacy of these drugs as antidepressants is increasingly questioned.[50] Atypical neuroleptics retain as an essential feature the major property of typical neuroleptics, dopamine receptor antagonism, tempered by additional properties, typically, serotonin receptor antagonism; they offer no new mechanism and very limited clinical advantage, and the prototype of this class of drug, clozapine (Clozaril®), was introduced as long ago as 1989. As indicated above, the early signs of efficacy of the mGlu$_{2/3}$ receptor agonist LY404039,[11] offers some hope of moving beyond dopaminergic compounds in the treatment of schizophrenia,[12] but this development is still at a very early stage. Acetylcholinesterase inhibition has been the standard treatment for dementia since the introduction of tacrine in 1993. Tacrine is hardly ever prescribed now: donepezil (Aricept®) is one of the drugs of choice, but even this "gold standard" is of limited effectiveness and duration.[51,52] Glutamatergic drugs offer some hope of a genuinely novel approach but the clinical efficacy of, in particular, memantine (Ebixa®/Namenda®) is extremely modest.[53,54] In Parkinson's disease, there has been no improvement, as monotherapy at least, on L-dopa. In contrast, new drugs have been approved for the treatment of reward deficit disorders such as alcoholism [naltrexone (Vivitrol®/Revia®) and acamprosate (Campral®)], nicotine abuse [varenicline (Chantix®/Champix®), bupropion (Zyban®)], and heroin abuse [methadone (Dolophine®), buprenorphine (Subutex®), and buprenorphine/naloxone (Suboxone®)]. These drugs, however, treat the symptoms of these disorders, and in the case of heroin abuse, the treatment is limited to replacement of heroin. We are still waiting for more effective drugs to be developed for all therapeutic indications surveyed in this book series.

And the certainties of 20–30 years ago have been questioned. Two major issues have emerged in the development and use of psychotherapeutics for the treatment of behavioral disorders: the placebo response, or the ability of certain patients to recover without medication,[50,55,56] and treatment-resistance,[57-59] which has led to initiatives such as the STAR*D trial.[60] For psychiatric indications the traditional triad of anxiety, depression, and schizophrenia are no longer viewed as self-contained entities: comorbidity is recognized as a major factor in the phenomenology of these disorders.[61] Traditional medications for one indication have now become drugs of choice for another. For example, selective serotonin reuptake inhibitor (SSRI) antidepressants such as fluoxetine (Prozac®), paroxetine (Paxil®), sertraline (Zoloft®), fluvoxamine (Luvox®), or escitalopram (Lexapro®) are all approved by the US Food and Drug Administration (FDA) for the treatment of various anxiety disorders. SSRIs as well as tricyclic antidepressants such as imipramine (Tofranil®) and desipramine (Norpramin®) indeed are now considered first-line treatment for general anxiety disorder.[62] Anti-epileptics such as lamotrigine (Lamictal®) are being used to treat depression, while antipsychotics such as olanzapine, as well as lamotrigine, are treatments of choice for bipolar disorder.[v] Research into previously under-treated disorders such as obsessive–compulsive disorder (OCD), ADHD, or autistic spectrum disorders has also contributed to a blurring of the boundaries of traditional psychiatry.[vi] The gradual realization that psychiatric disorders are etiologically complex,[63] and that it is unrealistic to take a simple view that one pill might "cure" depression, or anxiety, or schizophrenia, has important implications for the modeling of these disorders.

What has gone wrong? Perhaps the most frustrating thing of all is that there is no clear answer to this question. One potential explanation lies in the wide anatomical distribution of most drug receptors, and the likelihood that systemically administered drugs have multiple effects that may in some cases be mutually antagonistic. Studies in genomic models employing regionally specific conditional knockouts and other genetic techniques[64-71] may go some way to addressing this issue. However, another, more disturbing, potential explanation arises from a consideration of the validity of psychiatric diagnoses. The predominant contemporary approach to diagnosis, based on the use of diagnostic criteria, defines disorders in terms of lists of symptoms, with patients typically required to display one or more items from each of a list of core and subsidiary symptoms.[72,73] It has frequently been pointed out that this can lead to a situation in which two patients who share the same diagnosis may not share any symptoms in common.[74] There have been attempts to introduce a different approach based around a systematic focus on specific symptoms,[75-77] but the failure of this eminently sensible alternative testifies to the hegemony of diagnostic criteria in determining what constitutes permissible clinical research design.[vii]

There have, of course, been numerous instances where compounds are identified in animal models as having clinical potential. However, it is now almost routine for novel pharmacotherapies, identified in models that are assessed as having a high degree of validity, to fail in the clinic. Just as examples, ondansetron, a 5-HT$_3$ receptor antagonist, was reported to antagonize scopolamine-induced effects in marmosets[78] but not in humans;[79] talsaclidine, a muscarinic receptor agonist, did not exert the same effects on muscarinic M$_2$ and M$_3$ receptors in animals and humans,[80] while repinotan,

---

[v] Please refer to Large *et al.*, Developing therapeutics for bipolar disorder: From animal models to the clinic, in Volume 1, *Psychiatric Disorders*, for further discussion of psychotherapeutics for bipolar disorder.

[vi] Please refer to Joel *et al.*, Animal models of obsessive–compulsive disorder: From bench to bedside via endophenotypes and biomarkers; and Tannock *et al.*, An integrative assessment of attention deficit hyperactivity disorder: From biological comprehension to the discovery of novel therapeutic agents for a neurodevelopmental disorder, in Volume 1, *Psychiatric Disorders*.

[vii] Please refer to McEvoy and Freudenreich, Issues in the design and conductance of clinical trials, in Volume 1, *Psychiatric Disorders*; and Schneider, Issues in design and conduct of clinical trials for cognitive-enhancing drugs, in Volume 2, *Neurologic Disorders*, for further discussion regarding changes to standard clinical trial design.

a 5-HT$_{1A}$ receptor agonist, reduced the neurological deficit in animal models of stroke but not in humans.[81] Other 5-HT$_{1A}$ receptor agonists, flibanserin, and gepirone[23,82,83] were found to be active in the majority of animal models sensitive to antidepressants but failed in clinical trials. TCH346 and CEP1347 seemed very promising as antiparkinsonian agents in preclinical experiments but failed in clinical trials.[84] Tramiprosate (Alzhemed) was found to reduce β-amyloid brain and plasma levels in animals[85] and cerebrospinal levels in humans,[86] but failed to meet its primary endpoint in a Phase III clinical study,[87,viii] although there are claims that significant reductions in hippocampal atrophy were observed with Alzhemed and that the drug itself will be distributed as a food supplement.[88]

How are we to understand these predictive failures? They might represent a failure of the model to predict clinical efficacy, but there are several other potential explanations. One, suggested above, is that a clinical trial could fail to recognize a successful compound because the population of participants identified by the use of diagnostic criteria is clinically heterogeneous. Another explanation, given that drugs are usually administered to animals at much higher doses than they are to people, even after taking into account inter-species scaling factors, is that a clinical failure could reflect the use of an inefficient clinical dose.[23,25,28,84,89-93] Or there could be pharmacokinetic/metabolism issues; in particular, problems with bioavailability, which account for a high proportion of failures at an early stage of clinical testing.[89,91,93] Also, other considerations that go beyond scientific matters, involving corporate policies and politics, may contribute to these predictive failures.[94,95] On the other side of the coin, it is also important to recognize that successful clinical trials may not always be all they seem. In particular, recent meta-analyses of antidepressant efficacy have drawn attention to the fact that, for a variety of reasons, positive outcomes are much more likely to be published than negative outcomes, and that when all of the data are taken into account, antidepressants appear significantly less efficacious than has been generally assumed.[55,96,97] There is no reason to suppose that this is a problem peculiar to antidepressants.

In the search for alternative ways forward, two new concepts have been embraced within translational research: endophenotypes and biomarkers.[ix] Biomarkers are essential to follow the progress of a disorder and the effects of therapeutic intervention. In terms of translational research, the same biomarker of the disorder should be mirrored in the animal model. However, so far very few biomarkers have been validated and this remains a focus of intensive research and of great concern (cf.,[50,84,91,93,98-100]). As discussed in the preface to this volume, there is a notable proposal that the concept of validity for biomarkers should be deconstructed into face, predictive and construct dimensions, as used routinely to evaluate the validity of translational models.[101]

As discussed in many chapters of this book series, endophenotypes refer to the heritable, state-independent and family-associated characteristics of a disorder that

viii See Schneider, Issues in design and conduct of clinical trials for cognitive-enhancing drugs, in Volume 2, *Neurologic Disorders*, for further discussion on primary and secondary endpoints in Alzheimer clinical trials.

ix Please refer to McArthur and Borsini, preface to this volume, "What do *you* mean by translational research? An enquiry through animal and translational models for CNS drug discovery," and references within for further discussion on endophenotypes and biomarkers.

can be linked to a candidate gene or gene region, which can help in the genetic analysis of the disorder.[102-104] An endophenotypic approach to modeling requires as a first step the identification of "… critical components of behavior (or other neurobiological traits) that are more representative of more complex phenomena" ([102] p. 641). To date, there are very few putative behavioral endophenotypes that actually meet the five criteria proposed by Gottesman and Gould[102] of: (1) a specific association with the illness of interest; (2) heritability; (3) state-independence; (4) greater prevalence among ill relatives than in the general population (familial association) and (5) than in well relatives (co-segregation). For example, Hasler and colleagues[105] reviewed eight putative behavioral endophenotypes of depression, and concluded that only one of them, anhedonia, met all five of these criteria, as well as a sixth criterion, plausibility. (A second candidate, increased stress sensitivity, also scored highly in Hasler's analysis, but does not show a specific association with depression.) Two putative biological endophenotypes (REM sleep abnormalities and a depressive response to tryptophan depletion) also appeared to meet all six criteria.

For the purposes of the present book series, it is important to distinguish between clinical endophenotypes and translational models of clinical endophenotypes. Taking anhedonia as a putative endophenotype for depression, two distinct considerations clearly apply to a putative model of this putative endophenotype. Consider first Hasler's plausibility criterion. *The question of plausibility is reflected in Miczek's 1st principle for translational models, The translation of preclinical data to clinical concerns is more successful when the development of experimental models is restricted in their scope to a cardinal or core symptom of a psychiatric disorder.*[120] Plausibility is intimately related to construct validity, so it is also essential to verify the construct. The anhedonia endophenotype (an internal construct) is inferred in a translational model from the presence of a variety of different exophenotypes (observable behaviors) such as decreased sucrose intake, increased brain stimulation reward threshold, or impaired place conditioning;[106,107] therefore it is important to evaluate a range of appropriate behavioral endpoints rather than relying on a single procedure.[x] The second, and perhaps more obvious, but also more demanding, consideration is that the Gottesman and Gould criteria imply a change in the focus of model building, moving away from the traditional preoccupation with environmental precipitants of behavioral change to encompass a search for susceptible individuals. Strategies to achieve this objective include inbreeding[108,109] or genetic modification[110,111] to produce putatively anhedonic strains, and the identification of susceptible and resilient individuals within strains.[112,113] What needs to be recognized is that having identified susceptible individuals, a rigorous program of further research is needed to demonstrate face validity, which in this context means that the model conforms to the range of criteria that apply to a clinical endophenotype. For example, a genetically produced trait is by definition heritable, but may not show individual differences in response to stress; conversely, traits identified as individual differences may not be heritable; and both of these approaches raise questions of specificity and state-independence.

---

[x] See also Miczek's 3rd principle, *Preclinical data are more readily translated to the clinical situation when they are based on converging evidence from at least two, and preferably more, experimental procedures, each capturing cardinal features of the modeled disorder.*

While recognizing that the nature of translational modeling is changing, it remains important to retain the strengths of the traditional approach, such as the emphasis on validation of models. Indeed, as discussed in the preface to this volume, concepts of validity are also intimately involved in the establishment of human models of behavioral disorders in experimental medicine, as well as the establishment of biomarkers and endophenotypes.[101,114] There are several reasons to maintain this focus. Firstly, the use of a taxonomy of predictive, face and construct validity,[3,115] or similar alternative taxonomies,[116,117] ensures that when the merits of different models are compared, like is compared with like. Secondly, the practice of assessing validity along several dimensions challenges the predominant view within the pharmaceutical industry that pharmacological isomorphism is the paramount consideration, which incorporates the potentially unhelpful implication that novel agents must resemble known drugs in their spectrum of action. Thirdly, attention to validity forces the proponents of a particular procedure (perhaps one developed in their own laboratory) to engage a self-critical awareness of the model's weaknesses in addition to its strengths, and discourages the publication of over-zealous or biased claims that could be misleading to others. And fourthly, an overt discussion of validity will serve as a context for the selection and adoption of models by the increasing population of workers entering the field of translational modeling from molecular biology rather than from behavioral sciences.

In addition to the translational initiatives of training non-behavioral scientists in behavioral methods and analyses,[xi] a further issue that merits some reflection is the – largely unrecognized – increase in the volume of translational research emanating from the world's developing economics. This can be illustrated by the pattern of submissions to one of the major journals in the field, *Behavioral Pharmacology*, with similar trends in submissions to at least one other major journal (Personal Communication from the editor). In 2007, 20% of submissions to *Behavioral Pharmacology* were from four non-traditional sources: China, India, Brazil, and Iran, the majority of these papers reporting translational research. To take India as an example, submissions during the 1990s were only 0.2% of the total, rising to 2% in the 5 years from 2000 to 2004, and almost 4% in 2005–2007. The most dramatic change has been in submissions from China, mirroring the emergence of the Chinese economy, with submissions languishing at well below 0.5% for the 15 years to 2004 (and these largely from one laboratory), rising suddenly to well over 5% in 2005–2007. However, the growth of research in developing economies is not well integrated into the wider scientific community. With rare exceptions[118] scientists in developing countries have little direct contact with the mainstream scientific community, and therefore miss out on both the apprenticeship model of scientific training and the background of informal discourse, particularly the conversations that take place outside the formal sessions at scientific meetings. One important consequence of this dislocation is that claims made in the literature may be accepted more readily by scientists outside the mainstream, where investigators with access to the oral tradition and the informal chatter might be more

---

[xi] Please refer to http://www.ncrr.nih.gov/clinical_research_resources/clinical_and_translational_science_awards/index.asp, http://www.mrc.ac.uk/ApplyingforaGrant/InternationalOpportunites/fp7/index.htm for government-sponsored translational research training initiatives.

skeptical. Behavioral pharmacology in developing countries also is typically home grown, lacking the scientific cultural roots that come from a tradition of research and development in the area. There is a clear need for positive steps to enable engagement and integration between scientists in developing and developed economies. The European Behavioral Pharmacology Society has for many years achieved some success in meeting these objectives by offering financial support for attendance at scientific meetings to scientists in the developing economies of Eastern Europe. Models of outreach are now needed that can be applied globally, to support the development of behavioral pharmacology in general and translational research in particular, in emerging scientific communities. Academic institutions, scientific journals, learned societies, and the pharmaceutical industry will all have a role to play in shaping the new landscape.

Some considerations on the future DSM-V are also appropriate. Limitations to the current diagnostic paradigms described in the DSM-IV indicate that description of syndromes may never successfully uncover their underlying etiologies. Thus, in the agenda for preparing DSM-V (http://www.dsm5.org), a series of events is planned to try to overcome this limitation. First, a series of "white papers" is contemplated, with the aim of encouraging a research agenda that goes beyond our current thinking to integrate pieces of information from a wide variety of sources and technology. Neuroscience is the subject of one of these "white papers," aimed at developing a basic, clinical neuroscience, and genetics research agenda to guide the development of a future pathophysiological-based diagnostic classification. The working group focused on four main domains: (1) better animal models for the major psychiatric disorders; (2) genes that help determine abnormal behavior in animal models; (3) imaging studies in animals to understand better the nature of imaged signals in humans; and (4) functional genomics and proteomics involved in psychiatric disorders. Second, research conferences are planned to discuss several topics, among which is "stress-induced and fear circuitry disorders." A special session will also be dedicated to gender effects. Thus, we hope that the present series of books may also serve as another basis for discussion of how neuroscience can improve the diagnostic criteria of mental and nervous illnesses.

We end with some reflections on the scope of this project. Its predecessor[2] aimed to integrate academic, industrial, and clinical perspectives through a sequential construction process. Each section of the book had three chapters. The introductory chapter, which set out the concept of the project[1] was written first and forwarded to the academic authors in each therapeutic area, whose chapters were provided to the industrial authors, and finally, the academic and industrial chapters were forwarded to the clinical authors. The present project has taken a more adventurous approach, in which groups of academic, industrial, and clinical authors were established by the editors and were asked to write collaboratively. The introductory chapters to each volume, "What do *you* mean by translational research?" explain that this was done in order "to simulate the conditions of the creation of an industrial Project team" in which the combined talents and expertise of the project members are called together for a clearly defined goal. We can apply the, by now conventional, methodology to assess the validity of this attempt at simulation. There is certainly some face validity: in both the literary and industrial settings, the members of project teams "are all committed to achieving the goals set out by consensus" but "need not know each other …". Also, in some therapeutic areas "the authors were not able to establish an effective team", which reflects the reality that not all project teams are successful. In common with the majority of newly introduced models, predictive validity is less compelling, and only time will tell whether "what appears to be a novel and unusual way of working will become the norm." And as is so often the case, construct validity is elusive. The observation that "for many, this has been a challenging and exhilarating experience, forcing a paradigm shift from how they have normally worked" implies a theory of the role of paradigm shift in drug discovery. New paradigms are the bedrock of scientific revolutions[119] and the current explosion of knowledge that results from the transformations of psychopharmacology by systems neuroscience and behavioral genomics, as discussed earlier in this chapter, can certainly be understood in this light. We nurture the hope that adoption of the project-team approach might inject a comparable creative impetus into drug discovery!

REFERENCES

1. Willner, P. (1991). Behavioural models in psychopharmacology. In Willner, P. (ed.), *Behavioural Models in Psychopharmacology: Theoretical, Industrial and Clinical Perspectives*. Cambridge University Press, Cambridge, pp. 3–18.
2. Willner, P. (ed.) (1991). *Behavioural Models in Psychopharmacology: Theoretical, Industrial and Clinical Perspectives*. Cambridge University Press, Cambridge.
3. Willner, P. (1984). The validity of animal models of depression. *Psychopharmacology (Berl)*, 83(1):1–16.
4. Fendt, M. (2005). Animal models of fear and anxiety. In Koch, M. (ed.), *Animal Models of Neuropsychiatric Diseases*. Imperial College Press, London, pp. 293–336.
5. Koch, M. (2005). Animal models of schizophrenia. In Koch, M. (ed.), *Animal Models of Neuropsychiatric Diseases*. Imperial College Press, London, pp. 337–402.
6. Delay, J. and Deniker, P. (1955). Neuroleptic effects of chlorpromazine in therapeutics of neuropsychiatry. *J Clin Exp Psychopathol*, 16(2):104–112.
7. Delay, J., Deniker, P., and Harl, J.M. (1952). Therapeutic use in psychiatry of phenothiazine of central elective action (4560 RP). *Ann Med Psychol (Paris)*, 110(2:1):112–117.
8. Carlsson, A. (1977). Does dopamine play a role in schizophrenia? *Psychol Med*, 7(4):583–597.
9. Carlsson, M. and Carlsson, A. (1990). Schizophrenia: A subcortical neurotransmitter imbalance syndrome? *Schizophr Bull*, 16(3):425–432.
10. Carlsson, A. (1995). Neurocircuitries and neurotransmitter interactions in schizophrenia. *Int Clin Psychopharmacol*, 10(Suppl 3):21–28.
11. Patil, S.T., Zhang, L., Martenyi, F., Lowe, S.L., Jackson, K.A., Andreev, B.V. *et al.* (2007). Activation of mGlu2/3 receptors as a new approach to treat schizophrenia: A randomized Phase 2 clinical trial. *Nat Med*, 13(9):1102–1107.
12. Conn, P.J., Tamminga, C., Schoepp, D.D., and Lindsley, C. (2008). Schizophrenia: Moving beyond monoamine antagonists. *Mol Interv*, 8(2):99–107.
13. Rorick-Kehn, L.M., Perkins, E.J., Knitowski, K.M., Hart, J.C., Johnson, B.G., Schoepp, D.D. *et al.* (2006). Improved bioavailability of the mGlu2/3 receptor agonist LY354740 using a prodrug strategy: *In vivo* pharmacology of LY544344. *J Pharmacol Exp Ther*, 316(2):905–913.
14. Woolley, M.L., Pemberton, D.J., Bate, S., Corti, C., and Jones, D.N. (2008). The mGlu2 but not the mGlu3 receptor mediates the actions of the mGluR2/3 agonist, LY379268, in mouse models predictive of antipsychotic activity. *Psychopharmacology (Berl)*, 196(3):431–440.

15. Harich, S., Gross, G., and Bespalov, A. (2007). Stimulation of the metabotropic glutamate 2/3 receptor attenuates social novelty discrimination deficits induced by neonatal phencyclidine treatment. *Psychopharmacology (Berl)*, 192(4):511–519.

16. Greco, B., Invernizzi, R.W., and Carli, M. (2005). Phencyclidine-induced impairment in attention and response control depends on the background genotype of mice: Reversal by the mGLU(2/3) receptor agonist LY379268. *Psychopharmacology (Berl)*, 179(1):68–76.

17. Geyer, M.A. and Braff, D.L. (1987). Startle habituation and sensorimotor gating in schizophrenia and related animal models. *Schizophr Bull*, 13(4):643–668.

18. Robbins, T.W. (2002). The 5-choice serial reaction time task: Behavioural pharmacology and functional neurochemistry. *Psychopharmacology (Berl)*, 163(3–4):362–380.

19. Robbins, T.W. (2000). Animal models of set-formation and set-shifting deficits in schizophrenia. In Myslobodsky, M. and Weiner, I. (eds.), *Contemporary Issues in Modeling Psychopathology*. Kluwer Academic, Boston, MA, pp. 247–258.

20. Sams-Dodd, F. (1996). Phencyclidine-induced stereotyped behaviour and social isolation in rats: A possible animal model of schizophrenia. *Behav Pharmacol*, 7(1):3–23.

21. Lipska, B.K., Swerdlow, N.R., Geyer, M.A., Jaskiw, G.E., Braff, D.L., and Weinberger, D.R. (1995). Neonatal excitotoxic hippocampal damage in rats causes post-pubertal changes in prepulse inhibition of startle and its disruption by apomorphine. *Psychopharmacology (Berl)*, 122(1):35–43.

22. Jones, D.N.C., Gartlon, J.E., Minassian, A., Perry, W., and Geyer, M.A. (2008). Developing new drugs for schizophrenia: From animals to the clinic. In McArthur, R.A. and Borsini, F. (eds.), *Animal and Translational Models for CNS Drug Discovery: Psychiatric Disorders*. Academic Press, Elsevier, New York.

23. Cryan, J.F., Sánchez, C., Dinan, T.G., and Borsini, F. (2008). Developing more efficacious antidepressant medications: Improving and aligning preclinical and clinical assessment tools. In McArthur, R.A. and Borsini, F. (eds.), *Animal and Translational Models for CNS Drug Discovery: Psychiatric Disorders*. Academic Press, Elsevier, New York.

24. Steckler, T., Stein, M.B., and Holmes, A. (2008). Developing novel anxiolytics: Improving preclinical detection and clinical assessment. In McArthur, R.A. and Borsini, F. (eds.), *Animal and Translational Models for CNS Drug Discovery: Psychiatric Disorders*. Academic Press, Elsevier, New York.

25. Large, C.H., Einat, H., and Mahableshshwarkar, A.R. (2008). Developing new drugs for bipolar disorder (BPD): From animal models to the clinic. In McArthur, R.A. and Borsini, F. (eds.), *Animal and Translational Models for CNS Drug Discovery: Psychiatric Disorders*. Academic Press, Elsevier, New York.

26. Tannock, R., Campbell, B., Seymour, P., Ouellet, D., Soares, H., Wang, P. *et al.* (2008). Towards a biological understanding of ADHD and the discovery of novel therapeutic approaches. In McArthur, R.A. and Borsini, F. (eds.), *Animal and Translational Models for CNS Drug Discovery: Psychiatric Disorders*. Academic Press, Elsevier, New York.

27. Little, H.J., McKinzie, D.L., Setnik, B., Shram, M.J., and Sellers, E.M. (2008). Pharmacotherapy of alcohol dependence: Improving translation from the bench to the clinic. In McArthur, R.A. and Borsini, F. (eds.), *Animal and Translational Models for CNS Drug Discovery: Reward Deficit Disorders*. Academic Press, Elsevier, New York.

28. Markou, A., Chiamulera, C., and West, R.J. (2008). Contribution of animal models and preclinical human studies to medication development for nicotine dependence. In McArthur, R.A. and Borsini, F. (eds.), *Animal and Translational Models for CNS Drug Discovery: Reward Deficit Disorders*. Academic Press, Elsevier, New York.

29. Williams, W.A., Grant, J.E., Winstanley, C.A., and Potenza, M.N. (2008). Currect concepts in the classification, treatment and modelling of pathological gambling and other impulse control

disorders. In McArthur, R.A. and Borsini, F. (eds.), *Animal and Translational Models for CNS Drug Discovery: Reward Deficit Disorders*. Academic Press, Elsevier, New York.

30. Czachowski, C.L. and Samson, H.H. (1999). Breakpoint determination and ethanol self-administration using an across-session progressive ratio procedure in the rat. *Alcohol Clin Exp Res*, 23(10):1580–1586.

31. Goudie, A.J. (1991). Animal models of drug abuse and dependence. In Willner, P. (ed.), *Behavioural Models in Psychopharmacology: Theoretical, Industrial and Clinical Perspectives*. Cambridge University Press, Cambridge, pp. 453–484.

32. Cryan, J.F. and Holmes, A. (2005). Model organisms: The ascent of mouse: advances in modelling human depression and anxiety. *Nat Rev Drug Discov*, 4(9):775–790.

33. Holmes, A., le Guisquet, A.M., Vogel, E., Millstein, R.A., Leman, S., and Belzung, C. (2005). Early life genetic, epigenetic and environmental factors shaping emotionality in rodents. *Neurosci Biobehav Rev*, 29(8):1335–1346.

34. Nibuya, M., Nestler, E.J., and Duman, R.S. (1996). Chronic antidepressant administration increases the expression of cAMP response element binding protein (CREB) in rat hippocampus. *J Neurosci*, 16(7):2365–2372.

35. Blom, J.M., Tascedda, F., Carra, S., Ferraguti, C., Barden, N., and Brunello, N. (2002). Altered regulation of CREB by chronic antidepressant administration in the brain of transgenic mice with impaired glucocorticoid receptor function. *Neuropsychopharmacology*, 26(5):605–614.

36. Fujimaki, K., Morinobu, S., and Duman, R.S. (2000). Administration of a cAMP phosphodiesterase 4 inhibitor enhances antidepressant-induction of BDNF mRNA in rat hippocampus. *Neuropsychopharmacology*, 22(1):42–51.

37. Warner-Schmidt, J.L. and Duman, R.S. (2007). VEGF is an essential mediator of the neurogenic and behavioral actions of antidepressants. *Proc Natl Acad Sci USA*, 104(11):4647–4652.

38. Nestler, E.J., Gould, E., Manji, H., Buncan, M., Duman, R.S., Greshenfeld, H.K. *et al.* (2002). Preclinical models: Status of basic research in depression. *Biol Psychiatr*, 52(6):503–528.

39. Goldman-Rakic, P.S. (1987). Development of cortical circuitry and cognitive function. *Child Dev*, 58(3):601–622.

40. LeDoux, J. (2003). The emotional brain, fear, and the amygdala. *Cell Mol Neurobiol*, 23(4–5):727–738.

41. Clark, A.S., Schwartz, M.L., and Goldman-Rakic, P.S. (1989). GABA-immunoreactive neurons in the mediodorsal nucleus of the monkey thalamus. *J Chem Neuroanat*, 2(5):259–267.

42. Kuhn, R. (1958). The treatment of depressive states with G 22355 (imipramine hydrochloride). *Am J Psychiatr*, 115(5):459–464.

43. Kline, N.S. (1958). Clinical experience with iproniazid (marsilid). *J Clin Exp Psychopathol*, 19(2, Suppl 1):72–78. discussion 8–9.

44. Tobin, J.M., Bird, I.F., and Boyle, D.E. (1960). Preliminary evaluation of librium (Ro 5-0690) in the treatment of anxiety reactions. *Dis Nerv Syst*, 21(Suppl 3):11–19.

45. Kerry, R.J. and Jenner, F.A. (1962). A double blind crossover comparison of diazepam (Valium, Ro5-2807) with chlordiazepoxide (Librium) in the treatment of neurotic anxiety. *Psychopharmacologia*, 3:302–306.

46. Birkmayer, W. and Hornykiewicz, O. (1962). The *L*-dihydroxyphenylalanine (*L*-DOPA) effect in Parkinson's syndrome in man: On the pathogenesis and treatment of Parkinson akinesis. *Arch Psychiatr Nervenkr Z Gesamte Neurol Psychiatr*, 203:560–574.

47. Hornykiewicz, O. (1966). Dopamine (3-hydroxytyramine) and brain function. *Pharmacol Rev*, 18(2):925–964.

48. Hornykiewicz, O.D. (1970). Physiologic, biochemical, and pathological backgrounds of levodopa and possibilities for the future. *Neurology*, 20(12):1–5.

49. Bartus, R.T., Dean, R.L., Beer, B., and Lippa, A.S. (1982). The cholinergic hypothesis of geriatric memory dysfunction. *Science*, 217(4558):408–414.

50. Kirsch, I., Deacon, B.J., Huedo-Medina, T.B., Scoboria, A., Moore, T.J., and Johnson, B.T. (2008). Initial severity and antidepressant benefits: A meta-analysis of data submitted to the Food and Drug Administration. *PLoS Med*, 5(2(e45)):260–268.

51. Lindner, M.D., McArthur, R.A., Deadwyler, S.A., Hampson, R.E., and Tariot, P.N. (2008). Development, optimization and use of preclinical behavioral models to maximise the productivity of drug discovery for Alzheimer's disease. In McArthur, R.A. and Borsini, F. (eds.), *Animal and Translational Models for CNS Drug Discovery: Neurologic Disorders*. Academic Press, Elsevier, New York.

52. Schneider, L.S. (2008). Issues in design and conduct of clinical trials for cognitive-enhancing drugs. In McArthur, R.A. and Borsini, F. (eds.), *Animal and Translational Models for CNS Drug Discovery: Neurologic Disorders*. Academic Press, Elsevier, New York.

53. McShane, R., Areosa Sastre, A., and Minakaran, N. (2006). Memantine for dementia. *Cochrane Database Syst Rev*, 2. CD003154.

54. National Institute for Health and Clinical Excellence. (2006). NICE technology appraisal guidance 111. *Donepezil, Galantamine, Rivastigmine (Review) and Memantine for the Treatment of Alzheimer's Disease*. National Institute for Health and Clinical Excellence, London.

55. Kirsch, I. and Sapirstein, G. (1998). Listening to Prozac but hearing placebo: A meta-analysis of antidepressant medication. *Prev Treat*, 1(Article 0002a):1–13.

56. Khan, A., Kolts, R.L., Rapaport, M.H., Krishnan, K.R., Brodhead, A.E., and Browns, W.A. (2005). Magnitude of placebo response and drug-placebo differences across psychiatric disorders. *Psychol Med*, 35(5):743–749.

57. Peuskens, J. (1999). The evolving definition of treatment resistance. *J Clin Psychiatr*, 60(Suppl 12):4–8.

58. Souery, D., Oswald, P., Massat, I., Bailer, U., Bollen, J., Demyttenaere, K. *et al.* (2007). Clinical factors associated with treatment resistance in major depressive disorder: Results from a European Multicenter Study. *J Clin Psychiatr*, 68(7):1062–1070.

59. Fava, G.A., Ruini, C., and Rafanelli, C. (2005). Sequential treatment of mood and anxiety disorders. *J Clin Psychiatr*, 66(11):1392–1400.

60. Rush, A.J., Trivedi, M.H., Wisniewski, S.R., Nierenberg, A.A., Stewart, J.W., Warden, D. *et al.* (2006). Acute and longer-term outcomes in depressed outpatients requiring one or several treatment steps: A STAR*D report. *Am J Psychiatr*, 163(11):1905–1917.

61. Kessler, R.C., McGonagle, K.A., Zhao, S., Nelson, C.B., Hughes, M., Eshleman, S. *et al.* (1994). Lifetime and 12-month prevalence of DSM-III-R psychiatric disorders in the United States. Results from the National Comorbidity Survey. *Arch Gen Psychiatr*, 51(1):8–19.

62. Davidson, J.R. (2001). Pharmacotherapy of generalized anxiety disorder. *J Clin Psychiatr*, 62(Suppl 11):46–50. discussion 1–2.

63. Tsuang, M.T., Glatt, S.J., and Faraone, S.V. (2006). The complex genetics of psychiatric disorders. In: Runge, M.S. and Patterson, C. (eds.), *Principles of Molecular Medicine*, Humana Press, Totowa, NJ, pp. 1184–1190.

64. Zeller, A., Crestani, F., Camenisch, I., Iwasato, T., Itohara, S., Fritschy, J.M. *et al.* (2008). Cortical glutamatergic neurons mediate the motor sedative action of diazepam. *Mol Pharmacol*, 73(2):282–291.

65. Gaveriaux-Ruff, C. and Kieffer, B.L. (2007). Conditional gene targeting in the mouse nervous system: Insights into brain function and diseases. *Pharmacol Ther*, 113(3):619–634.

66. Monteggia, L.M., Luikart, B., Barrot, M., Theobold, D., Malkovska, I., Nef, S. *et al.* (2007). Brain-derived neurotrophic factor conditional knockouts show gender differences in depression-related behaviors. *Biol Psychiatr*, 61(2):187–197.

67. Chen, A.P., Ohno, M., Giese, K.P., Kuhn, R., Chen, R.L., and Silva, A.J. (2006). Forebrain-specific knockout of B-raf kinase leads to deficits in hippocampal long-term potentiation, learning, and memory. *J Neurosci Res*, 83(1):28–38.

68. Xiao, D., Bastia, E., Xu, Y.H., Benn, C.L., Cha, J.H., Peterson, T.S. *et al.* (2006). Forebrain adenosine A2A receptors contribute to *L*-3,4-dihydroxyphenylalanine-induced dyskinesia in hemiparkinsonian mice. *J Neurosci*, 26(52):13548–13555.

69. Nguyen, N.K., Keck, M.E., Hetzenauer, A., Thoeringer, C.K., Wurst, W., Deussing, J.M. *et al.* (2006). Conditional CRF receptor 1 knockout mice show altered neuronal activation pattern to mild anxiogenic challenge. *Psychopharmacology (Berl)*, 188(3):374–385.

70. Valverde, O., Mantamadiotis, T., Torrecilla, M., Ugedo, L., Pineda, J., Bleckmann, S. *et al.* (2004). Modulation of anxiety-like behavior and morphine dependence in CREB-deficient mice. *Neuropsychopharmacology*, 29(6):1122–1133.

71. Bingham, N.C., Anderson, K.K., Reuter, A.L., Stallings, N.R., and Parker, K.L. (2008). Selective loss of leptin receptors in the ventromedial hypothalamic nucleus results in increased adiposity and a metabolic syndrome. *Endocrinology*, 149(5):2138–2148.

72. American Psychiatric Association (ed.). (1994). *Diagnostic and Statistical Manual of Mental Disorders*. 4th edition. American Psychiatric Association, Washington, DC.

73. World Health Organization (2007). *International Statistical Classification of Diseases*, 10th revision, 2nd edition. World Health Organization, Geneva.

74. Fibiger, H.C. (1991). The dopamine hypotheses of schizophrenia and mood disorders: Contradictions and speculations. In Willner, P. and Scheel-Kruger, J. (eds.), *The Mesolimbic Dopamine System: From Motivation to Action*. John Wiley, Chichester, UK, pp. 615–638.

75. Costello, C.G. (ed.) (1993). *Symptoms of Depression*. John Wiley, New York.

76. Parker, G., Roy, K., Wilhelm, K., Mitchell, P., and Hadzi-Pavlovic, D. (2000). The nature of bipolar depression: Implications for the definition of melancholia. *J Affect Disord*, 59(3):217–224.

77. Parker, G., Hadzi-Pavlovic, D., Wilhelm, K., Hickie, I., Brodaty, H., Boyce, P. *et al.* (1994). Defining melancholia: Properties of a refined sign-based measure. *Br J Psychiatr*, 164(3):316–326.

78. Carey, G.J., Costall, B., Domeney, A.M., Gerrard, P.A., Jones, D.N., Naylor, R.J. *et al.* (1992). Ondansetron and arecoline prevent scopolamine-induced cognitive deficits in the marmoset. *Pharmacol Biochem Behav*, 42(1):75–83.

79. Broocks, A., Little, J.T., Martin, A., Minichiello, M.D., Dubbert, B., Mack, C. *et al.* (1998). The influence of ondansetron and m-chlorophenylpiperazine on scopolamine-induced cognitive, behavioral, and physiological responses in young healthy controls. *Biol Psychiatr*, 43(6):408–416.

80. Wienrich, M., Meier, D., Ensinger, H.A., Gaida, W., Raschig, A., Walland, A. *et al.* (2001). Pharmacodynamic profile of the M1 agonist talsaclidine in animals and man. *Life Sci*, 68(22–23):2593–2600.

81. Lutsep, H.L. (2002). Repinotan bayer. *Curr Opin Investig Drugs*, 3(6):924–927.

82. Blier, P. and Ward, N.M. (2003). Is there a role for 5-HT1A agonists in the treatment of depression? *Biol Psychiatr*, 53(3):193–203.

83. Scrip. (2007). *FDA Rejects Fabre Kramer Antidepressant Gepirone ER*. Scrip. 3310:24.

84. Merchant, K.M., Chesselet, M.-F., Hu, S.-C., and Fahn, S. (2008). Animal models of Parkinson's disease to aid drug discovery and development. In McArthur, R.A. and Borsini, F. (eds.), *Animal and Translational Models for CNS Drug Discovery: Neurologic Disorders*. Academic Press, Elsevier, New York.

85. Wright, T.M. (2006). Tramiprosate. *Drugs Today (Barc)*, 42(5):291–298.

86. Aisen, P.S., Gauthier, S., Vellas, B., Briand, R., Saumier, D., Laurin, J. *et al.* (2007). Alzhemed: A potential treatment for Alzheimer's disease. *Curr Alzheimer Res*, 4(4):473–478.

87. Scrip. (2007). *Neurochem Shares Fall after Alzheimer Disappointment*. Scrip. 3289/90:24.

88. Neurochem Inc. (2007). We are Neurochem Quarterly Report. Third Quarter ended September 30, 2007. Laval, Quebec, Canada.

89. Winsky, L. and Brady, L. (2005). Perspective on the status of preclinical models for psychiatric disorders. *Drug Discovery Today: Disease Models*, 2(4):279–283.

90. Dourish, C.T., Wilding, J.P.H., and Halford, J.C.G. (2008). Anti-obesity drugs: From animal models to clinical efficacy. In McArthur, R.A. and Borsini, F. (eds.), *Animal and Translational Models for CNS Drug Discovery: Reward Deficit Disorders*. Academic Press, Elsevier, New York.

91. Hunter, A.J. (2008). Animal and translational models of neurological disorders: An industrial perspective. In McArthur, R.A. and Borsini, F. (eds.), *Animal and Translational Models for CNS Drug Discovery: Neurologic Disorders*. Academic Press, Elsevier, New York.

92. McEvoy, J.P. and Freudenreich, O. (2008). Issues in the design and conductance of clinical trials. In McArthur, R.A. and Borsini, F. (eds.), *Animal and Translational Models for CNS Drug Discovery: Psychiatric Disorders*. Academic Press, Elsevier, New York.

93. Millan, M.J. (2008). The discovery and development of pharmacotherapy for psychiatric disorders: A critical survey of animal and translational models, and perspectives for their improvement. In McArthur, R.A. and Borsini, F. (eds.), *Animal and Translational Models for CNS Drug Discovery: Psychiatric Disorders*. Academic Press, Elsevier, New York.

94. Cuatrecasas, P. (2006). Drug discovery in jeopardy. *J Clin Invest*, 116(11):2837–2842.

95. McArthur, R. and Borsini, F. (2006). Animal models of depression in drug discovery: A historical perspective. *Pharmacol Biochem Behav*, 84(3):436–452.

96. Kirsch, I., Moore, T.J., Scoboria, A., and Nicholls, S.S. (2002). The emperor's new drugs: An analysis of antidepressant medication data submitted to the US Food and Drug Administration. *Prev Treat*, 5(1):1–23.

97. Turner, E.H., Matthews, A.M., Linardatos, E., Tell, R.A., and Rosenthal, R. (2008). Selective publication of antidepressant trials and its influence on apparent efficacy. *N Engl J Med*, 358(3):252–260.

98. Bartz, J., Young, L.J., Hollander, E., Buxbaum, J.D., and Ring, R.H. (2008). Preclinical animal models of autistic spectrum disorders (ASD). In McArthur, R.A. and Borsini, F. (eds.), *Animal and Translational Models for CNS Drug Discovery: Psychiatric Disorders*. Academic Press, Elsevier, New York.

99. Montes, J., Bendotti, C., Tortarolo, M., Cheroni, C., Hallak, H., Speiser, Z. *et al.* (2008). Translational research in ALS. In McArthur, R.A. and Borsini, F. (eds.), *Animal and Translational Models for CNS Drug Discovery: Neurologic Disorders*. Academic Press, Elsevier, New York.

100. Wagner, L.A., Menalled, L., Goumeniouk, A.D., Brunner, D.P., and Leavitt, B.R. (2008). Huntington disease. In McArthur, R.A. and Borsini, F. (eds.), *Animal and Translational Models for CNS Drug Discovery: Neurologic Disorders*. Academic Press, Elsevier, New York.

101. Lesko, L.J. and Atkinson, A.J.J. (2001). Use of biomarkers and surrogate endpoints in drug development and regulatory decision making: Criteria, validation, strategies. *Annu Rev Pharmacol Toxicol*, 41:347–366.

102. Gottesman, I.I. and Gould, T.D. (2003/4/1). The endophenotype concept in psychiatry: Etymology and strategic intentions. *Am J Psychiatr*, 160(4):636–645.

103. Bearden, C.E. and Freimer, N.B. (2006). Endophenotypes for psychiatric disorders: Ready for primetime?. *Trends Genet*, 22(6):306–313.

104. Cannon, T.D. and Keller, M.C. (2006). Endophenotypes in the genetic analyses of mental disorders. *Annu Rev Clin Psychol*, 2(1):267–290.

105. Hasler, G., Drevets, W.C., Manji, H.K., and Charney, D.S. (2004). Discovering endophenotypes for major depression. *Neuropsychopharmacology*, 29(10):1765–1781.

106. Willner, P. (1997). Validity, reliability and utility of the chronic mild stress model of depression: A 10-year review and evaluation. *Psychopharmacology (Berl)*, 134(4):319–329.

107. Willner, P., Muscat, R., and Papp, M. (1992). Chronic mild stress-induced anhedonia: A realistic animal model of depression. *Neurosci Biobehav Rev*, 16(4):525–534.

108. Bekris, S., Antoniou, K., Daskas, S., and Papadopoulou-Daifoti, Z. (2005). Behavioural and neurochemical effects induced by chronic mild stress applied to two different rat strains. *Behav Brain Res*, 161(1):45–59.

109. Pucilowski, O., Overstreet, D.H., Rezvani, A.H., and Janowsky, D.S. (1993). Chronic mild stress-induced anhedonia: Greater effect in a genetic rat model of depression. *Physiol Behav*, 54(6):1215–1220.

110. Martin, M., Ledent, C., Parmentier, M., Maldonado, R., and Valverde, O. (2002). Involvement of CB1 cannabinoid receptors in emotional behaviour. *Psychopharmacology (Berl)*, 159(4):379–387.

111. Mormede, C., Castanon, N., Medina, C., Moze, E., Lestage, J., Neveu, P.J. *et al.* (2002). Chronic mild stress in mice decreases peripheral cytokine and increases central cytokine expression independently of IL-10 regulation of the cytokine network. *Neuroimmunomodulation*, 10(6):359–366.

112. Bergstrom, A., Jayatissa, M.N., Mork, A., and Wiborg, O. (2008). Stress sensitivity and resilience in the chronic mild stress rat model of depression; an *in situ* hybridization study. *Brain Res*, 1196:41–52.

113. Strekalova, T., Gorenkova, N., Schunk, E., Dolgov, O., and Bartsch, D. (2006). Selective effects of citalopram in a mouse model of stress-induced anhedonia with a control for chronic stress. *Behav Pharmacol*, 17(3):271–287.

114. Littman, B.H. and Williams, S.A. (2005). The ultimate model organism: Progress in experimental medicine. *Nat Rev Drug Discov*, 4(8):631–638.

115. Willner, P. (1991). Methods for assessing the validity of animal models of human psychopathology. In Boulton, A., Baker, G., and Martin-Iverson, M. (eds.), *Neuromethods: Animal Models in Psychiatry I*, Vol. 18. Humana Press, Inc, pp. 1–23.

116. Geyer, M.A. and Markou, A. (1995). Animal models of psychiatric disorders. In Bloom, F.E. and Kupfer, D.J. (eds.), *Psychopharmacology, The Fourth Generation of Progress*. Raven Press, New York, pp. 787–798.

117. Geyer, M.A. and Markou, A. (2002). *The role of preclinical models in the development of psychotropic drugs*. American College of Neuropsychopharmacology, New York. pp. 445–455.

118. Li, Q., Zhao, D., and Bezard, E. (2006). Traditional Chinese medicine for Parkinson's disease: A review of Chinese literature. *Behav Pharmacol*, 17(5–6):403–410.

119. Kuhn, T.S. (1996). *The Structure of Scientific Revolutions*, 3rd edition. The University of Chicago Press, Chicago, IL.

120. Miczek, K.A. (2008). Challenges for translational psychopharmacology research – the need for conceptual principles. In McArthur, R.A. and Borsini, F. (eds.), *Animal and Translational Models for CNS Drug Discovery: Psychiatric Disorders*. Academic Press: Elsevier, New York.

Index

Printed and bound by CPI Group (UK) Ltd, Croydon, CR0 4YY

03/10/2024

01040312-0013